Introduction to Human Nutrition

The Nutrition Society Textbook Series

Public Health Nutrition, 2nd Edition
Judith L. Buttriss, Ailsa A. Welch, John M. Kearney, Susan A. Lanham-New

Nutrition Research Methodologies
Julie A. Lovegrove, Leanne Hodson, Sangita Sharma, Susan A. Lanham-New

Clinical Nutrition, 2nd Edition
Marinos Elia, Olle Ljungqvist, Rebecca J. Stratton, Susan A. Lanham-New

Sport and Exercise Nutrition
Susan A. Lanham-New, Samantha Stear, Susan Shirreffs, Adam Collins

Nutrition and Metabolism, 2nd Edition
Susan A. Lanham-New, Ian A. MacDonald, Helen M. Roche

Introduction to Human Nutrition

Third Edition

Edited on behalf of The Nutrition Society by

Susan A. Lanham-New
Head of the Department, Nutritional Sciences, University of Surrey, Guildford, UK

Thomas R. Hill
Professor of Nutrition, Newcastle University, Newcastle-Upon-Tyne, UK

Alison M. Gallagher
Head of the Doctoral College, Ulster University, Coleraine, NI

Hester H. Vorster
Emeritus Research Professor, North-West University, Potchefstroom, ZA

WILEY Blackwell

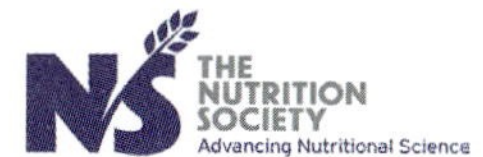

This edition first published 2020

Edition History
1e, 2002; 2e, 2009 The Nutrition Society

Registered Office(s)
John Wiley & Sons, Inc., 111 River Street, Hoboken, NJ 07030, USA
John Wiley & Sons Ltd, The Atrium, Southern Gate, Chichester, West Sussex, PO19 8SQ, UK

Editorial Office
111 River Street, Hoboken, NJ 07030, USA
101 Station Landing, Medford, MA 02155, USA
9600 Garsington Road, Oxford, OX4 2DQ, UK

For details of our global editorial offices, customer services, and more information about Wiley products visit us at www.wiley.com.

Wiley also publishes its books in a variety of electronic formats and by print-on-demand. Some content that appears in standard print versions of this book may not be available in other formats.

Library of Congress Cataloging-in-Publication Data

Names: Lanham-New, S. A., Editor-in-Chief. | Hill, T.R., Editor. |
Gallagher, A.M., Editor. | Hester H. Vorster Editor. | The Nutrition Society (UK)
Title: Introduction to Human Nutrition / edited on behalf of The Nutrition Society by
Professor Susan A. Lanham-New, Professor Thomas R. Hill,
Professor Alison M. Gallagher, Professor Hester H. Vorster.
Description: Third edition. | Hoboken, NJ : Wiley, 2020. | Series: Nutrition
Society Textbook Series | Includes bibliographical references and index.
Identifiers: LCCN 2019024477| ISBN 9781119476979 (paperback) |
ISBN 9781119477013 (adobe pdf) | ISBN 9781119477020 (epub)
Subjects: | MESH: Nutritional Physiological Phenomena | Food
Classification: LCC QP141 | NLM QU 145 | DDC 612.3–dc23 LC record available at
https://lccn.loc.gov/2019024477

Cover Design: Wiley
Cover Images: Abstract Curve © jxfzsy/iStock.com

Set in 10/12pt Minion by SPi Global, Pondicherry, India
Printed and bound in Singapore by Markono Print Media Pte Ltd

10 9 8 7 6 5 4 3 2 1

Contents

Contributors

Dr Cristina Arroyo
Food Safety Authority of Ireland, Dublin, Ireland

Professor David A. Bender
University College London, London, UK

Dr Declan J. Bolton
Teagasc Food Research Centre, Dublin, Ireland

Professor Dr Dr Anja Bosy-Westphal
Christian-Albrechts-University, Kiel, Germany

Dr Catherine M. Burgess
Teagasc Food Research Centre, Dublin, Ireland

Dr Angela Carlin
Ulster University, Jordanstown, Northern Ireland

Professor Kevin D. Cashman
University College Cork, Cork, Ireland

Professor Stephen C. Cunnane
Université de Sherbrooke, Quebec, Canada

Dr Martin Danaher
Teagasc Food Research Centre, Dublin, Ireland

Professor Paul Deurenberg
Nutrition Consultant, Philippines

Miss Cassandra H. Ellis
The Nutrition Society, London, UK

Professor Alison M. Gallagher
Ulster University, Coleraine, Northern Ireland

Dr James Gallagher
University College Dublin, Dublin, Ireland

Professor Bruce A. Griffin
University of Surrey, Guildford, UK

Professor Thomas R. Hill
Newcastle University, Newcastle upon Tyne, UK

Professor Susan A. Lanham-New
University of Surrey, Guildford, UK

Professor Georg Lietz
Newcastle University, Newcastle upon Tyne, UK

Professor Una E. MacIntyre
University of Pretoria, Pretoria, South Africa

Professor J. Alfredo Martínez
Universidad de Navarra, Pamplona, Spain
IMDEAfood CEI UAM + CSIC, Madrid, Spain

Professor Miguel A. Martínez-González
Univerisdad de Navarra, Pamplona, Spain

Professor John C. Mathers
Newcastle University, Newcastle upon Tyne, UK

Dr Aideen McKevitt
University College Dublin, Dublin, Ireland

Dr Marcela Moraes Mendes
University of Surrey, Guildford, UK

Professor D. Joe Millward
University of Surrey, Guildford, UK

Professor Dr med. Manfred James Müller
Christian-Albrechts-University, Kiel, Germany

Professor Marie H. Murphy
Ulster University, Jordanstown, Northern Ireland

Dr Lisa O'Connor
Food Safety Authority of Ireland, Dublin, Ireland

Dr Patrick J. O'Mahony
Food Safety Authority of Ireland, Dublin, Ireland

Dr Beluah Pretorius
University of Pretoria, Pretoria, South Africa

Professor Hettie C. Schönfeldt
University of Pretoria, Pretoria, South Africa

Professor JJ. Strain
Ulster University, Coleraine, Northern Ireland

Dr Christina Tlustos
Food Safety Authority of Ireland, Dublin, Ireland

Dr Estefania Toledo
Universidad de Navarra, Pamplona, Spain

Professor Hester H. Vorster
North-West University, Potchefstroom, South Africa

Dr Gareth A. Wallis
University of Birmingham, Birmingham, UK

Professor Friedeburg AM. Wenhold
North-West University, Potchefstroom, South Africa

Professor Gary Williamson
Monash University, Melbourne, Australia

Dr Alison J. Yeates
Ulster University, Coleraine, Northern Ireland

Dr Kate M. Younger
Technological University Dublin, Dublin, Ireland

Preface

I am absolutely delighted in my capacity as Editor-in-Chief (E-i-C) of the Nutrition Society Textbook Series to introduce the 3rd Edition of *Introduction to Human Nutrition* (IHN3e). The production of this Third Edition represents a significant milestone for the Society's Textbook Series, given that it is now exactly twenty years on since the production of the 1st Edition of IHN and a decade since the production of the 2nd Edition of IHN.

The Editorial Team of *Introduction to Human Nutriton* 3rd Edition, namely Professor Alison Gallagher (University of Ulster), Professor Thomas Hill (University of Newcastle) and Professor Hester Vorster (North-West University) have been absolutely fantastic; meticulously ensuring that each chapter is updated & accurate, and ensuring that new aspects of IHN3e are also brought into the Book including chapters on physical activity and phytochemicals. IHN3e comprises of a total of 17 chapters, each with their own unique summary of the take home messages. How indebted we are to have so many experts in the Field who have written chapters to make IHN3e a complete and thorough review of the area of Nutritional Sciences - a must read!

IHN3e is intended for those with an interest in nutritional science whether they are nutritionists, food scientists, dietitians, medics, nursing staff or other allied health professionals. We hope that both undergraduate and postgraduate students will find the book of great help with their respective studies and that the book will really put nutrition science as a *discipline* into context.

It is a great honour for our 3rd Edition of IHN to have the Foreword written by the The Earl of Selborne GBE FRS DL and we are most grateful to him for his support of our work at the Society, particularly given his position as Vice-President of the Foundation for Science and Technology and as a Fellow of the Royal Society. We are most grateful to the following individuals for their support and most generous Forewords in Public Health Nutrition2e, Sport and Exercise Nutrition1e, Clinical Nutrition2e and Nutrition Research Methods1e; namely – Her Royal Highness The Princess Royal; Professor Richard Budgett OBE, Chief Medical Officer for the London 2012 Olympic and Paralympic Games and now Medical and Scientific Director at the International Olympic Committee (IOC) based in Lausanne, Switzerland; Dame Sally Davies, Chief Medical Officer (CMO) for England, and the UK Government's Principal Medical Adviser; Professor Lord John Krebs, Principal, Jesus College, University of Oxford and our first Chairman of the UK Food Standards Agency. We are now planning ahead with respect to the production of the 3rd Edition of Nutrition and Metabolism and the 2nd Edition of Sport and Exercise Nutrition as well as bringing a *seventh* book to the Textbook Series!

The Society is most grateful to the Textbook publishers, Wiley-Blackwell for their continued help with the production of the textbook and in particular: James Watson – Senior Commissioning Editor; Jennifer Seward - Senior Project Editor; Baskar Anandraj - Production Editor. In addition, I would like to acknowledge formally my great personal appreciation to: Professor G.Q. Max Lu AO, FRSC, FIChemE, Vice-Chancellor & President of the University of Surrey; Professor Michael Kearney MA, PhD, CPhys, FInstP, CEng, FIET, FIMA, Provost & Executive Vice-President of the University of Surrey; Professor Helen Griffiths BSc, PhD, FRSB, Executive Dean of the Faculty of Health & Medical Sciences, University of Surrey for their respective great encouragement of the nutritional sciences field in general, especially in light of Surrey's success in the 2017/2018 Queen's Anniversary Prize for our work in *Food and Nutrition for Health*, and for their support of the Textbook Series production in particular.

Sincerest appreciation indeed to the Nutrition Society President, Professor Philip Calder (University of Southampton) and President-Elect, Professor Julie Lovegrove (University of Reading) for their great support and belief in the Textbook Series. With special thanks to past-Honorary Publications Officer, Professor Paul Trayhurn (just announced as the first recipient of the Nutrition Society Sir Frederick Gowland Hopkins Award) for his tremendous wise counsel to me during the six years we have worked together on the Textbooks and to the present-Honorary Publications Officer Professor Jayne Woodside (Queen's University, Belfast) for being such a great sounding board and I look forward to working with her going forward on the production of further Editions of the Textbooks. And finally an enormous thank you indeed to: Mark Hollingsworth MBA, FInstLM, Chief Executive Officer & Company Secretary of the Nutrition Society for his unstinting support of the Textbook Series and to Cassandra Ellis MSc RNutr (Public Health), Deputy Editor on the Textbook Series for her pivotal continued contribution to the development of the Series.

Finally, as I always write and absolutely do not forget (ever, ever!), the Textbook Series is indebted to the forward thinking focus that Professor Michael Gibney (University College Dublin) had at that time of the Textbook Series development. It remains such a tremendous privilege for me to continue to follow in his footsteps as the second E-i-C.

I really hope that you will find the textbook a great resource of information and inspiration .... please enjoy, and with so many grateful thanks to all those who made it happen!

With my warmest of wishes indeed

Professor Susan A. Lanham-New
RNutr, FAfN, FRSB
E-i-C, Nutrition Society Textbook Series
Professor of Human Nutrition and Head,
Department of Nutritional Sciences
School of Biosciences and Medicine,
Faculty of Health and Medical Sciences
University of Surrey

Series Foreword

In 1941, a group of leading physiologists, biochemists and medical scientists recognised that the emerging discipline of Nutrition needed its own Learned Society; hence The Nutrition Society was established. The mission was, and remains, "*to advance the scientific study of nutrition and its application to the maintenance of human and animal health*". The Nutrition Society is the largest Learned Society for Nutrition in Europe and is internationally respected for its scientific publications, conferences and training workshops.

The Society's first journal, *The Proceedings of the Nutrition Society* published in 1944, records the scientific presentations made to the Society. Shortly afterwards, in 1947, the *British Journal of Nutrition* was established for the publication of primary research on all aspects of human and animal nutrition by scientists from around the world. Recognising the needs of students and their teachers for authoritative reviews on topical issues in nutrition, the Society began publishing *Nutrition Research Reviews* in 1988. The journal *Public Health Nutrition*, the first international journal dedicated to this important and growing area, was subsequently launched in 1998. The Society's first open access journal, the *Journal of Nutritional Science*, was launched in 2012. The Society is constantly evolving in response to emerging areas of nutritional science and has most recently launched the journal *Gut Microbiome*, an open access journal published in partnership with Cambridge University Press.

The Nutrition Society Textbook Series, first established by Professor Michael Gibney (University College Dublin) in 1998 and now under the direction of the second Editor-in-Chief, Professor Susan Lanham-New (University of Surrey), continues to be an extraordinarily successful venture for the Society. This series of nutrition textbooks is designed for use worldwide and this has been achieved by translating the Textbook Series into many different languages including Spanish, Greek, Portuguese, Italian and Indonesian. The success of the Textbook Series is a tribute to the quality of the authorship, and the value placed on them in the UK and Worldwide as a core educational tool and a resource for practitioners.

I am very pleased to note Introduction to Human Nutrition is the most successful title in the Society's textbook series with over 28,000 copies sold to date across the World in all formats and translations. For many years I was involved in monitoring and determining science policy, whether as chair of a research council, as chair of the House of Lords Science and Technology Committee or as chair of the Foundation for Science and Technology. I have learned how important high-quality science is for underpinning sound policies, both in the UK and world-wide. This Textbook is uniquely placed in bringing together science and the practical application of methodologies in nutrition. It is a most valuable resource and I commend it to those working, studying and having an interest in the field of Nutritional Sciences.

The Earl of Selborne GBE FRS DL

About the Companion Website

www.wiley.com/go/lanham-new/humannutrition

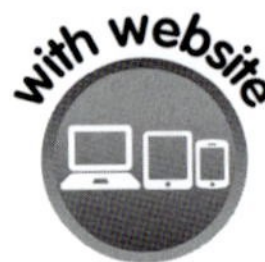

- Multiple choice questions
- Short answer questions
- Essay questions

1
Introduction to Human Nutrition: A Global Perspective on Food and Nutrition

Susan A. Lanham-New, Marcela Moraes Mendes, and Hester H. Vorster

Key messages

- Human nutrition is a complex, multifaceted scientific domain indicating how substances in foods provide essential nourishment for the maintenance of life.
- To understand, study, research, and practice nutrition, a holistic integrated approach from molecular to societal level is needed.
- Optimal, balanced nutrition is a major determinant of health. It can be used to promote health and well-being, to prevent ill-health, and to treat disease.
- The study of the structure, chemical and physical characteristics, and physiological and biochemical effects of the more than 50 nutrients found in foods underpins the understanding of nutrition.
- The hundreds of millions of food- and nutrition-insecure people globally, the coexistence of undernutrition and overnutrition, and inappropriate nutritional behaviors are challenges that face the nutritionist of today.
- Nutrition practice has a firm and well-developed research and knowledge base. There are, however, many areas where more information is needed to solve global, regional, communal and individual nutrition problems.
- The development of ethical norms, standards, and values in nutrition research and practice is needed.

1.1 Orientation to human nutrition

The major purpose of this series of four textbooks on nutrition is to guide the nutrition student through the exciting journey of discovery of nutrition as a science. As apprentices in nutrition science and practice students will learn how to collect, systemise, and classify knowledge by reading, experimentation, observation, and reasoning. The road for this journey was mapped out millennia ago. The knowledge that nutrition – what we choose to eat and drink – influences our health, well-being, and quality of life is as old as human history. For millions of years the quest for food has helped to shape human development, the organisation of society and history itself. It has influenced wars, population growth, urban expansion, economic and political theory, religion, science, medicine, and technological development.

It was only in the second half of the eighteenth century that nutrition started to experience its first renaissance with the observation by scientists that intakes of certain foods, later called nutrients, and eventually other substances not yet classified as nutrients, influence the function of the body, protect against disease, restore health, and determine people's response to changes in the environment. During this period, nutrition was studied from a medical model or

Introduction to Human Nutrition, Third Edition. Edited on behalf of The Nutrition Society by Susan A. Lanham-New, Thomas R. Hill, Alison M. Gallagher and Hester H. Vorster.

Companion website: www.wiley.com/go/lanham-new/humannutrition

paradigm by defining the chemical structures and characteristics of nutrients found in foods, their physiological functions, biochemical reactions and human requirements to prevent, first, deficiency diseases and, later, also chronic noncommunicable diseases.

Since the late 1980s nutrition has experienced a second renaissance with the growing perception that the knowledge gained did not equip mankind to solve the global problems of food insecurity and malnutrition. The emphasis shifted from the medical or pathological paradigm to a more psychosocial, behavioral one in which nutrition is defined as a basic human right, not only essential for human development but also as an outcome of development.

In this first, introductory text, the focus is on the principles and essentials of human nutrition, with the main purpose of helping the nutrition student to develop a holistic and integrated understanding of this complex, multifaceted scientific domain.

1.2 An integrated approach

Human nutrition describes the processes whereby cellular organelles, cells, tissues, organs, systems, and the body as a whole obtain and use necessary substances obtained from foods (nutrients) to maintain structural and functional integrity. For an understanding of how humans obtain and utilise foods and nutrients from a molecular to a societal level, and of the factors determining and influencing these processes, the study and practice of human nutrition involve a spectrum of other basic and applied scientific disciplines. These include molecular biology, genetics, biochemistry, chemistry, physics, food science, microbiology, physiology, pathology, immunology, psychology, sociology, political science, anthropology, agriculture, pharmacology, communications, and economics. Nutrition departments are, therefore, often found in Medical (Health) or Social Science, or Pharmacy, or Agriculture Faculties at tertiary training institutions. The multidisciplinary nature of the science of nutrition, lying in both the natural (biological) and social scientific fields, demands that students of nutrition should have a basic understanding of many branches of science and that they should be able to integrate different concepts from these different disciplines. It implies that students should choose their accompanying subjects (electives) carefully and that they should read widely in these different areas.

1.3 A conceptional framework for the study of nutrition

In the journey of discovery into nutrition science it will often be necessary to put new knowledge, or new applications of old knowledge, into the perspective of the holistic picture. For this, a conceptual framework of the multidisciplinary nature of nutrition science and practice may be of value. Such a conceptual framework, illustrating the complex interactions between internal or constitutional factors and external environmental factors which determine nutritional status and health, is given in Figure 1.1.

On a genetic level it is now accepted that nutrients dictate phenotypic expression of an individual's genotype by influencing the processes of transcription, translation, or post-translational reactions. In other words, nutrients can directly influence genetic (DNA) expression, determining the type of RNA formed (transcription) and also the proteins synthesised (translation). For example, glucose, a carbohydrate macronutrient, increases transcription for the synthesis of glucokinase, the micronutrient iron increases translation for the synthesis of ferritin, while vitamin K increases post-translational carboxylation of glutamic acid residues for the synthesis of prothrombin. Nutrients, therefore, influence the synthesis of structural and functional proteins, by influencing gene expression within cells.

Nutrients also act as substrates and cofactors in all the metabolic reactions in cells necessary for the growth and maintenance of structure and function. Cells take up nutrients (through complex mechanisms across cell membranes) from their immediate environment, also known as the body's internal environment. The composition of this environment is carefully regulated to ensure optimal function and survival of cells, a process known as homeostasis, which gave birth to a systems approach in the study of nutrition.

Nutrients and oxygen are provided to the internal environment by the circulating blood, which also removes metabolic end-products and harmful substances from this environment for

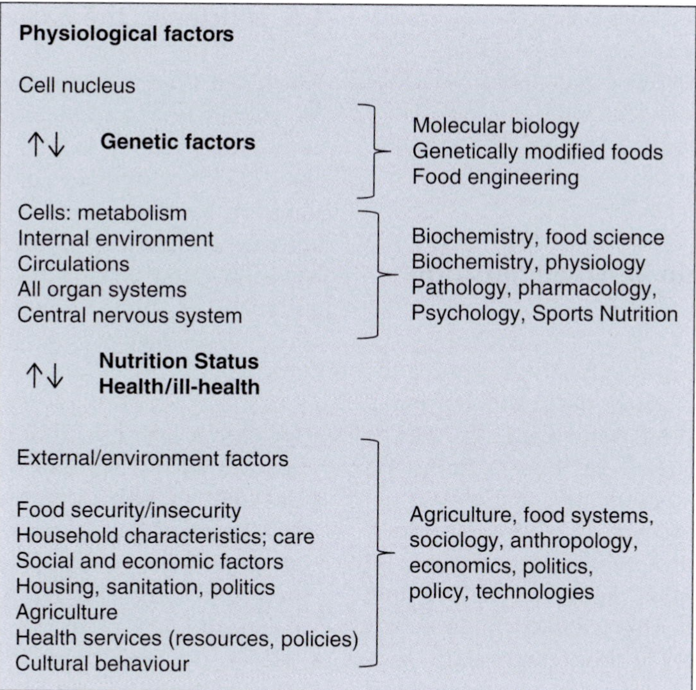

Physiological factors
Cell nucleus
↑↓ Genetic factors
Molecular biology
Genetically modified foods
Food engineering
Cells: metabolism
Internal environment
Circulations
All organ systems
Central nervous system
Biochemistry, food science
Biochemistry, physiology
Pathology, pharmacology,
Psychology, Sports Nutrition
↑↓ Nutrition Status
Health/ill-health
External/environment factors
Food security/insecurity
Household characteristics; care
Social and economic factors
Housing, sanitation, politics
Agriculture
Health services (resources, policies)
Cultural behaviour
Agriculture, food systems,
sociology, anthropology,
economics, politics,
policy, technologies

Figure 1.1 Conceptual framework for a holistic, integrated understanding of human nutrition.

excretion through the skin, the kidneys, and the large bowel.

The concerted function of different organs and systems of the body ensures that nutrients and oxygen are extracted or taken up from the external environment and transferred to the blood for transport and delivery to the internal environment and cells. The digestive system, for example, is responsible for the ingestion of food and beverages, the breakdown (digestion and fermentation) of these for extraction of nutrients, and the absorption of the nutrients into the circulation, while the respiratory system extracts oxygen from the air. These functions are coordinated and regulated by the endocrine and central nervous systems in response to the chemical and physical composition of the blood and internal environment, and to cellular needs.

The health or disease state of the different organs and systems will determine the nutrient requirements of the body as a whole.

The central nervous system is also the site or "headquarters" of the higher, mental functions related to conscious or cognitive, spiritual, religious, and cultural behaviors, which will determine, in response to the internal and external environments, what and how much will be eaten. What and how much is eaten will further depend on what is available, influenced by a host of factors determining food security. All of these factors, on an individual, household, community, national, or international level, shape the external environment.

During the first renaissance of nutrition, emphasis was placed on the study of nutrients and their functions. A medical, natural science, or biological model underpinned the study of the relationships between nutrition and health or ill-health. During the second renaissance, these aspects are not neglected, but expanded to include the study of all other external environmental factors that determine what and how much food and nutrients are available on a global level. These studies are underpinned by social, behavioral, economic, agricultural, and political sciences. The study of human nutrition therefore seeks to understand the complexities of both social and biological factors on how individuals and populations maintain optimal function and health, how the quality, quantity and balance of the food supply are influenced, what happens to food after it is eaten, and the way that diet affects health and well-being. This integrated approach has led to a better understanding of the causes and consequences of malnutrition including the double burden of over and under nutrition, and of the relationship between nutrition and health.

1.4 Relationship between nutrition and health

Figure 1.2 shows that individuals can be broadly categorised into having optimal nutritional status or being undernourished, overnourished, or malnourished. The major causes and consequences of these nutritional states are indicated. It is important to realise that many other lifestyle and environmental factors, in addition to nutrition, influence health and well-being, but nutrition is a major, modifiable, and powerful factor in promoting health, preventing and treating disease, and improving quality of life.

1.5 Nutrients: the basics

People eat food, not nutrients; however, it is the combination and amounts of nutrients in consumed foods that determine health. To read one must know the letters of the alphabet; to do sums one must be able to count, add, subtract, multiply, and divide. To understand nutrition, one must know about nutrients. The study of nutrients, the ABC and numeric calculations of nutrition, will form a major part of the student's nutrition journey, and should include:

- the chemical and physical structure and characteristics of the nutrient;
- the food sources of the nutrient, including food composition, the way in which foods are grown, harvested, stored, processed and prepared, and the effects of these on nutrient composition and nutritional value;
- the digestion, absorption, circulatory transport, and cellular uptake of the nutrient, as well as regulation of all these processes;

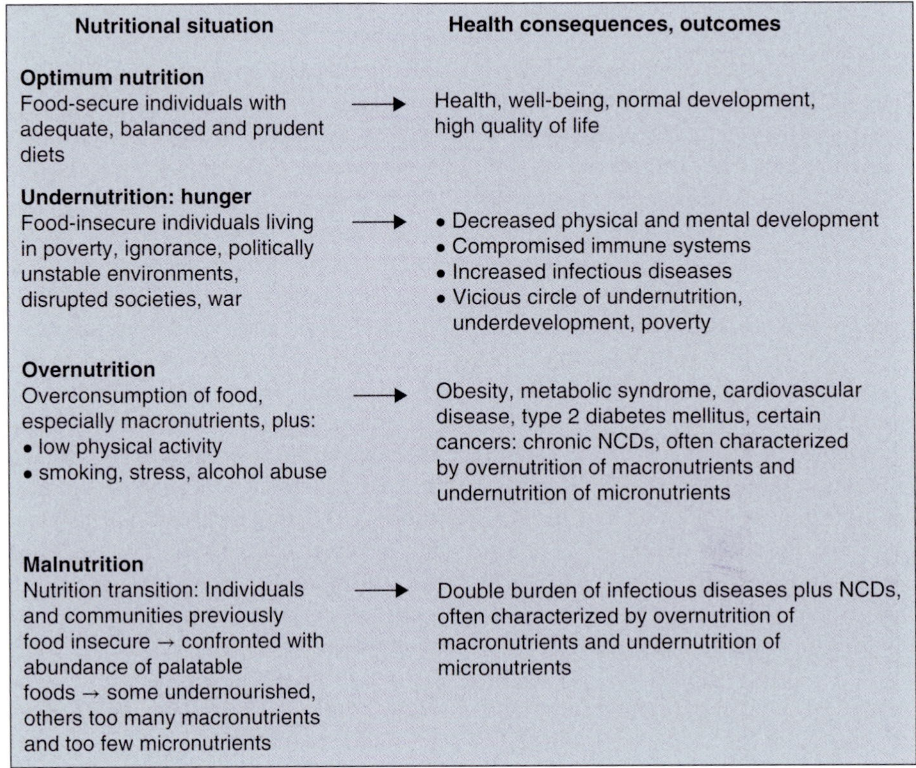

Figure 1.2 Relationship between nutrition and health. NCD, noncommunicable disease.

- the metabolism of the nutrient, its functions, storage, and excretion;
- physiological needs (demands or requirements) for the nutrient in health and disease, and during special circumstances (pregnancy, lactation, sport events), as well as individual variability (genetic factors);
- interactions with other nutrients, nonnutrients (phytochemicals), antinutrients, and drugs;
- the consequences of underconsumption and over-consumption of nutrients;
- the therapeutic uses of the nutrient;
- factors influencing food and nutrition security and food safety;
- dietary behavior and cultural patterns.

There are more than 50 known nutrients (including amino acids and fatty acids) and many more chemicals in food thought to influence human function and health (Box 1.1). Nutrients do not exist in isolation, except for water and others in some pharmaceutical preparations. In foods, in the gut during digestion, fermentation and absorption, in the blood during transport, and in cells during metabolism, nutrients interact with each other. Therefore, a particular nutrient should not be studied in isolation, but integrated with other nutrients and seen in the context of total body function. The study of nutrition also includes how to determine nutrient requirements to make recommendations for intakes and how nutritional status is monitored by measuring intakes, anthropometry, body composition, biochemical markers reflecting nutritional status, and the clinical signs of malnutrition.

This knowledge of nutrients and their functions will enable the nutritionist to advise individuals what and how much to eat. However, this knowledge is not sufficient to understand and address the global problem of malnutrition facing mankind today. This perception has resulted in the cultivation of social science disciplines to support knowledge from the biological sciences to address global malnutrition.

1.6 Global malnutrition

It is a major tragedy that millions of people currently live with hunger, and fear starvation. This is in spite of the fact that food security or "access for all at all times, to a sustainable supply of nutritionally adequate and safe food for normal physical and mental development and healthy, productive lives" is a basic human right embedded in the constitution of most developing countries. It is also despite the fact that sufficient food is produced on a global level (see Box 1.2). Food insecurity is an obstacle to human rights, quality of life, and human dignity. Chapter 15 provides a thorough overview of nutrition-related diseases in developed and developing countries.

The World Health Organization estimates that, during the last decade, around 1.9 billion adults are overweight or obese, while 850 million are undernourished. More than 52 million children under five years of age are wasted, 17 million are severely wasted and 155 million are stunted, while 41 million are overweight or obese. An estimated two billion people around

Box 1.1 Classes of nutrients for human nutrition

Class/category	Subclass/category	Nutrient examples
Carbohydrates (macronutrients)	Monosaccharides Disaccharides Polysaccharides	Glucose, fructose, galactose Sucrose, maltose, lactose Starch and dietary fibre
Proteins (macronutrients)	Plant and animal source proteins	Amino acids (n = 20): aliphatic, aromatic, sulfur-containing, acidic, basic
Fats and oils (lipids) (macronutrients)	Saturated fatty acids Monounsaturated fatty acids Polyunsaturated fatty acids (n-3, n-6, n-9)	Palmitic and stearic acid Oleic (cis) and elaidic (trans) fatty acids Linoleic, α-linolenic, arachidonic, eicosapentaenoic, docosahexaenoic acid
Minerals (micronutrients)	Minerals and electrolytes Trace elements	Calcium, sodium, phosphate, potassium, iron, zinc, selenium, copper, manganese, molybdenum, fluoride, chromium
Vitamins (micronutrients)	Fat soluble	Retinol (A), calciferols (D), tocopherols (E), vitamin K
	Water soluble	Ascorbic acid (C), thiamine (B_1), riboflavin (B_2), niacin (B_3), pyridoxine (B_6), folate, cobalamin (B_{12})
Water	Water	Water

Box 1.2

Food insecurity: when people lack secure access to sufficient amounts of safe and nutritious food for normal growth and development and an active and healthy life (FAO, 2011). Food security: when all people, at all times, have physical, social and economic access to sufficient, safe and nutritious food which meets their dietary needs and food preferences for an active and healthy life (FAO, 1996).

the world are at risk of iodine deficiency, iron anaemia affects around 800 million children and women, and vitamin A deficiency was endemic in 60 countries with 190 million preschool age children and 19.1 million pregnant women deficient. This has led to several global initiatives and commitments, spearheaded by a number of United Nations organisations, to reduce global undernutrition, food insecurity, hunger, starvation, and micronutrient deficiencies. Some progress has been made in reducing these numbers, but the problems are far from solved. Some of the initiatives are:

1990

The United Nations Children's (Emergency) Fund (UNICEF)-supported World Summit for Children, with a call to reduce severe and moderate malnutrition among children under five years of age by half the 1990 rate by the year 2000, including goals for the elimination of micronutrient malnutrition;

1992

the World Health Organization/Food and Agriculture Organization (WHO/FAO) International Conference on Nutrition that reinforced earlier goals and extended them to the elimination of death from famine;

1996

the FAO-supported World Food Summit during which 186 heads of state and governments pledged their political will and commitment to a plan of action to reduce the number of undernourished people to half their 1996 number by 2015;

1997

the establishment in of the Food Insecurity and Vulnerability Information and Mapping System (FIVIMS) and their Interagency Working Group (IAWG), which consists of 26 international organisations and agencies with a shared commitment to reduce food insecurity and vulnerability and its multidimensional causes rooted in poverty; information about these initiatives can be accessed at: http://www.fao.org/;

2000

Millennium Development Goals: the United Nations articulated eight goals, ranging from halving extreme poverty and hunger, halting the spread of the human immunodeficiency virus (HIV)/acquired immunodeficiency syndrome (AIDS) and providing universal primary education, to be reached by the target date of 2015; the blueprint of these goals was agreed to by all 191 United Nations member states at that time and 22 leading development institutions. Information about these initiatives can be accessed at: http://www.un.org/millenniumgoals/;

2015

Sustainable Development Goals: developed by the United Nations to succeed the Millennium Development Goals (MDGs), address global challenges including those related to poverty, inequality, climate, environmental degradation, prosperity, and peace and justice with 17 global goals to be achieved by 2030. Information about these initiatives can be accessed at: https://sustainabledevelopment.un.org/

The most recent report from the FAO, published in 2018 indicated that for the third year in a row, there has been a rise in world hunger. The absolute number of undernourished people (those facing chronic food deprivation) has increased to nearly 821 million in 2017, from around 804 million in 2016. These are levels equivalent to 1997–1999 numbers, over two decades ago, when there were 815 million undernourished people in the world. In 2017, a total of 155 million children were stunned (reduced growth rate due to malnutrition) and 52 million children under five were affected by wasting (low weight for height), consequently putting them at a higher risk of mortality. In contrast, adult obesity rates continue to rise each year, from 11.7 percent in 2012 to 13.2 percent in 2016. In 2017 more than one in eight adults (672 million) in the world was classified as obese.

Clearly, this is a huge challenge for food and nutrition scientists and practitioners. It would need a holistic approach and understanding of the complex, interacting factors that contribute to malnutrition on different levels. These include immediate, intermediate, underlying, and basic causes underlined in Figure 1.3.

To address these causes of undernutrition food-insecure and hungry communities and individuals must be empowered to be their own agents of food security and livelihood development. Complicating the task of fighting food insecurity and hunger are natural disasters such as droughts, floods, cyclones and extreme temperatures, ongoing wars and regional

Individual level or immediate causes	Household level or intermediate causes
• Food and nutrient intake • Physical activity health status, • Social structures • Care • Taboos • Growth • Personal choice	• Family size and composition • Gender equity • Rules of distribution of food within the household • Income • Availability of food • Access to food
National level or underlying causes	**International level or basic causes**
• Health, education, sanitation • Agriculture and food security • War • Political instability • Urbanisation • Population growth • Distribution and conflicts • War • Natural disasters • Decreased resources	• Social, economic and political structures • Trade agreements • Population size • Population growth distribution • Environmental degradation

Figure 1.3 immediate, intermediate, underlying, and basic causes that contribute to malnutrition.

conflicts, as well as the devastating impact of HIV and AIDS, especially in sub-Saharan Africa.

In many developing countries, indigenous people have changed their diets and physical activity patterns to those followed in industrialised countries. Supplementary feeding programmes in these countries have often been associated with increasing trends towards obesity, insulin resistance, and the emergence of chronic diseases of lifestyle in some segments of these populations, while other segments are still undernourished.

The coexistence of undernutrition and overnutrition, leading to a double burden of infectious and chronic, noncommunicable diseases, and the multifactorial causes of malnutrition, call for innovative approaches to tackle both undernutrition and overnutrition in integrated nutrition and health-promoting programmes, focusing on optimal nutrition for all.

1.7 Relationship between nutrition science and practice

The journey through the scientific domain of nutrition will, at a specialised stage, fork into different roads. These roads will lead to the different scopes or branches of nutrition science that are covered in the Nutrition Society Textbook Series. These different branches of nutrition science could lead to the training of nutrition specialists for specific practice areas.

The main aim of nutrition professionals is to apply nutrition principles to promote health and well-being, to prevent disease, and/or to restore health (treat disease) in individuals, families, communities and the population. To help individuals or groups of people to eat a balanced diet, in which food supply meets nutrient needs, involves application of nutrition principles from a very broad field to almost every facet of human life. It is therefore not surprising that these different branches or specialties of nutrition have evolved and are developing. They include clinical nutrition, community nutrition, public health, and public nutrition. It can be expected that there will be overlap in the practice areas of these specialties.

- The clinical nutritionist will counsel individuals from a biomedical–disease–behavioral paradigm to promote health, prevent disease, or treat disease. The clinical nutritionist will mostly work within the health service (facility-based settings such as hospitals, clinics, private practice).
- The community nutritionist, with additional skills from the psychosocial behavioral sciences, should be aware of the dynamics within

particular communities responsible for nutritional problems. These would include household food security, socioeconomic background, education levels, childcare practices, sanitation, water, energy sources, healthcare services, and other quality-of-life indicators. The community nutritionist will design, implement, and monitor appropriate, community-participatory programmes to address these problems.

- The public health or public nutritionist covers the health and care practice areas but will also be concerned with food security (agricultural) and environmental issues on a public level. The public health or public nutritionist will, for example, be responsible for nutrition surveillance, and the design, implementation, and monitoring of dietary guidelines that address relevant public health problems. A background knowledge in economics, agriculture, political science, and policy design is essential for the formulation and application of nutrition policy in a country.
- The sports nutritionist will work in sport and exercise nutrition, and will need to understand the specific science and physiology involved to apply into their practice with sports, athletes and other exercise enthusiasts.

Many developing countries will not have the capacity or the financial resources to train and employ professionals for different specialties. However, future specialised training and employment of different professionals could result in a capacity to address nutritional problems more effectively.

1.8 Nutrition milestones: the development of nutrition as a science

Ancient beliefs

Throughout human existence people have attributed special powers to certain foods and developed beliefs and taboos regarding foods. These were often based on climatic, economic, political, or religious circumstances and principles, but also on observations regarding the relationship between the consumption of certain foods and health.

Recorded examples are ancient Chinese and Indian philosophers who advised on the use of warming and cooling foods and spices for certain conditions and for "uplifting the soul," the Mosaic laws documented in the Old Testament which distinguished between clean and unclean foods, the fasting and halal practices of Islam, and the Benedictine monks from Salerno who preached the use of hot and moist versus cold and dry foods for various purposes. Hippocrates, the father of modern medicine, who lived from 460 to about 377 BC, and later Moses Maimonides, who lived in the twelfth century, urged people to practice abstemiousness and a prudent lifestyle. They, and others, advised that, for a long and healthy life, one should avoid too much fat in the diet, eat more fruit, get ample sleep, and be physically active – advice that is still incorporated in the modern, science-based dietary guidelines of the twenty-first century!

Cultural beliefs

The perception that food represents more than its constituent parts is still true. Eating together is an accepted form of social interaction. It is a way in which cultural habits and customs, social status, kinship, love, respect, sharing, and hospitality are expressed. Scientists and nutrition professionals realise that, when formulating dietary guidelines for traditional living people, cultural beliefs and taboos should be taken into account and incorporated. There are numerous examples of traditional food habits and diets, often based on what was available. Today, with the world becoming a global village, cultures have learned from each other, and dietary patterns associated with good health, such as the Mediterranean diet, are becoming popular among many cultures.

The first renaissance: development of an evidence base

The knowledge of the specific health effects of particular diets, foods, and nutrients is now firmly based on the results of rigid scientific experimentation. Nutrition developed gradually as a science, but advanced with rapid strides during the twentieth century. There are numerous meticulously recorded examples of how initial (often ancient and primitive) observations about diet and health relationships led to the discovery, elucidation of function, isolation, and synthesis of the different nutrients. Perhaps the most often quoted example is James Lind's description in 1772 of how citrus fruit could cure and prevent scurvy in seamen on long voyages. The anti-scurvy factor (ascorbic acid or vitamin C) was only isolated in 1921, characterised in 1932, and chemically synthesised in 1933. Other examples of nutritional milestones are the induction of beriberi in domestic fowl by Eijkman in 1897, the observation of Takaki in 1906 that beriberi in Japanese sailors could be prevented by supplementing their polished rice diets with wheat bread, and, eventually, the isolation of the responsible factor, thiamine or vitamin B_1, by Funk in 1911. Others are the Nobel Prize-winning discovery by Minot and Murphy in 1926 that pernicious anemia is a nutritional disorder due to a lack of vitamin B_{12} in the diet, the description of kwashiorkor as a protein-deficiency state by Cecily Williams in 1935, and the discovery of resistant starch and importance of colonic fermentation for humans by nutritionists of the Dunn Clinical Nutrition Centre in the 1980s.

The history of modern nutrition as practised today is an exciting one to read, and students are encouraged to spend some time on it. It is often characterised by heartbreaking courage and surprising insights. An example of the former is the carefully documented clinical, metabolic, and pathological consequences of hunger and starvation by a group of Jewish doctors in 1940 in the Warsaw ghetto: doctors who were themselves dying of hunger. An example of the latter is the research by Price, an American dentist, who tried to identify the dietary factors responsible for good dental and overall health in people living traditional lifestyles. He unwittingly used a fortigenic paradigm in his research, examining the strengths and factors that keep people healthy, long before the term was defined or its value recognised.

At present, thousands of nutrition scientists examine many aspects of nutrition in laboratories and field studies all over the world and publish in more than 100 international scientific nutrition journals. This means that nutrition science generates new knowledge based on well-established research methodologies. The many types of experiments, varying from molecular experimentation in the laboratory, through placebo-controlled, double-blinded clinical interventions, to observational epidemiological surveys, and experiments based on a health (fortigenic) or a disease (pathogenic) paradigm, will be addressed in this volume (Chapter 13). The peer-review process of published results has helped in the development of guidelines to judge how possible, probable, convincing, and applicable are the results from these studies. New knowledge of nutrients, foods, and diet relationships with health and disease is, therefore, generated through a process in which many scientists examine different pieces of the puzzle all over the world in controlled scientific experiments. Therefore, nutrition practice today has a firm research base that enables nutritional professionals to practice evidence-based nutrition.

The second renaissance: solving global malnutrition

There is little doubt that improved nutrition has contributed to the improved health and survival times experienced by modern humans. However, global figures on the prevalence of both undernutrition and overnutrition show that millions of people do not have enough to eat, while the millions who eat too much suffer from the consequences of obesity. It is tempting to equate this situation to the gap between the poor and the rich or between developing and developed countries, but the situation is much more complex. Obesity, a consequence of overnutrition, is now a public health problem not only in rich, developed, food-secure countries but also in developing, food-insecure countries, especially among women. Undernutrition, the major impediment to national development, is the biggest single contributor to childhood death rates, and to impaired physical growth and mental development of children in both developing and developed countries. Moreover, a combination of undernutrition and overnutrition in the same communities, in single households, and even in the same individual is often reported. Examples are obese mothers with undernourished children and obese women with certain micronutrient deficiencies. The perception that these global problems of malnutrition will be solved only in innovative, multidisciplinary, and multisectorial ways has led to the second, very recent renaissance in nutrition research and practice.

1.9 Future challenges for nutrition research and practice

Basic, molecular nutrition

The tremendous development in recent years of molecular biology and the availability of sophisticated new techniques are opening up a field in which nutrient–gene interactions and dietary manipulation of genetic expression will receive increasing attention. The effects of more than 12 000 different substances in plant foods, not yet classified as nutrients, will also be examined. These substances are produced by plants for hormonal, attractant, and chemoprotective purposes, and there is evidence that many of them offer protection against a wide range of human conditions. It is possible that new functions of known nutrients, and even new nutrients, may be discovered, described, and applied in the future.

Clinical and community nutrition

Today, the focus has moved from simple experiments with clear-cut answers to studies in which sophisticated statistics have to be used to dissect out the role of specific nutrients, foods, and diets in multifactorial diseases. Nutrition epidemiology is now established as the discipline in which these questions can be addressed. A number of pressing problems will have to be researched and the results applied, for example:

- the biological and sociological causes of childhood obesity, which is emerging as a global public health problem;
- the nutrient requirements of the elderly: in the year 2017, more than 962 million of the Earth's inhabitants were older than 60 years and the number is expected to double by 2050 reaching nearly 2.1 billion (WHO,2017); to ensure a high-quality life in the growing elderly population, much more needs to be known about their nutrient requirements;
- the relationships between nutrition and immune function and how improved nutrition can help to defend against invading microorganisms; in the light of the increasing HIV/AIDS pandemic, more information in this area is urgently needed;
- dietary recommendations: despite sufficient, convincing evidence about the effects of nutrients and foods on health, nutritionists have generally not been very successful in motivating the public to change their diets to more healthy ones. We need to know more about why people make certain food choices in order to design culturally sensitive and practical dietary guidelines that will impact positively on dietary choices. The food-based dietary guidelines that are now being developed in many countries are a first step in this direction.

Public health nutrition

The single most important challenge facing mankind in the future is probably to provide adequate safe food and clean water for all in an environmentally safe way that will not compromise the ability of future generations to meet their needs. In addition to the hundreds of millions not eating enough food to meet their needs for a healthy, active life, an additional 80 million people have to be fed each year. The challenge to feed mankind in the future calls for improved agriculture in drought-stricken areas such as sub-Saharan Africa, the application of biotechnology in a responsible way, interdisciplinary and intersectorial cooperation of all involved, and a better distribution of the food supply so that affordable food is accessible by all. The need for sustained economic growth in poor countries is evident.

Nutritionists have an important part to play in ensuring food security for all, a basic human right, in the future. One of their main functions would be to educate and inform populations not to rely too heavily on animal products in their diet, the production of which places a much heavier burden on the environment than plant foods. A major challenge would be to convince political leaders and governments that addressing undernutrition (the major obstacle in national development) in sustainable programmes should be the top priority in developing and poor communities. Another challenge is to develop models based on the dynamics within communities and, using a human rights approach, to alleviate undernutrition without creating a problem of overnutrition. There are examples where such models, incorporated

Microbial contamination Bacteria and Mould (fungi) producing toxins and aflatoxins Toxins cause "food poisoning" and aflatoxins are carcinogenic	
Natural toxins Such as cyanide in cassava, solanine in potatoes; can be produced by abnormal circumstances, could be enzyme inhibitors or antivitamins	**Agricultural residues** Pesticides such as DDT or hormones used to promote growth such as bovine somatotrophin
Environmental contamination Heavy metals and minerals Criminal adulteration, industrial pollution Substances from packaging materials Changes during cooking and processing of foods	**Intentional additives** Artificial sweeteners Preservatives Phytochemicals Modified carbohydrates (for functional foods)

Figure 1.4 Potential hazardous substances in food. DDT, dichloro-diphenyl-trichloroethane.

into community development programmes, have been very successful (e.g., in Thailand).

Functional foods: a new development

Functional foods are new or novel foods, developed to have specific health benefits, in addition to their usual functions. Examples are spreads with added phytosterols, to lower serum low-density lipoprotein cholesterol and the risk of coronary heart disease, and the development of starchy products with resistant starch and lower glycemic indices, to help control blood glucose levels. The development and testing of functional foods is an exciting new area. These foods may help to improve or restore nutritional status in many people. However, much more should be known about suitable biomarkers to test their efficacy, variability in human response to specific food products, safety, consumer understanding, and how their health messages must be formulated, labeled, and communicated.

Food safety

The continued provision of safe food, free from microorganisms, toxins, and other hazardous substances that cause disease, remains a huge challenge (see chapter 15 for more on food safety). Recent experiences with animals suffering from bovine spongiform encephalopathy (BSE or mad cow disease) or from foot-and-mouth disease, or birds infected with the influenza A virus (bird flu), have shown how quickly a national problem can become an international one because of global marketing of products.

The list of possible hazardous substances in foods emphasizes the need for continuous monitoring of the food supply by health officials (Figure 1.4).

Supplements and food fortification

A dietary or nutritional supplement is defined as a product with the purpose of supplementing the diet, providing additional nutrients that may be missing from it or not being consumed in sufficient quantities. Dietary supplements might contain vitamins, minerals, herbs, amino acids, enzymes, fibre, and fatty acids. They are available in a variety of forms, including traditional tablets, capsules, powders, drinks and supplement bars. It has been estimated that millions of people around the world take vitamins and dietary supplements to achieve good health, ease our illnesses and defy ageing. In 2009 the market for dietary supplements and vitamins was worth more than £670 million in the UK alone.

Food fortification increases the content of an essential micronutrient (i.e. vitamins and minerals) in a food to improve the nutritional quality of the food and provide a public health benefit with minimal risk to health. Bio-fortification is the process by which the nutrient levels in crops during plant growth, rather than through manual means as in conventional fortification, by agronomic practices, conventional plant breeding, or modern biotechnology. Food fortification in general provides a potentially effective strategy to improve the nutritional status of populations.

1.10 Perspectives on the future

Nutrition research and practice, although it has been around for many years, is in its infancy as a basic and applied scientific discipline. The present and future nutrition student will take part in this very exciting second renaissance of nutrition and see its maturation. However, to influence effectively the nutrition and health of individuals and populations, the nutritionist will have to forge links and partnerships with other health professionals and policy-makers, and will have to develop lateral thinking processes. The magnitude and complexity of nutritional problems facing mankind today demand concerted multidisciplinary and multisectorial efforts from all involved to solve them. Therefore, the principal message to take on a nutrition science journey is that teamwork is essential: one cannot travel this road on one's own; partners from different disciplines are needed. Another essential need is the continuous development of leadership in nutrition. Leaders on every level of research and practice are necessary to respond to the existing challenges of global malnutrition and to face future challenges.

The modern advances in molecular biology and biotechnology on the one hand, and the persistence of global malnutrition on the other, increasingly demand a re-evaluation of ethical norms, standards, and values for nutrition science and practice. Direction from responsible leaders is needed (Box 1.3). There is an urgent need for ethical guidelines and a code of conduct for partnerships between food industries, UN agencies, governments, and academics. These partnerships are necessary for addressing global malnutrition in sustainable programmes.

The student in nutrition, at the beginning of this journey of discovery of nutrition as a science, must make use of the many opportunities to develop leadership qualities. May this be a happy, fruitful, and lifelong journey with many lessons that can be applied in the research and practice of nutrition to make a difference in the life of all.

Box 1.3 Future challenges that require exceptional leadership

- Basic molecular nutrition
  - Nutrient–gene interactions
  - Role of phytochemicals in health
  - New nutrients? New functions?
- Community and public health nutrition
  - Childhood obesity
  - Requirements of the elderly
  - Dietary recommendations
  - Nutrition of patients with human immunodeficiency virus/ acquired immunodeficiency syndrome
  - Noncommunicable diseases including cardiovascular diseases (like heart attacks and stroke), cancer, chronic respiratory diseases (such as chronic obstructed pulmonary disease and asthma) and diabetes.
- Public nutrition
  - To feed mankind
  - Food security
- Functional foods
  - To ensure that novel foods are effective and safe
  - Food safety
  - Continuous monitoring
- Partnerships with other disciplines to offer multidisciplinary approaches
- Nutrition research
- Leadership

Further reading

Websites

http://www.who.int/nutrition/en
https://www.un.org/nutrition/
www.fao.org/nutrition/en/
http://www.ifpri.org

2
Measuring Dietary Intake

Una E. MacIntyre and Friedeburg AM. Wenhold

Key messages

- Measuring the dietary intake in free-living individuals is a complex task.
- The dietary assessment method used depends on the purpose of the study, the target group and the setting.
- All measurements of food intake are subject to sources of error.
- The existence of error means that it is always important to be aware of and, whenever possible, to assess the nature and magnitude of the error.
- To increase our understanding of the error associated with measurements of food intake it is also necessary to use physiological and biochemical markers of dietary intake.
- To evaluate dietary intake data effectively it is important to collect sufficient additional data to allow individuals to be identified not only by age and gender, but also by body mass index, physical activity, and supplement use.
- Dietary assessment is a growing field. New formats, tools, techniques, and strategies are constantly emerging.

2.1 Introduction

The purpose of this chapter is to describe the various ways in which one can determine what people eat. The task may be to find out about the national food supply, the usual intake of a group or a household, or the intake of a given individual over a specified period.

The many reasons for finding out about the food that people eat fall into three broad categories:

- Public Health: to evaluate the adequacy and safety of the food that people eat at national or community level, to formulate national or local food production and/or supply policies and to identify the need for or to evaluate nutrition-based intervention programmes.
- Clinical: to assist with the prevention, diagnosis, and management of diet-related conditions.
- Research: to study the interrelationships between dietary intake and physiological function or ill-health under controlled (experimental) or in real life (field) conditions. The kind and amount of dietary intake data required differ in each situation and may be at the national, community, household, or individual level.

Assessment of nutritional status

Nutritional health is maintained by a state of equilibrium in which nutrient intake is balanced by nutritional requirements. Malnutrition occurs when net nutrient intake is less than requirements (undernutrition) or exceeds requirements (overnutrition). Both under- and overnutrition lead to metabolic changes which have acute and chronic consequences for health.

There is no ideal tool to measure a person's nutritional status accurately. Attempts to predict the influence of malnutrition based on single measurements fail to consider the many interacting factors between nutrition and disease state. For this reason, it is necessary to look at several different measurements in order to

Introduction to Human Nutrition, Third Edition. Edited on behalf of The Nutrition Society by Susan A. Lanham-New, Thomas R. Hill, Alison M. Gallagher and Hester H. Vorster.

Companion website: www.wiley.com/go/lanham-new/humannutrition

Box 2.1

Food intake: Foods and beverages consumed by a population, community, household or individual.
Nutrient intake: The energy and individual macro and micronutrient intake, whether provided by foods and beverages consumed and derived from either direct analysis or food composition tables/databases or from nutritional supplements.
Dietary intake: The sum of the food, beverage and nutritional supplement intake and the macro- and micronutrients, non-nutrient components and water derived therefrom.

assess a person's nutritional status. This process is known as the A, B, C, D of nutritional assessment:

- **a**nthropometry (discussed in detail in Chapter 5)
- **b**iochemical and haematological variables
- **c**linical and physical assessment
- **d**ietary intake.

Dietary intake refers to both the consumption of food, beverages, including water, and supplements (when relevant) and the energy, nutrients, and non-nutrient components provided by these foods, beverages, and supplements. Box 2.1 gives definitions of the components of dietary intake. Figure 2.1 shows the relationships between the components of dietary intake, dietary requirements, and the nutritional status of an individual.

The rest of this chapter will concentrate on the measurement of diet, that is, measuring food intake, the conversion of food intake data to energy and nutrients and methods for summarising and reporting food and/or nutrient intake information. More detailed descriptions of the assessment of nutritional status, at the population and individual level can be found in the *Public Health Nutrition* and *Clinical Nutrition* textbooks in this series.

Challenges of dietary assessment

Obtaining data on dietary intake is probably the most difficult aspect of nutritional assessment and is associated with several problems:

- "Dietary intake" is not a simple measure of one variable, such as weight or height, but requires data on the intake of many different food and beverage items.
- Dietary intake data are subject to many sources of variability, since even the same individuals eat different foods, at different times, in different places, in many different combinations, and with many different preparation methods. The net effect of all these sources of variability is that more data are needed to generate reliable results than would be the case with a less variable measure.
- We are rarely in a position to know the truth about dietary intake. With many biological measurements it is possible to check the results obtained against a reference method that is known to give accurate results or by means of an independent measure. For example, we can check an infant's birth weight by using a standard weight to confirm the accuracy of the scale or, if the information was obtained by means of a questionnaire, we may be able to check the data from official records. When assessing dietary intake, we have to rely on the individuals who eat the food to provide us with the answers to our questions. We ask individuals to remember what and how much they ate, to estimate how often they eat particular foods, or even, in some situations, to weigh or measure their food intake for a number of days. Furthermore, we rely on the individuals' ability to describe or record their food intake in detail. For this reason one of the most important considerations, when obtaining information on dietary intake from individuals, is to take all possible steps to obtain their full cooperation. It is also extremely important that individuals understand the purpose of the process and what is expected of them. This may well involve much time and effort on the part of the nutrition professional(s), but is essential for high-quality data.
- There are a number of different methods to obtain dietary intake data. Each method has its purposes, strengths, and limitations. It is, therefore, essential that the purpose of collecting dietary intake data is clearly defined, so that the most appropriate dietary assessment method is used.

It is also essential to recognise that finding out what people eat requires adequate resources. Appropriately trained personnel must be employed not only for the period of data

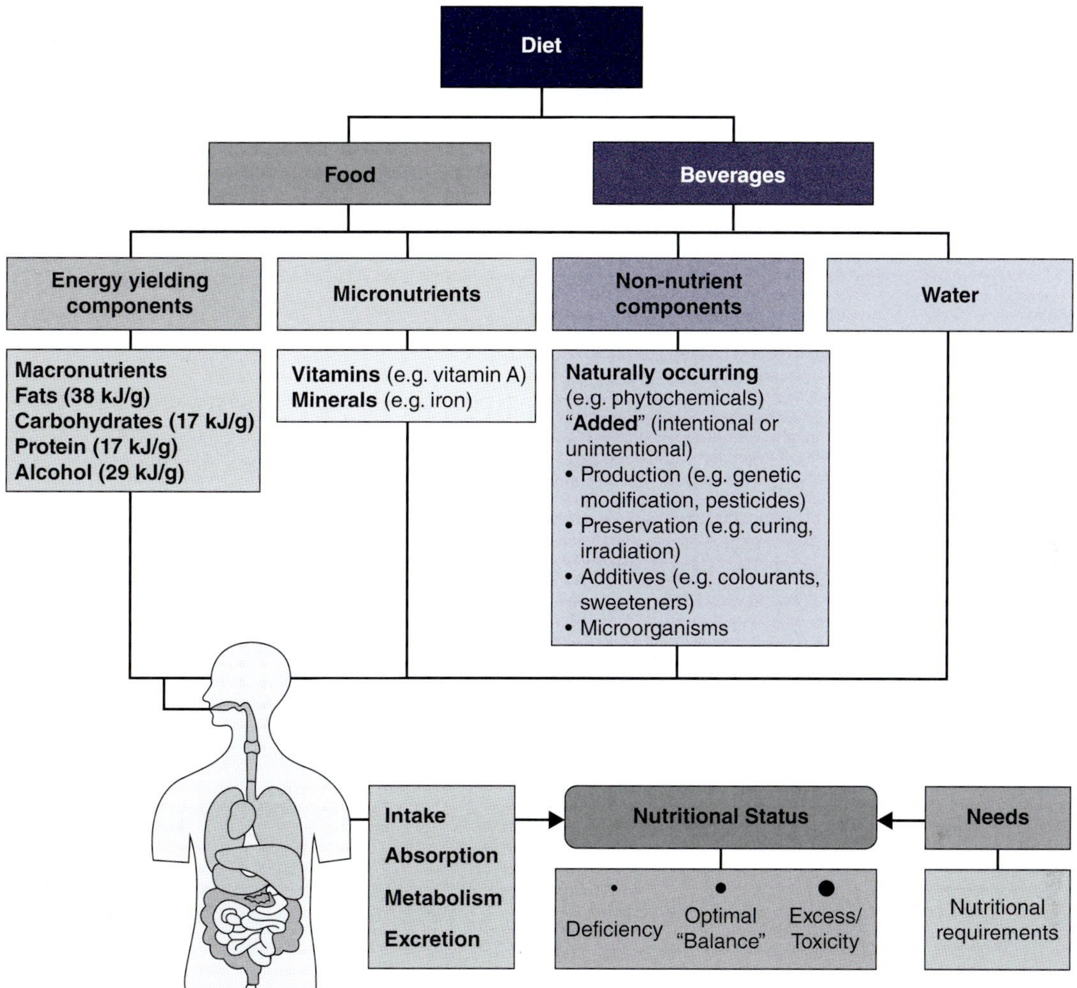

Figure 2.1 The relationship between the components of diet, nutritional requirements and the nutritional status of an individual. Source: Wenhold F.A.M, Faber M. Beverage intake: Nutritional role, challenges, and opportunities for developing countries. In: Grumezesu A.M. (ed). Nutrients in beverages. (Woodhead Publ/Elsvier, Duxford, 2019).

collection but also for the time it takes to review, enter, and analyse the data. It may not always be necessary to obtain detailed data on food intake in order to answer a particular question. When resources are limited it is probably more useful to collect limited data of high quality than to attempt to collect comprehensive dietary data with inadequate resources. Being able to recognise this situation is important for maximising available resources. Table 2.1 lists the different approaches to measurement of food intake that are described in this chapter.

Finally, it is important that the interpretation and application of data derived from dietary intake studies take into account the limitations of the data. This clearly does not improve the quality of the data per se, but maximises their usefulness for the purpose for which they were originally collected. Recognition of the limitations of dietary data involves more than simply stating the limitations. External comparisons to check whether the data are consistent with independent sources of information on food intake and to determine the likely direction and magnitude of any bias are an integral part of the interpretation of dietary data. Relevant sources of comparative information may include food supply and expenditure data and physiological or biochemical measures related to nutrient intake.

Table 2.1 Approaches to the measurement of food intake in population groups, households, and individuals

Type and nature of data	Name of method	Used for describing and/or assessing differences between
Indirect data		
Commodity-level food supply data, e.g., production, imports and exports	Food balance sheets	Countries and regions of the world
Product-level food supply data, e.g., retail and wholesale sales data	Food disappearance data	Country, locality, and season
Household food acquisition and expenditure, e.g., money spent on food	Household consumption and expenditure surveys	Country, locality, season, and type of household
Household food acquisition, e.g., amount of food entering the household	Household food account Household food procurement Household food inventory	Country, locality, season, and type of household
Direct data		
Household food consumption	Household food records	Country, locality, season, and type of household
Qualitative record of foods (but not amounts) eaten over the course of one or more days by individuals	Menu records	Geographical, seasonal, and demographic subgroups and individuals
Quantitative record of food intake, e.g., record of foods eaten over the course of one or more days by individuals	Weighed records and records estimated in household measures	Geographical, seasonal, and demographic subgroups and individuals
Quantitative recall of foods eaten on the previous day, usually obtained from individuals by interview	Single or multiple 24 hour recalls	Geographical, seasonal, and demographic subgroups and individuals (if multiple recalls obtained)
Qualitative, semi-quantitative or quantitative recall, usually of a specified list of foods, eaten in the previous month to year by individuals	Food frequency questionnaires	Geographical, seasonal, and demographic subgroups and individuals
Quantitative recall of habitual intake in the immediate past obtained from individuals by interview	Diet history	Temporal and demographic subgroups and individuals

Source: Adapted from: Gibney, M.J., Lanham-New, S.A., Cassidy, A. *et al. Introduction to Human Nutrition, 2e.* (Wiley Blackwell, Chichester, 2009)

2.2 Indirect measurement of food intake

Indirect measurements of food intake make use of information on the availability of food at national, regional, local or household levels to estimate food intakes, rather than using information obtained directly from the individuals who consume the food. Indirect methods are most useful at population and household levels for determining the amount and types of foods that are:

- available for consumption at national level (commodity-level food supply data).
- traded at wholesale or retail levels (product-level food supply data).
- purchased or otherwise acquired at household level (household acquisition and expenditure data).

Commodity level food supply data

Food supply data are usually produced at national level from compilations of data from multiple sources. The primary sources of data are records of agricultural production and food exports and imports adjusted for changes in stocks and for agricultural and industrial use of food crops and food products. National food supply data are usually referred to as "food balance sheets" or as "apparent consumption" data. Food balance sheets give the total production and utilisation of reported food items and show the sources (production, stocks, and imports) and utilisation (exports, industrial use, wastage, and human consumption) of food items available for human consumption in a country for a given reference period. The amount of each food item is usually expressed per caput (per person) in grams or kilograms per year by dividing the total amount of food available for human consumption by relevant population statistics. An analysis of the energy, protein, and fat provided by the food item may also be given.

The Food and Agriculture Organization (FAO) has compiled and published food balance sheet data for most countries in the world since 1949. Regularly updated food balance sheet data are available for most countries for about 100 primary crop, livestock, and fishery commodities and some products such as sugar, oils, and fats derived from them. Food balance sheets may be downloaded in Excel format from the FAO website (http://www.fao.org/faostat/en/#data/FBS) with options to select the country or region, the commodities and required output.

The accuracy of food balance sheets and apparent consumption data depends on the reliability of the basic statistics used to derive them, i.e., population, supply, utilisation, and food composition data. These can vary markedly between countries in terms not only of coverage but also of accuracy.

Several internal and external consistency checks are built into the preparation of the FAO food balance sheets, but users still need to evaluate the data in terms of the purpose for which they are being used. One of the crucial factors in using the data appropriately is to understand the terminology used. Box 2.2 provides "in principle" definitions of the key terms (FAO, 2002).

Food balance sheets provide important data on food supply and availability in a country and show whether the food supply of the country as a whole is adequate for the nutritional needs of its population. Over a period of years, food balance sheets show trends in national food supply and food consumption patterns and can be used to predict future supply needs, set agricultural production targets, and set and evaluate national food and nutrition policies. They may be used for population comparisons such as comparing population estimates of fat intake with cardiovascular disease rates.

In practice, the data needed to compile food balance sheets are not always available and estimates may have to be made at each stage in the calculation of per caput food and nutrient availability. In most countries reliable data are usually available on primary commodities, but this is not necessarily the case for the major processed products. For example, data may be available on flour but not on products such as bread and other cereal products made from flour having quite different nutrient characteristics. The overall impact of incomplete data will vary from country to country. It has been suggested that, in

Box 2.2

Commodity coverage: all potentially edible commodities whether used for human consumption or for non-food purposes.
Exports: all movements out of the country during the reference period.
Feed: the quantity of the commodity available for feeding livestock and poultry.
Food quantity: the amounts of the commodity and any commodity derived therefrom available for human consumption during the reference period, e.g., for maize includes maize, maize meal, and any other products derived from maize that are available for human consumption.
Imports: all movements of the commodity into the country, e.g., commercial trade, food aid, donated quantities, and estimates of unrecorded trade.
Industrial uses: commodities used for manufacture for non-food purposes, e.g., oils for soap.
Per caput supply: adjustments are made when possible to the resident population for temporary migrants, refugees, and tourists. The figures represent only the average supply available for the population as a whole and not what is actually consumed by individuals. Many commodities are not consumed in the primary form in which they are reported in food balance sheets. To take this into account the energy, protein and fat content shown against primary commodities are derived by applying appropriate food composition factors to the relevant amounts of processed foods, and not by multiplying the quantities shown in the food balance sheet by food composition factors relating to the primary commodity.
Production: total domestic production whether produced inside or outside the agricultural sector, i.e., includes non-commercial production and production from home gardens.
Seed: quantity of the commodity set aside for sowing or planting or any other form of reproduction for animal or human consumption.
Stock variation: changes in stocks occurring during the reference period at all levels between the production and retail levels, i.e., stocks held by the government, manufacturers, importers, exporters, wholesale and retail merchants, and distributors. In practice, the available information often only relates to government stocks.
Waste: commodities lost through all stages between post-harvest production and the household, i.e., waste in processing, storage, and transportation, but not domestic waste. Losses occurring during the manufacture of processed products are taken into account by means of extraction/conversion rates.

general, underestimation of per caput availability of nutrients is more likely in middle and low income countries and overestimation in industrialised countries where most of the food supply is consumed in the form of processed products.

It is also very important to keep in mind that food balance sheets show only data on foods available for consumption, not the actual consumption of foods; nor do they show the distribution of foods within the population, for example among different regions or among different socioeconomic, age, and gender groups. Food balance sheets also do not provide information on seasonal variations in food supply.

Product-level food supply data

In most industrialised as well as middle and low income countries data on *per caput* food availability are prepared from information on raw and processed foods available at the retail or wholesale level (also known as food disappearance data). Such data are derived mainly from food industry organisations and firms engaged in food production and marketing such as supermarkets. Errors arise mainly from inappropriate conversion factors for processing, the absence of data for some processed products, and the lack of data on food obtained from non-commercial sources such as home gardens, subsistence farming, fishing, and hunting.

Commercial databases and reports such as those produced by market research companies, e.g., the international Nielsen Corporation (formerly the AC Nielsen Company) (http://www.nielsen.com), and the electronic stock-control records from supermarket chains or individual supermarkets from which they are compiled, have the potential for monitoring national, regional, and local trends in the food supply, at a product-specific level. Their principal disadvantage at present lies in the costs associated accessing, on a regular basis, the very large amounts of data that are involved.

FAO food balance sheets and similar sources of information are primarily useful for formulating agricultural and health policies, for monitoring changes in national food supplies and food security over time, and as a basis for forecasting food consumption patterns. They can also be used to make intercountry comparisons of food and nutrient supplies, provided that potential differences in data coverage and accuracy are taken into account.

Household acquisition and expenditure data

Household-based surveys determine the foods and beverages available for consumption at family, household, or institutional levels. Some surveys such as household consumption and expenditure surveys (HCES) determine the amount of money spent on food for a given period, while others, such as the food account, food inventory and food record methods, attempt to describe the food available and/or consumed by a household or institution.

Household consumption and expenditure surveys

HCES refer to a range of national surveys undertaken, not only by industrialised but also middle and low income countries, primarily to describe living standards, calculate consumer price indices and inform national statistics. HCES include, among others, Household Income and Expenditure Surveys (HEIS), Household Budget Surveys (HBS), and Living Standards Measurement Surveys (LSMS). Typically, HCES contain questions on the types and quantities of foods acquired and expenditure on food by households over a given recall period. Although HCES do not measure food consumption directly, food related data derived from HCES may be used to describe and compare food consumption patterns at national, regional and local levels and according to socio-economic levels and season. When HCESs are carried out at regular intervals, the data are useful for monitoring changes in food consumption patterns over time. If of satisfactory quality and appropriately analysed, HCES data may further be used to measure poverty levels, calculate food security indicators such as household dietary diversity scores (HDDS), identify high risk groups for nutrition related conditions, compile food balance sheets, identify needs for, plan and monitor food-based nutrition interventions including food fortification programmes and provide food consumption information to the private sector (Fiedler *et al.*, 2012).

HCES have several advantages:

- they are usually conducted at regular intervals of between two and five years.
- they are conducted on representative samples of households.
- data collection is usually over a 12-month period.
- food-related information may be classified by socio-demographic characteristics, geographic region and season.

Previous limitations of HCES were their failure to collect data on foods acquired from sources other than purchases and on foods consumed out of the home. Over the last number of years, these concerns have been addressed by the inclusion of questions on the acquisition of foods from:

- market-place purchases
- the household's own production
- in-kind wages, gifts or donations
- consumption outside the home and places of consumption such as work cafeteria, restaurants, fast-food outlets and another's home.

Nevertheless, obtaining reliable information on food obtained from sources other than purchases and foods consumed outside the home is extremely complex and requires great skill in both the design and administration of the questionnaire.

Other limitations of the information provided by HCES which must be considered include:

- differences in the number of food items recorded and in the type of information collected from different countries
- food coding systems differ between countries making inter-country comparisons difficult
- most surveys do not collect information on domestic wastage such as food given to pets, spoiled food and plate waste, or food provided for guests
- no information is given regarding the distribution of foods within the household.

In 2006, the International Household Survey Network (IHSN) was established to provide leadership and technical assistance, particularly to middle and low income countries, to improve the availability, quality, standardisation and use of HCES data. The IHSN website (http://www.ihsn.org/food) is a rich resource providing a database of HCES conducted throughout the world, guidance on survey and questionnaire design, criteria for assessing the quality of HCES information and mathematical methods for deriving food and nutrient intakes from survey information.

Three conclusions can be drawn about the use of HCES to measure food intakes. First, despite efforts to harmonise instruments and procedures of HCES, data are not necessarily comparable between countries. Second, obtaining sufficient data to provide an accurate assessment of the total food supply available at household level is complex and must be interpreted within the context in which it has been collected. Third, provided that the HCES methodology remains consistent, HCES can provide a great deal of valuable information about food patterns over time, in different socio-demographic groups, and in different parts of the country, and how these relate to social, economic, and technological changes in the food supply.

Household food account method

In the food account method, the household member responsible for the household's food keeps a record of the types and amounts of all food entering the household including purchases, gifts, foods produced by the household itself such as from vegetable and fruit gardens, foods obtained from the wild, or from other sources. Amounts are usually recorded in retail units (if applicable) or in household measures. Information may also be collected on brand names and costs. The recording period is usually one week but may be as long as four weeks.

This method is used to obtain food selection patterns from populations or subgroups within a population. It has the advantage of being fairly cost-effective and is particularly useful for collecting data from large samples. It may also be repeated at different times of the year to identify seasonal variations in food procurement.

The food account method does not measure food consumption, wastage, or other uses, nor does it account for foods consumed outside the home. It assumes that household food stocks stay constant throughout the recording period, which may not necessarily be the case. For example, food purchases may be done once a month and therefore stocks may be depleted in the days preceding the purchase. It also does not reflect the distribution of food within the household and therefore cannot be used to determine food consumption by individuals within the household. Since the method relies on the respondents being literate and cooperative, bias may be introduced in populations with high levels of illiteracy. The fact of having to record the acquisition may lead to respondents changing their procurement patterns either to simplify recording or to impress the nutrition professional.

Household food procurement questionnaire/interview

A food procurement questionnaire or interview may be used as an alternative method to the food account method. In this method, the respondent indicates, from a list of foods, which are used, where these are obtained, the frequency of purchase, and the quantities acquired for a given period. The uses of the food procurement method are similar to those of the food account: to describe food acquisition patterns of populations or subpopulations. In contrast to the food account method, it does not require the respondent to be literate as it may be administered as an interview and it does not influence purchasing or other procurement patterns.

The food procurement questionnaire/interview does not provide information on actual food consumption or distribution within the household. As the method relies on recalled information, errors may be introduced by inaccurate memory or expression of answers.

Household food inventory method

The food inventory method uses direct observation to describe all foods in the household on the day of the survey. The nutrition professional/investigator records the types and amounts of foods present in a household, whether raw, processed, or cooked, at the time of the visit. Information may also be collected on how and where food is stored.

A food inventory may be combined with the food account to determine the changes of food stocks during the survey period. It may also be used together with a food procurement questionnaire to describe the acquisition of foods in the household. This method is time-consuming for the investigator and very intrusive for the respondent, but is useful when foods are procured by means other than purchase and when levels of food security in vulnerable households need to be assessed.

Household food record

All foods available for consumption by the household are weighed or estimated by household measures prior to serving. Detailed information such as brand names, ingredients, and preparation methods are also recorded over a specific period, usually one week. This method provides detailed information on the food consumption patterns of the household, but it is very time-consuming and intrusive and relies heavily on the cooperation of the household. As for the other household methods, it does not provide information on distribution of food within the household or on individual consumption. When details of the household composition are given, estimates of individual intakes may be calculated. The method also does not determine foods eaten away from the home nor does it take into account food eaten by guests to the home.

2.3 Direct measures of dietary intake

Information on dietary intake can be obtained directly from consumers in a number of different ways. Direct measures are usually used to obtain food intake data from individuals but may also be used to obtain data from households. For example, in societies where it is usual for members of the household to eat out of the same pot this may be the only practical approach because it does not disrupt the normal pattern of food intake. Unlike indirect measures of food intake, direct measures provide sufficient information on food consumption to convert the food intake into energy and nutrient intakes.

Irrespective of the method used, the process of obtaining food intake information and converting this to energy and nutrient data is the same. The procedure for measuring food and nutrient intake involves five steps (Figure 2.2):

- obtaining a report of all the foods consumed by each individual
- quantifying the portion sizes and frequency with which each food is eaten (food frequency questionnaires (FFQ) and diet history)
- describing foods in sufficient detail to choose an appropriate item in the food composition database
- calculating the nutrient intake from the food composition database
- evaluating the food and/or energy and nutrient intakes against a reference standard.

To convert the information on food intake into nutrient intake, the nutrient content of each food eaten is calculated from food database as:

$$\text{Portion size}\left(g\right)\times\text{nutrient content per gram}$$

and summed for all foods eaten by each individual during the study period.

It must be kept in mind, as indicated in Figure 2.2, that the calculation of nutrient intakes may not necessarily be the only or the desired outcome of the measurement of food intakes. Depending of the purpose of the dietary intake assessment, food intakes may be reported as individual food items or food groups consumed, food patterns or scores calculated to reflect the overall quality of the diet.

Direct measurement of food intake can be divided into two basic approaches:

- reports of foods consumed on specified days: menu records, weighed food records, estimated food records and 24 hour recalls
- reports of food intake over a period in the past: FFQ and diet histories.

Food records are usually limited to fairly short periods, usually not longer than seven consecutive days, while recalls may relate to a single period of 24 hours or occasionally 48 hours. FFQ and diet histories relate to longer periods in order to obtain an assessment of habitual intake over the period in question rather than a detailed day-to-day recall of what was eaten. Each of these approaches has specific strengths and limitations. No single method of measuring food intake can be regarded as the ideal method for all situations.

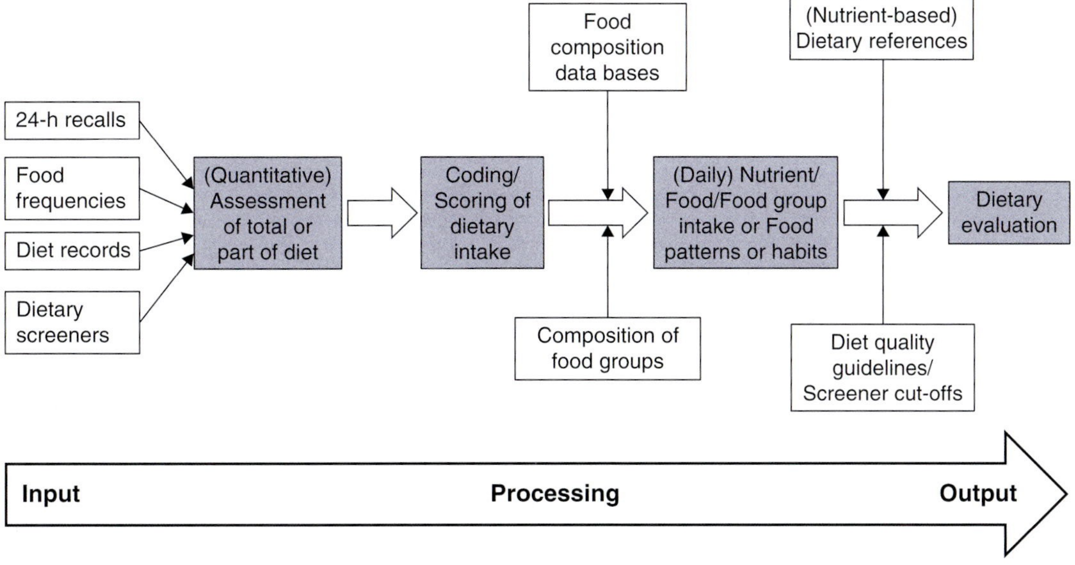

Figure 2.2 The dietary assessment process. Source: Wenhold FAM. Technology in dietary assessment. Public Health Nutrition 2018;21(2):257–9. https://www.cambridge.org/core/journals/public-health-nutrition/article/technology-in-dietary-assessment/5DC9AE6C1728DE4E76CC067A1D67E619

In the past, weighed intake recorded over a seven day period was taken as the reference method against which less detailed methods were compared. It has, however, been realised that this method has its limitations and that it is not only desirable but also necessary to use physiological and biochemical measures to determine whether any method of measuring food intake is actually measuring what it sets out to measure. This will be discussed in more detail in Section 2.9.

2.4 Basic concepts

Before describing the most commonly used direct dietary assessment methods, it is appropriate to introduce four fundamental concepts relevant to the process of dietary assessment and evaluation. A brief definition of terms related to these concepts is given in Box 2.3. Terms are listed in the box in alphabetical order for ease of reference.

Habitual intake

The objective of virtually all dietary assessments is to obtain an estimate of the habitual or average long-term intake for the group or the individual of interest. Habitual intake represents what is "usual" in the long term and not simply at a specific moment in time. It is this level of intake that is relevant for the maintenance of energy balance and nutrient status, and for the assessment of relationships between nutrient intake and health in the long term. Habitual intake, however, is difficult to measure because food intake varies widely from day to day and, to a lesser extent, from week to week and month to month. Figure 2.3 illustrates the energy intake of one individual who maintained a weighed food record every sixth day for one year. The horizontal line indicates the overall average intake over the year in MJ per day. The open circles show the intake on individual days and the solid circles the average intake over seven day periods. It is obvious that intake on a single day does not provide a reliable estimate of habitual intake and that even average intake over seven days can differ by as much as 20% from the overall mean.

Box 2.3

Accuracy: a statistical term which describes the extent to which a set of measurements is close to the true value.
Bias: the extent by which a set of estimates differs from the true value.
Coefficient of variation: the standard deviation of a set of observations expressed as a percentage of their mean.
Habitual intake: an estimate of the long-term average intake of an individual.
Random errors: errors that are randomly distributed about the true value. Random errors increase the variability of a set of observations but do not affect their mean.
Repeatability: repeatability is part of the process of establishing the reproducibility of a method (Nelson, 1997).
Reproducibility: a method is reproducible when it gives the same result on repeated measurements of the same individuals under the same circumstances.
Systematic errors: errors that are not randomly distributed about the true value. Systematic errors can increase or decrease the variability of a set of observations and also affect the estimate of their mean. The effect on the mean is referred to as bias.
Validity: a method is valid if it measures what it is intended to measure:

- **Absolute validity:** the extent to which a method measures the true value. It is not possible to determine the absolute validity of the measurement of habitual intake by comparison with another dietary assessment method.
- **Face validity:** a measure of the extent to which, for example, the food list of a food frequency questionnaire or questions in a diet history reflect the food intake of the target population.
- **Comparative (relative) validity:** the extent to which a test method performs in relation to a criterion or reference method, i.e., a dietary assessment method judged to provide the "best" available measure of the true value.
- **Content validity:** a measure of the extent to which the questions, e.g., in a diet history questionnaire, cover all aspects of the habitual diet of an individual.

Variance: statistical term to describe the variation that occurs in a set of observations. It is equal to the square of the standard deviation of the individual observations:

- **Between-person (inter-individual) variance:** the variance arising from differences between individuals.
- **Within-person (intra-individual) variance:** the variance arising from differences within individuals.

The nature of error

There is not, and probably never will be, a method that can estimate dietary intake without error. This does not mean that we should stop collecting dietary data but rather that dietary data need independent validation. Methods need to be developed to assess the error

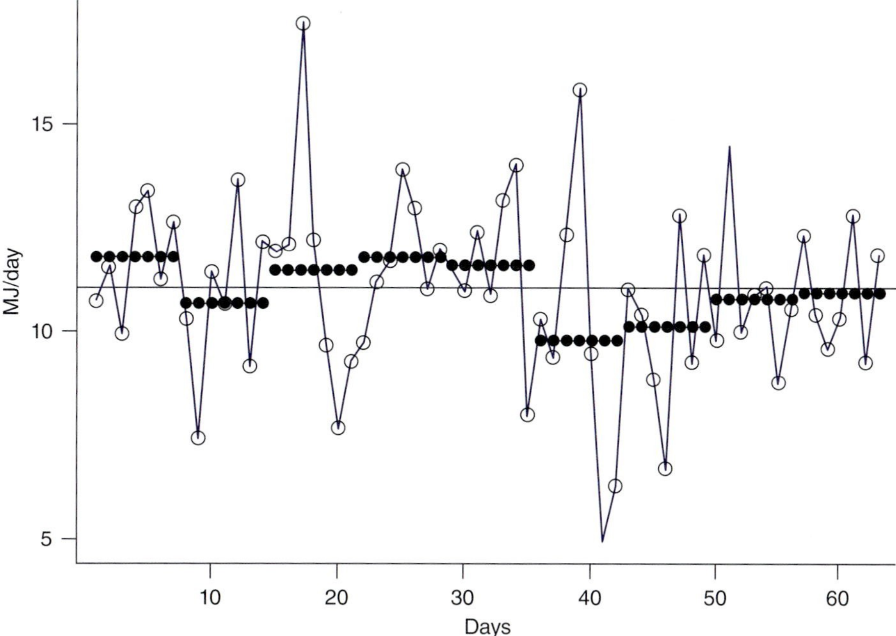

Figure 2.3 Energy intake of one individual from weighed records obtained for 1 day every sixth day over 1 year. —, overall mean; ●●●, weekly mean; ○○○, intake on individual.

structure of dietary datasets so that it can be taken into account in analysing and evaluating the data. Basically, there are two types of error: random error and systematic error.

Random error increases the variance of the estimates of intakes derived from a dietary assessment method. Day-to-day variation in the dietary intake of individuals is one example of a random error. The effect of random errors introduced by day-to-day variations can be reduced by increasing the number of days of observation, recording or the number of 24 hour recalls. Figure 2.3 illustrates how the large day-to-day variation in energy intake (MJ) of an individual who kept weighed records for one day every sixth day for year can be reduced when the number of recording days is increased.

In contrast, the effects of systematic error cannot be reduced by increasing the number of observations. Systematic error arises from errors that are not randomly distributed in the group or in the data from a given individual. For example, an inappropriate portion size estimation aid will have a greater effect on the food intake data of individuals who consume the food more frequently. Likewise, inappropriate nutrient data for some food items will not affect the nutrient intake data for all individuals in the same way but will have a greater effect on nutrient intake data of individuals who consume the food in large amounts than on the data of those who consume only small amounts of the food. Systematic error leads to bias in the estimates of intake obtained.

Reproducibility

In the laboratory the precision of a method is given by the coefficient of variation (CV) of repeated determinations on the same sample made under the same conditions. In the context of dietary studies we determine whether the same method gives the same answer when repeated in the same individuals. The term reproducibility is commonly used to describe the extent to which similar results are obtained from repeated measurements by a dietary assessment method (Box 2.3). It is important to note that it is possible for a method to be reproducible yet not provide a valid estimate of intake.

Validity

A valid method is one that measures what the method intends to measure, i.e., the "truth." In the context of dietary studies the truth represents the actual intake over the period of the study. For example, a valid diet record is a complete and accurate record of all the food and drink consumed over the period that the record is kept. To be a valid record of habitual intake it also needs to reflect what would have been consumed had the individual not been keeping a record. If the process of recording influenced what was eaten then the record is not a valid record of habitual intake, although it may be a true record of actual intake over the period. Similarly, a valid 24 hour recall is a complete and accurate account of all food and drink consumed during the specified period if it reflects all foods and drinks in the amounts that they were actually consumed. It may not, however, be a valid reflection of habitual intake if the items consumed were not typical of the individual's usual intake.

Determining the absolute validity of a dietary assessment method is not possible in the absence of external markers of intake or of direct observation, for example, of the 24 hour period prior to a 24 hour recall or of an individual meal.

2.5 Methods for measuring intake on specified days

Menu records

Menu records are the simplest way of recording information on food intake. They only require the respondent to write down descriptions of the food and drink consumed at each meal and snack throughout the day for the specified days without quantifying the portions. A menu record is useful when information on food patterns rather than intake is required over a longer period or when respondents have difficulty in providing quantitative information. For example, elderly people may have difficulty in measuring food portions. To derive information on nutrient intake from menu records nutrition professionals also need to obtain information on portion sizes of commonly eaten foods. Information on portion sizes may be derived from existing data or collected in a preliminary study.

Menu records work well when the diet is relatively consistent and does not contain a great variety of foods. The method can be used to distinguish differences in the frequency of use of specific foods over time, to determine whether quantitative short-term intake records are likely to be representative of habitual intake and as a way of assessing compliance with special diets.

Weighed food records (food diaries)

Weighed food records require the respondent, or a nutrition professional/fieldworker, to weigh each item of food or drink before it is consumed and if necessary, any of the food/beverage not eaten and to write down a description and the weight of this item in a booklet specially designed for this purpose (sometimes referred to as a food diary). Weighed records are usually kept for three, four, five, or seven days. A seven consecutive day recording period has the advantage of including all days of the week and less frequently consumed foods. However, the longer recording period may result in respondent fatigue where respondents may record foods and quantities less accurately, miss out foods, or skip meals or days. Shorter recording periods of three or four days have a lower respondent burden and therefore better compliance and. provided that recording days across the sample are planned in such a way as to include both week and weekend days, can provide an estimate of habitual diet. As food intake on consecutive days may be related, e.g., eating leftovers, respondents may be asked to record intakes on single non-consecutive days spread over one week to a month or longer. Weighed records (usually three-day) may be kept at monthly or seasonal intervals to provide information on seasonal variations in intakes.

To obtain accurate information it is necessary to use trained nutrition professionals/fieldworkers to collect the data or to demonstrate the procedures and to provide clear instructions to the respondents not only on how to weigh foods, but also on how to describe and record foods and recipes. When respondents are responsible for weighing, the nutrition professional or fieldworker needs to make regular visits to the respondent during the recording period to ensure that the equipment is used correctly and that information is recorded accurately in sufficient detail and to encourage the respondent.

Weighing can be carried out in two different ways:

- the ingredients used in the preparation of each meal or snack, as well as the individual portions of prepared food, are weighed. Any food waste occurring during preparation and serving or food not consumed is also weighed
- all food and beverage items are weighed, in the form in which they are consumed, immediately before they are eaten. Any previously weighed food that is not consumed is also weighed.

The first approach is sometimes referred to as the precise weighing technique and is usually carried out by trained fieldworkers rather than the respondents themselves. It is thus very labour intensive, time consuming, and expensive to carry out. It is most appropriate when the food composition databases available contain limited data on cooked and mixed dishes or if exposure to non-nutrients, e.g., contaminants is being assessed. It should be noted, however, that the precise weighing technique does not allow for nutrient losses in cooking. To take these into account information on cooking losses for the most commonly used cooking methods must also be available.

The second procedure, which is more widely used, involves weighing all food eaten in the form in which it is consumed. Using this method the nutrient content of the diet can be determined from the appropriate food composition database. An alternate method for is for the respondent to weigh duplicate portions of all foods consumed which are then chemically analysed for their nutrient content. Scales used for weighing food need to be robust and able to weigh up to 2 kg, accurate to at most 5 g and preferably to 1–2 g. Digital scales are preferred as these are more accurate and easier to read than spring-balance scales. Record books (food diaries) must have clear instructions, be easy to use, and of a convenient size. They should contain guidelines for weighing and examples illustrating the level of detail required. Addendum 2.1 shows an extract from the instructions and example record sheets of a seven day weighed food diary used in a South African dietary intake study.

The strengths of the weighed record are that it provides the most accurate measurement of portion sizes, as food is recorded as it is consumed, it does not rely on memory, and it gives an indication of food habits such as the number and times of meals and snacks. Depending on the purpose of the study, weighed records kept for three or more days and which include weekend days may be considered to represent habitual intake.

Limitations are that weighed records are time consuming and require a high level of motivation and commitment from both the nutrition professionals/fieldworkers and respondents. Respondents may change their food habits to simplify measuring and recording or may not measure and record food items accurately. Samples of respondents who keep weighed records may not be representative of the population for three reasons:

- because of the high respondent burden, respondents must be volunteers and thus random sampling cannot be used.
- respondents are limited to those who are literate and who are willing to participate.
- those who volunteer may have a specific interest in food intake, e.g being very health conscious, and thus may not be representative of the population.

Metabolic studies carried out to determine absorption and retention of specific nutrients from measurements of intake and excretion are a specialised application of the weighed food record and are normally conducted under controlled conditions in a metabolic unit. In metabolic studies all foods consumed by the respondents are usually either preweighed or weighed by the investigators at the time of consumption. The foods consumed are usually also chemically analysed for the nutrient constituents of interest or prepared from previously analysed ingredients.

Estimated food records

This method of recording food intake is essentially similar to weighed records except that the amounts of food and beverages consumed are measured by volume rather than by weight, i.e., they are described in terms of cups, spoons, teaspoons, or other commonly used household measures, dimensions, or units. Measuring equipment such as cups and spoons may be provided by the nutrition professional or respondents make use of their own household utensils. Food portion photographs, models, or other portion size estimation aids (PSEAs) may be used to assist quantification. These descriptive terms have then to be converted to weights by the nutrition professional, using appropriate conversion data when available, or by obtaining the necessary information when not. For example, the nutrition professional can determine the volume of the measures commonly used in a given household and then convert these to weights by weighing food portions of appropriate size or using information about the density (g/ml) of different kinds of foods. A record book (food diary) for this kind of study is similar to that for a weighed record study. In some situations a precoded record form that lists the commonly eaten foods in terms of typical portion sizes may be appropriate, but an open record form is generally preferred.

Although respondents do not have to weigh foods, it is still necessary for the nutrition professional/fieldworker to demonstrate how to measure, describe, and record food items and to provide detailed instructions. Nutrition professional/fieldworker visits during and immediately after the recording period are needed to ensure that respondents are performing and recording estimations correctly and to encourage respondents to continue keeping the record. In some situations, for example, where a large number of respondents are distributed over a large geographic area, it may be more practical to provide record forms and instructions by mail, electronically or online rather than via individual interviews. In this case, personal contact via telephone and/or electronically, before, during and on completion of the recording period, is essential to ensure that all information is measured and recorded correctly.

The strengths and limitations of estimated records are similar to those of the weighed record, but the method has a lower respondent burden and thus a higher degree of cooperation. Loss of accuracy may occur during the conversion of household measures to weights, especially if the nutrition professional is not familiar with the utensils used in the household.

Weighed records are used in countries where kitchen scales are a common household item and quantities in recipes are given by weight, e.g., the United Kingdom. Estimated records are favoured in countries where it is customary for recipe books to give quantities by standard spoons and cups, e.g., the United States of America and Canada. The dietary literature frequently uses the phrase "diet record" without specifying how portions were quantified. In these instances, estimated records are most likely to have been used.

Recalled intake

Information on dietary intake over a specified period can also be obtained by asking individuals to recollect the types and amounts of food they have eaten. This approach therefore does not influence the type of food actually consumed in the way that a food record may do. Response rates in short-term recall studies tend to range from 65% to 95% and depend largely on how, under what conditions, and from whom the information is obtained. A recall may consist of a face-to-face or telephone interview or of a self-completed paper, automated computer, or web-based questionnaire.

The 24 hour recall is probably the most widely used method of obtaining information on food intake from individuals. It is often used in national surveys because it has a relatively high response rate and can provide the detailed information required for representative samples of different population subgroups.

The 24 hour recall is an attempt to reconstruct quantitatively the amount of food consumed either in the previous 24 hours or on the previous day. This period is considered to provide the most reliable recall of information. With longer periods memory becomes an increasing limitation. Incomplete recalls are more likely with self-completed records unless these records are subsequently checked with the respondent by the nutrition professional. An example of an interviewer administered 24 hour recall sheet is shown in Addendum 2.2.

Traditionally, the food intake has been reviewed chronologically, i.e., starting from the time the respondent wakes up and going through the day until the following morning. Recalling daily activities often assists the respondent to remember food intakes. Problems encountered in estimating the amounts of foods consumed are similar to those encountered with estimated records. Recalls conducted by means of a face-to-face interview often use PSEAs such as food portion photographs, food models, and household utensils to help the respondent to describe how much food was eaten. Examples of food labels, packets, boxes or other containers and/or photographs of locally available food and beverage products may also assist respondents to identify specific types and amounts of commercial food products consumed. Telephone and self-administered recalls may provide pictures or other two-dimensional PSEAs while automated and web-based recalls include digital photographs of food portions and utensils to help respondents describe the types and amounts of foods consumed. There is, however, very little information on how effective these aids are. Irrespective of the way in which the 24 hour recall is administered, a standardised protocol and record sheet, based on a thorough knowledge of local food habits and commonly used foods, is essential.

In its simplest form, the 24 hour recall consists of foods and the amounts consumed over a 24 hour period. In order to obtain sufficient information to quantitatively analyse food intakes from a 24 hour recall, a skilled interviewer will use several "passes" or stages in questioning the respondent. This procedure has become known as the multiple-pass 24 hour recall. This is an interviewing technique consisting of three to five steps which take the respondent through the previous day's food consumption at different levels of detail. All multiple-pass 24 hour recalls commence with the respondent simply listing all foods and beverages consumed during the previous 24 hours. The content and number of further steps differ from study to study. The US Department of Agriculture (USDA) has developed a five-step multiple pass method comprising the following passes (steps) (Conway *et al.*, 2003).

Pass 1 Quick list: the respondent lists all food and beverages consumed during the preceding 24 hours in any order without any prompting or interruptions from the interviewer.

Pass 2 Forgotten foods list: the interviewer asks about categories of foods, such as snacks and sweets, which are frequently forgotten.

Pass 3 Time and occasion: the interviewer asks for details of the times and names of the eating occasions at which foods were consumed.

Pass 4 Detail: the interviewer asks for details, such as descriptions and preparation methods, and amounts of foods consumed.

Pass 5 Review: the interviewer goes through the information probing for any foods which may have been omitted.

A simplified version of the multiple-pass 24 hour recall consists of three steps:

Pass 1 the respondents provide a list of all foods eaten on the previous day using any recall strategy they desire, not necessarily chronological.

Pass 2 the interviewer obtains more detailed information by probing for amounts consumed, descriptions of mixed dishes and preparation methods, additions to foods such as cream in coffee, and giving respondents an opportunity to recall food items that were initially forgotten.

Pass 3 in a third pass the interviewer reviews the list of foods to stimulate reports of more foods and eating occasions.

The multiple-pass approach is thought to assist recall more effectively than chronological cues and thus provide more accurate and complete information. This approach, however, is more time-consuming than the traditional 24 hour recall and may irritate respondents by seemingly asking about the food intake over and over again. Irrespective of the approach used, it is essential that the approach is tested in the target population prior to the study, that all interviewers are thoroughly trained and that the same procedure is used by all interviewers with all respondents throughout the study.

Automated computer and web-based 24 hour recalls simulate the multiple pass approach. Examples of such 24 hour recalls are the Automated Self-administered 24 hour dietary assessment tool (ASA24) (National Cancer Institute, 2016) and Myfood24 (Nutritional Epidemiology Group, School of Food Science & Nutrition, University of Leeds).

The 24 hour recall provides information for only a single day and therefore does not take account of day-to-day variation in the diet. In large cross-sectional studies in which the aim is to determine average intakes of a group of individuals, a single 24 hour recall may be sufficient. When the diets of individuals are assessed or when sample sizes are small, repeated 24 hour recalls are required. This method is known as multiple 24 hour recalls. The number of recalls depends on the aim of the study, the nutrients of interest, and the degree of precision needed. For example, when diets consist of a limited variety of foods, two 24 hour recalls may be sufficient whereas four or more recalls may be required when diets are complex. Recalls may also be repeated during different seasons to take account of seasonal variations. (Note that multiple 24 hour recalls must not be confused with the multiple-pass 24 hour recall technique. The multiple-pass 24 hour recall refers to an interviewing technique, whereas the multiple 24 hour recall method refers to repeated 24 hour recalls conducted per respondent.)

The strengths of the 24 hour recall method are that it has a low respondent burden in comparison to food records and thus compliance is high, it does not require respondents to be literate (if interviewer administered), it does not alter usual food intake, and it is relatively quick and inexpensive to administer and may therefore be cost-effective when large numbers of respondents are involved. It is most successful in populations with limited dietary variety, when respondents are able to accurately recall and express the types and amounts of foods consumed and when interviewers are skilled in the interview technique.

A major drawback of the 24 hour recall is that it does not give an accurate reflection of habitual dietary intake if only a single 24 hour recall is conducted. This may be overcome to some extent by conducting repeated 24 hour recalls. Another difficulty is that the 24 hour recall relies on the respondent to accurately recall and report the types and amounts of foods consumed. There is a tendency for respondents to overestimate low intakes and underestimate high intakes. This is known as the flat slope syndrome. Respondents may omit certain foods that are considered "bad" or include foods not consumed but considered "good" (phantom foods) in order to impress the interviewer. Respondents may also provide inaccurate or incomplete information if they do not understand what is expected of them, cannot express themselves clearly or cannot recall aspects of their intakes.

Of the methods so far described weighed records should contain the least error as they report all food consumed on specified days with weighed portions. Estimating the size of portions increases error and, if menu records are quantified with average portions, then the error at the individual level is further increased. If food that has already been eaten has to be recalled then poor memory can introduce an additional source of error. All methods that report intake on specified days are also subject, in individuals, to the error associated with day-to-day variation in intake, but this error can be reduced by increasing the number of days studied.

2.6 Methods for measuring intake over the longer term

Food frequency questionnaires

Food frequency questionnaires (FFQ) consist of a list of foods and options to indicate how frequently each food is consumed. FFQ may be self-administered in paper, automated computer or web-based formats or interviewer administered either by face-to-face or telephonic interviews.

The food lists may contain only a few food items or up to 200 foods. Food items may be listed individually, for example, butternut, or similar foods may be grouped together, for example, dark yellow and orange vegetables. The type and number of foods included are determined by the purpose of the study and the target population. For example, an FFQ designed to determine calcium intake would contain only foods which provide calcium, while a questionnaire to measure overall dietary adequacy would need to contain all foods known to be consumed by the target population. Likewise, an FFQ designed to assess dietary intakes of a homogeneous target population with a diet of limited variety would be shorter than one designed to assess food intakes of a heterogeneous population with a variety of food intake patterns.

There are several types of FFQ, which are defined in Box 2.4. Figure 2.4 shows examples of the three most frequently used FFQ formats. The type of FFQ used depends on the purpose of the study, the target population, and the required level of accuracy of food portion estimation.

The period of recall or reference period depends on the study objectives. In the past, most FFQs used the preceding year or six months as the reference period. Theoretically, this should take account of the effects of the season. In practice, however, respondents tend to answer according

Box 2.4

Food frequency questionnaire (FFQ) (simple/nonquantitative): respondents report usual consumption of foods and beverages from a set list of items for a specific period. Portion sizes are not determined.
Semi-quantitative food frequency questionnaire (SFFQ): an FFQ which includes a reference portion size.
Quantitative food frequency questionnaire (QFFQ): an FFQ which includes a reference portion size and options for respondents to estimate their portion size as small, medium, or large in relation to the reference.
List-based food frequency questionnaire: food items are listed according to groups or categories of similar foods or foods usually eaten together.
Meal-based food frequency questionnaire: foods are asked about according to meals or the time of day at which they are consumed.
Culture-sensitive food frequency questionnaire: an FFQ that takes account of the food values, beliefs, and behaviours of a specific population or cultural group.

to what is currently in season or available at the time of the study. For example, intake of oranges was found to be higher when interviews were carried out during the citrus season than at other times of the year. Information may be more reliable when the recall period is shorter. If annual intakes are required, the FFQ should be repeated in different seasons. It is very important that the respondent understands what the recall period is and that only this period should be considered when giving frequencies of intake.

The frequency of consumption is usually indicated by options such as: more than once a day; daily; three to four times per week; one to two times per week; one to two times per month; occasionally; never. This type of response format requires only that the appropriate columns be marked and is most suitable for self-administered questionnaires. When appropriately designed,

(a)	Average use during the past year					
Food item	<1 month	1–3 month	1–4 week	5–7 week	2–4 day	5+ day
Rice						
Brown bread						
Muffin						

(b)	Average use during the past year					
Food item	<1 month	1–3 month	1–4 week	5–7 week	2–4 day	5+ day
Rice (1/2 cup)						
Brown bread (1 slice)						
Muffin (1 medium)						

(c)		Your portion size			How often?				
Food item	Medium portion	S	M	L	Day	Week	Month	Year	Never
Rice	1/2 cup								
Brown bread	1 slice								
Muffin	1 medium								

Figure 2.4 Examples of 3 food frequency questionnaire formats: (a) – the simple or nonquantitative format; (b) – the semi-quantitative format; (c)- the quantitative format. (Adapted from Lee R.D. Nieman D.C. *Nutritional assessment.* 7th edn. Mc Graw Hill, St Louis, 2019. Figure 3.3 pg 74.)

such questionnaires can be optically scanned, which saves time on data entry and checking procedures. With increasing computer and internet availability and use, automated and web-based versions of FFQ which include digital food portion photographs to aid portion size estimation and which may be linked directly to food composition databases further reduce the time needed for the administration, coding, and analysis of FFQ data. Addenda 2.3 and 2.4 are examples of two formats of scanable or automated FFQ.

Closed response options, however, treat the frequency of consumption as a categorical variable and assume that frequency of consumption is constant throughout the recall period. The choice of categories may bias the results: too few categories may underestimate frequencies whereas too many may overestimate frequencies. Respondents may have difficulty in matching their food intake to the available categories. For example, when food is purchased monthly, food items such as fresh fruit and vegetables, may be consumed every day while stocks last, but, once used up, will not be consumed until purchased in the following month.

An alternative open response format for recording responses is to provide space to record the number of times a food is consumed per day, the number of days per week on which the food is consumed, and the number of weeks during the month on which the food is consumed. From this, the average frequency of consumption and the amount of food consumed per day can be calculated. The advantage of this response format is that it allows the respondent to describe the frequency of consumption in detail. The disadvantages are that clear instructions must be given, making this method more appropriate for interviewer-administered questionnaires than self-administered questionnaires, trained skilled interviewers are needed and the interview takes longer and requires more writing and calculations than the closed format, making more room for recording errors. Addendum 2.5 is an extract of such an FFQ.

Most FFQs obtain information only on the frequency of consumption of a food over a given period and not on the context in which the foods were eaten, i.e., on meal patterns. Meal-based food frequency questionnaires have been used on the basis that it may be easier for respondents to provide the information in the context of meals. The information on meal patterns obtained from such questionnaires is, however, more limited than that which can be obtained from a dietary history.

Some FFQs also attempt to quantify the frequency information by obtaining data on portion size. Semi-quantitative FFQs (SFFQs) provide a standard portion size (usually derived from food records or 24 hour recalls in the target population) to guide the respondent in estimating the frequency of consumption (Figure 2.4b). In quantitative FFQs (QFFQs) more detailed information on the quantity of each food consumed is obtained by asking respondents to indicate whether their usual portions are small, medium, or large relative to a standard portion size (Figure 2.4c; Addendum 2.6). A variation of the QFFQ is to provide food portion photographs, food models, or other PSEA to allow the respondents to select their own portion size. Addendum 2.5 is an example of an open response format QFFQ which used food portion photographs and household measures to estimate portion sizes. When portion sizes are used, it is important that these reflect the consumption patterns of the population.

Depending on the purpose of the FFQ, additional questions may be included to obtain information such as brand names, types of margarine or milk used, the addition of salt to food, preparation methods, recipes of mixed dishes and the use of nutrient supplements. An "other" category may be included to record items consumed but not specified on the food list.

FFQs are mainly used in studies designed to look for associations between food intake and disease or risk of disease, particularly when specific foods rather than the level of consumption of a nutrient are thought to be the important factor. They are also useful for classifying food and/or nutrient intakes of individuals in relation to of the distribution of intakes of the sample. FFQs do not affect usual dietary intakes and may give a better picture of habitual intake than single recalls or records. Since the cost of administration and respondent burden are relatively low, they are suitable for use when sample sizes are large, particularly if a postal, electronic, or web-based method is used.

The success of an FFQ depends on how closely the food list and portion size descriptions reflect the food patterns of the target population. This is sometimes referred to as being culture sensitive. Much time and care must be put into the development of an FFQ in order to ensure that it provides an accurate reflection of the dietary intakes of a population. Preliminary studies, using 24 hour recalls, food records, or indirect methods may be needed to obtain information on food items, frequency of consumption, and portion sizes in the target population. Since FFQs are usually developed for use in specific target populations, an FFQ developed for use in one population may not be appropriate for use with another population with different food intake patterns. It is also extremely important that the questionnaire be tested for reproducibility and validity in the target population before being used, even if it has been previously tested in a different population. Detailed instructions and training and standardisation of interviewers are essential to ensure that data of good quality are obtained.

Since recalling and estimating frequency and quantities (for SFFQ and QFFQ) of foods consumed are complex cognitive tasks, FFQs are not suitable for populations with low literacy levels, children, and the elderly. Even when used in literate populations, when self-administered, information may be incomplete.

The Nutritools website (https://www.nutritools.org) and the dietary assessment website of the National Cancer Institute (https://dietassessmentprimer.cancer.gov//profiles/questionnaire/) are useful resources for examples of, and guidelines for the development, use and analysis of FFQs.

Diet history

The principal objective of the diet history is to obtain detailed information on the habitual intake of an individual. It is usually used in the clinical setting. The method had several components:

- an interview to obtain usual diet
- a cross-check of this information by food group
- a three day record of food consumed in household measures.

The three day record is now seldom used as a regular component of a diet history. Its purpose originally was as a way of checking the data obtained from the diet history interview. A diet history is usually obtained by an experienced nutrition professional by means of an open interview followed by some kind of cross-check using a standard list of commonly consumed foods. The interview begins with a review of the food that was eaten in a specific time-frame (e.g., yesterday) or on a typical day, and then moves on to explore the variations in food intake that occur for each meal over a given period. Information on the usual size of food portions is obtained with the aid of food models or photographs in the same way as for a 24 hour recall. The time-frame for a diet history can range from the previous month to the previous year.

In practical terms it is easier for respondents to reconstruct the immediate past, but the past year is often used to capture seasonal variation. Whatever the time-frame used, it must be clearly specified. In the literature the term "diet history" is sometimes used loosely to describe any form of diet recall, including the 24 hour recall and FFQ, as well as interviewer-administered recalls of habitual or longer term intake. This broader use can be confusing and is best avoided. The dependence of the diet history on both respondent and interviewer skills may make the results obtained less comparable between individuals than those obtained from other methods. For this reason it is often considered more appropriate to categorise diet history data (e.g., as high, medium or low intake of a food or nutrient) rather than to treat them as intakes expressed in terms of absolute units per day (e.g., mg calcium).

The diet history is favoured in Scandinavia and the Netherlands, where a structured interview may be used. The structured interview is more standardised but may miss elements specific to the individual or bore the respondents with irrelevant questions. The open-ended interview allows for tailoring to the individual, but risks missing important items and inter-rater reproducibility may be compromised.

2.7 Dietary screeners

Short dietary assessments or dietary screeners are becoming increasingly popular. Screening in this context refers to the early detection of dietary behaviours or intakes (risk factors), known to be associated with malnutrition or nutrition-related ill-health. Any trained health professional should be able to perform it, in any setting. It should be clearly interpretable and, above all, cost-effective. In public health and clinical nutrition it is intended to identify those who should be followed-up by a comprehensive nutritional assessment and /or early intervention.

Dietary screeners can focus on a specific group of people (e.g., elderly) in a certain setting (e.g., people living with a specific diagnosis), at risk of a particular nutritional problem (e.g., protein energy under-nutrition). The instruments can be of a general nature, yet often a specific food group (e.g., fruit and vegetables) or nutrient (e.g., calcium), or combinations thereof, is targeted. Sometimes the basic dietary assessment methods (e.g., FFQ) are abbreviated or simplified, but novel thinking is also emerging. Screening protocols may include other aspects of nutritional assessment (e.g., anthropometry).

Whilst screening can be administered by any trained professional or by the respondent him/herself using traditional (e.g., paper-based) approaches or new technology, the development (including the implementation and interpretation guidelines), as well as the validation of a dietary screener are the responsibility of the nutrition professional. The validation typically includes application of the principles of diagnostic accuracy testing. A screener that is not valid will not achieve its aim nor be effective. A register of validated short dietary assessment tools is available on the website of the Epidemiology and Genomics Research Program of the National Cancer Institute (https://epi.grants.cancer.gov/diet/shortreg/register.php).

Against the backdrop of the labour and time-intensity of comprehensive dietary assessments, open-mindedness in exploring new approaches and methods is needed. Combined with sound science and validation, this may pave the way for assessments matched to current times.

2.8 Portion size estimation and portion size estimation aids

A major source of error in dietary assessment is related to the quantification of intakes. Whilst weighing food and beverage intakes - as in food records or diaries - theoretically represents the most accurate approach, this is often not practical and may introduce a selection bias: participants who complete such assessments may differ significantly from the general population. It follows that nutrition professionals usually rely on portion size estimation, as opposed to measurement.

Estimating food quantities involves cognitive processes, in addition to remembering the eating occasion. Mindful eating or routine consumption with limited variation or choice may make reporting amounts consumed easier. The cognitive ability of quantification is age-related, and consequently young children can usually not be expected to provide detailed information. Different strategies may be used by respondents for expressing quantities. For certain foods they may report intake as counts or number of units of food, e.g., 1 packet of crisps or 10 grapes. This may be coupled with current societal norms such as "small", "medium", "large" or "jumbo" in a particular setting. For other foods visualisation may be employed or intakes are reported relative to familiar household utensils or common reference objects. The shape and form of the food may play a role in the cognitive process used. In this regard solid foods may differ from amorphous food (i.e. those that take on the shape of the container in which they are served) and fluids. Some of the factors that may be related to portion size estimation are listed in Table 2.2, yet at this stage generalisations and final conclusions are illusive.

Apart from the respondent's ability to recall and express the amounts consumed, the nutrition professional should have knowledge of local eating habits, and be able to accurately convert reported intakes (e.g., volume or units) into quantities suitable for analysis.

Due to the complexity of expressing food quantities, nutrition professionals often make use of PSEAs. PSEAs are tools to assist respondents to recall and report the amount of food consumed. Two- or three-dimensional or digital PSEAs can be distinguished. Examples of the former two are given in Table 2.3.

The choice of PSEAs depends on the target population and setting, available resources, and the purpose of the dietary assessment. Practical considerations such as user acceptability and bulkiness are also important. In many countries kits have been developed. Ideally the PSEA should be validated in the target group and for the food(s) of interest.

Table 2.2 Factors that may be related to portion size estimation

Food characteristics	Food type	Solids, liquids, amorphous masses or pieces
	Container size, shape and colour	Optical illusions (e.g. the vertical-horizontal illusion in tall thin glasses compared to short fat glasses, or the Delbouff illusion in plates with and without rims) may lead to over- or underestimation
	Familiarity or routine consumption	
	Energy density and perceived healthiness	Underestimation of low energy density foods and overestimation of high energy density foods
	Portion size	A flat slope syndrome may result in over-reporting small portions and under-reporting large portions
Personal characteristics	Age	The very young may be cognitively not able to quantify amounts, but exact age cut-offs are unknown, and conflicting
	Socio-economics	Literacy and numeracy as part of educational level may play a role, yet training may counter the effect
	Sex	Earlier studies suggested that women as primary users of recipes may be better able to quantify food amounts
	Body weight	The tendency of obese persons to under-report, may in part be attributed to portion size under-estimation

Table 2.3 Examples of 2- and 3-dimensional portion size estimation aids

2D PSEA's	3D PSEA's
Photographs, life-size or small; single reference or series	Household utensils (plates, bowls, cups, glasses)
Drawings	Geometric and amorphous shapes, e.g. sponges, bean bags
Geometric and irregular shapes	Food models, e.g. commercial kits or single items, home-made or 3D printed
Wrappers of commercial foods	

2D: Two dimensional; 3D: Three dimensional; PSEA: Portion size estimation aids

2.9 Technology in dietary assessment

In this chapter many challenges associated with dietary assessment are highlighted. The aim of technology should be to address at least some of these challenges. Technology may be applied in one or more of the stages of the process of dietary assessment (Figure 2.2). This may start with the *input stage* during which technology may be used to collect the intake data, e.g., in an automated 24 hour recall, a web-based FFQ or with digital food photography. Technology that improves food description (e.g., types of spread used), quantification of intakes (portion size estimation) or completeness of intake data (under-reporting), represents major advances. Methods for capturing the food intake data may rely on text (the user selects food from a list and enters amounts consumed), be image-assisted (pictures or photographs are added to text) or image-based (photographs of food consumed are primary sources of information), or use video clips.

Technology may also be used in the *coding and processing stage* of dietary assessment, when the raw intake data are entered into food composition databases. Software packages facilitating this have been available for many years (Chapter 3), yet these have come closer to the end-user by being included in some of the technology types or devices listed below or by being part of a more integrated process. From a scientific perspective, the most important part of any software package is the comprehensiveness and relevance of the database. User friendliness and error reduction during coding and data entry, as well as adaptability of data output to research or practice settings are features that attract potential users.

Lastly, technology may aid in the *interpretation stage* of the process of evaluating dietary intake. This is critical for making a final judgement about dietary adequacy by comparing the data to nutrient or food intake guidelines, references, standards or cut-offs. Visual appeal of the findings (e.g., colour and pie-charts) may translate the hard, scientific findings into a more understandable message for the client, and create a bridge between the dietary assessment step of nutrition care and nutrition education.

The devices that may assist the recording of dietary intake may be grouped into:

- personal digital assistant (PDA) technologies
- mobile phone-based technologies
- interactive computer-based technologies
- web-based technologies
- camera and tape-recorder-based technologies
- scan and sensor-based technologies.

Each technology type has its inherent strengths and limitations, and this may be mediated by the setting in which the dietary assessment is applied. When new technologies are considered the following criteria may guide decision making:

- accuracy (validity and reproducibility), including the likelihood of reporting bias and potential of standardisation
- applicability to the setting and target group, and participant usability
- cost (of development, equipment, administration)
- logistics and organisation (time and complexity of each stage of the dietary process)
- comparison to conventional methods.

The above implies that a researcher or nutrition professional has to carefully take stock of resources at hand and what the technology has to achieve. In the first place the technology has to be appropriate for the purpose, setting, and population. Currently the most important limitation of new technologies is the lack of evidence of their validity. Improving, complementing, or replacing the stages in the traditional methods can be strived for, but rigorous validation should be applied.

2.10 Sources of error in dietary studies

Sources of error in dietary studies can be divided into those that are common to all studies involving the measurement of food intake and those which are associated with specific dietary assessment methods. Errors common to dietary studies can be minimised by careful study design and execution including the implementation of quality control measures at all points of the study and adequate pretesting and piloting of the study instruments and procedures. The following are examples:

- sampling and nonresponse bias
- respondent bias
- investigator or interviewer error
- inappropriate coding of foods
- limitations of food composition databases.

In contrast, the errors that are associated with specific methods are generally much more dependent on the nature of the method and the abilities of the interviewers and respondents, and therefore less easy to control. Errors of this type include:

- estimation of portion size
- recall or memory
- day-to-day variation in intake
- effect of assessment method on food intake.

Sampling and nonresponse bias

A randomly selected sample, with a sufficiently large sample size, which represents the population from which it is drawn (target population) is essential to draw conclusions about the diet of the target population. However, even if a sample has been randomly selected, those respondents who provide usable data may not represent the target population.

Some selected respondents may not be willing to participate in dietary assessment due to the time and commitment needed. The proportion of the sample which agrees to participate (the response rate) can vary considerably even with the same method. It can vary with the group and the circumstances of study. For example, respondents who are employed or who have many demands on their time, may be less willing to participate in a lengthy FFQ, keep food records, or be available for multiple 24 hour recalls than those who are unemployed or retired. In general, the response rate is higher for 24 hour recalls and FFQ (which make fewer demands on the respondents) than for estimated and weighed records which demand much time, effort, and commitment from the respondents.

In methods which collect data over a number of days, such as food records and multiple 24 hour recalls, respondents may not complete all recording days or recalls, with the number who drop out increasing with the number of days recoding days or recalls. This will further reduce the number of respondents who supply usable data, and hence the representativeness of the data. For example, in a study of rural males using four 24 hour recalls, 95% of the sample completed two recalls while only 73% completed all four recalls. Particularly with food records, respondents may skip meals or days during the recording period. As a result the record may appear complete, but on close examination may not be usable.

The major concern about nonresponse is that those who participate may have different characteristics to the nonresponders. For example, when data are collected during working hours, the proportion of unemployed and retired individuals in the sample may be greater than in the target population, or those who are willing to commit to keeping a food record or to multiple recalls may be more health and diet conscious or have specific reasons for participating and thus their diets may differ from those of others in the target population.

Steps to reduce the number of nonresponders and drop-outs must be planned into and followed during the study. Such steps include providing potential respondents with detailed and honest explanations about the purpose and procedures of the study and what is expected of them, allowing respondents to ask questions or raise concerns before and during the study, streamlining and simplifying data collection procedures, providing specific assistance if required, giving telephonic and/or electronic reminders, allowing the respondents as much flexibility as possible within the context of the study and providing appropriate and ethical incentives, such as dietary feedback at the conclusion of the study.

Respondent bias

Respondent bias occurs when the respondents, consciously or unconsciously, provide incomplete or inappropriate information. Unconscious errors occur when respondents misunderstand what is expected or a specific question, do not remember details or amounts of foods consumed or are not be able to express their responses clearly. Respondents may deliberately report foods which they consider "healthy" or "desirable" even if not consumed and under report or miss out foods which they consider "bad" or "unhealthy". In long food frequency or diet history interviews, respondents may lose concentration or become impatient and give answers without thinking or which they hope will speed up the interview.

Respondent bias can be reduced by giving clear and well-presented instructions, giving opportunities for respondents to ask questions, providing adequate support and encouragement and checking questionnaires and record forms for completeness.

Since all dietary methods engage the cognitive processes of respondents, an appreciation of the properties of human cognition and its limitations is fundamental to improving the accuracy of dietary assessments. Some of the important issues in this area that are relevant to improving the quality of dietary data include identification of:

- factors that improve communication between respondent and nutrition professional/interviewer (e.g., language usage)
- the most effective cues for recall over different periods (e.g., events during the 24 hour recall period)
- factors that influence retention of dietary information over time
- ways in which individuals conceptualise foods and food quantities.

Investigator/Interviewer bias

The nutrition professional (investigator) or interviewer can him/herself introduce bias into the data collection process. Personal characteristics or the way in which the interviewer approaches the respondent may influence the way in which the interviewee responds. For example, an older respondent may be less comfortable being interviewed by a young interviewer than an older interviewer, or an interviewer who comes across as authoritative or impatient may cause the respondent to withdraw or provide answers which the respondent believes he/she is expected to give. Interviewers may introduce bias by incorrect interviewing techniques such as asking leading questions or inappropriate use of probing questions, omitting questions, not listening to, misunderstanding or making assumptions about responses, or incorrectly recording responses. Furthermore, distractions, lack of privacy, or discomfort in the interview setting may affect both the interviewer and the respondent and the level of trust and rapport between interviewer and respondent. Although interviewer bias is considered mostly in the interview setting, the way in which the nutrition professional approaches, trains, follows up and supports respondents who keep food records may influence the detail, completeness, and accuracy of the record.

Interviewer bias may be reduced by having standardised interview procedures, well designed questionnaires or recall sheets which require a minimum of writing, adequate training before the study, checking completed questionnaires, and debriefing and re-training sessions during data collection. The use of standard procedures, however, can also introduce systematic error; for example, if one interviewer is assigned to interview all respondents in areas of low socioeconomic status and another to interview all respondents in areas of high socioeconomic status. Thus, allocation of interviewers to respondents should be random. In cross cultural or multi-ethnic studies, interviewers should be from the target population, speak the language/s and understand the social structure and food culture of the target population.

Coding errors

Coding refers to the allocation of a specific code to each food item prior to the nutrient analysis of the food intake data. Since the nutritional content of a food varies with different processing and preparation methods, it is vital that the correct codes be assigned to each food item. Coding errors arise when the food that has been consumed is not described in sufficient detail to enable unambiguous allocation, by the nutrition professional, to a food item in a food composition table or database. FFQs are often precoded to reduce the time needed for coding and the possibility of coding errors. Making it easy for respondents to describe foods with the level of detail required is therefore an important consideration in all dietary assessment methods. This is increasingly difficult, particularly in industrialised countries where the food supply consists of thousands of different manufactured foods, of ever-changing composition, the names of which are often not a good guide to their nutrient content.

Coding errors are likely to arise when more than one person is involved in coding and there is no agreed procedure and/or comprehensive coding manual. Coding errors arising exclusively from inadequate description of foods have resulted in coefficients of variation ranging from 3% to 17% for different nutrients. On the other hand, standard procedures for coding foods, while minimising differences between coders (random error), can also introduce bias if the coding decisions are not based on up-to-date knowledge of the local food supply and food preparation methods. Gross errors associated with weights of foods can be checked, before analysis, by means of computer routines that identify values outside a prescribed range and by using data-checking techniques such as duplicate data entry.

Automated computer and web-based 24 hour recalls and FFQ provide drop-down lists from which users select the relevant food item. This removes the need for coding and, if directly linked to the appropriate food composition database, greatly reduces the time needed for analysis. Great care however must be taken to ensure that the programming of such links is correct. The risk of errors remains if incorrect food items are selected.

Use of food composition tables/ databases

Most dietary studies use food composition tables or databases rather than chemical analysis to derive the nutrient content of the foods consumed. Chapter 3 describes the way in which data on food composition are derived and compiled. The purpose of this section is to review briefly the kinds of error that can arise as a consequence of using food composition tables/databases to calculate nutrient intake, compared with chemical analysis of the diet, thereby introducing both systematic and random errors.

Systematic error can result from:

- the way in which results are calculated or expressed
- the analytical method used
- the processing and preparation methods in common use.

Food composition databases for different countries often use different ways of expressing results and different analytical methods. The ways in which food items are processed or prepared are also likely to differ. Thus different databases will not necessarily provide comparable data for the same foods. Systematic differences, which may not necessarily be errors (e.g., when foods are prepared differently in different countries), often only become evident when different food composition databases are used to evaluate the same diets.

Random error arises from the fact that most foods vary in their composition as a result of changes associated with the conditions of production, processing, storage, preparation, and consumption. The random error associated with the use of food composition databases generally decreases as the size of the sample group increases. This may not be true, however, in institutional settings where everyone is likely to be consuming food from the same source.

To compare calculated and analysed data without the complication of other sources of error it is necessary that the diets are analysed by collecting a duplicate of what has been eaten at the same time as a food record. At group level it has been observed that mean intakes calculated from food databases are generally within approximately 10% of the mean analysed value for energy and macronutrients, but not for micronutrients. However, a large proportion of individuals have values that fall outside this range.

In general, calculated and analysed values for nutrients agree more closely:

- for groups than for individuals
- for macronutrients than for micronutrients
- when data for locally analysed foods are used.

Estimation of portion size

As discussed in Section 2.5, the quantification of portion sizes is a major source of error in all assessment methods which estimate amounts of foods consumed. The type and extent of the error varies with the characteristics of both the food and the respondents (Table 2.2). In an attempt to reduce portion size estimation errors, a variety of PSEAs have been developed to assist respondents to describe portion sizes.

Each PSEA has strengths and limitations. The type of PSEA chosen will depend, among others, on the type of study, the target population, whether interviewers go from house to house or respondents go to a research centre, available resources, and the availability of appropriate PSEAs. Probably the most effective method is a combination of PSEAs such as food photographs and household utensils. Irrespective of the type of PSEA used, it is essential that respondents are able to identify and relate to the PSEAs, that PSEAs are tested in the target population prior to their use, and that PSEAs are used consistently throughout the study.

Recall errors

Factors that have been studied in relation to the accuracy of dietary recall include food consumption patterns, weight status, gender, and age. Many other characteristics, such as intelligence, mood, attention, and salience of the information, however, have also been demonstrated to influence performance tests of general recall, but have not been studied in the context of dietary recall.

Short-term memory

Like the ability to estimate portion size, the ability to remember what was eaten varies with the individual. Studies that have compared the abilities of different groups to remember what they have eaten conclude that women are generally better than men and that younger adults are better than older adults. In short-term recalls of intake (e.g., 24 hour recalls) individuals more often tend to omit an item or items that they have consumed than to include ones that they have not consumed. The size of the error incurred by the omission of one or more food items clearly depends on what is omitted and not only on the proportion of food omitted. For example, the effect, on 24 hour energy intake, of omitting a cup of black coffee, a glass of milk, or a bar of chocolate is quite different.

The omission of food items in 24 hour recall studies can be reduced by appropriate probing by the interviewer in relation to meals, between-meal snacks, and other activities on the previous day, but even when respondents have previously weighed their food the average energy intake may still be underestimated by as much as 20%.

Long-term memory

The diet history and most FFQs set out to measure the habitual intake of an individual over a period of weeks or months. Individuals are not asked to recall their food intake on specific days, but to construct a picture of their "usual" food consumption pattern over a specified reference period. To provide good quality information individuals need to remember the range of foods that they usually consume, to judge the frequency of consumption on a long-term basis, and to estimate correctly the average amount that is usually consumed. These are complex cognitive tasks.

As in the case of 24 hour recalls, no attempt is usually made to assess how well individuals are able to perform these various tasks. From the limited amount of data available from comparative studies between diet histories and long-term diet records, it appears that the two methods do not give concordant results in individuals. FFQ are subject to the same difficulties, and have the added problem that estimates of portion size are usually based on standard measures, especially in the case of SFFQ.

When respondents are asked to report their intake over a period of weeks they rely largely on generic knowledge of their diet and tend to report items that they are likely to have eaten or items that they routinely eat, rather than items that they specifically remember having eaten during the reference period. This tendency increases with the length of the reference period. While individuals appear to report more frequently eaten foods with greater accuracy than less frequently eaten foods, there are differences between individuals in the way that they report the same frequency of consumption. Ranking of individuals on the basis of the usual frequency of intake is thus likely to lead to misclassification.

Day-to-day variation in intake

We have already seen that individuals vary considerably in their intake of food and nutrients from day to day (Figure 2.3). In addition, the extent of day-to-day variation differs between nutrients. The implication of the first observation is that short-term intake data (e.g., 24 hour recall data) are unlikely to provide a good estimate of habitual intake for most individuals. The implication of the second observation is that the length of time for which dietary data need to be collected, in order to estimate habitual intake with any given level of confidence, varies with the nutrient of interest.

Table 2.4 expresses the impact of this variation in terms of the number of days of dietary information needed to classify 80% of individuals into the correct third of the distribution. It is clear from this table that not only 24 hour recalls but also seven day records are likely to be inadequate to classify 80% of individuals correctly into the appropriate third of the distribution for most micronutrients. This is an important reason, although not the only reason, why short-term records are rarely used for epidemiological studies, in preference to FFQs, despite the loss of detail and precision inevitably associated with the use of the latter.

Table 2.4 Number of days of records required to enable 80% of men to be assigned into their correct third of the intake distribution

Nutrient	British civil servants	Random sample of British men	Random sample of Swedish men
Energy	7	5	7
Protein	6	5	7
Fat	9	9	7
Carbohydrate	4	3	3
Sugar	2	2	–
Dietary fiber	6	10	–
P:S ratio	11	–	–
Cholesterol	18	–	–
Alcohol	4	–	14
Vitamin C	–	6	14
Thiamin	–	6	15
Riboflavin	–	10	–
Calcium	–	4	5
Iron	–	12	9

P:S ratio, ratio of polyunsaturated to saturated fatty acids in the diet. Source: Reproduced from Margetts, B.M., Nelson, M. (eds.) *Design Concepts in Nutritional Epidemiology* 2e. Oxford University Press, Oxford,1997, with permission from Oxford University Press. p144.

Effect on usual diet

Recall methods clearly cannot change what has already been eaten, but what has been eaten can be misreported either consciously or unconsciously. When individuals are asked to keep records, however, they may alter their habits as a consequence of the recording process. One obvious reason for doing so would be to simplify the process of recording. Other reasons may include a desire to eat less in order to lose weight or to be seen to conform to dietary recommendations. If this is what happens in practice, then what is measured in short-term dietary records may be actual intake or desired intake, but not usual intake.

Studies have demonstrated that there is a tendency, in most population subgroups, for short-term dietary records to provide estimates of energy and protein intake that are on average around 15% lower than would be expected on the basis of measured and/or estimated levels of energy expenditure. The fact that for some groups measurements of energy intake and energy expenditure agree quite closely indicates that it is possible to obtain a food a food record without a concomitant change in diet when there is full cooperation from respondents. It also highlights the importance of efforts to achieve such cooperation.

2.11 Choosing a dietary assessment method

It is not possible to decide which dietary method and specific dietary assessment tool to use until the purpose of the study has been clearly defined, since this will determine the kind of information and the length of time for which it needs to be collected from each individual. Often, the purpose of the study also determines the level of precision that is required to meet the study objectives and therefore the sample size. While these two considerations are most important in determining the method to be used, other factors which influence the choice of the method and specific dietary assessment tool include: the characteristics of the target population, the availability and suitability of dietary assessment tools to address the research objectives, the ways in which the dietary data will be analysed and presented, the potential sources of bias related to the chosen method and the human, financial and other resources required to implement the method. Cade *et al.* (2017) have published Best Practice Guidelines for the selection of an appropriate dietary assessment method and tool for a given research study. These guidelines can be accessed at www.nutritools.org.

Purpose of the study

There are generally four purposes of dietary assessment which determine both the type of data to be collected and the way in which the data are analysed (Gibson, 2005):

- to describe intakes of a group and/or to compare intakes of two or more groups
- to identify the proportion of a population at risk of dietary deficiency or excess of specific nutrients in relation to a reference or standard
- to rank usual intakes of food or nutrients of individuals within a group, often to determine an association between level of intake and risk of disease or other outcome
- to determine associations between food or nutrient intakes and other variables such as biochemical markers.

Table 2.5 summarises the characteristics of the various dietary assessment methods in relation to the purpose of the study. When deciding on the most appropriate method to meet the study purpose, the nutrition professional must not only ensure that the method will provide the appropriate data, but also that it can be implemented efficiently in the target population within limitations of time, personnel, and other resources. It is also vital to consult a statistician to ensure that the data collected can be used for the planned statistical analyses.

Type of information and time frame

Single day food records or 24 hour recalls will provide information on actual/current or short term intakes when used in a large sample, e.g., in a national or regional study. When individual intakes are needed or when sample sizes are small, three or more days of recording or multiple 24 hour recalls are needed. Although these methods are likely to identify most frequently consumed foods, they may miss infrequently consumed foods or under report nutrients that are present in large amounts in less frequently consumed foods (e.g., vitamin A in liver) unless the number of recording/recall days is sufficiently large. Diet histories can also reflect habitual food patterns, but are too complex and time consuming for research purposes.

If information on meal patterns only is required, a simple method, e.g., menu records is preferable to food records or 24 hour recalls.

When the objective is to identify long term/habitual/usual intakes, an FFQ is the most appropriate choice. FFQ are also able to identify infrequently consumed foods, provided that the food list has been planned to do so and that the reference period is long enough to cover foods, possibly consumed once a month or less.

Level of detail

When the purpose of a study is to quantify food or report nutrient intakes, methods which measure or estimate portion sizes such as food records, 24 hour recalls or QFFQs are needed. SFFQs are adequate if less precise information on portion sizes is needed. Nonquantitative methods such as menu records/recalls and nonquantitative FFQs will provide information on food patterns and food choices.

Characteristics of the target population

As previously discussed, respondent characteristics such as age, gender, education level, employment,

Table 2.5 Choice of dietary assessment methods according to sample size, level of detail, type of information and purpose of study

	Sample			Level of detail			Type of information		Purpose			
Dietary assessment method	Individual	Small	Large	Meal patterns	Food choices	Quantitative food and nutrient intakes	Actual/ current/ short term	Habitual/ long term	Describe / compare intakes	Identify proportion 'at risk'	Rank individuals	Identify associations
Menu record												
Single day			√	√	√		√		√			
Multiple days	√	√	*	√	√		√		√			
Weighed/estimated food record												
Multiple days (< 7)	√	√	√	√	√	√	√		√			
Increased number of days and recording period	√	√	*	√	√	√		√	√	√	√	√
24 Hour recalls												
Single recall			√	√	√	√	√		√	√		
Multiple recalls	√	√	*	√	√	√	√		√	√		
Food frequency questionnaires												
Nonquantitative	√	√	√		√	**		√	**			
Semi-quantitative	√	√	√		√	√		√	√	√	√	√
Quantitative	√	√	√		√	√√		√	√	√	√	√
Diet history	√	√		√	√	√	√	√	√			

* The cost and logistics of carrying out multiple days menu/weighed/estimated records and multiple 24 hour recalls in large samples may be prohibitive.
** If predefined population-based portion sizes are used; √√ Increased detail

socio-economic status and weight status may affect the way in which respondents report dietary intakes. A key question is whether respondents are able to report their intakes themselves or whether, as for children, a parent or other responsible adult is be required. When the literacy level of the target population is low, interviewer administered recalls or FFQs are needed. Likewise, the complex cognitive skills required for FFQs, even when interviewer administered, may make them unsuitable for low literacy populations, children, or the elderly who may have difficulty in recalling and expressing frequencies of intake. The availability of and familiarity with computer and internet technology are essential if automated methods of administration are to be used. Irrespective of the method chosen, care must be taken to ensure that the method is culturally acceptable, in the language of the respondent and that time and effort demands on the participant are reasonable.

Resources

It is inevitable that the resources available, both financial and human, also influence the choice of method. They should not, however, be the primary consideration. The method used should be determined by the question to be answered. If the method or methods needed to answer the question are beyond the resources available it is better either to abandon the study or to redefine the question than to collect inadequate data.

Choice of dietary assessment tool

Once the dietary assessment method has been decided upon, the nutritional professional must decide whether to use an existing dietary assessment tool or to develop a tool from scratch. Within each method, there are numerous tools which vary in format (design, layout, question wording, instructions), mode of administration (self or interviewer administered, paper, automated computer, or web-based), the use and type of PSEAs and the support available (expertise, manuals, online help). Websites such as Nutritools (www.nutritools.org) and the National Cancer Institute (https://dietassessmentprimer.cancer.gov/ and https://epi.grants.cancer.gov/diet/shortreg/register.php) provide catalogues of dietary assessment tools and guidance for selecting, modifying, and developing tools. A thorough search of the recent literature will provide information, including pitfalls and limitations, on tools used in studies and populations similar to those of a planned study.

If no suitable tool is available, the nutrition professional may need either to extensively modify an existing tool or develop a tool from scratch. Cade *et al.* (2002) and Willet (2013) provide detailed guidelines specifically for the development of FFQs, arguably the most complex dietary assessment tool to develop. Regardless of the dietary assessment method and tool selected, input from experienced nutrition professionals and thorough pretesting and piloting of the tool in the target population are essential if high quality data are to be obtained.

2.12 Measuring reproducibility and validity

This section looks at ways in which the reproducibility and validity of dietary assessment methods can be assessed. For a more detailed overview, see the Nutrition Research Methodology textbook.

Measuring reproducibility

Assessing the reproducibility of a laboratory method is relatively straightforward because, with care, it is possible to reproduce both what is measured and the conditions of measurement. This is almost always impossible for a dietary intake measurement. Individuals do not eat exactly the same quantities or the same foods on different days or weeks. Additionally, their willingness and the way in which they respond may differ from one occasion to the next.

All measures of reproducibility obtained by applying the same method to the same individuals, on more than one occasion, include not only measurement error but also real day-to-day or week-to-week variability in intake.

While at first sight it might appear easier to measure the reproducibility of recall methods such as 24 hour recalls and food frequencies, this process introduces additional sources of variation since the interviews have to be conducted at different times and possibly by different interviewers. Measures of reproducibility for all dietary assessment methods will thus tend to overestimate the extent of measurement error because they will always include an element of variation due to real differences in dietary intakes and in the conditions under which measurements were done.

Usually, the reproducibility of a dietary assessment method is determined by repeating the same method on the same individuals on two separate occasions, that is, by a test–retest study. The interval between administrations of the method depends on the time-frame of the dietary method being assessed, but should generally be short enough to avoid the effects of seasonal or other changes in food habits and long enough to avoid the possibility of the first interview or recording period influencing the second.

The different measures of reproducibility provide different information. The correlation coefficient is widely quoted but is not a good measure since a strong correlation may be obtained even if one set of measurements has been systematically biased and has a different mean from the other set. The mean difference is not a good measure of reproducibility in individuals since it depends primarily on whether the differences are random or systematic. Measures that reflect the differences between repeated measurements within individuals (intra-individual) and between individuals (inter-individual) are to be preferred and are summarised in Table 2.6.

Measuring comparative (relative) validity

Demonstrating that a dietary method measures what it is intended to measure is even more difficult than demonstrating that a method is reproducible, because in effect it "requires that the truth be known."

This is almost always impossible unless it is possible to observe, surreptitiously, what is consumed over short periods such as 24 hours or at most a few days. Observation is usually only feasible in institutional settings or in situations specially set up to allow unobtrusive observation of what people eat.

For methods that are designed to obtain information on habitual longer-term intake, such as the diet history or FFQ, unobtrusive observation is impossible. This is a problem that has been faced by all investigators of dietary assessment methods and has usually been "solved" by assessing one dietary assessment method in relation to a more detailed and established method, known as the reference method. This latter method is considered to provide better estimates of the dietary intake of a study population. Reference methods include weighed or estimated food records, kept from seven consecutive days to three or four day records kept at monthly intervals over a given period of up to a year and multiple (3 to 24) 24 hour recalls conducted on non-consecutive days during a given period.

Table 2.6 Statistical test and interpretation criteria for reproducibility and validation of dietary assessment methods

Statistical test	Aspect of validity / reproducibility reflected	Interpretation criteria	
		Acceptable - good outcome	Poor outcome
Correlation coefficient	Strength and direction of association at individual level	$r \geq 0.3$	$r < 0.3$
Paired t test (normally distributed data) / Wilcoxon signed rank test (non normally distributed data)	Agreement at group level	$P > 0.05$	$P \leq 0.05$
Percent difference	Agreement at group level; size and direction of error	< 10%	>10%
Cross-classification (tertiles/quartiles)	Agreement, including chance, at individual level	>50% in same; <10% in opposite tertile/quartile	>50% in same; <10% in opposite tertile/quartile
Weighted Kappa statistic	Agreement, excluding chance, at group level	Kw > 0.2	Kw ≤ 0.2
Bland-Altman analysis: Limits of agreement (LOA) and correlation between mean and mean difference	Extent of error at group level Presence, extent and direction of bias at group level.	Narrow LOA $P > 0.05$	Wide LOA $P \leq 0.05$

r: Correlation coefficient; P: Probability value; Kw: Weighted Kappa statistic; LOA: Limits of agreement; P: probability value. Source: Adapted from Lombard *et al.* Application and interpretation of multiple statistical tests to evaluate validity of dietary assessment methods. *Nutrition Journal* 2015;14:40. Table 1 pg 2.

Comparison with another dietary method provides at best a comparative or relative form of validity and at worst information that is unrelated to validity but reflects either real differences or similar errors between the methods. For example, comparison of data from a single 24 hour recall or a FFQ with data from a seven day weighed record for the same individuals does not compare the same information because the time periods are not concurrent.

In the past, a method was judged to have acceptable reproducibility or validity if the mean intakes, as measured by both administrations or methods, did not differ significantly and if correlations for nutrient intakes in individuals exceeded 0.3 (Willett, 2009). Although these statistics are frequently reported, it is now recognised that these tests alone do not fully describe the all aspects of reproducibility or comparative validity. Table 2.6 summarises the statistical tests most frequently reported for reproducibility and comparative validity studies.

More advanced statistical techniques such as the correction of nutrient intakes for energy intake and adjustment of correlation coefficients for within- and between- person variations are described by Willett (2013).

Biological measures to validate energy and nutrient intake

It is now recognised that to assess the validity of any dietary assessment method, including weighed records, it is necessary to compare the dietary data with one or more objective measures that reflect but are independent of dietary intake. At the group level such measures include food supply or food expenditure data, and at the individual level biochemical or physiological measures that reflect energy and nutrient intake. The latter are often referred to as biological or biochemical markers and include energy expenditure, urinary breakdown products of protein, sodium, and potassium, plasma levels of vitamins, tissue levels of minerals, and the fatty acid composition of subcutaneous adipose tissue.

Biological markers are assumed to be objective, i.e., they do not rely on memory, or the respondents' ability to express themselves, and are free of biases introduced by the presence of the interviewers. These measures are also subject to errors of measurement and classification, but these errors are not related to the errors inherent in dietary intake assessment methodologies.

The three most widely used measures to assess the validity of dietary intake data are urinary nitrogen to validate protein intake, energy expenditure as measured by the doubly labelled water (DLW) method to validate energy intake in weight-stable individuals, and the ratio of energy intake to basal metabolic rate to identify "plausible" records of food intake.

Urinary nitrogen

One of the first to suggest an external measure as a means of validating dietary intake data was Isaakson (1980), who proposed urinary nitrogen as an independent measure of protein intake according to the equation:

$$\text{Reported protein intake (g)} \\ = (24 \text{ hour urinary N} + 2) \times 6.25 (\text{g})$$

where N is the urinary nitrogen output in grams and 2 is a constant representing nitrogen losses via the faeces and skin (note that some more recent equations give a constant of 4 or estimate extra urinary losses using body weight). Like the 24 hour recall, a single 24 hour urine collection does not necessarily reflect what is "usual." However, it appears that urinary nitrogen excretion is less variable from day to day than dietary protein intake, and that while 16 days of food intake are needed to assess habitual protein intake only eight 24 hour urine collections are needed to assess nitrogen excretion with the same level of confidence.

Although fewer 24 hour urine collections may be needed they are, in general, no more acceptable to respondents than 24 hour food records and require access to laboratory facilities. Nevertheless, they can provide a practical independent assessment, not only of protein but also of potassium and sodium intake.

Doubly labelled water method

The DLW technique, described in Chapter 6, allows the measurement of energy expenditure in free-living respondents over several days with minimal inconvenience to the respondent and with a high level of accuracy and precision.

Using the DLW technique several investigators have compared self-reported dietary energy intake with energy expenditure based on the equation:

$$\text{Energy expenditure}(\text{EE}) = \text{Energy intake}(\text{EI}) \pm \text{Change in the body energy store}$$

The main advantage of the DLW method is that it makes minimal demands on the respondents and does not interfere with their normal daily activities and therefore their habitual level of energy expenditure. Its main disadvantage is that the cost of the DLW required for each estimate is exceedingly high. The method also requires access to sophisticated laboratory equipment for mass spectrometric analysis. It is, therefore, not available for use on a routine basis for the validation of dietary intake data.

Ratio of energy intake to basal metabolic rate

Because of the limitations of the DLW method, another approach that is used compares the energy intake (EI) derived from the dietary intake data with the presumed requirements for energy expenditure, both intake and expenditure being expressed as multiples of the basal metabolic rate (BMR). The relevant equation is:

$$\text{EI:BMR} = \text{EE:BMR}\,(\text{PAL})$$

where PAL is the physical activity level. To determine whether reported energy intake is a "plausible" measure of actual diet during the measurement period (i.e., represents either the habitual diet or is a low/high energy intake obtained simply by chance) an equation was developed by Goldberg and colleagues (1991) to calculate the 95% confidence limits of agreement between EI:BMR and PAL. This equation allowed for variation in EI, BMR, and PAL and also for the length of the dietary assessment period and study sample size.

For a group, a mean reported EI:BMR below the lower 95% confidence limit (cut-off) for the given study period and sample size, suggests that there is bias towards the underestimation of energy intake.

However, the identification of individual under and over reporters is much more difficult, since reported EI can deviate quite markedly from energy expenditure (EE) before it can be considered implausible.

- The equations for the estimation of BMR have been derived for Western populations and their application to other populations must be done with caution.
- The equations require an estimation of physical activity levels.
- Using a single cut-off point to identify under reporters has been found to have poor sensitivity for underreporting (fails to identify under reporters), especially at high levels of energy intake.
- Cut-off values differ among studies. Thus it is difficult to select an appropriate value and to compare studies.
- Cut-off values apply only to individuals in energy balance. They cannot be applied to growing children or to adults trying to lose weight (Gibson, 2005).
- There is no cut-off value above which an intake can be considered implausible. Thus it is not possible to identify over reporters.

An alternate method to the EI:BMR method, proposed by Rennie *et al.* (2009) and Mendez *et al.* (2011) uses the Food and Nutrition Board, Institute of Medicine's (IOM) (2005) formula to calculate the estimated energy requirement (EER). The percentage by which an individual under or over reports energy intake is then calculated using the formula

$$\%\text{under-/over reported} = \left[100 \times \left(\text{EER - Reported EI}\right) / \text{EER}\right)\right]$$

Sample specific cut-off values can then be applied to identify possible under- or over reporters. This method has the advantages of being easier to interpret than the EI:BMR method, using a single EER equation, thereby allowing for between study comparisons and identifying over as well as under reporters.

Evaluation of dietary intake data

As previously indicated, dietary studies are often conducted in order to describe the current or habitual intake of individuals, to compare food and nutrient intake between different groups in the population, to determine the proportion of individuals at risk of dietary inadequacy or excess, or to investigate associations between dietary components and risk of disease or disease states.

In each case it is important first to assess the reproducibility and validity of the data. If the results of the reproducibility and validity analyses fall below the levels considered "acceptable" (Table 2.6) for some or all of the nutrients tested, the nutrition professional may need to consider modifying or changing the dietary assessment method. Steps which could be taken to improve the reproducibility and validity of a dietary assessment method include revising and clarifying instructions given to the respondents, improving the of training of interviewers, adding or changing PSEA and implementing strict quality control measures during the collection, processing and analysis of the data. Changes to the dietary assessment tool or data collection procedures may necessitate re-assessing the reproducibility and validity of the dietary assessment method.

Although techniques for handling biased dietary data have been developed, most are complex. Furthermore, most techniques address under reporting and very little guidance is provided in the literature regarding over-reporting. Nevertheless, the following suggestions serve to promote critical examination of data and wariness in drawing conclusions.

If the proportion of individuals who report extreme low or high intakes of energy differs between groups being compared, then any comparisons that do not take this into account will be biased. One way to draw attention to the possibility of bias between groups is to report not only the mean or median energy intake of the groups being compared but also the EI:BMR ratio or the percentage under/over reporting. If differences are evident, then the groups should be compared both with and without the extreme values included. One problem that arises is that by subdividing the groups the sample size is reduced and imprecision increased, so that a difference of biological significance may be missed, not because it does not exist but because the sample size is too small to detect it statistically.

When dietary inadequacy or excess is the question of interest, it is again important to consider extreme values separately. Energy intake is highly correlated with the intake of many nutrients and, consequently, intake of nutrients is also likely to be under or overestimated. An alternative approach is to compare nutrient intake per unit energy for both groups (e.g., mg thiamin/1000kJ). Likewise, when diet – disease associations are investigated, it is advisable to perform analyses and present results with and without extreme values.

For detailed explanations of the various techniques for managing bias in dietary data, the reader is referred to Willett (2013).

2.13 Assessment of dietary adequacy

Methods for evaluating dietary adequacy are described in Chapter 4. This section draws attention to the limitations of these methods.

The first limitation is that the evaluation of nutrient intake can provide only an estimate of the risk of nutrient inadequacy for a population or an individual. None of the methods can identify the specific individuals who have a nutrient deficiency. Individuals with a nutrient deficiency or excess can be identified only on the basis of biochemical and/or clinical measures of nutritional status.

The second limitation is that all estimates of dietary adequacy/inadequacy obtained by comparison with reference values for nutrient requirements depend on how the estimate is derived.

However, irrespective of the approach that is used to assess dietary adequacy, unless the extent of under- or over-reporting is known and taken into account, the proportion of individuals at risk of inadequacy will be over- or underestimated. While it may become possible to distinguish more reliably in population-based studies valid from invalid reports of dietary intake, this still does not enable population-based estimates of inadequacy to be made unless those who provide valid intakes are also representative of the population as a whole. All the evidence available to date suggests that this is highly unlikely.

When the principal objective of a dietary survey is to identify the proportion of the population who may have inadequate intakes of energy and nutrients, it is essential that the dietary intake information is interpreted in the light of appropriate biological measures of nutritional status.

2.14 Assessing food intake

Nutrition professionals usually analyse dietary intake data by converting the information on food intake into nutrient intake using relevant food composition databases. This approach simplifies the process of analysis and enables the resulting data to be compared with energy and nutrient requirements. Describing dietary intake in terms of foods rather than nutrients presents three practical difficulties that do not exist when food intake is analysed in terms of nutrients. First, the variety of foods consumed is much greater than the range of nutrients for which food composition data are available. Second, while essentially all individuals in a group contribute to nutrient intake data, not all individuals contribute food data for all foods, i.e. not all individuals are "consumers" of the same foods. Third, since foods consumed by different populations and subgroups of populations vary widely, comparisons between and even within populations may not be possible.

There are, however, several uses for which information on food intake is more relevant or for which information on food intake is needed in conjunction with data on nutrient intake. Although, as discussed in section 2.2, indirect approaches to measuring food intake at national, community and household level, provide information for planning and monitoring food and nutrition policies and identifying food consumption trends, they do not provide data on individual food intake patterns or differences between intakes of subgroups of the population, nor can they be used to determine food intake – disease risk associations at an individual level.

Food intake data are needed to develop food-based dietary guidelines and to monitor the extent to which these guidelines are met in different segments of the population. Information on both food and nutrient intake is necessary to address food and nutrition security needs of specific communities and households, and to address micronutrient deficiencies through fortification programmes. For example, in South Africa, data on food intakes obtained from a national food consumption survey were used to identify the most suitable vehicles for food fortification (maize meal and bread), while nutrient data identified the specific micronutrients which required fortification to reduce the risk of micronutrient deficiencies at national level. Similarly, nutritional epidemiologists are interested in the relationship of different foods and dietary patterns to specific health outcomes. The use of dietary data in the context of epidemiological studies is covered in the textbook *Public Health Nutrition* (Butriss *et al.* 2018).

The analysis and presentation of food intake data depends on the objectives of the study. When the purpose is to examine the intake of specific foods, the intake of foods may be presented as the total number of times a food is recorded, the number or percentage of individuals who consume a food, the total amount of the food consumed, mean or median daily intakes of the food, either per caput (for the whole sample) or for only those consuming the food, or the percentage contribution of the food to the total energy or nutrient of interest intake. Since not all members of a sample consume a given food, it is always important to clearly indicate whether the total sample size or only the number of respondents consuming the food has been used in statistical calculations. Table 2.7 summarises the ways in which food intake data can be reported.

Although intakes of individual food items may be reported, food intake data are usually reduced to more manageable proportions by grouping foods into appropriate categories. While this can be done in different ways, for example in terms of composition, biological origin, or cultural use, the process is relatively straightforward within a given culture or country. It is more difficult, however, to develop a classification that can be used consistently across different countries or food cultures. National food classification systems tend to differ not only because the type and range of foods differs, but also because the same foods are used in different ways. For the purpose of comparing food intake patterns between countries or regions, it is, therefore, necessary to develop a food classification or coding system that allows food data from individual regions or countries to be assigned in a consistent way. Guidelines for reporting and interpreting food intake data to allow for comparisons across studies, can be found in Faber *et al.* (2013).

Tracking changes in the food sources of nutrients and nonnutrients is particularly important in the context of technological developments in food production and manufacture that result in the addition of nutrients to foods, in the development of foods for specific functional purposes, and in the genetic modification of foods.

Table 2.7 Options for ranking and identifying the "most important" foods

Number of times each food was recorded
- reflects the frequency of consumption;
- does not take into account the number of consumers, portion size or number of times consumed per day;
- is influenced by dietary methodology:
  24-hr recall/record: one person may consume a given food several times during the recording period, while another may not consume the item at all, leading to overestimation of consumption within the sample;
  food frequency questionnaire: the number of responses to an item reflects the number of individuals who consume the food, but does not differentiate between frequent and infrequent consumers (e.g. daily or monthly consumption);
- may exceed the total number of study respondents (24-hr recalls / records) for frequently consumed foods.

Percentage of individuals reporting consumption of a food
- reflects the percentage of consumers (and not "importance" by quantity or frequency);
- does not distinguish between true non-consumers (who never eat the specific food) and occasional consumers (who do eat the specific food, but did not do so during the reference period for dietary intake) amongst non-consumers;
- provides a good indication of the most commonly consumed foods making it useful to identify the most / least consumed foods;
- does not reflect the frequency of consumption or the amount consumed;
- can be misleading if amounts consumed are small or if consumption is occasional.

Total intake (e.g. in grams of food) by sample studied
- favours foods consumed in large quantities and discriminates against foods consumed in small (but sometimes nutritionally important) quantities
- is not a good representation of the number or percentage of consumers

Mean daily intake (e.g. in grams of food) per consumer
- can be used to identify the proportion of low or high consumers, e.g. for fruit and vegetable intake relative to a standard;
- is restricted to those who consumed the food item during the reference period.
- is affected by respondent characteristics such as age and sex, thus affecting comparability

Per capita intake
- includes the whole sample regardless of whether the food item was consumed or not;
- is comparable to daily intake for consumers of commonly consumed foods;
- may differ substantially from daily intake of consumers for foods consumed by only a small number of respondents.

Energy and/or nutrient contribution by foods and/or food groups
- identifies food sources of nutrients;
- aids interpretation, total energy / nutrient intake must be given;
- must specify whether this refers to foods or dishes e.g., if the aim is to report energy intake from potatoes, margarine added to e.g., mash potatoes should not be included.

Source: Reproduced from Faber *et al.* Presentation and interpretation of food intake data: factors affecting comparability across studies. *Nutrition* 2013; 29: 1286-1992. Table 1 pg 1287.

A specific example of the need for individual food, rather than nutrient, intake data is provided by exposure assessments to dietary non-nutrients such as food additives, pesticide residues, and other possible food contaminants.

2.15 Dietary quality indicators

Traditionally dietary intakes have been analysed and reported as mean or median intakes of energy and individual nutrients or the distribution of nutrient intakes below or above a predefined cut-off point indicative of the risk of deficient or excessive intakes. This approach however has two drawbacks. On the one hand, the expertise, time, and resources needed to collect, analyse, and report energy and nutrient data may not be available. In such instances, a way to assess and report the quality of diets with minimal resources and which is easy to interpret is needed. On the other hand, as epidemiologic research has identified the many dietary and non-dietary factors associated with the risk of disease, the need for a single numeric value to summarise the overall quality of a diet and, in some instances, of the diet and other life style factors such as physical activity, has arisen.

In response to the need for a single value to reflect the complexity of the diet, many diet quality indicators have been developed, with the numbers increasing dramatically over the last two decades. In addition, many indicators have been revised in line with changes to dietary guidelines or modified for use in different populations. For example, the Healthy Eating Index (HEI) originally developed from the 1995 Dietary Guidelines for Americans has been revised three times, in 2005, 2010 and 2015 to incorporate new knowledge regarding dietary risk in relation to non-communicable diseases. The Mediterranean Diet Score (MDS), also created in 1995, to assess adherence to the Mediterranean dietary pattern has been modified for use in different regions, age groups and physiological status.

Some dietary quality indicators are based on nutrient intakes only. Examples are the Deficient and Excess Indices developed by Thiele *et al.* (2004) and the Mean Adequacy Ratio (MAR) derived from the ratio of nutrient intakes to nutrient requirements. Other indicators are based on food intakes only, for example, dietary diversity (DDS) and food variety scores (FVS). Lastly, some indicators include criteria for both food and nutrient intakes. The majority of diet quality indicators fall into the last group, among which the HEI, the Dietary Quality Index (DQI), the Healthy Diet Indicator (HDI) and the MDS are the most frequently reported (Gil *et al.*, 2015). A fourth group of indicators comprises diet quality indices which are combined with healthy life style indicators such as physical activity and social habits. The Mediterranean Lifestyle Index (MEDLIFE) is an example of this type of indicator.

Dietary quality indicators use established criteria such as Dietary Reference Intakes (DRI) and country specific food based guidelines to score individual intakes as either "healthy" or "unhealthy". For most indicators a higher score indicates a more healthy diet. There are however indicators, such as the DQI and DQI revised (DQIr), where lower scores are associated with a better quality of intake. Scoring varies according to the indicator. Scores may be assigned according the number of servings of specific foods or food groups per day, average intake in relation to a standard or median intake of the sample, percentage of energy provided by macronutrients or ratios of healthy to less healthy foods, e.g., white to red meat and monounsaturated to saturated fats.

The DDS and FVS are the simplest indicators to calculate and require only a count of the number of food groups (DDS) or different food items (FVS) collected from a single, nonquantitative 24 hour recall. The DDS and FVS have been shown to provide an acceptable reflection of dietary adequacy and are particularly useful in populations who consume unvaried diets and where expertise and resources are limited.

Since dietary quality indicators provide a summary of the quality of habitual diet, the most appropriate dietary assessment methods are multiple 24 hour recalls, food records or QFFQ if food intake is scored according to portion sizes or nonquantitative FFQ or menu records if only frequency of intake is scored. Calculation of indices which require both food and nutrient data may be complex, requiring that food intake data be analysed as food, food group, and nutrient intake. Since many indicators are based on population specific food based guidelines, their use in other populations is limited to those with similar food patterns. Comparisons between diet quality indicators are not possible because of the difference in components and scoring. An understanding of the rationale of the indicator and the components making up the score are essential if diet quality indicator results are to be correctly interpreted.

Diet quality indicators are useful for comparing total diet quality of groups within the same population, for tracking changes in diet quality over time, assessing the impact of an intervention programme on diet quality and for determining associations between total diet and disease or disease risk. Most frequently reported associations of diet quality have been with obesity, cardiovascular disease, and certain cancers.

2.16 Food safety assessments

Safety assessments for food additives, other than those classified as "generally recognised as safe (GRAS)" by the US Food and Drug Administration, are expressed in terms of the acceptable daily intake (ADI) estimated on the basis of lifetime exposure. While it is clearly not possible to collect food consumption data over the lifetimes of individuals, it is important that the dietary data used for the purpose of estimating acceptable levels of intake over a lifetime reflect, as far as is possible, the habitual level of intake of the foods being assessed.

For the purpose of food safety assessments only the intake of "consumers" is of interest. It follows, therefore, that the dietary data need to be adequate to obtain both an accurate estimate of the proportion of the population who are consumers and of the average habitual intake of consumers. Because the frequency of consumption varies between foods (some foods are eaten by most people on most days, but many other foods are eaten less frequently), the duration of the dietary recording period influences both the estimate of the proportion of consumers and the average intake of consumers. Intake data for one day will inevitably underestimate the true number of consumers for most foods and overestimate the average habitual intake of those consumers because not all foods are eaten every day. However, it appears that 75% or more of household menu items are normally consumed within a 14 day period and that a 14 day diary provides a good estimate of the habitual intake of most foods by consumers.

Most studies of the food intake of individuals, however, do not last for 14 days because of the increased cost and nonresponse associated with such a long study period. For the purpose of food safety assessment an approach that combines a three day food intake record with a FFQ has the potential to give estimates for the intake of consumers that are similar to those obtained from 14 day records.

2.17 Perspectives on the future

It is unlikely that either the measurement or the evaluation of food intake will become less complex in future. If anything, the reverse is likely to be true given the increasing diversity in the food supply and the increasing recognition of the need to be able to assess accurately not only the intake of foods and nutrients but also the intake of nonnutrient constituents of foods and dietary supplements. While the existence of errors in association with measurements of food intake is now widely appreciated, much work still remains to be done in this area.

Other aspects of food intake measurement that also require further development in the immediate future are likely to include the following:

As all direct methods of food intake measurement involve interaction between nutrition professionals and individuals and our understanding of the cognitive aspects of these interactions is still limited, more work is needed to improve the communications aspect of dietary assessment. Similarly, with the increased use of technology in dietary assessment, information is needed on how individuals interact with automated assessment tools and how technology affects the way in which dietary intakes are reported.

As the food supply becomes more complex individuals will no longer be able to describe the foods they have eaten in adequate detail unless technological developments such as the use of barcodes and similar systems of food identification become an integral part of dietary assessment.

As the number of food constituents of interest, in relation to health, increases it is important that appropriate physiological and biochemical markers are also developed for these constituents, as well as for the nutrient constituents of foods.

Finally, since dietary intake data serve no useful purpose unless they can be appropriately evaluated, it is essential that dietary studies include sufficient ancillary information to allow this to occur. This means routinely collecting information not only on age, gender, body size, and physiological status, but also on key aspects of lifestyle such as physical activity and the consumption of nonfood items such as supplements (both nutrient and nonnutrient) and drugs (both social and medicinal).

Diet is an integral part of health. It follows that measuring diet is essential for health promotion and disease prevention. Nutrition professionals must take the challenge to refine measurement. This requires openness and critical analysis of current methods and tools, and of new developments.

Addendum 2.1 Respondent instructions and example record sheet for a 7 day food record from a South African study

SEVEN DAY FOOD DIARY
INSTRUCTIONS

1 Please use this booklet to write down everything you eat or drink for the following seven days: ____________
As you will see, each day is marked into sections, beginning with the first thing in the morning and ending with bedtime. For each part of the day write down everything that you eat or drink, how much you eat or drink, and a description if necessary. If you do not eat or drink anything during that part of the day, draw a line through the section.
2 You have been provided with: a scale to weigh food, a measuring jug to measure liquids and a set of measuring spoons to measure small amounts of foods and liquids.
3 Write down everything at the time you eat or drink it. Do not try to remember what you have eaten at the end of the day.
4 Before eating or drinking, the **prepared** food or drink must be weighed or measured and written in the diary. If you do not consume all the food or drink, what is left must also be weighed or measured and recorded in the diary.
5 Please prepare foods and drinks as you always do. Also eat and drink in the same way as normal: eat the foods and drink in the amounts and at the times that you always eat and drink. Try not to change the way you eat and drink at all.
6 We need to know **ALL** the food and drink you take during these seven days. So, if you eat away from home, (e.g., at work, with friends, at a cafe or restaurant) please take your measuring equipment with you so you can still measure your food. Also do not forget to measure food bought at takeaways.
7 Please write down the recipes of home-made dishes such as stews, soups, cakes, biscuits, or puddings. Also, say how many people can eat from them or how many biscuits or cakes you get from the recipe.
8 On the next page is a list of popular foods and drinks. Next to each item is the sort of thing we need to know so that we can tell how it is made and how much you had. This list does not contain all foods, so if a food that you have eaten is missing, try to find a food that is similar to it. Please tell us as much about the food as you can.
9 Please tell us the amount and type of oil or fat that you use for cooking, frying, or baking
10 Most packet and tinned foods, like Simba chips, Niknaks, corned meat, tinned pilchards have weights printed on them. Tins, bottles, and boxes of cold drinks and alcoholic drinks also have weights printed on them. Please use these to show us how much you ate or drank. When possible, please keep the empty packets, bottles or tins.
PLEASE NOTE: we need to know the amount **YOU** eat or drink. So, if you do not eat the whole packet or tin of food, or drink the whole bottle of cold drink, please **measure** the amount you eat or drink.
11 At the end of each day there is a list of snacks and drinks that can easily be forgotten. Please write any extra items in here if you have not already written them down in some part of the day.
12 The research assistant will visit you during the record days to help you if you have any questions or problems. She will collect the equipment and diary after the seven days.

ALL THE INFORMATION YOU GIVE US IS STRICTLY CONFIDENTIAL. IT WILL ONLY BE USED FOR RESEARCH PURPOSES. ONLY YOUR PARTICIPANT NUMBER APPEARS ON THE DIARY. NOBODY WILL BE ABLE TO IDENTIFY YOU WITH THE DIARY.

EXAMPLE

Breakfast				Office use	
Food/Drink	**Description and Preparation**	**Amount served**	**Amount left**	**Amount eaten**	**Code**
Mealie meal porridge	*Iwiza. Soft, 1 cup meal and 3 cups water*	*300 g*	–		
Milk	*Fresh, full cream Clover*	*300 ml*			
Bread	*Brown*	*1x60 g*			
Margarine	*Rama, soft*	*10 ml*			
Tea	*Glenn tea bags*	*1 cup*			
Milk	*Fresh, full cream Clover*	*25 ml*			
Sugar	*White*	*2 heaped teaspoons*			

Addendum 2.2 An extract of a record sheet for an interviewer administered 24 hour recall

24 – HOUR RECALL

Study Number:___________ **Date:**__________
Recall Number:____________ **Day:**___________
Interviewer:______________

I want to find out about everything you ate or drank yesterday, including water, snacks, sweets or food eaten away from home. Please tell me **everything** you ate from the time you woke up yesterday morning until you went to sleep last night. I will also ask you where you ate the food and how much you ate.

Place (home, work, friends etc)	Food / drink	Description/brand/ preparation	Amount (HHM)	Amount (g) (office use only)	Code (office use only)
	Did you eat or drink anything when you got up yesterday? Yes No **If Yes,** what did you have?				
	Did you eat or drink anything during the morning (before about midday/ lunch time)? Yes No **If Yes,** what did you have?				
	Did you eat or drink anything in the middle of the day (lunch time)? Yes No **If Yes,** what did you have?				

Addendum 2.3 Typical layout of a nonquantitative food frequency questionnaire suitable for optical scanning (reproduced with permission of Anti Cancer Council of Victoria, Melbourne, Australia).

Please completely fill one oval in every line. Please MARK LIKE THIS: ○●○○	NEVER	1 time	2 times	3 or more times	1 time	2 times	3 or 4 times	5 or 6 times	Less than once	1–3 times
		per month			per week				per day	
Flavoured milk drink (cocoa, Milo™ etc.)	○	○	○	○	○	○	○	○	○	○
Nuts	○	○	○	○	○	○	○	○	○	○
Peanut butter or peanut paste	○	○	○	○	○	○	○	○	○	○
Corn chips, potato crisps, Twisties™ etc.	○	○	○	○	○	○	○	○	○	○
Jam, marmalade, honey or syrups	○	○	○	○	○	○	○	○	○	○
Vegemite™, Marmite™ or Promite™	○	○	○	○	○	○	○	○	○	○
Dairy products, meats and fish										
Cheese	○	○	○	○	○	○	○	○	○	○
Ice cream	○	○	○	○	○	○	○	○	○	○
Yoghurt	○	○	○	○	○	○	○	○	○	○
Beef	○	○	○	○	○	○	○	○	○	○
Veal	○	○	○	○	○	○	○	○	○	○
Chicken	○	○	○	○	○	○	○	○	○	○
Lamb	○	○	○	○	○	○	○	○	○	○
Pork	○	○	○	○	○	○	○	○	○	○
Bacon	○	○	○	○	○	○	○	○	○	○

Addendum 2.4 Alternate layout of a quantitative food frequency questionnaire suitable for optical scanning or automated computer administration (Cancer Council Victoria http://www.cancervic.org.au/research/epidemiology/nutritional_assessment_services. Accessed 13 May 2018)

12. In the last 12 months, how many slices of bread did you usually eat each day? Please include all types of bread, fresh or toasted. Count one bread roll as 2 slices.
    - o None – (Go to Q.14)
    - o Less than 1 slice per day
    - o 1 slice per day
    - o 2 slices per day
    - o 3 slices per day
    - o 4 slices per day
    - o 5 to 7 slices per day
    - o 8 or more slices per day

13. What types of bread and rolls did you usually eat? You may choose more than 1 type.
    - o White (include Turkish and white sourdough)
    - o High fibre white
    - o Wholemeal
    - o Multi-grain
    - o Rye (include rye sourdough)
    - o Soy and linseed
    - o Gluten free

14. In the last 12 months, how many eggs did you usually eat each week? Include eggs that are fried, boiled, scrambled, poached and used in omelettes.
    - o None
    - o Less than 1 egg per week
    - o 1 to 2 eggs per week
    - o 3 to 5 eggs per week
    - o 6 or more eggs per week

Addendum 2.5 An extract from a quantitative food frequency questionnaire (Reproduced from https://faunalytics.org/ffq/)

How often, in the past 3 months, did you eat the following?	never	Less than 1 time per week	1-3 times per week	4-6 times per week	1 time per day	2-3 times per day	4 or more times per day	What was your usual serving size, relative to thє following?
Fruit (apples, bananas, oranges, etc.)								½ cup raw fruit; ½ medium applє large orange
Vegetables (carrots, mushrooms, potatoes, etc.)								½ cup cooked or raw; 1 carrot oı stalk celery
Chicken (fried chicken, in soup, grilled chicken, etc.)								3-4 oz; ½ large or 1 small breast drumsticks
Turkey (turkey dinner, turkey sandwich, in soup, etc.)								3-4 oz; 6-8 very thin slices; 1-3 tł slices
Fish and Seafood (tuna, shrimp, crab, etc.)								3-4 oz; 1 can of tuna; 6 medium shrimp
Pork (ham, pork chops, ribs, etc.)								3-4 oz; 1 pork chop; 2 ribs; 3-4 s bacon
Beef (steak, meatballs, in tacos, etc.)								3-4 oz; ¼ lb burger; 3-6 slices ro beef
Other Meat (duck, lamb, venison, etc.)								3-4 oz; a piece about the size of palm
Nuts (almonds, cashews, walnuts, etc.)								¼ cup or 1 handful; 20 almonds; tbsp nut butter
Beans (tofu, chickpeas, chili, etc.)								½ cup cooked beans; ¼ cup hur or tofu
Dairy (cheese, milk, yogurt, etc.)								3 slices cheese; 1 cup milk; 1 cu yogurt
Eggs (omelet, in salad, in baked goods, etc.)								1 egg; ¼ cup scrambled eggs or cup egg salad
Grains (breads, pasta, rice, etc.)								1 slice bread or pizza; ½ cup ricє pasta
Sweets (candy, cookies, pie, etc.)								2 small cookies; 1 slice cake or ꞃ
Caffeinated Soft Drinks (cola, diet cola, energy drinks, etc.)								1 can (12 oz) soda; small founta drink
Coffee and Tea (hot coffee, iced coffee, black tea, etc.)								6 oz hot coffee or tea; small icec coffee

Addendum 2.6 An extract from a quantitative food frequency questionnaire with open ended response options used in a rural South African population

Food	Description	Amount (g /HHM)	Number of				Code*	Amount/Day
			Times eaten in a day	Days food is eaten in a week	Weeks food is eaten in a month	Not eaten in previous month		
A. CEREALS AND BREAD								
Maize meal: stiff porridge	Home grown						4406	
	Shop bought: Brand:						4411	
Maize meal: soft porridge	Home grown						4405	
	Shop bought: Brand:						4410	
Maize meal: sour porridge	Home grown						4406	
	Shop bought: Brand:						4411	
Sorghum (Mabelle) porridge	Home grown						3999	
	Shop bought: Brand:						3241	

* Food item code from the South African Food Composition Tables (van Graan *et al.* 2017)

References

Cade, J., Thompson, R., Burley, V. *et al.* (2002). Development, validation and utilisation of food-frequency questionnaires: a review. *Publ Health Nutr* 2002; **5**: 567–587.

Cade, J., Warthon-Medina, M., Albar, S. *et al.* DIET@NET: Best practice guidelines for dietary assessment in health research. *BMC Medicine* 2017; **15**: 202–217.

Cancer Council, Victoria. Dietary questionnaire (DQES V3.2). Available from http://www.cancervic.org.au/research/epidemiology/nutritional_assessment_services. (Accessed 15 April 2018).

Conway, J.M., Ingwersen, L.A., Vinyard, B.T. *et al.* (2003). Effectiveness of the US Department of Agriculture 5-step multiple-pass method in assessing food intake in obese and nonobese women. *Am J Clin Nutr* 2003; **77**: 1171–1178.

Faber, M., Wenhold, F.A.M., MacIntyre, U.E. *et al.* (2013). Presentation and interpretation of food intake data: factors affecting comparability across studies. *Nutrition* 2013; **29**: 1286–1992.

Fiedler, J.L., Lividini, K., Bermudez, O.I. *et al.* (2012). Household consumption and expenditure surveys (HCES): a primer for food and nutrition analysts in low- and middle-income countries. *Food and Nutrition Bulletin* 2012; **33** (Suppl 3):S170–S184.

Food and Agriculture Organisation (FAO). (2002). *Food balance sheets. History, sources, concepts and definitions.* Paper no. 5. Training in the preparation of food balance sheets. Available at http://www.fao.org/elearning/course/fa/en/pdf/5_fbs_concepts.pdf. (Accessed 25 April 2018).

Food and Nutrition Board, Institute of Medicine of the National Academies. (2005). *Dietary reference intakes for energy, carbohydrate, fiber, fat, fatty acids, cholesterol, protein and amino acids.* Washington DC: The National Academies Press.

Gibson, R.S. (2005). *Principles of Nutritional Assessment*, 2e. Oxford: Oxford University Press.

Gil, A., Martinez de V.E., and Olza, J. (2015). Indicators for the evaluation of diet quality. *Nutr Hosp* 2015; **31**(Suppl 3): 128–144.

Goldberg, G.R., Black, A.E., Jebb, S.A. *et al.* (1991). Critical evaluation of energy intake data using fundamental principles of energy physiology. I. Derivation of cur-off limits to identify under-recording. *Eur J Clin Nutr* 1991; **41**: 569–581

Isaksson, B. (1980). Urinary nitrogen output as a validity test in dietary surveys. *Am J Clin Nutr* **33**: 4–5.

Lee, R.D. and Nieman, D.C. (2019). *Nutritional assessment*, 7e. St Louis: Mc Graw Hill.

Lombard, M., Steyn, N.P., Charlton, K.E. *et al.* (2015). Application and interpretation of multiple statistical tests to evaluate validity of dietary assessment methods. *Nutrition Journal* **14**:40. DOI 2.1186/s12937-015-0027-Y

Mendez, M.A., Popkin, B.M., Buckland, G. *et al.* (2011). Alternative intake-obesity relations. *Am J Epidemiol* **173**: 448–458.

National Cancer Institute. (2016). Automated Self-administered 24 hour dietary assessment tool (ASA24). Available at https://epi.grants.cancer.gov/asa24/ (Accessed 30 April 2018).

Nelson, M. (1997). The validation of dietary assessment. In: *Design concepts in nutritional epidemiology*, 2e. (ed. B.M. Margetts and M. Nelson). Oxford: Oxford University Press.

Nutritional Epidemiology Group, School of Food Science & Nutrition, University of Leeds (2018). Myfood24. Available at https://www.myfood24.org/web/. (Accessed 30 April 2018).

Rennie, K.L., Coward, A., and Jebb, S.A. (2007). Estimating under-reporting of energy intake in dietary surveys using an individualised method. *BJN* **97**: 1169–1176

Thiele, S., Mensink, G.B.M., and Beitz, R. (2004). Determinants of diet quality. *Publ Health Nutr* **7**: 29–37.

Van Graan, A.E., Chetty, J.M., and Links, M.R. (2017). *Food Composition Tables for South Africa*, 5e. Parow: Medical Research Council.

Wenhold, F.A.M. and Faber, M. (2019). Beverage intake: Nutritional role, challenges, and opportunities for developing countries. In: *Nutrients in beverages*.(ed. A.M. Grumezesu). Duxford: Woodhead Publ/Elsvier.

Willett, W. (2009). Foreword. *BJN* **102**(Suppl): S1–S2.

Willett, W., ed. (2013). *Nutritional Epidemiology*, 3e. Monographs in Epidemiology and Biostatistics. New York: Oxford University Press.

Further reading

Castro-Quedzada, I., Ruano-Rodriguez, C., Ribas-Barba, L. *et al.* (2015). Misreporting in nutritional surveys: methodological implications. *Nutr Hosp* **31**(Suppl 3): 119–127.

Food and Agricultural Organisation of the United Nations. (2001). Food balance sheets. A handbook. Rome: FAO. Available from: http://www.fao.org/3/a-x9892e.pdf. (Accessed 12 April 2018).

Illner, A.-K., Freisling, H., Boeing, H. *et al.* (2012). Review and evaluation of innovative technologies for measuring diet in nutritional epidemiology. *Int J Epidemiol* **41**: 1187–1203.

Matt, G.E., Rock, C.L., and Johnson-Kozlov, M. (2006). Using recall cues to improve measurement of dietary intakes with a food frequency questionnaire in an ethnically diverse population: an exploratory study. *J Am Diet Assoc* **106**: 1209–1217.

Molag, M.J., de Vries, J.H.M., Ocke, M.C. *et al.* (2007). Design characteristics of food frequency questionnaires in relation to their validity. *Am J Epidemiol* **166**: 1468–1478.

Smith, L.C., Dupriez, O., and Troubat, N. (2014). Assessment of the reliability and relevance of the food data collected in national household consumption and expenditure surveys. *IHSN Working Paper* No. 8. Available at http://www.ihsn.org/sites/default/files/resources/IHSN_WP008_EN.pdf. (Accessed 25 April 2018).

Stumbo, P.J. (2013). New technology in dietary assessment: a review of digital methods in improving food record accuracy. *Proceedings of the Nutrition Society* **72**: 70–76.

Websites

Cancer Council, Victoria. Dietary questionnaires: http://www.cancervic.org.au/research/epidemiology/nutritional_assessment_services

Food and Agricultural Organization: Food balance Sheets: http://www.fao.org/faostat

Food Standards Agency Scotland. INTAKE24 Online 24 hour recall tool: https://intake24.co.uk/

Nielsen corporation: http://www.nielsen.com

International Household Survey Network: http://www.ihsn.org/food

Automated Self-administered 24 hour dietary assessment tool (ASA24) (National Cancer Institute, 2016): https://epi.grants.cancer.gov/asa24/)

Myfood24: https://www.myfood24.org/web/

University of Cambridge EPIC – Norfolk: Nutritional methods: http://www.srl.cam.ac.uk/epic/images/ffq.jpg

Nutritools: https://www.nutritools.org

National Cancer Institute Dietary Assessment Primer: https://dietassessmentprimer.cancer.gov

Epidemiology and Genomics Research Program of the National Cancer Institute: https://epi.grants.cancer.gov/diet/shortreg/register.php

3
Food Composition

Hettie C. Schönfeldt and Beluah Pretorius

Key messages

- Reliable good-quality composition data of foods for human consumption are critical resources for a variety of applications.
- These data are required for a spectrum of users ranging from international to national, regional, household, and individual levels.
- In general, data obtained on food intake by individuals, or groups of individuals, are used to estimate the consumption of nutrients and to establish nutritional requirements and health guidelines.
- The determination of the consumption of nutrients can be achieved either by analysing the foods consumed directly (by far the most accurate, but also the most costly method) or by using food composition tables/databases.
- The food described in the food composition table should be recognisably similar to that being consumed by the individual or group.
- Factors such as sampling, variability, and analytical methods involved must be considered when developing such tables.
- Inadequacies of food composition tables can be minimised by calculating nutrient losses and gains during food processing and preparation.

New activities in food composition include:

- future composition tables could include bioavailability and the glycemic index
- harmonizing food composition tables regionally
- focusing on biodiversity within species
- investigation of the composition of specific traditional and ethnic foods
- bioactives in foods and their effect on health and well-being
- food composition data and their role in nutrition and health claims.

3.1 Introduction

Although the amount, quality, and availability of food composition data vary among countries and regions, in general most developing countries still do not have adequate and reliable data. This is despite the fact that the components of specific foods have been published for over 150 years. Over time food composition data have assumed more scientific, academic, and political importance owing to their utility. Refer to Table 3.1 for practical examples of the uses of food composition data. It was only in 1961 that a regional food composition table was developed and published for Latin America, followed by a food composition table for Africa (1968), the Near East (1970), and Asia (1972). The data in these tables were based on a very limited number of samples, a limited number of nutrients and, in today's terms, outdated analytical methodologies. However, these tables are still being used today as there are limited up-to-date tables available. Worldwide, there are currently over 150 food composition tables or nutrient databases, or their electronic/magnetic equivalents, in use. Many tables are based on the data from the United States Department of Agriculture's (USDA) National Nutrient Database for Standard Reference, SR, available on the Nutrient Data Laboratory's web site: www.ars.usda.gov/nutrientdata. Public

Introduction to Human Nutrition, Third Edition. Edited on behalf of The Nutrition Society by Susan A. Lanham-New, Thomas R. Hill, Alison M. Gallagher and Hester H. Vorster.

Companion website: www.wiley.com/go/lanham-new/humannutrition

Table 3.1 Examples of the uses of food composition data

Level	Examples
International	Role of food in the provision of nutrients and/or the estimation of adequacy of the dietary intake of population groups Investigation of relationships between diet, health, and nutritional status, e.g., epidemiologists correlate patterns of disease with dietary components Evaluation of nutrition education programs Nutrition intervention and food fortification programs such as in food assistance programs; foods are distributed or enriched to address the specific nutritional needs of populations, e.g., iodine or vitamin A In food trade nutritional labeling
National	Monitoring at governmental level, the availability of foods produced and estimating the individual intake for specific dietary requirements, e.g., protein and energy Food balance sheet data are used to provide data on food available nationally for the whole population and are useful in monitoring trends in food consumption over time Researchers work to improve the food supply by selecting or developing new strains or cultivars, improving cultivation, harvesting, preservation, and preparation Estimation of adequacy of the dietary intake of groups within populations Investigation of relationships between diet, health, and nutritional status Evaluation of nutrition education programs Food and nutrition training Nutrition education and health promotion Nutrition intervention and food fortification programs Food and nutrition regulation and food safety Nutrition labeling of foods
Regional (influenced by meal patterns and food preferences)	Institutions such as hospitals, schools, dormitories, and troops/armies (ration scale) formulate nutritionally balanced diets to the individuals in their care Food industries regulate the quality of their foods by routinely analyzing the components in their products Food industries change and improve their products to appeal to new customers by improving nutrient content or sensory appeal through the change in ingredients Product development
Household	Household food surveys provide data on household food consumption Household budget surveys Household food economics
Individual	Dietary intake of the individual is assessed to understand present health and to monitor changes in dietary intake Impact of interpretation of choice and preference via data composition Individual energy expenditure is the only true measurement of energy need, e.g., in the management of a sportsman's diet or in obesity Personal dietary needs and goals with associated likes and dislikes can be assessed on an individual basis Individual nutritional balance studies Therapeutic or restricting diets with specific nutrient contents, e.g., management of diabetes and hypertension, can only be described on an individual basis Individual shoppers scan the ingredient list and nutrient content on the labels of packaged foods Sports nutrition

Health England is responsible for maintaining up-to-date data on the nutrient content of the United Kingdom (UK) food supply through the the Composition of Foods Integrated Dataset (CoFID), available on: https://www.gov.uk/government/publications/composition-of-foods-integrated-dataset-cofid. A comprehensive list of the food composition tables available can be obtained from the Food and Agriculture Organizsation of the United Nations (FAO) homepage on the World Wide Web (http://www.fao.org/infoods/directory). EuroFIR, the European Food Information Resource Consortium, is a partnership between universities, research institutes, and small to-medium-sized enterprises from European countries. EuroFIR aims to develop and integrate a comprehensive cohort and validated network of databanks of food composition data.

There is still a continued need to carry out food analyses as the number of foods consumed all over the world, especially unique foods, is still several times greater than the number for which analytical data exist. The Cross Cutting Initiative on Biodiversity for Food and Nutrition led by the FAO and Biodiversity International focused on genetic diversity within species and of underutilized, uncultivated, and indigenous foods. The investigation has highlighted the need for composition data of foods, not only at species level, but also at subspecies level. The limited amount of composition data for underutilised, uncultivated, and indigenous foods playing important roles in the consumption patterns in underdeveloped and developing countries increases this need for food composition analysis. Food analyses are also needed under the following circumstances:

- when the data in existing tables are based on a single or very limited number of samples
- when the content of a nutrient or other food component is not available in an existing food table
- when there is no information available on which foods are important sources of a nutrient or another food component of interest
- when there is no information on the loss or gain of nutrients in foods during preparation by the methods being used by the population under investigation
- when it is necessary to check the comparability of the various food composition tables being used in a multicentre study
- when the method available to determine a particular nutrient is considerably improved
- when scientific evidence is found correlating newly recognized food components to health
- when new policies are adopted for public health initiatives which dictate reformulations
- when new foods are produced or existing foods are reformulated.

3.2 Foods

Food composition tables normally consist of a list of selected foods with data on the content of selected nutrients in each food. For a food composition table to be of value in estimating nutrient content, a significant portion of the foods consumed by the group or individual being studied, as well as the nutrients of interest, should be present in the table. To a large extent this relationship is critical in determining the quality of the information obtained by using the tables, assuming that the data in the tables are of a desirable quality.

Criteria for inclusion in tables

The identification of potential contributions of foods to the diet of the population group being studied is unquestionably the first step in identifying and selecting which foods should and should not be included in the production of a database. However, common sense dictates that it is unreasonable to expect that all foods consumed by all individuals at all times be included in a specific food composition table at any one time. Therefore, most tables aim to include all foods that form a major part of the food supply and that are major contributors to the diet in the forms most commonly obtained or consumed, and as many as possible of the less frequently consumed foods. For instance, in the USA the number of foods contributing to quartiles of critical nutrient intakes was identified as the following: nine foods contribute to 25% of food intake, 34 foods to 50%, 104 to 75%, and 454 to approximately 100%.

Databases can be compiled directly, where the compiler initiates sampling and analyses to obtain the data, or indirectly by drawing on the following sources of data, in order of preference:

- original analytical values
- imputed values derived from analytical values from a similar food, e.g., values for "boiled" used for "steamed"
- calculated values derived from recipes, calculated from the ingredients and corrected for preparation factors
- borrowed values (refers to using data originally generated or gathered by someone else) from other tables and databases.

Today, database compilers normally draw on a combination of the direct and indirect methods.

Description of foods

The food described in the food composition table should be recognizably similar to that being consumed by the individual or group. The precise description of foods is a difficult task and much is required to ensure that foods are described adequately. The introductory material (description and explanation) in a printed table may be almost as important as the data values. By using several words to describe a food, called an extended or multifaceted description, the chance of misinterpreting the data is reduced. As internationalization of food composition data continues, linguistic aspects of defining foods, with one definition meaning different things in different cultures and even from place to place within countries, are highlighted. For instance, sorbet or sherbet is made by beating whisked egg whites into the partly frozen mixture such as in apple sorbet and lemon sorbet. However, the term sorbet is preferred to sherbet, since the latter can also refer to a flavored, sweet, sparkling powder or drink, or a drink of sweet diluted fruit juice. The name tortilla is also applied to a variety of foods in Latin America. In Africa morogo is a collective term used for a variety of indigenous green leafy vegetables harvested from the veld. Using scientific names for food items is not necessarily a solution, since the relationship between common name and scientific name is neither consistent nor universally unique, for example the German tables group pears and apples in the same genus, while the British and US tables separate them.

In 1975 the Food and Drug Administration (FDA) of the USA developed a controlled vocabulary for food description, based on the principle of a faceted thesaurus, where each food indexed is described by a set of standard terms grouped in facets, characteristic of the product type of a food source and process applied to food ingredients. Examples are the biological origin, the methods of cooking and conservation, and technological treatments. It is an automated method for describing, capturing, and retrieving data about food, adapted to computerized national and international food composition and consumption databanks, and is therefore language independent. In Table 3.2 an example of the application of LanguaL is presented. More information can be obtained from the LanguaL (Langua aLimentaria or "language of food") homepage (www.langual.org). LanguaL is an international framework for food description, which the European LanguaL Technical Committee has administered since 1996. The thesaurus is organized into 14 facets of the nutritional and/or hygienic quality of foods. These include the biological origin, the methods of preparation or conservation. The European LanguaL Technical Committee has linked LanguaL to other international food categorizing and coding systems including the CIAA Food Catgorizing System, Codex Classifications, and E-numbers used for additive identifications.

Table 3.2 Example of the international use of LanguaL

Facet	Code	English term	French term	Danish term	Hungarian term
Product type	A0178	Bread	Pain	Brød	Kenyér
Food source	B1418	Hard wheat	Blé de force (Triticum aestivum)	Hård hvede (Triticum aestivum)	Kemény búza (Triticum aestivum)
Part of plant or animal	C0208	Seed or kernel, skin removed, germ removed (endosperm)	Graine ou grain sans enveloppe et sans germe	Frø eller kerne, skaldele (pericarp/caryopse) fjernet, kim fjernet (endosperm)	Szénhidrát vagy hasonló vegyület
Physical state, shape, or form	E0105	Whole, shape achieved by forming, thickness 1.5–7 cm	Entier façonné épais de 1.5–7 cm	Hel, facon dannet ved formning, tykkelse 1.5–7 cm	Egész, formázott, 1.5–7 cm közötti vastagság
Extent of heat treatment	F0014	Fully heat treated	Transformation thermique complète	Fuldt varmebehandlet	Teljesen hókezelt
Cooking method	G0005	Baked or roasted	Cuit au four	Bagt eller ovnstegt	Sütött vagy piritott
Treatment applied	H0256	Carbohydrate fermented	Fermenté au niveau des glucides	Kulhydratfermenteret	Szénhidrátos fermentált
Preservation method	J0003	No preservation method used	Sans traitement de conservation	Igen konservering	Tartósitási eljárást nem alkalmaztak
Packing medium	K0003	No packing medium used	Sans milieu de conditionnement	Intet pakningsmedium anvendt	Csomagoló eszközt nem alkalmaztak
Consumer group/ dietary use/ label claim	P0024	Human food, no age specification	Alimentation humaine courante	Levnedamiddel uden aldersspecifikation	Emberi fogyasztásra szánt élelmiszer, kormeghatározás nélkül

Since, many structured food description systems have been proposed. These systems should be adapted to the specific purpose (e.g., nutrient content, pesticide regulation) for which they are intended. For example, the FAO Committee report, INFOODS Guidelines for Describing Foods: A Systematic Approach to Describing Foods to Facilitate International Exchange of Food Composition Data, published in 1991, was designed to facilitate interchange of food composition data between nations and cultures. The system is a broad, multifaceted, and open-ended description mechanism using a string of descriptors for foods. The International Food Data System Project (INFOODS) Nomenclature and Terminology Committee has developed guidelines for describing foods to facilitate international exchange of food composition data. INFOODS is a comprehensive effort, begun within the United Nations University Food and Nutrition Program to improve data on the nutrient composition of food from all parts of the world. In line with the FAO's lead role in classification of agricultural activities and products, and to facilitate international data comparability and exchange, FAOSTAT has developed and standardized the Harmonized Commodity Description and Coding System in 1996. The coding system has developed multipurpose goods' nomenclature used as the basis for trade statistical nomenclatures all over the world.

In 2008, the European Food Safety Authority (EFSA) developed a standardised detailed Food Classification and Description System (FoodEx or FoodEx1). It consists of about 1700 terms (food groups) organized in a hierarchical system based on 20 main food categories that are further divided into subgroups up to a maximum of four levels; each term is identified by a unique code. In the following years, based on the experience gathered in the use of FoodEx1, a more detailed Food Classification and Description System (FoodEx2) was released in 2015. FoodEx2 is a comprehensive food classification and description system for exposure assessment applicable across different food safety domains including food consumption, chemical contaminants, pesticide residues, zoonoses and food composition. A browser to support navigating the classification and encoding was developed for users of the FoodEx1 and has been progressively improved based on suggestions received by the users of FoodEx2 in the European Member State organisations providing data to EFSA or in international organisations like FAO, as well as EFSA staff. The latest revision of the FoodEx2 browser is made available for free download in the EFSA website (http://www.efsa.europa.eu/en/data/data-standardisation). FAO, EFSA and other organizations aim to code existing and future data using FoodEx2, e.g., food composition, food consumption, food safety, food prices, and other food-related data to facilitate national and international data linkages across domains.

Classification of foods

Most food composition tables are organized according to the classification of foods into food groups, with food items listed alphabetically within each food group. For example, the fruit group could start with apples and end with tangerines. A simple coding system could supplement the alphabetically listed foods (used in the British tables), but it presents a problem when a new food is introduced and all the codes have to change. Although food groups of different countries and organizations are never completely identical, they are usually recognizably similar. However, problems normally arise with the description of cooked mixed dishes where a dish can be equally well described by one or more food group. In some tables, particularly those for educational purposes, there are subgroups based on the content of specific nutrients such as high-fat and low-fat dairy products. Table 3.3 provides an example of major food groups that are used by the FAO for their food balance sheets and regional food composition tables.

Table 3.3 Major food groups that are utilised by the Food and Agriculture Organization

Cereals and grain products
Starchy roots, tubers and fruits
Grain legumes and legume products
Nuts and seeds
Vegetables and vegetable products
Fruits
Sugars and syrups
Meat, poultry, and insects
Eggs
Fish and shellfish
Milk and milk products
Oils and fats
Beverages
Miscellaneous

Sampling of foods for inclusion in tables

Food sampling concerns the selection of the individual units of foods, food products, or bulk foodstuffs from the food supply or source, whether it be the marketplace, manufacturing outlet, field, or the homes of the members of the study population. (Sampling also concerns the selection of the representative aliquot from the individual unit or homogenized mixture in the laboratory just before analysis.) In-context sampling can be defined as the selection and collection of items of food defined in number, size, and nature to represent the food under consideration. The objectives for sampling will, in the large part, determine the type and nature of the sampling plan. One of the major objectives of food sampling is to provide representative mean values for individual components in foods. The sampling process is described in detail in Table 3.4.

Food sampling is a critical step in any food composition program. For any research project, personnel, and financial resources are always limited. The selection, procurement, shipping, and storage of sample units require a significant portion of available resources. Therefore, sampling must follow a specific and detailed statement of the objectives and procedures to ensure that the selection of units is sufficient in number and weight and representative of the foods of interest. If sampling or sample preparation is done incorrectly then all subsequent analyses are a waste of time and money, as a mistake in sampling can only be corrected by repurchasing and repreparing of a new sample. Pilot studies, conducted by the investigator(s) or published in the scientific literature, can be used as the basis of sampling decisions for the current study.

Variability in foods: regional and other differences

Foods are biological materials and, as such, have a naturally variable composition. Even processed foods produced under highly controlled circumstances show some variability. Therefore, a database must be able to predict the composition of a single sample of food within the limits defined by its natural variability. Variability may be contributed by one or more of the following factors: brand, cultivars or species, season, climate, geographical location (e.g., soil type), fertilizer treatment, method of husbandry, harvesting, preservation state, stage of maturity, enrichment/fortification standards, preparation methods, food colour, variation in recipes and formulations, distribution and marketing practices, and other factors. For critical components variability may affect the sufficiency, deficiency, or excess of the intake of a given component. Estimates of variability must be based on sampling and analyses specifically planned to yield such data. The intended use of the data should determine the specificity and level of precision for the estimates.

For instance, it was found that the nutrient composition of whole milk in South Africa differed among the five localities investigated between winter and summer, with the fat-soluble vitamins showing the greatest variation of all the nutrients. Vitamin A is commonly regarded as one of the micronutrients that are deficient in most developing countries and specifically in disadvantaged schoolchildren in South Africa. Considering the results of the nutrient composition of whole milk, a recommendation was made to the health authorities to fortify summer milk with retinol in the South African school-feeding intervention program, where milk is served as a mid-morning snack to five million primary school children.

There is a growing recognition that the composition of commodities such as meat and cereals tends to change over time. This necessitates updating food composition data every 5–10 years. In most countries this has not been possible. Changes in nutrient composition of red meat consumed are due to consumer demand for leaner cuts, changes in breeding for faster growth, and higher proportions of marketable meat as well as changes in feed to meet scientific standards or due to economic reasons.

3.3 Nutrients, nonnutrients and energy

Analytical methods

Judgement should be made on the availability of suitable methods of analyses for nutrients and whether the resources, laboratory equipment, and experience are adequate before deciding which nutrients should be included in a nutrient database. If the methods available are not well

Table 3.4 Sampling process of foods for food composition data

1 *Prioritising foods for inclusion*

May be based on:
- type
- frequency and
- amount of specific foods or products consumed
- quality and quantity of existing data
- appropriateness of prior analytical methods or
- perceived benefit/risk of particular foods as sources of components of interest

May be affected by:
- changes in the forms of foods or
- levels of components, including reformulation or fortification Levels of available resources will impact on the process of setting priorities

2 *Defining prioritised foods*

Within the context of the objective, define the specific characteristics of the food that may contribute to the variability of the estimate:
- uncooked or raw foodstuffs versus cooked forms of the food
- composition of prepared or multicomponent foods (i.e., mixed dishes)
- individual brands or cultivars or generic value

3 *Definition of sampling unit*

Collection of units (packages, bunches, or items) representative of the total population of food units:
- sample units must be taken from the available types and forms of the food for which the composition estimates are being determined. Production, consumption or sales statistics may be used. The population of items may be supplied to or distributed through an entire nation or region or be only typical of a particular subpopulation (e.g., ethnic group or tribe)
- select sample units from all the various types of food and geographical or manufacturing locations of food consumed by the population of interest. The units may be selected according to the relative importance (e.g., frequency of consumption) for given types
- sample units that are collected can be analyzed as individual units or may be combined together or composited and analyzed. The analysis of composite samples reduces the costs associated with the analysis of individual samples, but information about the variability of the component in that food will be lost

4 *Definition of sampling size*

Amount of material required:
- objective of analyses
- analyses of individual samples or composite samples of the food
- number of components to be measured; determine the number and weight of aliquots needed as required by the chemical methods
- policy for saving reserve or archive aliquots

5 *Protocol for sample collection*

Foods should be typical of the usual preparation and consumption practices

Correct units of foods should be selected

Protocols should be tested for the adequacy of food storage and transportation facilities, sample unit documentation and labeling, and packaging and short-term preservation requirements

Policies for the substitution of units should be in place in the event of unavailable sample units

Sampling among ethnic or native populations may impose additional restrictions owing to cultural or religious customs

Samples should be clearly coded for identification. Documentation should start from the planning stage, throughout purchasing, transporting, preparation and the combining of samples, to analyses including storage condition, use of reference samples, recording of data obtained (duplicate or triplicate values), as well as manipulation of the data, e.g., expression of the data on a wet (as eaten) basis, as opposed to the content of a freeze-dried sample. Correction factors applied or calculations (e.g., N × Jones factor = protein) should be recorded for each foodstuff analyzed

Documentation and handling of sample units should be under the careful control of the principal co-coordinator and all laboratory personnel should be informed before the start of the project of the reasons for handling the samples in a specific manner. The samples should preferably be marked with three-digit random codes for analysts to ensure that analyses are unbiased. Values should only be decoded as results become available, by the principal investigator. This will improve the reliability of the results if performed on a double-blind basis

developed, one should reconsider the importance of the nutrient and whether it justifies using limited resources, in most instances and countries, to develop the method and train the staff accordingly. It will not be cost-effective to analyse food for a particular nutrient, however high in priority, if methods yield conflicting values. This implies that, as new or improved methods for measuring a nutrient emerge, foods that are important in the food supply and are known or suspected to be a good source of that nutrient should be analyzed or reanalyzed. Food regulation sometimes limits the choice of methods.

The choice of method selected should be that which most closely reflects the nutritive content of the foodstuff analyzed. A basic understanding of the chemistry of the nutrients, the nature of the food substrate (the way in which the nutrient is distributed and held in the food matrix) to be analyzed, the effect of processing and preparation on both the food matrix and the nutrient, and the expected range of concentration of the nutrient determine the choice of method. An understanding of the role of the nutrient in the diet of individuals or populations is also a prerequisite.

The basic principle is that the method used should provide information that is nutritionally appropriate. For instance, traditionally, carbohydrate was estimated by difference, that is, by directly measuring the percentage of protein (from the nitrogen content), fat, ash, and water, and deducting these from 100 to provide the percentage of carbohydrate. This method is inadequate for all nutritional purposes as it combines in one value all of the different carbohydrate species: sugars, oligosaccharides, and polysaccharides (starch and non-starch), together with all of the errors in the other determinations, as the physiological effects of all of the components are quite different. Therefore, the sum of the individually analyzed carbohydrates is widely recommended today.

In studying the relationship between particular foods and health or disease, the biological action of related nutrients may be crucial information for particular uses of food composition data. For example, a study on the role of vitamin A and carotenoids in lung cancer requires more information than the vitamin A activity expressed in retinol equivalents. At the very least, vitamin A and provitamin A activity are required separately. Information on provitamin A could be divided into the various provitamin A carotenoids, and it may also be desirable to have information on other carotenoids present. This is also true for the vitamers of other vitamins, including vitamin B_6 (pyridoxal, pyridoxal phosphate, and pyridoxamine), folic acid (with a side-chain with one, three, or seven glutamic acid residues), vitamin D (D_2, D_3 and 25(OH) D_3), vitamin E (various tocopherols and tocotrienols) and vitamin K (with various numbers of saturated and unsaturated isoprene units in the side-chain).

The EuroFIR BASIS bioactives database includes critically assessed composition data on the bioactives present in edible plants and plant-based foods as well as compilation of critically assessed data on their biological effect (http://www.eurofir.net).

Criteria for inclusion in tables

As the number of nutrients is reasonably infinite, it is to some extent easier to choose and prioritize food items. Core nutrients for a nutritional database include the major proximate constituents, those that are essential, and those for which there are recommended intakes. The inclusion of micronutrients, especially trace elements, fatty acid profiles, amino acid composition and the various forms of vitamins is normally limited by the resources available. Many databases give limited coverage of the carbohydrates and carotenoids in foods, but methods are available and this limitation will probably disappear in the future.

Nutrients to be included in the food composition table will depend on the proposed use of the table. For instance, when assessing nutrient intake, two types of nutrients can often be distinguished: those nutrients that are found in small quantities in a large number of foods, such as iron and most of the B vitamins, and those that are found in large quantities in a small number of foods, such as cholesterol and vitamin A. The FAO limits the inclusion of nutrients in the table for group feeding schemes to 11 nutrients per 100 g of edible portion. The nutrients that have been selected by the FAO as the most important for developing countries are energy, protein, fat, calcium, iron, vitamin A, thiamine, riboflavin, niacin, folate, and vitamin C. Iodine can also be included as a nutrient of concern in developing countries.

Complete coverage of all nutrients in a single food database is unlikely, as priorities are set according to the importance of a food in the provision of a nutrient, resulting normally in analyses of proximates and major nutrients. However, with the growing interest in the role of biologically active compounds, residues, and toxicants in food there is increased pressure to include these in special-purpose food composition tables. Phytochemicals or phytoprotectants, often used in functional foods, are bioactive compounds found in food that may have benefits to human health.

A provisional database for food flavonoid composition has been developed and is maintained by the United States Department of Agriculture (USDA) on its National Nutrient Databank website (http://www.ars.usda.gov/nutrientdata). The database contains values for 385 food items for five subclasses of flavonoids namely flavonols, flavones, flavanones, flavan-3-ols, and anthocyanidins.

A European network established to compile and evaluate data on natural food plant toxicants, the EU AIR Concerted Action NETTOX, has previously identified 31 major compound classes called the NETTOX: a list of toxicant classes with 334 major food plants listed in Europe. This list, now known as the EuroFIR NETTOX plant list (http://www.eurofir.net) has recently been published after being updated to include additional plant parts. The list now includes 550 beneficial biological effect outputs of the bioactive compounds of the edible plants. This list facilitates calculations of exposure to bioactive compounds such as flavanols, phenolic compounds, phytosterols, carotenoids, isoflavones, and lignans.

For a food composition database to include all these substances will imply that there may be an over-emphasis on "nonnutrients." In general, levels of pesticides, residues, toxicants, and additives in food, with the exception of those that contribute to energy and nutrients, are often not reported in food composition tables.

Modes of expression

An increasing amount of attention is being paid to how data are presented in food composition tables. Interchange and compatibility of food composition databases are only possible if the data are uniformly expressed. To overcome ambiguities in the naming of nutrients and also to allow for the transfer of data among food composition tables, INFOODS has developed a system for identifying food components, referred to as tags. The term "tag" refers to the significant part of a generic identifier. Generic identifiers are predefined word-like strings of characters used to distinguish one element type from another. An example of a tagname and its definition is presented in Table 3.5. The latest information on this system is available on the World Wide Web via the INFOODS home page (http://www.fao.org/infoods). As already mentioned, LanguaL is a multilingual system that provides a standardized language for describing food products using faceted classification. Each food is described by a set of standard, controlled terms chosen from facets characteristic of the nutritional and/or hygienic quality of a food, for example the biological origin, method of cooking and conservation, and technological treatments.

Other problems related to the method of expression of nutrients may arise from the long-standing convention of using protein values derived by applying a factor to measured total nitrogen values and from the calculation of energy values using energy conversion factors. Calculation of total carbohydrate content by difference as

Table 3.5 Example of an INFOODS tagname and its definition for a food component

<ENERC>

Energy, total metabolisable; calculated from the energy-producing food components

Unit: kJ. The value for <ENERC> may be expressed in kilocalories instead of the default unit of kiloJoules. However, if expressed in kilocalories, kcal must be explicitly stated with the secondary tagname <Unit>

Note: It would be confusing and would imply additional information that does not exist if two <ENERC> values, i.e., one expressed in kilocalories and the other expressed in kiloJoules, were included for a single food item when one value has simply been calculated from the other using the conversion equation: 1 kcal = 4184 kJ. Consequently, one or the other should be used, but not both

Synonyms: kiloJoules; kilocalories; calories; food energy

Comments: In addition to a value for the quantity of total metabolisable energy, <ENERC> includes a description or listing of the conversion factors used to calculate this energy value from the proximate quantities. The conversion factors may be described by a keyword, or the conversion factors may be listed using secondary tagnames within <ENERC>. (More than one <ENERC> tagname may exist for a single food item if the values were calculated from the proximate components using different conversion factors.)

opposed to the sum of the individual carbohydrates is no longer the norm. The bases of expression in databases are the most commonly used units (such as g) per 100 g of edible portion. In some instances unit per 100 g of dry mass is presented, or unit per 100 ml. However, some tables list nutrient content per serving size or household measure, either as purchased or as prepared.

Quality of data

The quality of food composition data is critical for the accuracy of the estimates of compounds in food. In particular, analytical data obtained from scientific literature and laboratory reports can be evaluated for quality. The quality of the analytical data is affected by various factors, including how the food samples were selected (sampling plan) and handled before analysis, use of appropriate analytical method and analytical quality control, and adequacy of number of samples to address variability. In addition, complete food description and identification of the components analyzed are also important.

The data quality evaluation system developed by the USDA is based on the evaluation of five categories: sampling plan, sample handling, analytical method, analytical quality control, and the number of individual samples analyzed. Detailed documentation of all the steps within each category is important for evaluating that category. Each category gets a maximum rating of 20 rating points. A quality index (QI) is generated by combining points of all the five categories and confidence codes (CCs) ranging from A to D indicating relative confidence in the data quality are assigned. These confidence codes could be released with the data and thus provide an indication of the data quality to the user of the data. Confidence code "A" indicates data of the highest quality, while confidence code "D" suggests data of questionable quality. These procedures can be used to guide the planning and conducting of food analysis projects.

3.4 Information required on sources of data in tables

It is important to have information on the source of the data in a food composition table to be able to check its appropriateness for the study and to confirm its authenticity. The four major categories of sources of data are:

- primary publications, e.g. peer-reviewed articles in scientific literature
- secondary publications, e.g. reviews or published compilations with compositional data
- unpublished reports ranging from analytical records to documents prepared with limited circulation, e.g. confidential reports for clients or internal use within a company
- unpublished analytical data that can be either specifically commissioned analyses for the generation of nutrient data or analytical data that were not particularly generated for the purpose of generating food composition data.

Data in food composition tables may be original analytical values, imputed, calculated, or borrowed. Original analytical values are those taken from published literature or unpublished laboratory reports. Unpublished reports may include original calculated values, such as protein values derived by multiplying the nitrogen content by the required factor, energy values using energy conversion factors for some constituents of food, and "logical" values, such as the content of cholesterol in vegetable products, which can be assumed to be zero. Imputed values are estimates derived from analytical values for a similar food or another form of the same food. This category includes those data derived by difference, such as moisture and, in some cases, carbohydrate and values for chloride calculated from the sodium content. Calculated values are those derived from recipes by calculation from the nutrient content of the ingredients corrected by the application of preparation factors. Such factors take into account losses or gain in weight of the food or of specific nutrients during preparation of the food. Borrowed values are those derived from other tables or databases without referring to the original source. When a value for the content of a specific nutrient in a food is not included, there is a "–" or "0" value and, when a table has no values for a particular nutrient, the value is regarded as being "not included." In some tables, e.g., the National Nutrient Database for Standard Reference, SR, of the USDA, "0" value is a true zero, meaning the particular nutrient

Table 3.6 Proportion of various types of data in food composition tables

Types of data	McCance and Widdowson tables, UK (developed country)	South African food composition table (developing country)
Analyses	70%	41% in 1999 (improved from 18% in 1991)
Borrowed	10%	49%
Calculated	15%	10%
Estimated	5%	–

was not detected by the analytical method used; "–" indicates a missing value.

The proportion of the various types of data differs between tables and for different nutrients (Table 3.6). Details on food tables can be obtained from the Food and Agriculture Organization (http://www.fao.org/infoods). In other tables, such as those in the Netherlands, where sources of the data are given in the references, information on how the data have been obtained can also be found. However, this is not the case for all tables of food composition.

3.5 Overcoming the inadequacies of food composition tables

Nutrient losses and gains during food processing and preparation

In the absence of analytical data for all forms of foods, nutrient values can be estimated by calculation using standard algorithms that have been experimentally derived. Since the content of nutrients per unit mass of food changes when foods are prepared, such losses and gains can be classified in two ways. The first can be described by a food yield factor, when the weight of the primary ingredients at the precooking stage is compared with the weight of the prepared food at the cooking stage and also with the final weight of the food as consumed at the post-cooking stage. The weight of the food can be increased due to the hydration of the dry form of a food (e.g., rice, macaroni) with cooking liquid, (e.g., water or broth) or increased due to the absorption of fat during frying of the food (e.g., potato). Alternatively, the weight of the food can decrease due to dehydration during cooking as a result of evaporative and drip losses.

The second, the nutrient retention factor, is related to changes in the amount of specific nutrients when foods are prepared. Changes in the nutrient levels can occur due to partial destruction of the nutrient as a result of the application of heat, alkalization, etc. Also, for some dietary components (e.g., β-carotene) the amount of available component may increase due to the breakdown of cell walls in the plant-based sample. Although original analytical data would be the most desirable type of data for foods at all stages of preparation, they are seldom available. Efforts are in progress in several regions to revise the nutrient losses and gain factors, including nutrient retention and yield factors, in order to compare and harmonize them and thereby improve the quality of food composition data calculated.

As food composition data are frequently lacking for cooked foods, estimates based on the use of these factors for calculating the nutrient content of prepared foods from raw ingredients are made. Thus, the nutrient composition of a prepared or cooked food is calculated from the analytical data of uncooked food by applying suitable nutrient retention and yield factors. To obtain the nutrient content per 100 g of cooked food, the nutrient content per 100 g of raw food is multiplied by the percentage retained after cooking, and this is divided by the percentage retained after cooking, divided by the percentage yield* of the cooked product

$$\text{Nutrient content of cooked food per 100 g} = [(\text{nutrient content of raw food} \times \text{retention factor}) / \text{yield of cooked food}] \times 100$$

*Yield of cooked food (%) = (weight of edible portion cooked food/weight of raw food) × 100

The retention factor accounts for the loss of solids from foods that occurs during preparation and cooking. The resulting values quantify the nutrient content retained in a food after nutrient losses due to heating or other food preparations. This is called the true retention method and is calculated as follows:

%True retention = [(nutrient content per g of cooked food × g cooked food)/(nutrient content per g of raw food/g of food before cooking)] × 100

The following example uses only the yield factor to predict the nutrient content of the cooked food. The yield factors for different foods are reported in the USDA Agriculture Handbook 102 and for cooked carrots it is 92%. Selected nutrient values in SR 21 for 100 g of raw carrots are 0.93 g of protein, 33 mg of calcium and 5.9 mg of ascorbic acid. Using the yield factor the composition of 100 g of cooked carrots is calculated as 0.93 g/0.92 = 1.01 g protein, 33 mg/0.92= 36 mg calcium and 5.9 mg/0.92 = 6.4 mg of ascorbic acid. This compares favorably to the determined values for carrots of 0.76 g of protein and 30 mg of calcium, but less so for ascorbic acid at a value of 3.6 mg, probably because it is heat sensitive; therefore, applying the nutrient retention factor for ascorbic acid (70%) would have resulted in a more accurate prediction (5.9 × 0.7/0.92 = 4.9) of 4.9 mg/100 g) (http://www.ars.usda.gov/nutrientdata).

Missing values in food composition tables

In general, original analytical data provide information of the highest quality for inclusion in a food composition table or nutrient database. However, it is seldom possible to construct a food composition table with only such data. A plan of action should be developed by the compilers of the database to deal with missing food items and values for particular nutrients. Very often, values of a biologically similar food are used. For composite or mixed dishes the composition of the dish is estimated by calculation from a standard recipe and applying appropriate nutrient retention factors and, in some cases, adjusting for changes in moisture content due to cooking loss or gain in the different cooking procedures. If a food item forms an important part of the population's diet and analysis is not possible, existing food composition databases should be searched to see whether data on the same or a similar food item could be borrowed. If a value for a nutrient is missing, a similar approach can be followed, as it is more desirable to have a slightly incorrect estimated value of lower quality than no value at all. A value of "–" or "0" assigned to missing nutrient values may lead to underestimation of nutrient intake, especially if those nutrients make a significant contribution to the diet.

Bioavailability and glycemic index

Nutrient composition information in food composition tables indicates the amount of nutrients as analyzed in that specific food sample and does not give an indication of the absorption or bioavailability of the nutrient from that food item. However, when dietary reference intakes such as recommended dietary allowances (RDAs) are drawn up, the recommendation makes provision for the amount of ingested nutrient that may not be absorbed. The concept of bioavailability has developed from observations that measurements of the amount of a nutrient consumed do not necessarily provide a good index of the amount of a nutrient that can be utilized by the body. The bioavailability of a nutrient can be defined as the proportion of that nutrient ingested from a particular food that can be absorbed and is available for utilization by the body for normal metabolic functions. This is not simply the proportion of a nutrient absorbed, and cannot be equated with solubility or diffusibility in *in vitro*-simulated physiological systems. Bioavailability is not a property of a food or of a diet per se, but is the result of the interaction between the nutrient in question, other components of the diet and the individual consuming the diet. Owing to the many factors influencing bioavailability, tables of food composition cannot give a single value for a nutrient's bioavailability. Most research until now has centered upon inorganic constituents, particularly iron, but the concept is applicable to virtually all nutrients. Iron incorporated into heme is more readily absorbed than iron in the nonheme form, and these two forms of iron are sometimes listed separately in food composition tables. Yet, such information does not take into account, for example, the effect of ascorbic acid (vitamin C) and organic acids (citric, malic, tartaric, and lactic acid) on nonheme iron absorption. Iron absorption is also increased in a state of iron deficiency and research has shown that vitamin A and iron intake has to be increased simultaneously to alleviate anemia. In the coming years, it can be expected that much more work will be carried out on bioavailability than in the past, because of its key role in relating functional nutritional status to nutrient intake.

Future research will probably also focus more on the measurement of the bioavailability of food constituents. Several vitamins and minerals, such as calcium, iron, zinc, and a number of B vitamins, are already being studied, with limited attention to carotenoid bioavailability. Inhibitors of absorption and the effects of processing and storage on the foodstuffs must be determined. As bioavailability is also influenced to a large extent by the meal in which a food constituent is consumed, this means that more information will be needed not only on daily food consumption but also on intake of other constituents at individual meals.

There is an increasing demand from users of food composition tables for information on the glycemic index (GI) of food, which is used as a tool in the selection of food in the management of diabetes, as opposed to the previous system of carbohydrate exchange. The GI is a food-specific measure of the relative tendency of carbohydrate in food to induce postprandial glycemia. The body's response to a 50 g carbohydrate dose induced by either glucose or white bread is taken as the reference and assigned a value of a 100. Responses to all other foods are rated in comparison and listed in tabular format. New datasets with complementary values, based on the GI and available carbohydrate content of food, have been proposed, of which one is a measure of the relative glycemic response to a given mass of whole food and the other is the mass of a food responsible for a given specific glycemic response. A more recently proposed identification of a food's GI value lies in indicating the specific food's category of GI as high, medium, or low. Accurate numerical values of a food's GI are difficult to obtain as various factors, including human subject variability both between and within subjects during analysis as well as response during ingestion of the food, can differ significantly.

Both bioavailability and GI are food indices that are influenced not only by the characteristics of the food, but also by the response of the individual to the food (i.e., absorption, metabolism, and excretion of the metabolites). For example, quantitative analysis of carotenoids alone could lead to a misinterpretation of vitamin A value. Therefore, the bioavailability of test foods in a single mixture may be investigated using the digestive system of nutrient-depleted rats (i.e., measuring retinol accumulation factor as a measure of total carotenoid bioavailability), or in humans using the relative dose–response test. Advances in analytical chemistry such as improvements in analytical methods, information science, computer hardware and software will assist in filling these gaps in special-purpose databases in the future.

How to calculate a recipe not included in the database

If the composition of a composite or mixed dish is not known, it can be estimated by calculation from a standard recipe and applying appropriate nutrient retention factors and, in some cases, adjusting for changes in moisture content due to cooking loss or gain during cooking. The following guidelines are suggested:

- Identify the ingredients of the recipe from the most appropriate foods available in the food composition database table.
- Quantify the ingredients in mass (g).
- Calculate the nutrient values for the specific amount of each ingredient.
- Add up the nutrient values of the individual ingredients.
- Calculate the nutrient composition for 100 g of the recipe.
- Apply suitable retention factors to the mineral and vitamin nutrient values if the recipe food is cooked. Note that if individual ingredients are in a cooked form this step is not necessary.
- Compare the moisture content of the calculated recipe with a similar cooked composite dish. If the moisture content differs by more than 1%, adjust the moisture content of the recipe food. All of the nutrients of the recipe food must be adjusted (concentrated or diluted) according to either the decrease or increase in moisture content.
- Assign to a suitable food group and list.

This is only an estimation of the make-up of a composite or mixed dish of unknown composition. Refer to Table 3.7 for an example of the calculation of the composition of a dish from a recipe. However, if this dish is a very important part of the diet of an individual or group and the information is crucial in assessing the adequacy of the diet, analysis should be considered.

Table 3.7 Calculation of the composition of a dish from a recipe

Recipe for scrambled eggs with onions
2 large eggs
1/6 cup whole milk
1/8 teaspoon salt
1/4 cup chopped raw onions
2 teaspoons oil
Add milk and salt to eggs and beat with a fork. Fry onions in the oil. Pour egg mixture into frying pan with the onions, and stir mixture with a fork while cooking until it solidifies. Makes one serving.

Calculation of nutrient content of scrambled eggs from nutrient values for raw ingredients

Step 1: Add nutrient levels for the specified quantities of ingredients. The nutrients in the raw eggs, whole milk, salt, raw onions and oil are added together.

Step 2: Readjust quantities of those nutrients in the raw ingredients that are lost during cooking due to evaporation or heat.

Nutrient loss on cooking	Eggs	Milk	Onions
Thiamin (%)	15	10	15
Riboflavin (%)	5		
Niacin (%)	5		
Ascorbic acid (%)		25	20
Folacin (%)			30

Step 3: Determine weight of the recipe before cooking
1 large egg = 57 g; 57 g × 2 eggs = 114 g; refuse factor to calculate weight without shell of 11%;
1 14 g × 0.89 = 101.46 g
1 cup whole milk = 244 g × 1/6 = 40.66 g
1 teaspoon salt = 5.5 g × 1/8 = 0.69 g
1 cup chopped raw onions = 170 g × 0.25 = 42.5 g
1 teaspoon oil = 4.53 g × 2 = 9.06 g
Total weight = 194.37 g

Step 4: Determine weight of recipe after cooking
Weight loss during cooking due to evaporation is estimated to be 8%
Weight of recipe after cooking = 194.37 g × 0.92 = 179 g

Step 5: Determine the nutrient levels of the recipe per 100 g and per serving
Divide the nutrient levels by 1.79 to determine the nutrient content of 100 g scrambled eggs
The calculated nutrient levels represent the nutrient content of one serving

Accurate estimation of portion size

Food composition tables and databases are mainly used in nutritional epidemiology to estimate the composition of foods consumed by individuals. All subjects have difficulties in estimating the exact portion sizes of food consumed. This issue is further complicated by the difference between the weight of a product as purchased and that of the actual item consumed (e.g., in meat after cooking there is at least a 25% cooking loss, without bone and with or without visible fat). Standardized portion sizes for individual foods within countries may help, but a set of standard food models (small, medium, and large) for use in dietary assessment may be of more value.

3.6 Description of food composition tables and databases and how to retrieve data

A food composition table or database is easier to use if the format allows easy access to the data available. Advances in information technology have led to more and more food composition tables being available in electronic form, progressively replacing the printed format. Printed food composition tables, although limited by physical proportions such as the size of both the written text and the printed table, continue to be popular in developing and underdeveloped countries. The printed word is seen as authoritative and only a limited level of literacy or knowledge on nutrition is necessary to be able to access the data. Electronic data and access to them are more limited in remote areas in these countries, and a higher level of computer literacy and equipment is necessary, which is generally seen as a luxury and not a necessity.

However, electronic databases have many advantages over printed tables, including virtually unlimited capacity to store information, rapid access to individual data items, and easy sorting and manipulation of data for use in a wide range of calculations. However, the ease of accessing data in an electronic or a computerized database is dependent on the database access software and not only on the way in which data are stored. The development of relational databases has led to the opening up of possibilities to link different databases in regions and countries with each other. This has led to the identification of new challenges such as food identification, compatibility of data, data interchange and data quality.

3.7 Converting foods to nutrients

Entering data

Before the computer age, the conversion of food consumption into nutrient intake had to be done manually, which was a laborious and time-consuming task. Later, much of the work, especially for larger surveys, was done on mainframe computers, and has since passed on to microcomputers, because of their ready accessibility and ease of use. Data on food and nutrient intakes were often subsequently transferred to a mainframe computer, where they were combined with other survey data for further analysis. Today, there is little that cannot be done on a microcomputer, including data manipulation such as sorting and calculations.

Before proceeding to calculate nutrient intake from data on food consumption, it is necessary to ensure that mistakes that have crept into the data set during acquiring, coding, merging, transcription, and storage are reduced to an acceptable level. Regardless of the method used for the collection of data on food consumption, consideration should be given to how the data will be entered into the computer. Suitable forms should be designed for the collection of data. These can be on paper or in a personal computer-based program that can save time and eliminate errors associated with the transcription of data from paper to the computer. The use of carefully prepared forms, with information to guide those collecting the data, can reduce the chance of error during the collection of data and, if a separate process, during entry into the computer. The collection and entry of data are subject to human and computer error; therefore, procedures must be developed to ensure that the quality of data is as high as possible. Editing and error checking routines should be incorporated in the data entry process and subsets of data entered into the computer should be compared with the original written records. Where mistakes are found, the extent of the error should be determined, because it could involve data for the previous (or next) subject or day, or those previously (or subsequently) entered by the operator involved. In addition to such checks, frequency distributions of all amounts of food and food codes should be carried out. The Food Surveys Research Group of the Agricultural Research Service of the USDA has developed an automated method for collecting and processing dietary intake data. The three computer systems, Automated Multiple Pass Method (AMPM), Post-Interview Processing System (PIPS) and Survey Net collect, process, code, review, and analyze data for nutrient intakes. The system has been used for the National Health and Nutrition Examination survey since 2002.

Converting data in food intake to nutrient intake

A crucial aspect of food composition research is the transmission of information from those working in food composition and analysis to those working in food monitoring, to scientists trying to improve the food supply, to workers in epidemiological, training and nutrition programs, and to regulators. Yet there is little discussion in the scientific literature of the issues relating directly to the compilation of food composition databases, which are the primary means of transmission of food composition data to most professionals in the field. If good food statistics are available in a country, as well as access to food intake and food composition databases, estimates of a higher quality can be made regarding the nutrient intake of the individual or population as a whole. However, few data on food composition exist for the 790 million people in developing countries who are chronically undernourished and where malnutrition in the form of deficiencies of iron, iodine, and vitamin A is rife.

3.8 Perspectives on the future

No universal food database system has been developed that fulfills all of the needs of compilers and users of food databases, despite the fact that it would represent the primary scientific resource from which all other nutritional studies flow. However, recent international collaboration has considerably improved the development and compatibility of food composition data. It is essential for the development of nutritional sciences that this resource be maintained and improved to serve at both national and international levels. The quest for continued improvement in quality of representative food composition data are at the core of most food composition programs.

3.9 Recent advances in food composition

Harmonizing of regional food composition tables

High-quality, comprehensive food composition data for foods commonly consumed is important across an ever increasing list of applications, e.g., in epidemiological research studying the effect of specific foods on health and well-being. Integrated, comprehensive, and validated food composition databanks from individual countries within a region will contribute immeasurably towards shifting the barriers of current scientific understanding. Towards this end Europe has moved much closer to obtaining this goal, preceded by the ASEAN Food Composition Tables (2000) (www.fao.org/infoods/tables_asia_en.stm).

Focusing on biodiversity within species

The FAO has begun a study on the development of baseline data for the Nutritional Indicators for Biodiversity – 1. food composition. The aim is to collect food composition data at the inter- and intra-species level for regions and countries. The process includes obtaining information on food composition data at the interspecies level (variety, cultivar, breed) and on underutilized and wild foods at the species level, as well as reviewing all available food composition data at national, regional, and international levels. The data collected are reported in a template, naming the country and the INFOODS regional data centre. Table 3.8 gives an example of the format of reporting at the national level. For the baseline reporting, at the beginning of 2008 data from 254 publications from 49 countries were included.

Table 3.8 Template for reporting on the nutritional indicator of biodiversity in the food composition literature

			Number of foods on subspecies level with following number of components			
Publication	Material examined	References	1	2–9	10–30	>30
1. Food composition databases (FCDB) Reference database of national FCDB User database of national FCDB Other national FCDB						
2. Literature						
National peer-reviewed journals	Indicate journals and years					
National laboratory reports	Indicate laboratories and years					
Reports from national research institutes	Indicate research institutes and years					
National conference presentations (incl. posters)	Indicate conferences and years					
Theses	Indicate universities and years					
Other (specify)	Indicate publication and years					
Material examined						
Letter	Material examined					
A						
B						
References						
Number	Full reference				DOI, CiteXplore ID, other international publication code	
1						
2						

Investigating specific traditional and ethnic foods

Traditional and ethnic foods reflect cultural inheritance and in many cases form key components in the dietary patterns in many countries. In many instances traditional foods include underutilized vegetable species and in the current evolved world there are still many of these species and subspecies of which the nutrient information is lacking. Traditional and ethnic foods contribute considerably to the diet of many populations, and may have significant health contributions. Research and analysis on these foods has slowly emerged as a matter of great interest, but with financial constraint on such type of research, much is still to be done.

Ethnic minority populations have become significant parts of the population in many countries, and similarly in many developing countries traditional foods form a major component of these populations' diet. Inequalities in health status are observed in these subpopulations compared with the general population. These inequalities, which could be due to socio-economic status, have highlighted the need for the expansion of nutrient data on ethnic and traditional foods. A limited budget is mostly all that is available for the analysis of these foods, which is one of the main reasons why there are limited data available. Often composition data for ethnic foods are derived or borrowed from other food composition tables or derived from recipes. Variation and modification in recipes and cooking practices between individuals are also some of the complications to consider when the composition of ethnic and traditional foods is investigated.

Bioactives in foods and their effect on health and well-being

Dietary constituents commonly found in foods with health-promoting or beneficial effects when ingested are part of the emerging evidence that drives consumers, researchers, and the food industry in their quest for validated information. It is generally recognized that a diet high in plant foods is associated with decreased incidence of certain diseases such as cancers and cardiovascular disease. One of the several plausible reasons for this decrease in incidence of disease is the antioxidant properties of plant-derived foods, which may prevent some of the processes involved in the development of cancer (protecting DNA from oxidative damage) and cardiovascular disease (inhibiting oxidative damage to low-density lipoprotein cholesterol). Apart from containing antioxidants, plant foods contain other compounds, not classified as traditional essential nutrients, but as bioactives. These bioactives, backed up with substantial evidence, may play a role in health promotion.

Thousands of plant bioactives have been identified and the major classes of plant bioactives are flavonoids and other phenolic compounds, carotenoids, plant sterols, glucosinolates, and other sulfur-containing compounds (http://www.eurofir.net). The USDA has prepared several Special Interest databases on flavonoids, proanthocyanidins, isoflavones, and ORAC (antioxidant powers assayed by oxygen radical absorption capacity assay). The ORAC database contains values for total phenols also.

Nutrition and health claims

Focusing on the relationship between diet and health, consumers are demanding more information on the food they purchase and consume. Not only has there been an increase in demand for nutrition information, but the increased prevalence of non-communicable diseases such as cardiovascular disease and diabetes mellitus, as a consequence of obesity, has led to increase in the need for nutrition communication and guidance in making healthy food choices. Food labeling has become an important communicator to the consumer, with the provision that it is based on the truth and not misleading. The Codex Alimentarius Commission (http://www.codexalimentarius. net) aims to strengthen local and regional efforts towards harmonizing and simplifying the process of making a nutritional or health claim.

Towards this end they proposed the following areas for further development:

- labeling to allow consumers to be better informed about the benefits and content of foods
- measures to minimize the impact of marketing on unhealthy dietary patterns

- more detailed information about healthy consumption patterns including steps to increase the consumption of fruits and vegetables
- production and processing standards regarding the nutritional quality and safety of products.

Nutrition and health claims are used to present products as having an additional nutritional or health benefit. In most cases, consumers perceive products carrying certain claims to be better for their health and well-being. Nutrient profiling is the first step towards a possible health claim. At present, different systems for the setting of nutrient profiling range from a simple algorithm to a scientifically complicated approach. It is difficult to develop a single system that reflects both the nutrition contribution of a food or food group to the diet and the effect of the matrix on nutrient bioavailability. This discussion is continuing.

Acknowledgement

With grateful appreciation of the outstanding work of Joanne Holden (1946–2014), formerly of the Nutrient Data Laboratory, Maryland, USA. We would like to acknowledge Clive West (1939 - 2004), formerly from Wageningen University, Netherlands, for his high-quality research contributions.

Further reading

Brussard, J.H., Löwik, M.R.H., Steingrímsdóttir, L. *et al.* (2002). European food consumption survey method - conclusions and recommendations. *European Journal of Clinical Nutrition* **56** (Suppl. 2): S89–S94.

Food and Agriculture Organization of the United Nations (2008). *Expert Consultation on Nutrition Indicators for Biodiversity 1.* Rome: *Food Composition.*

Greenfield, H. and Southgate, D.A.T. (2003). *Food Composition Data. Production. Management and Use.* Rome: Food and Agriculture Organization of the United Nations.

Greenfield, H. (1990). Uses and abuses of food composition data. *Food Australia* **42** (8), (Suppl.).

Gry, S. and Holden, J. (1994). Sampling strategies to assure representative values in food composition data. *Food. Nutrition and Agriculture* **12**: 12–20.

Ireland, J., Van Erp-Baart, A.M.J., Charrondière, U.R. *et al.* (2002). Selection of food classification system and food composition database for future food consumption surveys. *European Journal of Clinical Nutrition* **56** (Suppl. 2): S33–S45.

Klensin, J.C. (1992). *INFOODS Food Composition Data Interchange Handbook.* Tokyo: United Nations *University* Press.

Rand, W.M., Pennington, J.A.T., Murphy, S.P. *et al.* (1991). *Compiling Data for Food Composition Data Bases.* Tokyo: United Nations University Press.

Southgate, D.A.T. (2000). Food composition tables and nutritional databases. In: *Human Nutrition and Dietetics, 10e* (ed. J.S. Garrow, W.P.T. James, A. Ralph), 303–310. Edinburgh: Churchill Livingstone.

Truswell, A.S., Bateson, D.J., Madafiglio, K.C. *et al.* (1991). INFOODS guidelines for describing foods: a systematic approach to describing foods to facilitate international exchange of food composition data. *Journal of Food Composition and Analysis 1991* **4**: 18–38.

Verger, P., Ireland, J., Møller, A. *et al.* (2002). Improvement of the comparability of dietary intake assessments using currently available individual food consumption surveys. *European Journal of Clinical Nutrition* **56** (Suppl. 2): S18–S24.

Websites

Codex Alimentarius Commission: http://www.codexalimentarius.net

European Food Safety Authority: http://www.efsa.europa.eu

Eurocode2: http://www.eurofir.org/eurocode

EuroFIR: http://www.eurofir.net

Food and Agriculture Organization of the United Nations: http://www.fao.org

INFOODS: United Nations University of International Food Data Systems Project: http://www.fao.org/infoods/directory

LanguaL: http://www.langual.org

United States Department of Agriculture National Nutrient Databank: http://www.ars.usda.gov/nutrientdata

4 Dietary Reference Standards

Kate M. Younger

Key messages

- This chapter discusses the development of terminology and the change in conceptual approaches to setting nutrient recommendations from adequate to optimum nutrition.
- The interpretation and uses of dietary recommendations are discussed.
- The chapter describes how reference values can be used to assess the adequacy of the nutrient intakes of population groups.
- The methods used to determine requirements are discussed. These include depletion–repletion studies, isotope studies, balance studies, factorial methods, measurement of nutrient levels in biological tissues, biochemical and biological markers, and animal experiments.

4.1 Introduction

The first attempt to set standards for nutrient intakes was by the Food and Nutrition Board of the National Research Council of the USA in 1941, which published recommended dietary allowances (RDAs) in 1943 to "provide standards to serve as a goal for good nutrition." The first UK RDAs followed in 1950, published by the British Medical Association, and many other countries and international agencies now publish dietary standards that are intended to allow the adequacy of the nutrient intake of groups or populations to be assessed by comparison with the standards.

As the amount known about human requirements and nutrient functions has increased, so too has the size of the documents describing the recommendations, from a mere six pages dealing with 10 nutrients in 1943, to the comprehensive UK dietary reference values (DRVs) from COMA published in 1991, closely followed by EC recommendations published in 1993, to the series of weighty books, each dealing with only a few of more than 30 nutrients, published by the Institute of Medicine (IOM, now the National Academy of Medicine) in the USA, and the series of detailed Scientific Opinions on single nutrients published by the European Food Safety Authority (EFSA). Furthermore, continuing research and the development of more informed interpretations of the expanding body of data available necessitate the regular revision and updating of the recommendations. Thus, the "standards" of the past become obsolete as they are replaced by new figures based on new data or new interpretations of existing data, for example the updates published by the UK Scientific Advisory on Nutrition (SACN) on energy requirements (2011), carbohydrates (2015) and vitamin D requirements (2016).

4.2 Terminology and conceptual approaches to setting nutrient recommendations

From the time of their first issue in the 1940s and throughout the next 50 years, the concepts

Introduction to Human Nutrition, Third Edition. Edited on behalf of The Nutrition Society by Susan A. Lanham-New, Thomas R. Hill, Alison M. Gallagher and Hester H. Vorster.

Companion website: www.wiley.com/go/lanham-new/humannutrition

and terminology of RDAs remained unchanged. The basis on which these RDAs were built was the statistical distribution of individual requirements to prevent deficiency criteria for the target nutrient. The peak of the curve of the Gaussian distributions of such requirements is the "average requirement," with half the population having requirements above this value and the other half having lower requirements. The RDA was taken to be a point on that distribution that was equal to the mean or "average requirements" plus two standard deviations (SDs) (Figure 4.1). By setting the recommendation close to the upper end of the distribution of individual requirements, the needs of most of the population would be met. If the standards were set to meet the apparent needs of almost everyone, the resultant value would be so high as to be unattainable at population level. If the standards were set at the point of the average of all individual requirements, then half the population would have requirements in excess of the standard. In a normal distribution, some 2.5% of points lie at the upper and lower tails outside that range of the mean plus or minus two SDs.

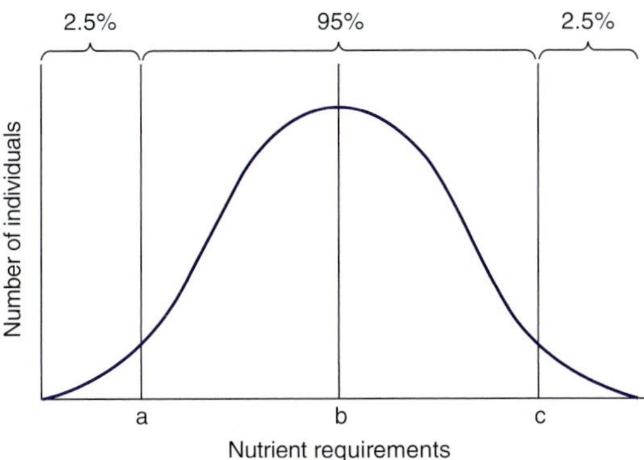

Figure 4.1 Frequency distribution of individual requirements for a nutrient. (a) The mean minus a notional two standard deviations (SDs); intakes below this will be inadequate for nearly all of the population. (b) The mean; the midpoint of the population's requirement. (c) The mean plus a notional two SDs; the intake that is adequate for nearly all of the population. Note that, in practice, because insufficient data exist to establish reliable means and SDs for many nutrient requirements, the reference intake describing the points (a) and (c) on the curve are generally set, in the case of (a), at the level that is judged to prevent the appearance of signs of deficiency (biochemical or clinical) and, in the case of (c), at the level above which all individuals appear to be adequately supplied. Thus, it is unlikely that even 2.5% of the population would not achieve adequacy at intake level (c).

Thus, by setting the RDA to this point of the mean plus two SDs, we are setting the standard for 97.5% of the population. The consumption of most nutrients at levels somewhat greater than actually required is generally not harmful; hence, setting recommendations at the population average requirement plus a notional two SDs is logical if the aim is to describe an intake that is adequate for almost everyone. However, this is spectacularly inappropriate in the case of recommendations for energy intake, since even relatively small imbalances in energy intake over expenditure will lead, over time, to overweight and ultimately obesity, an increasing problem in most populations. Recommendations for energy intake are therefore given only as the estimated population average requirement (EAR).

Thus, for almost half a century, these were the terms used and the underlying conceptual approaches. However, since the 1980s, changes have occurred in both of these areas.

Changes in terminology

Two basic changes occurred with regard to terminology. The first was that new terms were introduced so that the adequacy of diets could be evaluated from several perspectives. These "umbrella" terms include the full set of nutrient recommendations (as described by the points (b) and (c), and sometimes (a), in Fig 4.1); for example the UK and then EFSA adopted the "umbrella" term dietary reference values (DRV), the USA the term dietary reference intakes (DRIs) and Australia and New Zealand the term nutrient reference values (NRVs).The second change was that the term "recommended dietary allowance" was often replaced, in order to re-emphasise some of the basic concepts underlying the term RDA. "Recommended" has a prescriptive air about it and there were concerns that consumers might see this as something that had to be met daily and met precisely. The term "allowance" reinforces the perception of a prescriptive approach. Thus, the UK adopted the term "reference nutrient intake" (RNI), whilst the EU introduced the term "population reference intake" (PRI), whereas Australia and New Zealand use the term "recommended dietary intake" (RDI). All are precisely equivalent to the original concept of the RDA, a term still used in many countries, including the US and Canada.

Several new terms were introduced. The minimum requirement represents the average requirement minus two SDs (point (a) in Figure 4.1). A definition describing this point is given in Figure 4.1 along with the various terms used to define this point (Box 4.1). The concept of an upper safe limit of intake has gained importance in view of the increased opportunity for people to consume high levels of nutrients from fortified foods or supplements. The US DRIs set "tolerable upper intake" levels (ULs) that are judged to be the highest average daily intake level of a nutrient that is likely to pose no risk of adverse health effects in almost all individuals in a group. The current European and UK recommendations also address this concern in the case of those nutrients for which toxic levels have been reported. Where there is insufficient evidence to set precise recommendations, the term "adequate intake" (AI) may be used (EFSA and USA). The World Health Organization/Food and Agriculture Organisation (WHO/FAO) revises and publishes nutrient requirements and dietary guidelines for groups of nutrients at different times; these may include ULs, also sometimes "protective nutrient intakes" for some micronutrients where higher amounts may be protective against a specified health or nutritional risk (e.g., in the case of vitamin C to enhance iron absoption).

The terms used by different recommending bodies to describe the various points on the

Box 4.1 Terms used to describe points a, b, and c on the frequency distribution (shown in Figure 4.1)

	a	b	c
US Food and Nutrition Board, National Academy of Sciences, National Research Council **Recommended dietary allowances (RDA)** (1989)			Recommended dietary allowance (**RDA**)
British Committee on Medical Aspects of Food Policy (COMA) now the Scientific Advisory Committee on Nutrition (SACN) **Dietary reference values (DRV)** (1991)	Lower reference nutrient intake (**LRNI**)	Estimated average requirement (**EAR**)	Reference nutrient intake (**RNI**)
European Communities Scientific Committee for Food **Population reference intakes (PRI)** (1993)	Lowest threshold intake (**LTI**)	Average requirement (**AR**)	Population reference intake (**PRI**)
US Food and Nutrition Board, Institute of Medicine, National Academies of Health, Canada now the National Academy of Medicine **Dietary reference intakes (DRI)** (1997–2010)		Estimated average requirement (**EAR**)	Recommended dietary allowance (**RDA**)
National Health and Medical Research Council (NHMRC), Australia and New Zealand **Nutrient reference values (NRV)** (2006)		Estimated average requirement (**EAR**)	Recommended dietary intake (**RNI**)
United Nations University (UNU) **Nutrient intake values (NIV)** (2007)		Average nutrient requirement (**ANR**)	Individual nutrient level (**INL**$_x$ where x is the percentage of the population whose needs are met by the recommendation; in this case **INL**$_{98}$ would cover the needs of 98% of the population)
European Food Safety Authority (EFSA) **Dietary reference values (DRV)** (2010–2019)	Lower threshold intake (**LTI**)	Average requirement (**AR**)	Population reference intake (**PRI**)
World Health Organization/Food and Agriculture Organization (WHO/FAO) **Recommended Nutrient Requirements**		Estimated average requirement (**EAR**) and Average nutrient requirement (**ANR**)	Recommended dietary allowance (**RDA**) and recommended nutrient intake (**RNI**)

Box 4.2 Additional terms used

US recommended daily allowance (**RDA**) (1989)	Safe intake and adequate intake
British dietary reference value (**DRV**) (1991)	Safe and adequate intake Individual minimum and maximum and population average intakes
European population reference intake (**PRI**) (1993)	Acceptable range of intakes
World Health Organization (1974–1996)	Recommended intake
WHO/FAO (1996)	Basal, normative, and maximum population requirement ranges, mean intake goals Acceptable macronutrient distribution range (**AMDR**) Adequate intake (**AI**) Tolerable upper limit (**UL**)
US dietary reference intake (**DRI**) (1997–2010)	Acceptable macronutrient distribution range (**AMDR**) Adequate intake (**AI**) Tolerable upper intake level (**UL**)
Australia and New Zealand National Health and Medical Research Council (**NRV**) (2006)	Acceptable macronutrient distribution range (**AMDR**) Suggested dietary target (**SDT**) Upper level of intake (**UL**)
United Nations University (**NIV**) (2007)	Adequate macronutrient distribution range (AMDR) Upper nutrient level (**UNL**)
European dietary reference value (**DRV**) (2010)	Reference intake ranges for macronutrients (**RI**) Adequate intakes (**AI**) Tolerable upper intake level (**UL**)

distribution of individual requirements for a nutrient are given in Box 4.2, while precise definitions may be found in the relevant publications referred to.

In 2007, the United Nations University (UNU) published a suggested harmonised approach and methodologies for developing nutrient recommendations, together with proposed terminology (Boxes 4.1 and 4.2). Their preferred term, nutrient intake value (NIV), refers to dietary intake recommendations based on research data; the term "nutrient" was chosen in order to distinguish these from dietary components such as cereals, and the term "value" is intended to emphasise the potential usefulness for both assessing dietary adequacy (and hence dietary planning) and policy-making. The individual nutrient level (INL_x) is flexible, in that x refers to the chosen percentile of the population for whom this intake is sufficient; for example 98% (mean or median requirement + two SDs), written as INL_{98}, but it could be set lower in the case of certain nutrients.

Changes in conceptual approach

When a committee sits to make a recommendation for a standard in relation to nutrient intakes, it begins with a distribution of requirements. In the past, although the choice of criteria for requirement might vary between committees, the orientation was always the same: requirements were set at a level that should prevent deficiency symptoms. More recently, the concern for health promotion through diet has led to the introduction of the concept of optimal nutrition, in which the optimal intake of a nutrient could be defined as that intake that maximises physiological and mental function and minimises the development of degenerative diseases. It should be borne in mind that, although this may appear simple enough to define in the case of single nutrients, things clearly become more complex when considering all nutrients together, in all possible physiological situations. Genetic variability may also, increasingly, be taken into account; for example, the requirement for folate of those carrying certain variants of the *MTHFR* gene (for example in North America, Europe and Australia approximately 8-20% of the population is homozygous for *MTHFR* C677T) might, arguably, need to be set higher than for the rest of the population.

It is now recognised that there are several levels for considering the concept of optimal nutrition, i.e., the level that:

- prevents deficiency symptoms, traditionally used to establish reference nutrient intakes
- optimises body stores of a nutrient
- optimises some biochemical or physiological function
- minimises a risk factor for some chronic disease
- minimises the incidence of a disease.

In the USA, the reference value for calcium is based on optimising bone calcium levels, which is a move away from the traditional approach of focusing on preventing deficiency symptoms.

An example of attempts to set the reference standard for optimising a biochemical function is a level of folic acid that would minimise the plasma levels of homocysteine, a potential risk factor for cardiovascular disease. Another might be the level of zinc to optimise cell-mediated immunity. An example of a possible reference standard to optimise a risk factor for a disease is the level of sodium that would minimise hypertension or the level of n-3 polyunsaturated fatty acids (PUFAs) to lower plasma triacylglycerols (TAGs). The amount of folic acid to minimise the population burden of neural tube defect would be an example of a reference value to minimise the incidence of a disease. At present, there is much debate as to the best approach to choosing criteria for setting reference standards for minerals and vitamins, and this is an area that is likely to continue to court controversy. An important point to note in this respect is that, while minimising frank deficiency symptoms of micronutrients is an acute issue in many developing countries, any evolution of our concepts of desirable or optimal nutrient requirements must lead to a revision of the estimate of the numbers of those with inadequate nutrition.

4.3 Interpretation and uses of dietary recommendations

When using dietary recommendations, several important points need to be considered.

The nutrient levels recommended are per person per day. However, in practice this will usually be achieved as an average over a period of time (days, weeks, or months) owing to daily fluctuations in the diet. As stated above, the setting of a range of dietary recommendations should encourage appropriate interpretation of dietary intake data, rather than the inappropriate assumption that the value identified to meet the needs of practically all healthy people is a minimum requirement for individuals. If an individual's nutrient intake can be averaged over a sufficient period then this improves the validity of the comparison with dietary recommendations. However, in the case of energy intakes, such a comparison is still inappropriate: dietary reference values for energy (defined as the EAR) are intended only for use with groups, and it is more useful to compare an individual's energy intake with some measure or calculation of their expenditure in order to assess adequacy.

In the case of a group, the assumption can be made that the quality of the diet can be averaged across the group at a given time-point, and therefore that apparently healthy individuals within a group may compensate for a relative deficiency on one day by a relative excess on another. It should also be remembered that allowances may need to be made for body size, activity level, and perhaps other characteristics of the individual or group under consideration, since the recommended intakes are designed for "reference" populations.

Another assumption made when setting recommendations for a particular nutrient is that the intake of all other nutrients is adequate, which in an apparently healthy population eating a varied diet is probably reasonable.

Recommendations are not intended to address the needs of people who are not healthy: no allowance is made for altered nutrient requirements due to illness or injury. For example, patients confined to bed may require less energy owing to inactivity, and may require higher micronutrient intakes because of an illness causing malabsorption by the gut. Certain nutrients may also be used as therapeutic agents, for example n-3 fatty acids can have anti-inflammatory effects. These clinical aspects are considered elsewhere in these texts.

One complication arising in the formulation of dietary recommendations is caused by the fact that various groups of people within a population may have different nutrient requirements. Therefore, the population is divided into subgroups: children and adults by age bands, and by gender. For women, allowances are also made for pregnancy and lactation.

Infants are generally recommended to be exclusively breast-fed for the first six months of life (WHO, 2001). This poses a problem for the bodies setting the dietary recommendations, which have to set standards for those infants who are not breast-fed. The dietary recommendations for formula-fed infants are based on the energy and nutrients supplied in breast milk, but, because the bioavailability of some nutrients is lower in formula than in breast milk, the amounts stated appear higher than those that might be expected to be achieved by breast-feeding. This should not therefore be interpreted as an inadequacy on the part of human (breast) milk compared with formula milks, but rather the reverse.

The dietary recommendations for infants post-weaning and for children and adolescents are generally based on less robust scientific evidence than those for adults, for whom much more good information is available. In the absence of reliable data, values for children are usually derived by extrapolation from those of young adults. The calculation of nutrient requirements is generally based on energy expenditure because metabolic requirements for energy probably go hand in hand with those for nutrients in growing children. In the case of infants post-weaning on mixed diets, values are obtained by interpolation between values known for infants younger than six months and those calculated for toddlers aged one to three years. Thus, the dietary recommendations for children and adolescents need to be approached with some caution, being more suitable for planning and labeling purposes than as a description of actual needs.

Finally, assessment of the dietary adequacy of people at the other end of the population age range is made difficult by the lack of data on healthy elderly people. One of the normal characteristics of aging is that various body functions deteriorate to some extent, and disease and illness become more common as people age. Until more data are available, the assumption is made that, except for energy and a few nutrients, the requirements of the elderly (usually defined as those over 65 years old) are no different from those of younger adults.

Bearing the above points in mind, dietary recommendations can be useful at various levels.

- Governments and non-government organisations (NGOs) use dietary recommendations to identify the energy and nutrient requirements of populations and hence allow informed decisions on food policy. This could include the provision of food aid or supplements (or rationing) when the diet is inadequate, fortification of foods, providing appropriate nutrition education, introducing legislation concerning the food supply, influencing the import and export of food, subsidies on certain foods or for producers of food, and so on.
- The food industry requires this information in the development and marketing of products. The industry is aware of consumers' increasing interest in the nutritional quality of the food that they buy, and has responded by providing foods to address particular perceived needs, and more informative food labels.
- Researchers and the health professions need to assess the nutritional adequacy of the diets of groups (or, cautiously, of individuals) by comparing dietary intake survey data with the dietary reference values (see below). Once the limitations of the dietary assessment data have been taken into account (see Chapter 2), this information can be used to attempt to improve people's nutrient intakes by bringing them more into line with the dietary recommendations. The formulation of dietary advice or guidelines depends on an appreciation of the existing situation: the solution can only be framed once the problem is characterised.
- Institutions and caterers use dietary recommendations to assess the requirements of groups and devise nutritionally adequate menus. This is a great deal more easily said than done, mainly because of the financial constraints involved and, often, the food preferences of the population being catered for.
- The public needs this information to help in the interpretation of nutrition information on food labels that may describe nutrient content in both absolute terms (g, mg, etc.) and as a percentage of the recommended intake (% reference intake, RI in Europe (previously guideline daily amount, GDA); or, in the US, % Daily Value) for that nutrient (usually per 100 g or per "serving"). It is thought that the latter is more meaningful to consumers, even though the concepts involved in setting the dietary recommendations are rather complex (making it difficult to judge which level of recommendation should be used as the standard) and they can be open to misinterpretation (see above). Unless consumers are provided with nutrition information in the most appropriate form on food labels, they cannot make informed choices as to what foods to buy and eat to meet their own perceived needs. At the very least, consumers should be able to compare products to get their money's worth.

4.4 The use of reference values to assess the adequacy of the nutrient intakes of population groups

Ideally, this is accomplished by discovering the distribution of intakes of a nutrient in the population group (e.g., by carrying out a dietary survey), and comparing these intakes with the distribution of requirements for that nutrient within the same population. In practice, reliable data with which to plot the second of these distributions have rarely been collected, and therefore what must be used is an estimation of the average requirement together with an estimation of the variance in that requirement, i.e., the standard deviation (based on whatever scientific evidence is available), that is used to plot the population distribution of requirements as shown in Figure 4.1.

When considering how to assess the adequacy of nutrient intakes of populations it is important to compare the intakes with the most appropriate level of requirement as defined in dietary recommendations.

It is not useful to compare usual intakes with the RDA/PRI/RNI (i.e., the average requirement plus a notional two SDs) at the population level since this approach leads to overestimates of the prevalence of inadequacy; it may, however, be justified to compare an individual's intake with the RDA/PRI/RNI. Furthermore, this approach might be seen to encourage the consumption of higher intakes, which could be toxic in the case of certain nutrients (for example retinol, Vitamin D).

Comparison of the population intake with the average requirement (AR or estimated average requirement, EAR) is now considered to be the best estimation of dietary adequacy; if the average intake is less than the average requirement, then it is clear that there could be a problem of inadequacy in that population. Accordingly, using the average requirement as a cut-off point, the proportion of individuals in the group whose usual intakes are not meeting their requirements can be calculated, allowing the problem to be quantified. However, this approach cannot be used in the case of energy since energy intakes and requirements are highly correlated (the effects of an imbalance being quickly obvious to the individual).

The lowest defined intake level (LTI/LRNI, i.e., the average requirement minus a notional two SDs) is not regarded as being useful in the context of assessing the adequacy of population nutrient intakes. This is because it would identify only those individuals who were almost certainly not meeting their requirement, and by the same token would omit to include many in the population who would be at appreciable risk of nutrient inadequacy (in other words, those whose intake was below the average requirement).

Finally, the tolerable upper levels of intake defined for certain nutrients (for example iodine, fluoride) can also be used as cut-off points to identify those individuals at risk of consuming toxic levels of a nutrient.

4.5 Methods used to determine requirements and set dietary recommendations

In order to derive the most accurate and appropriate dietary recommendations, committees of experts are established that look at the scientific evidence and use their judgment to decide which nutrients to consider and then, for each nutrient, make decisions in respect of the:

- criterion by which to define adequacy
- estimation of the average amount required to meet that criterion of adequacy
- estimated standard deviation of requirement in the population under consideration (i.e., the shape of the frequency distribution over the range of requirements: broad, narrow, skewed, etc.).

The problem of different committees identifying different criteria of adequacy is illustrated by vitamin C (ascorbic acid). Experimental evidence (the Sheffield and Iowa studies) has shown that an intake of approximately 10 mg/day is required to prevent the deficiency disease scurvy in adult men. At intakes below 30 mg/day, serum levels are negligible, rising steeply with intakes of between 30 and 70 mg/day, after which they begin to plateau (and urinary excretion of the unmetabolised vitamin increases). The question facing the committees drafting dietary reference values is whether to choose a level of intake that allows some storage of the vitamin in the body pool (e.g., UK EAR 25 mg/day for adults) or one that more nearly maximises plasma and body pool levels (e.g., US EAR 60 and 75 mg/day for women and men, respectively). Similarly, variations in calcium recommendations exist because some committees choose to use zero calcium balance as the criterion of adequacy, while others use maximum skeletal calcium reserves.

In some cases, one recommending body will include a nutrient among its dietary recommendations while others will not; for example, vitamin E, the requirement for which depends directly on the dietary intake and tissue levels of PUFAs, which are highly skewed. The vitamin E requirement corresponding to the highest levels of PUFA intake would be much higher than that needed by those with much lower (but adequate) intakes. To set the high value as the recommendation might suggest to those with lower polyunsaturate intakes that they should increase their intake of vitamin E (unnecessarily). Thus, in Britain and Europe, only "safe" and "adequate" intakes have been set respectively, based on actual intakes in healthy populations. In contrast, the US set both an EAR of 12 mg/day and an RDA of 15 mg/day for adults as α-tocopherol, based on induced vitamin E deficiency studies in humans and measures of lipid peroxidation.

There are some examples of dietary components that have not traditionally been regarded as essential nutrients having recommendations set for them, as in the case of choline. The US (and subsequently EFSA) defined adequate intakes for choline (US AI of 450 and 550 mg/day for women and men, respectively; EFSA AI of 400 mg/day for adults) on the basis that endogenous synthesis of this compound is not always adequate to meet the demand for it (for the synthesis of acetylcholine, phospholipids, and betaine). Dietary intake data for choline and the scientific evidence for inadequacy are limited; thus, dose–response studies would need to be undertaken before an average requirement could be derived. It is probable that further dietary components will be included in dietary recommendations as research data accumulate. Potential candidates include the flavonoids and some other antioxidant compounds.

4.6 Methods used to determine requirements

Depletion-repletion studies

This is the most direct method and involves removing the nutrient from the diet, observing the symptoms of deficiency, and then adding back the nutrient until the symptoms are cured or prevented. Difficulties with this approach are as follows. First, that the experiment may need to continue for several years owing to the presence of body stores of the nutrient, and often requires a very limited and therefore boring dietary regimen. Second, unpredicted long-term adverse consequences may result. Third, such experiments are not ethical in vulnerable groups such as children (often the most relevant for study). In some cases, epidemiological data may be available; for example, the deficiency disease beriberi occurs in populations whose average thiamin intake falls below 0.2 mg/4.2 MJ (1000 kcal).

Isotope studies

This approach makes use of a known amount of the labelled nutrient (containing a radioactive or heavy isotope), which is assumed to disperse evenly in the body pool, allowing the estimation of the total pool size by dilution of the isotope in samples of, for instance, plasma or urine (i.e., if the body pool is large, then the dilution will be greater than if the body pool is small). Specific activity, that is radioactivity per unit weight of the nutrient in the samples, can be used to calculate pool size as long as the total dose administered is known. The rate of loss can then be monitored by taking serial samples, allowing calculation of the depletion rate. In the case of vitamin C, the average body pool size of a healthy male was found to be 1500 mg, which, on a vitamin C-free diet, depleted at a rate of approximately 3% (of the body pool) per day. This fractional catabolic rate was independent of body pool size, and symptoms of scurvy appeared when the body pool fell below 300 mg. The estimated replacement intake needed to maintain the body pool above 300 mg was therefore 3% of 300 mg, i.e., 9 mg (similar to the 10 mg found to be needed to prevent scurvy in the earlier Sheffield experiment).

Balance studies

These rely on the assumption that, in healthy individuals of stable body weight, the body pool of some nutrients (e.g., nitrogen, calcium and sodium) remains constant. Compensation mechanisms equalise the intake and output of the nutrient over a wide range of intakes, thereby maintaining the body pool. Thus, day-to-day variations of intake are compensated for by changes in either the rate of absorption in the gut (generally in the case of those nutrients of which the uptake is regulated) or the rate of excretion in the urine (in the case of very soluble nutrients) or faeces, or both. However, there comes a point beyond which balance cannot be maintained; therefore, it can be proposed that the minimum intake of a nutrient at which balance can be maintained is the subject's minimum required intake of that nutrient. However, this approach would need to be extended over time to investigate possible adaptive responses to reduced intakes, e.g., absorption efficiency could eventually be increased. In the case of calcium, the European consensus (EFSA, 2015) is that the mean value at which intake equals excretion is 715 mg/day (taking into account efficiency of absorption in the gut), and adding an allowance for dermal losses of calcium of 40 mg/day gives an AR of 750 mg/day for adults, and a PRI of 950 mg/day, whereas the 2011 US EAR for adults is 800 mg/day and the RDA is 1000 mg/day.

Factorial methods

These are predictions, rather than measurements, of the requirements of groups or individuals, taking into account a number of measured variables (factors, hence "factorial") and making assumptions where measurements cannot be made. For example, the increased requirements during growth, pregnancy, or lactation are calculated by this method; this approach is necessitated by the lack of experimental data in these physiological situations owing to ethical problems. The rationale is that the rate of accumulation of nutrients can be calculated and hence the amount required in the diet to allow that accumulation can be predicted. In the case of pregnancy, the requirement is estimated to be the amount of the nutrient needed to achieve balance when not pregnant plus the amount accumulated daily during the pregnancy, all multiplied by a factor accounting for the efficiency of absorption and assimilation (e.g., 30% for calcium). For lactation, the calculation for energy is based on the amount in the milk secreted daily, which is increased by a factor accounting for the efficiency of conversion from dietary energy to milk energy (estimated to be 95%), from which total is subtracted an allowance for the contribution from the extra fat stores laid down during pregnancy, which it is desirable to reduce in this way. The difficulty with this approach is that the theoretical predictions do not necessarily take account of physiological adaptations (e.g., increased efficiency of absorption in the gut) that may reduce the predicted requirement. This would apply particularly in the case of pregnancy, as shown by the ability of women to produce normal babies even in times of food shortage.

Measurement of nutrient levels in biological tissues

Some nutrient requirements can be defined according to the intakes needed to maintain a certain level of the nutrient in blood or tissue. For many water-soluble nutrients, such as vitamin C, blood levels reflect recent dietary intake, and the vitamin is not generally measurable in plasma at intakes less than about 40 mg/day. This level of intake has therefore been chosen as the basis for the reference in some countries such as the 1991 UK DRVs. This approach is not, however, suitable for those nutrients of which the plasma concentration is homeostatically regulated, such as calcium. In the case of the fat-soluble vitamin retinol, the dietary intake required to maintain a liver concentration of 20 μg/g has been used as the basis of the reference intake. To do this, the body pool size needed to be estimated; assumptions were made as to the proportion of body weight represented by the liver (3%) and the proportion of the body pool of retinol contained in the liver (90%). The fractional catabolic rate has been measured as 0.5% of the body pool per day, so this would be the amount needing to be replaced daily. The efficiency of conversion of dietary vitamin A to stored retinol was taken to be 50% (measured range 40–90%), giving an EAR of around 500 μg/day for a 74 kg man.

Biochemical markers

In many respects, biochemical markers represent the most satisfactory measure of nutrient adequacy since they are specific to the nutrient in question, are sensitive enough to identify subclinical deficiencies, and may be measured precisely and accurately. However, such markers are available at present for only a few nutrients, mostly vitamins. One well-established example of a biochemical marker is the erythrocyte glutathione reductase activation test for riboflavin status. Erythrocytes are a useful cell to use for enzyme assays since they are easily obtainable and have a known life-span in the circulation (average 120 days), aiding the interpretation of results. Glutathione reductase depends on riboflavin and, when activity is measured in both the presence and absence of excess riboflavin, the ratio of the two activities (the erythrocyte glutathione reductase activation coefficient, EGRAC) reflects riboflavin status: if perfectly sufficient, the ratio would be 1.0, whereas deficiency gives values greater than 1.0.

Biological markers

These are measures of some biological function that is directly dependent on the nutrient of interest; again, not always easy to find, hence the recent suggestion that some functional indices be considered that are not necessarily directly dependent on the nutrient. Iron status is assessed according to a battery of biological markers, including plasma ferritin (which reflects body iron stores), serum transferrin saturation (the amount of plasma transferrin in relation to the amount of iron transported by it is reduced in deficiency), plasma-soluble transferrin receptor (an index of tissue iron status), and the more traditional tests such as blood hemoglobin (now considered to be a rather insensitive and unreliable measure of iron status since it indicates only frank anemia, and also changes as a normal response to altered physiological states such as pregnancy).

Vitamin K status is assessed by measuring prothrombin time (the length of time taken by blood to clot), which is increased when vitamin K levels fall since the synthesis of prothrombin in the liver depends on vitamin K as a cofactor. This test is clinically useful in patients requiring anticoagulant therapy (e.g., using warfarin, which blocks the effect of vitamin K), in whom the drug dosage must be closely monitored.

Animal experiments

These are of limited use in defining human nutrient requirements because of species differences (e.g., rats can synthesise vitamin C, so it is not a "vitamin" for them), differences in metabolic body size (i.e., the proportions of metabolically active tissue, such as muscle, and less active tissue, such as adipose tissue, gut contents), and differences in growth rates (young animals generally grow far more rapidly than humans, e.g., cattle reach adult size in about one year). However, animals have provided much of the information on the identification of the essential nutrients, and their physiological and biochemical functions. Furthermore, animals can be used in experiments that would not be possible in humans, such as lifelong modifications in nutrient intake; it is merely the setting of human requirements for which they are inappropriate.

4.7 Perspectives on the future

As the amount known about human requirements and nutrient functions increases, so too will the complexity of dietary recommendations. It is probable that further dietary components will be included in dietary recommendations as research data accumulate. Potential candidates include the flavonoids and some other antioxidant compounds. New techniques may be implemented for measuring nutrient status, including molecular methods (e.g., "omics"), or functional indices (e.g., immune function, arterial compliance). Furthermore, continuing research and the development of more informed interpretations of the expanding body of data available necessitate the regular revision and updating of the recommendations. The size of the task now means that most revised recommendations are now reviewed and published for only one or a few nutrients at a time, usually every 10 to 15 years. Summary tables for all the nutrients may be produced when a cycle is complete, for example the EFSA summary report published in 2017.

Further reading

Committee on Medical Aspects of Food Policy (COMA) (1991). *Dietary Reference Values for Food Energy and Nutrients for the United Kingdom*. Report on Health and Social Subjects 41. London: HMSO.

EC Scientific Committee for Food Report (1993). *Nutrient and Energy Intakes for the European Community*. 31st Series. Director General, Industry, Luxembourg, available at; https://ec.europa.eu/food/sites/food/files/safety/docs/sci-com_scf_out89.pdf

European Food Safety Authority webpage *Dietary Reference Values and Dietary Guidelines - with links to updated DRVs* https://www.efsa.europa.eu/en/topics/topic/drv

European Food Safety Authority *Dietary Reference Values for Nutrients Summary Report*, 2017, available at: http://www.efsa.europa.eu/en/supporting/pub/e15121

European Food Safety Authority *Tolerable Upper Intake Levels for Vitamins and Minerals*, 2006, available at https://www.efsa.europa.eu/sites/default/files/assets/ndatolerableuil.pdf

Expert Group on Vitamins and Minerals. *Safe Upper Limits for Vitamins and Minerals*. Food Standards Agency, London, 2003, available at; https://cot.food.gov.uk/committee/committee-on-toxicity/cotreports/cotjointreps/evmreport

Food and Agriculture Organization website for FAO and joint FAO/WHO publications http://www.fao.org/ag/humannutrition/nutrition/63160/en/

Institute of Medicine *Dietary Reference Intakes* separate texts from 1997 - available at https://ods.od.nih.gov/Health_Information/Dietary_Reference_Intakes.aspx

Institute of Medicine of the National Academies *Dietary Reference Intakes: the essential guide to nutrient requirements*, JJ Otten, JP Hellwig, LD Meyers (Eds) The National Academies Press, Washington DC, 2006, available at https://www.nap.edu/catalog/11537/dietary-reference-intakes-the-essential-guide-to-nutrient-requirements

Institute of Medicine Dietary reference intakes for calcium and vitamin D, 2011, available at https://www.nap.edu/catalog/13050/dietary-reference-intakes-for-calcium-and-vitamin-d

National Health and Medical Research Council. *Nutrient Reference Values for Australia and New Zealand*, available at https://www.nrv.gov.au/introduction

National Research Council, Food and Nutrition Board, Commission on Life Sciences. *Recommended Dietary Allowances*, 10th edn. National Academy Press, Washington, DC, 1989.

Public Health England. *Government Dietary Recommendations* PHE gateway number 2016202 pdf, 2016 available at https://www.gov.uk/government/uploads/system/uploads/attachment_data/file/547050/government__dietary_recommendations.pdf

Scientific Advisory Committee on Nutrition (SACN) reports and position statements on Vitamin D, Carbohydrates, Energy,etc available at: https://www.gov.uk/government/collections/sacn-reports-and-position-statements

United Nations University. International harmonisation of approaches for developing nutrient-based dietary standards. In: King JC, Garza, C, eds. *Food and Nutrition Bulletin*, vol. 28, no. 1 (supplement). International Nutrition Foundation for The United Nations University, Tokyo, 2007. Available online at http://archive.unu.edu/unupress/food/FNBv28n1_Suppl1_final.pdf

World Health Organization website for WHO and joint FAO/WHO publications *Nutrient Requirements and Dietary Guidelines* http://www.who.int/nutrition/publications/nutrient/en/

World Health Organization. *Global Strategy for Infant and Young Child Feeding: the Optimal Duration of Exclusive Breastfeeding*. World Health Organization, Geneva. 2001. Available online at http://apps.who.int/iris/handle/10665/78801

5
Body Composition

Anja Bosy-Westphal, Paul Deurenberg, and Manfred James Müller

Key messages

- Body composition data are used to evaluate health risk associated with overweight, malnutrition, and specific disease states (e.g., obesity, sarcopenia, cachexia), growth and development, to characterise changes in energy balance and water homeostasis, to adjust body mass-related metabolic functions (e.g., energy expenditure) and to indirectly calculate energy intake from changes in energy stores.
- Human body composition is studied at atomic, molecular, cellular, tissue, and anatomical levels. The levels are interrelated.
- Several techniques are available to measure body composition. The availability of methods depends on the target outcome parameter and is influenced by the required accuracy and precision of methods and techniques, the availability of suitable reference values, invasiveness, and cost.
- Interpretation of body composition data should take into account the limitations and underlying assumptions of the method used, the inter-relationships between individual body components as well as their functional correlates (e.g., resting energy expenditure).
- Body composition analysis (BCA) is a prerequisite for detailed phenotyping of individuals providing a sound basis for in depth biomedical research and clinical decision making.

5.1 Introduction

With progress in the development of analytical chemical methods in the twentieth century, scientists such as Mitchell, Widdowson, and Forbes performed the most important work of chemical analyses in adult cadavers during the 1940s and 1950s. Today, organ and tissue masses as well as the physical properties of the body can be studied *in vivo* using dual energy X-ray absorptiometry (DXA), dilution methods, densitometry and imaging technologies like Computer Tomography (CT) and Magnetic Resonance Imaging (MRI).

Application of body composition analysis

Besides anatomy, body composition analysis (BCA) applies concepts of molecular and cellular physiology, biochemistry and experimental approaches to understand the relationship between organ and tissue masses and their related functions. Information on body composition is required for normalisation or interpretation of body functions (e.g., energy expenditure, glucose turnover, and protein synthesis in relation to muscle mass and/or secretion of adipokines, inflammation, and insulin resistance in relation to fat mass (FM) and fat distribution).

Chronic diseases such as cancer and disorders associated with inflammation are characterised by tissue catabolism leading to weight loss and malnutrition-associated changes in body composition (e.g., a loss in skeletal muscle and FM). In obesity, BCA is indispensable for the diagnosis of both metabolic risks (related to visceral adipose tissue (VAT) and liver fat) and malnutrition that can manifest as sarcopenic obesity in frail elderly people or "hidden cachexia" in obese

Introduction to Human Nutrition, Third Edition. Edited on behalf of The Nutrition Society by Susan A. Lanham-New, Thomas R. Hill, Alison M. Gallagher and Hester H. Vorster.

Companion website: www.wiley.com/go/lanham-new/humannutrition

cancer patients. Other diseases (such as diseases of liver and kidneys) are related to abnormalities in total body water and the distribution of body water across the intracellular and extracellular space. Disturbances in hydration remain a particular challenge to BCA because many techniques require a normal hydration to give valid results.

BCA-data can also be used to reduce radiation exposure with (CT; McLaughlin *et al.*, 2018) and to improve pharmacokinetic modeling for predicting drug absorption, distribution, metabolism and excretion. It can thus improve drug dosage and limit drug toxicity, for e.g., of chemotherapy in cancer patients (Prado *et al.*, 2007, and Prado *et al.*, 2009). In addition, skeletal muscle mass may also serve as a basis to calculate protein needs (Geisler *et al.*, 2015).

Of the many methods available to measure body composition, a few are highlighted and a short description of each is given. For more detailed information, the books by Forbes (1987), Heymsfield *et al.* (2005) and Lukaski *et al.* (2017) on human body composition and comprehensive reviews (Baracos *et al.*, 2012; Prado and Heymsfield, 2014; Müller *et al.*, 2013 and 2016b, Lemos and Gallagher, 2017; Teigen *et al.*, 2017) are recommended for further reading.

5.2 Different levels of body composition

The classical concept of (BCA) is about models and so-called compartments. At the "chemical level" a two-compartment model (or 2C-model) divides the body into FM, and fat-free mass (FFM) (Forbes, 1987; Withers *et al.*, 1999; Heymsfield *et al.*, 2005; Figure 1). FM refers to total body lipids (mainly tri-acyl-glycerol (TAG) accounting for about 60%–90% of adipose tissue; essential structural lipids such as the phospholipids (cell membranes) and sphingomyelin (nervous system) form only a minor part of the total lipids in the body).

In a "normal weight" healthy adult, the amount of body fat varies between 10% and 25% in men and between 15% and 35% in women. In normal weight subjects, essential fat accounts for 2.1 kg (or 3.0% of body weight) in males and 6.8 kg (or 12%) in females with the sex difference related to childbearing and reproduction. In severe obesity FM can be as high as 60–70% of body weight. "Over-fatness" is defined by a FM >25% and >35% body weight in males and females, respectively. In elderly women this *cut-off* is slightly increased. By contrast, in thin subjects FM is below 20%, the leanest women in a population have an FM of about 10 to 12%. The lowest level of FM compatible with survival is assumed to be in the order of 3 or 12% in males and females, respectively. In elite female athletes in ballet, gymnastics, track running or triathlon and also in body builders body fat is between 8 and 15% of body weight.

FFM comprises all non-fat components and includes water, protein, and minerals within adipose tissue. The total amount of water in the body is high and, depending on the body fat content, can be as high as 60–70% of total body weight. The water content in the body varies with age. In a foetus, body water slowly decreases from more than 90% after conception to about 80% at seven months of gestation. A newborn has about 70% body water, which is about 82% of the FFM. This value slowly decreases further to 72% of the FFM at the age 15–18 years. In general, males have more body water (related to body weight) than females, as their body fat content is lower.

Both FM and FFM can be adjusted for height and are expressed as the FM-index (FMI) and the FFM-index (FFMI) as kg/m^2. This is because both body compartments scale to height rounded to a power of 2 as the nearest integer. Height is the most important factor contributing to the magnitude of FFM across the lifespan. FFMI allows comparing nutritional status in subjects differing in height. FM and FFM are also be normalised for body size by expressing it as a percentage of body weight (%FM and %FFM, respectively).

Body protein varies between 10% and 15% of body weight. It is higher in males than in females, as males generally have more skeletal muscle mass. There is no protein storage in the body and, generally speaking, loss of protein coincides with a loss of functionality given the high protein content and high protein turnover rates in vital organs. The amount of minerals in the body varies between 3% and 5%, again dependent on body fat. Calcium and phosphorus are the two main minerals and are found mainly in bones. When compared with FFM, lean soft tissue (LST) is the sum of all lean compartments, organs and tissues except bone, and includes non-adipose tissue lipids. LST is mostly water in both, adipose and muscle tissues. When compared with LST, lean body mass (LBM) also includes bone mass (i.e., LBM = body weight - FM).

At the **atomic level** the body can be divided into eleven major elements, H, O, N, C, Na, K, Cl, P, Ca, Mg, S), whereas the "**molecular level**" relates to six components, lipid, water, protein, bone minerals, soft tissue minerals and carbohydrates. Carbohydrates are found in the body as plasma glucose (blood sugar) and glycogen, a polysaccharide mainly prevalent in muscle and liver cells that serves as a short-term energy store. The amount of carbohydrates (i.e., glycogen) stored in the body rarely exceeds 500 g and is not assessed by current methods for body composition analysis. A "normal weight" human body consists of approximately 43.0 kg oxygen, 16.0 kg carbon, 7.0 kg hydrogen, 1.8 kg nitrogen, and 1.0 kg calcium; of 60–70% water, 10–35% fat (depending on gender), 10–15% protein, and 3–5% minerals.

At the "**cellular level**" body composition can be described in terms of three or four components, body cell mass (BCM, which does not include storage fat), extracellular fluid (ECF), extracellular solids. BCM includes cells with all their contents, such as intracellular water (ICW), proteins, and minerals. ECF contains about 95% water (extracellular water, ECW), which is plasma in the intravascular space and interstitial fluid in the extravascular space. Extracellular solids are organic and inorganic, i.e., mainly proteins (e.g., collagen) and minerals (bone minerals and soluble minerals in ECF). Body composition at the cellular level is not easy to measure. *In vivo* determination of total body potassium (by total ^{40}K counting, WBC, or *in vivo* neutron activation analysis, IVNAA) can be used to assess BCM because most of the body potassium is known to be intracellular. Dilution techniques, for example the combination of deuterium and bromide dilution, can be used to differentiate extracellular water from total body water.

The "**tissue-organ level**" comprises major tissues such as adipose tissue, skeletal muscle, bone, and organs (brain, liver, kidneys, heart, spleen). Adipose tissue contains about 80% triglycerides and some 1–2% protein, and the remaining part is water plus electrolytes. Bones consist mainly of hydroxyapatite, $[Ca_3(PO_4)_2]_3Ca(OH)_2$, bedded in a protein matrix. At the anatomic level, a young man (body weight 78.1 kg, height 178 cm) has a FM of 14.5 kg with masses of skeletal muscle, brain heart, liver, kidneys and spleen of 31.6, 1.613, 0.366, 1,602, 0.312, and 0.263 kg, respectively (Later *et al.*, 2010). For comparison, a young female (67.4 kg, 169cm) has corresponding values for FM, muscle mass and masses of brain, heart, liver, kidneys and spleen of 23.3, 21.7, 1.456, 0.261, 1.433, 0.254 and 0.194 kg, respectively. (Later *et al.*, 2010).

When compared with the 2C-model all these models are considered as multi-component or multi-compartment models (Heymsfield *et al.*, 2005 and 2015; Müller *et al.*, 2016b; Figure 5.1).

The different levels of body composition are interrelated. Thus, information at one level can be translated to another level (e.g., after determining the amount of calcium in the body by, IVNAA (atomic level), or bone mineral content by DXA (molecular level) the amount of bone can be calculated assuming that a certain amount of total body calcium or bone minerals is in the skeletal tissue.

5.3 Body composition techniques

Densitometry

The densitometric method assumes that the body consists of two components, an FM, in which all "chemical" fat (including storage fat and essential fat, e.g., in the central nervous system and bone marrow) is located, and the FFM, which consists of (fat-free) bones, muscles, water, and organs. Chemically, the FFM consists of water, minerals, protein, and a small amount of carbohydrate, the last often being neglected. The density of the FM is 0.900 kg/l and, from carcass analysis data, the density of the FFM can be calculated as 1.100 kg/l, depending on the relative amount of minerals, protein, and water in the FFM. The density of FFM is lower in

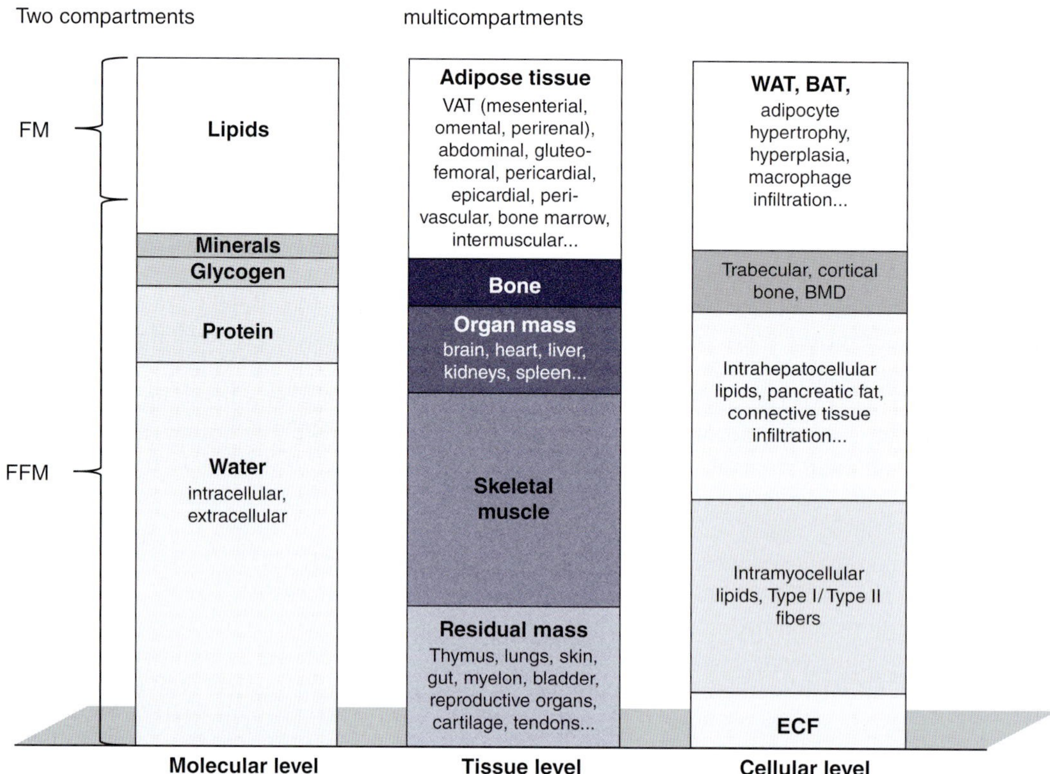

Figure 5.1 Compartment models of body composition at different levels. The first bar represents compartment models of body composition at the molecular level. In the second bar, body compartments at the tissue level are shown. The third bar represents body compartments at the cellular level. BAT, brown adipose tissue; BMD, bone mineral density; ECF, extracellular fluid; FM, fat mass; FFM, fat free mass; VAT, visceral adipose tissue; WAT, white adipose tissue. Reproduced from Müller *et al.*, 2016b.

children than in adults due to relatively higher water content. In females the density of FFM is lower at each age compared to males which is explained by a higher water but lower mineral content of FFM in females.

The density of the whole body depends on the ratio of FM to FFM. Once the density of the body has been determined, the percentage of fat in the body (BF%) can be calculated by Siri's formula:

$$\mathrm{BF\%} = \left(495/\text{body density}\right) - 450$$

Body density can be determined by several techniques, the oldest being underwater weighing (UWW; see Figure 5.2). Behnke (1963, 1966) first used the technique, showing that excess body weight in American football players was not the result of excess fat but of enlarged muscle mass. Today, body density is more conveniently measured by Air-displacement Plethysmography (ADP; see Figure 5.3). Using UWW or ADP body density can be accurately measured within 0.004 kg/l.

In underwater weighing, the weight of the subject is first measured in air and then while totally immersed in water. The difference between weight in air and weight under water is the upwards force, which equals the weight of the displaced water (Archimedes' law), from which, after correction for the water temperature (density), the displaced water volume (and thus the body volume) can be calculated. Corrections must be made for residual lung volume and air in the gut. Figure 5.2 shows a modern underwater weighing device. The technique gives very reproducible results within about 1% of BF%. The absolute error in determined body fat is assumed to be maximal 3% of BF%. This error is mainly due to violation of the assumption that the density of the FFM equals 1.100 kg/l in the subject under study (Box 5.1). It can

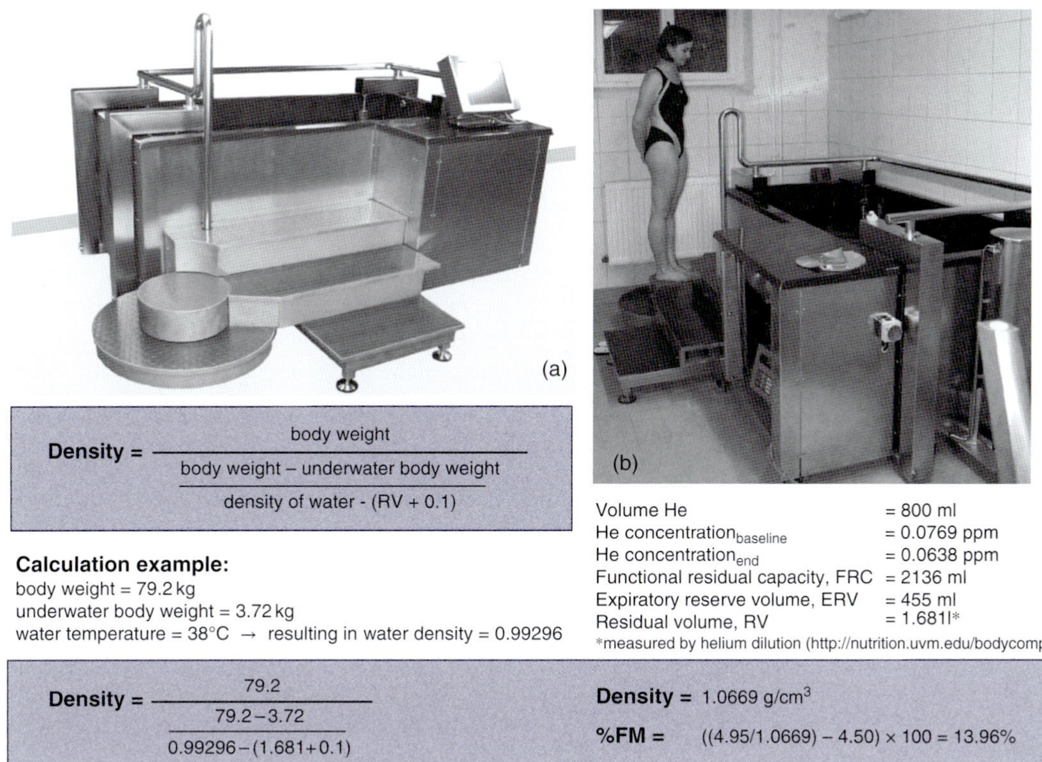

(a)
(b)
Density = body weight / ((body weight – underwater body weight) / density of water - (RV + 0.1))
Calculation example:
body weight = 79.2 kg
underwater body weight = 3.72 kg
water temperature = 38°C → resulting in water density = 0.99296
Volume He = 800 ml
He concentration baseline = 0.0769 ppm
He concentration end = 0.0638 ppm
Functional residual capacity, FRC = 2136 ml
Expiratory reserve volume, ERV = 455 ml
Residual volume, RV = 1.681l*
*measured by helium dilution (http://nutrition.uvm.edu/bodycomp/)
Density = 79.2 / ((79.2 – 3.72) / 0.99296 – (1.681 + 0.1))
Density = 1.0669 g/cm3
%FM = ((4.95/1.0669) – 4.50) × 100 = 13.96%

Figure 5.2 (a) Underwater weighing device (Borngässer Waagenbau, Grebbin, Germany); (b) subject standing on the scale to measure body weight before entering the underwater scale. This device is used at the Reference Center of Body Composition which is part of the Institute of Human Nutrition and Food Science of the Christian-Albrechts-University, Kiel, Germany.

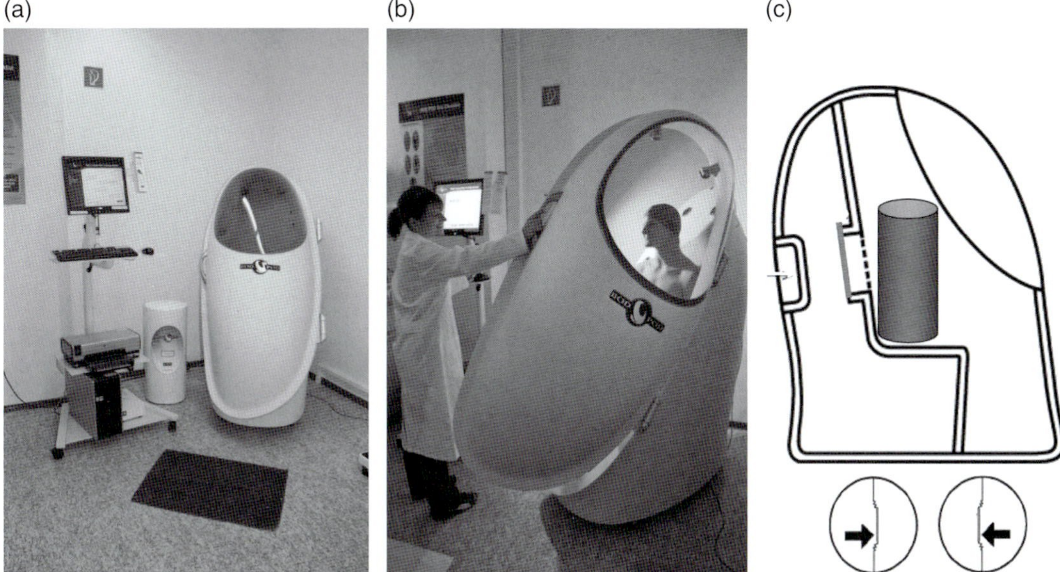

Figure 5.3 (a) Air displacement plethysmography (ADP) device (BodPod®, Cosmed, Italy); (b) ADP measurement; (c) 2-point calibration: chamber volume with and without 50l cylinder.

Box 5.1

The density of the FFM can be calculated if its composition is known. In the calculation example it is assumed that the FFM consists of 73.5% water, 19.6% protein, and 6.9% minerals with densities (at 37°C) of 0.993, 1.340, and 3.038 kg/l, respectively. In addition, it is assumed that the volumes of the separate compartments can be added up to the total volume of the FFM. Thus, the volume of the FFM equals the sum of the other compartments:

$$\mathrm{FFM_{volume}} = \mathrm{Water_{volume}} + \mathrm{Mineral_{volume}} + \mathrm{Protein_{volume}}$$

As volume is weight/density, the equation can be written as:

$$100/\mathrm{Density_{FFM}} = 73.5/0.993 + 6.9/3.038 + 19.6/1.340$$

From this, the density of the FFM can be calculated as 1.0999 kg/l. It is obvious that differences in composition of the FFM will result in a different density.

Box 5.2

Siri's formula can be derived assuming that the body consists of FM and FFM. If bw is assumed to be 100% and body fat is *x*%, then FFM is 100 – *x*%. It is assumed that the volumes of these two compartments can be added up to total body volume. Then:

$$\mathrm{Body_{volume}} = \mathrm{FM_{volume}} + \mathrm{FFM_{volume}}$$

As volume is weight/density, the equation can be written as:

$$100/\mathrm{body\ density} = x/0.9 + (100 - x)/1.1$$

From this, body fat percentage (BF%) can be calculated as:

$$\mathrm{BF\%} = 495/\mathrm{density} - 450$$

The general formula to calculate BF% from body density (D_b) is:

$$\mathrm{BF\%} = \frac{1}{D_b} \times \left(\frac{D_{FFM} \times D_{FM}}{D_{FFM} - D_{FM}}\right) - \left(\frac{D_{FFM}}{D_{FFM} - D_{FM}}\right)$$

In general, a lower density of the FFM than 1.1 kg/l will result in an overestimation of BF% if Siri's formula is used. It is likely that the density of the FFM is lower in elderly people, owing to bone mineral loss (osteoporosis).

be argued that in certain subjects or groups of subjects this assumption may be violated, as for example in young children, very obese patients and in pregnant women. Use of Siri's formula (Box 5.2) will then lead to biased conclusions.

An air-displacement plethysmographic measurement device to assess body volume has been commercially available since 1995. Today, two different systems, the PEA POD^{TM} and the BOD POD^{TM}, allow the measurement of subjects with a wide range of body weight from <1 kg in infants to 150 kg in adults. The plethysmograph consists of two airtight chambers with a known empty volume (Figure 5.3).

The subject is located in the one chamber and the other air filled chamber is located in the rear of the instrument. Between the two chambers a diaphragm oscillates and creates sinusoidal volume perturbations in the two chambers that are equal in magnitude but opposite in sign and cause slight pressure changes. The ratio of the pressure perturbations in the two chambers is equal to the inverse ratio of the chambers' volumes. The decrease in the chamber volume due to the subject reveals the volume of the subject. The operating principle is based on the relationships between pressure and volume expressed by Boyle's Law and Poisson's Law (Box 5.3).

Research to date has generally shown good agreement between underwater weighing and air displacement. Air displacement is better accepted by the volunteers, but some experience difficulties because of claustrophobia.

Dual energy X-ray absorptiometry

During DXA (previously described as DEXA), the body or part of the body is scanned with X-rays of two distinct levels of energy. The attenuation of the tissues for the two different levels of radiation depends on its chemical composition and is detected by photocells. The ratio of the attenuation at higher and lower energy is specific for fat, bone mineral, and lean soft tissue. The instrument's software generates a two-dimensional picture of the body or the body compartment under study. Each pixel of the image has a measured attenuation ratio that can be resolved into two components, fat and LST or bone mineral content (BMC) and total soft tissue. The software uses assumptions on the composition of total soft tissue in pixels containing bone minerals and can thus calculate several body components: BMC and bone mineral density (BMD), LST and FM. These calculations are possible for each of the body parts, e.g., for legs, trunk, spine, femur, and arms. However, the method cannot distinguish between subcutaneous adipose tissue (SAT) and discrete adipose tissue sites such as visceral and/or perirenal

Box 5.3

Boyle's Law states that the pressure exerted by air is inversely proportional to the volume it occupies if the temperature remains unchanged (isothermal conditions). When air is allowed to change temperature in response to volume changes (adiabatic conditions), Poisson's Law expresses its behavior as follows:

$$P1/P2 = (V2/V1)^{1.4}$$

P1 and V1 are pressure and volume at an initial condition and P2 and V2 are pressure and volume at a final condition. For a known reference chamber volume, and assuming adiabatic conditions, varying test chamber volumes are a linear function of the ratios of the pressure perturbations in the two chambers. However, air close to the subject's surface and in the lungs behaves isothermally because it is warmed-up by body temperature. Under adiabatic conditions P2 is approximately 40% larger than P2 under isothermal conditions. A subject's volume would be underestimated by 40% of the subject's volume at the surface and in the thorax. The subject therefore needs to wear tight fitting swimsuit and a swimming cap to keep the layers of isothermal air as low as possible. In addition, the measurement needs to be corrected for calculated body surface area and measured thoracic gas volume.

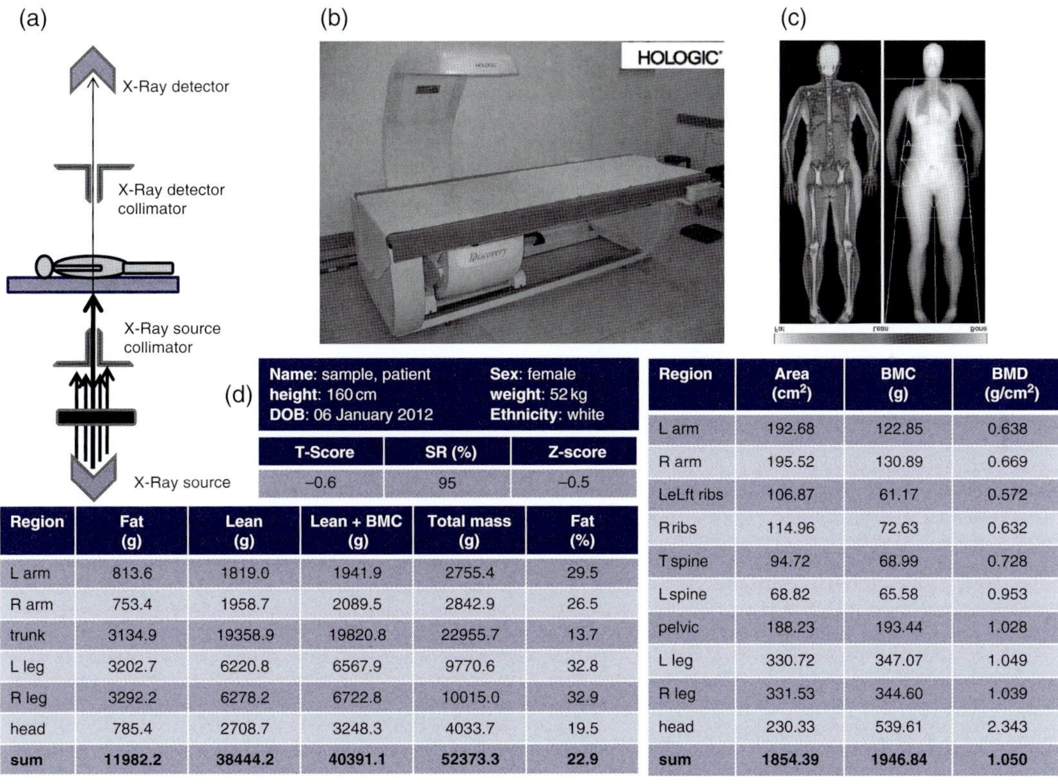

Name: sample, patient | Sex: female
height: 160 cm | weight: 52 kg
DOB: 06 January 2012 | Ethnicity: white

T-Score	SR (%)	Z-score
−0.6	95	−0.5

Region	Fat (g)	Lean (g)	Lean + BMC (g)	Total mass (g)	Fat (%)
L arm	813.6	1819.0	1941.9	2755.4	29.5
R arm	753.4	1958.7	2089.5	2842.9	26.5
trunk	3134.9	19358.9	19820.8	22955.7	13.7
L leg	3202.7	6220.8	6567.9	9770.6	32.8
R leg	3292.2	6278.2	6722.8	10015.0	32.9
head	785.4	2708.7	3248.3	4033.7	19.5
sum	**11982.2**	**38444.2**	**40391.1**	**52373.3**	**22.9**

Region	Area (cm^2)	BMC (g)	BMD (g/cm^2)
L arm	192.68	122.85	0.638
R arm	195.52	130.89	0.669
LeLft ribs	106.87	61.17	0.572
Rribs	114.96	72.63	0.632
T spine	94.72	68.99	0.728
L spine	68.82	65.58	0.953
pelvic	188.23	193.44	1.028
L leg	330.72	347.07	1.049
R leg	331.53	344.60	1.039
head	230.33	539.61	2.343
sum	**1854.39**	**1946.84**	**1.050**

Figure 5.4 (a) Schematic Dual Energy X-Ray (DXA) measurement principle; (b) DXA device (Hologic Discovery A, Bedford, MA, USA); (c) whole body DXA scan; (d) subject result tables. Images and data are taken from the Reference Center of Body Composition which is part of the Institute of Human Nutrition and Food Science of the Christian-Albrechts-University, Kiel, Germany.

adipose tissue. Figure 5.4 shows a typical output of the DXA measurement.

The reproducibility of DXA is very high, varying from about 0.5% for bone mineral density to about 2% for total body composition. The reproducibility for regional body composition is less. The method is quick and easy to perform and places very few demands on the subject. The radiation dose (0.02-mSv) is only a fraction of the radiation dose of a normal chest radiograph, and hardly higher than the normal background. Apart from repeated scanning, the radiation dose should not be a limiting factor in terms of volunteers being exposed to hazardous levels of

Box 5.4

As a limitation to DXA, only two components can be distinguished in one pixel using the attenuation ratio of two different X-ray energies. Despite being based on a two-compartment model, the DXA output consists of 3 components: bone, fat, and lean soft tissue. The information about the third compartment can therefore only be obtained by calculation based on assumptions. Because the composition of soft tissue cannot be measured in those pixels containing bone, soft tissue composition in bone pixels has to be extrapolated from adjacent areas. This procedure may however be invalid if (i) the composition of soft tissue in front of or behind the bone differs in composition from soft tissue next to the bone (i.e., *extra-osseous soft tissue effect*) or (ii) if the composition of bone marrow differs from an average or standard (i.e., *intra-osseous soft tissue effect*). In pixels not containing bone, dissolving one pixel into fat mass and lean soft tissue also requires assumption on the composition (e.g., hydration) of lean soft tissue.

Box 5.5

A subject with a body weight of 75 kg is given an exactly weighed dose of 15 g deuterium oxide. This deuterium oxide is allowed to be equally distributed in the body water compartment for about three to five hours. Then, blood is taken and the deuterium concentration in the sample is determined. Assuming the plasma level to be 370 mg/ kg, the "deuterium space" can be calculated as 15 000/370 = 40.5 kg. As deuterium exchanges in the body with hydroxyl groups from other molecules, the deuterium space has to be corrected for this non-aqueous dilution (4–5%). Thus, total body water is 0.95 × 15 000/370 = 38.5 kg. Assuming a hydration of the FFM of 73%, the body fat percentage of this 75 kg weight subject would be: 100 × [75 − (38.5/0.73)/75] = 29.7%. For the computation of body composition from dual X-ray absorptiometry, especially body fat and lean tissue, several assumptions are made, one of which is a constant hydration of the (FFM).

radiation. A disadvantage of the method is that the attenuation of the X-rays depends on the thickness of the tissue. Therefore, correction for the body size has to be made. Compared with traditional methods, DXA scanning is easy and widely available which, in turn, leads to prediction equations for body composition based on DXA. However, as with other methods, DXA relies on certain assumptions and there are many publications showing that the bias in body composition measurements using DXA can be considerable. Although DXA is not considered as a two-compartment method because it measures FM, bone mineral content, and lean soft tissue, every pixel of the DXA image can only be resolved into two components and therefore requires assumptions (Box 5.4). Moreover, devices from different manufacturers or using different software versions, can give different results in scanning the same person.

Dilution techniques

In adult subjects, carcass analyses revealed that the amount of water in the FFM is relatively constant at about 73%. Total body water (TBW) can be determined by dilution techniques. Dilution techniques are generally based on the equation:

$$C_1 \times V_1 = C_2 \times V_2 = \text{Constant}$$

where C is the tracer (deuterium oxide, or ^{18}O water) concentration and V is the volume.

When a subject is given a known amount of a tracer ($C_1 \times V_1$), which is known to be diluted in a given body compartment, the volume of that body compartment can be calculated from the dose given and the concentration of the tracer in that compartment after equilibrium has been reached. Suitable tracers for the determination of TBW are deuterium oxide (D_2O), and ^{18}O-labeled water ($H_2{}^{18}O$). Other tracers can also be used, such as tritium, alcohol, and urea, but they are less suitable because they are unstable and radioactive (tritium), partly metabolised (alcohol) or because they are actively excreted from the body (urea) during the dilution period. After giving a subject the tracer and allowing around 3–5 hours for equal distribution throughout the body, determination of the concentration of deuterium in blood, saliva, or urine allows the calculation of TBW (see Box 5.5 for an example).

Alternatively, the tracer can be given intravenously, which is advantageous when the subject has gastrointestinal disorders. The reproducibility of the method is 1–3%, depending on the tracer used and the analytical method chosen. From TBW, the FFM, and hence FM, can be calculated, assuming that 73% of the FFM is water:

$$BF\% = 100 \times \left(\text{Weight} - TBW / 0.73\right) / \text{Weight}$$

The accuracy for estimations of body fat is about 3–4% of body weight. As with the densitometric method, this bias is due to violations of the assumption used (i.e., that the relative amount of water in the FFM is constant and equals 73% of the FFM). In subjects with a larger than 73% water content in the FFM (e.g., pregnant women, morbid obese subjects, and patients with edema), the factor 0.73 will result in an overestimation of the FFM. A three-compartment model of the body that contains FM, water, and dry FFM has a lower bias than a 2C-model because it avoids the assumption of a constant hydration of FFM is higher. Based on measurements of TBW (by D_2O-dilution) and FFM (by ADP) is higher during early compared to adult life, i.e., in the newborn, hydration of FFM is about 80%, going down to about 77% in infants and 75%, respectively at age of 120 months. These changes are associated with age-related increases in BMD resulting in an increase in FFM-density during childhood and adolescence.

The use of tracers that do not cross the cell membrane enables the determination of extracellular water (ECW). Commonly used tracers in this respect are bromide salts or sodium-24. Intracellular water (ICW) cannot be determined directly and is calculated as the difference between TBW and ECW.

Multi-compartment models

Most body composition techniques that are in use today are based on assumptions, often derived from carcass analyses or experimentally derived from observational studies. Violation of these assumptions leads to biased results. Patients with chronic heart, liver or renal failure, and morbid obesity often have an increased water content of FFM that violates the underlying assumptions of two-compartment methods for body composition analysis. An increase in hydration will thus lead to an overestimation of FFM by deuterium dilution (and also by Bioelectrical Impedance Analysis (BIA), see below) and an underestimation by densitometry or DXA. A combination of techniques often results in more valid estimates, as is the case when, for example, body density and body water are combined. In this particular case, the body is divided into three compartments:

$$\text{Body weight} = \text{Fat mass} + \text{Body water} + \text{Dry fat-free mass}$$

In a three-compartment model the variation of the water content in the FFM is accounted for by measuring TBW. There are fewer assumptions in this model, leading to more valid results.

In osteoporosis the mineral content of FFM is low and leads to an overestimation of FM by densitometry. DXA enables the measurement of bone mineral, from which total body mineral can be estimated. When the mineral content of the body is combined with body density and body water, a four-compartment model of the body is generated:

$$\text{Body weight} = \text{Fat mass} + \text{Water} + \text{Minerals} + \text{Protein}$$

In a four-compartment model, most of the variation in the amounts of the chemical components is accounted for, resulting in a very accurate body composition measure. The four-compartment model shown has only minor assumptions and provides body composition data that are very accurate. Four-compartment models can also be obtained using other techniques. For example, the measurement of calcium, phosphorus, and nitrogen with IVNAA in combination with TBW provides information for a model consisting of fat, minerals, protein, and water. In the literature, models based on six compartments are also described. However, they do not provide much additional information and the increased technical error negates the methodological advantage.

Compartment models can be obtained at different levels of body composition that extend beyond the molecular level and are adapted to specific research questions or clinical applications.

Imaging technologies

Medical imaging by using CT or MRI is a rapidly advancing field that allows the measurement of anatomical structures as well as tissue function (Prado and Heymsfield, 2014). Using either CT or MRI the thickness of the obtained slices can vary, but is usually 5 mm. During CT scanning a source of X-rays rotates perpendicularly around the body or a body segment, while

Box 5.6

The Houndsfield unit scale is used to calibrate the gray-scale applied to the X-ray attenuation of the tissue in every image. The gray level of the pixels in every image thus resembles the attenuating properties of the measured voxels (volume elements). Volumes that contain a homogeneous tissue have the HU typical for this tissue. The interval from -1001 to 191 HU covers air, gas and lung, −190 to −30 HU reflects adipose tissue, and yellow bone marrow, −29 to +150 HU covers soft tissue and the interval between +151 and +2001 HU defines cortical bone and spongiosa (Müller et al., 2002). Volumes which contain a mixture of tissues with different attenuating properties, e.g., at the interfaces between fat and muscle, will have an averaged HU. This effect is called partial volume artifact and may influence the accuracy and reproducibility of the method. Software enables the calculation of the amounts of tissues with different attenuation, for example adipose tissue against non-adipose tissue. The precision of the calculation of a tissue area or tissue volume from the same scan(s) is very accurate, with an error rate of about 1%.

photo-detectors, opposite to the source, register the attenuation of the X-rays after they have passed through the body in the various directions. The information received by the photo-detectors is used to generate images. CT attenuation is expressed in Houndsfield Units (HU) and is representative of tissue density, with water represented as 0 HU and air as −1000 HU (with principally no attenuation) (Box 5.6).

A single CT scan provides only relative data, for example in a scan of the abdomen the relative amount of VAT to abdominal subcutaneous adipose tissue. Multiple CT scanning allows the calculation of tissue volumes. The advantages of CT are a fast acquisition time, moderate cost, and a very high structural resolution. CT scanning however involves a relatively high level of radiation that is a limitation for repeated measurements and leads to the assessment of single slices instead of tissue volumes.

In contrast to CT, MRI has the advantages of excellent soft tissue contrast and involves no ionising radiation. During MRI, the signals emitted when the body is placed in a strong magnetic field are collected and, as with CT scanning, the data are used to generate a visual cross-sectional slice of the body in a certain region (Figure 5.5 A and B). The determination of adipose tissue versus non-adipose tissue is based on the shorter relaxation time of adipose tissue than of other tissues that contain more protons or differ in resonance frequency. The time necessary to make an MRI image is higher compared to CT, which has implications for the quality of the image. Any movement of the subject, even the movements of the intestinal tract when making images in the abdominal region, will decrease the quality of the image. In addition, intensity inhomogeneity artifacts occur where the intensity level of a single tissue class varies gradually over the extent of the image. These shading effects over the images affect the segmentation result when simple grey level based segmentation techniques are used.

Figure 5.5 shows an example of whole body MRI including evaluation of subcutaneous and visceral adipose tissue as well as skeletal muscle mass.

Imaging technologies today are indispensable for measurement of VAT and SAT as well as other specific fat depots like perirenal, pericardial, or perivascular adipose tissue. In addition, imaging technologies are reference methods for the assessment of organ masses and skeletal muscle mass. Whole body MRI provides an accurate and non-invasive assessment of total skeletal muscle mass, but is very time consuming and expensive. Single slice CT or MRI images are often available in cancer patients for staging of tumors. A single slice at the level of lumbar vertebra L3 has shown to provide the best estimates for SAT, and VAT volume whereas total skeletal muscle mass was best represented by a single area at the mid-thigh. The limited validity of single slices to assess changes in these tissue volumes with weight loss reveals the limitation of this approach (Schweizer *et al.*, 2015; Shen *et al.*, 2012)

In addition to quantitative analysis of body compartments, imaging technologies allow the assessment of tissue quality. CT-derived skeletal muscle density is examined as an index for muscle quality that is impaired by fatty infiltration and myosteatosis and has been shown to be a prognostic indicator in cancer and critically ill patients. Ectopic fat in lean tissue like skeletal muscle, heart, liver, or pancreas that is related to the development of insulin resistance can be measured using proton (^1H) Magnetic Resonance Spectroscopy (MRS) determines: (i) intracellular fat in relation to tissue water in liver

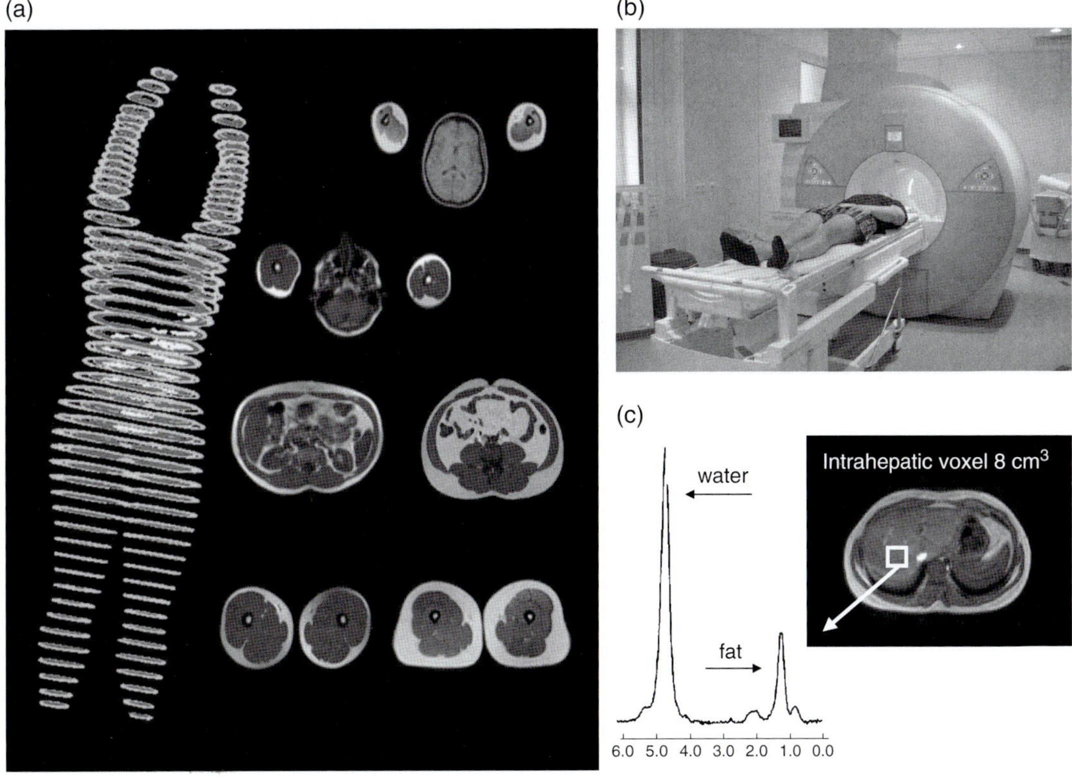

Figure 5.5 Magnetic Resonance Imaging (MRI); (a) segmented whole body MRI slices (SliceOmatic 4.3, TomoVision Inc. Montreal, Canada); (b) MRI device (Siemens Avanto 1,5 T, Erlangen, Germany); (c) intrahepatic (ectopic) fat measurement using Magnetic Resonance Spectroscopy (MRS). Images and data are taken from the Reference Center of Body Composition which is part of the Institute of Human Nutrition and Food Science of the Christian-Albrechts-University, Kiel, Germany.

(Figure 5.5C), skeletal muscle and pancreas; or (ii) the creatinine signal in a defined voxel in muscle. With this technique water and fat signals are uniquely identified by their chemical shift locations along the frequency spectrum and in muscle, intramyocellular lipids can be discriminated from extramyocellular lipids due to a small difference in resonance frequency between these two lipid components. Single-voxel MRS approaches (5-20 ml volume per voxel) have however limitations to be representative due to inhomogeneous fat infiltration of tissues. By contrast, multi-voxel Chemical Shift Imaging (CSI) is based on multiple and smaller voxels (about 1ml volume) and thus captures heterogeneous fat accumulation across the organ. The method has however a lower spatial resolution. The advantage of spectroscopy is the accurate quantification of very low amounts of fat. As an alternative to spectroscopy in single or multiple voxels, Chemical-Shift-Encoded Water-Fat MRI integrates two-component water-fat spectral detection with high spatial resolution MRI. In 1984, the method was initially proposed by Dixon, and simultaneously acquires water and fat signals that are subsequently separated based on chemical-shift-encoding and mathematical fat spectrum modeling. Water and fat signals can thus be separated on a voxel-wise basis, allowing to compute proton-density fat fraction maps that allow the quantification of ectopic fat in the whole image.

The variety of disease-related outcome parameters and wide distribution of CT and MRI scanners in clinical use, as well as the improvements in software and growing availability of automated protocols for data analysis, has led to an increased application of these techniques in clinical practice as well as in epidemiologic studies on large populations.

Bioelectrical impedance analysis (BIA)

BIA has been commercially available since the mid-1980s and today is widely used for the estimation of body composition in health and disease because the technology is relatively inexpensive, quick, and noninvasive and generates a range of clinically meaningful outcome parameters. Despite a general public perception that BIA measures "body fat," the technology determines the electrical impedance of body tissues, which primarily provides an estimate of total body water (TBW). Therefore a small alternating current (I), of about 800 μA, most often at a frequency of 50 kHz is applied to the body and conducted by electrolyte containing body water. TBW is calculated using the impedance index (Ht^2/Z) (Box 5.7).

Calculating TBW from Ht^2/Z requires a uniform cross-sectional area and homogenous conductivity of the conductor. However, in reality the human body is not a homogenous cylinder but consists of trunk and extremities and there is biological variability in the amount and kind of electrolytes in body fluids (pure water does not conduct the current), and the temperature of the solution and the temperature of the skin (current is mainly conducted at the surface and a higher blood flow decreases impedance of the skin) (Box 5.8). Therefore a statistical relationship between Ht^2/Z and TBW measured by deuterium dilution accounts for some of the population differences in these influencing factors. These prediction equations derived by multiple regression analysis include age, sex, and sometimes even body mass index (BMI) or ethnicity because these variables partly account for the variance in these influencing variables. As body water in healthy subjects is an assumed fixed part (73%) of the FFM, bioelectrical impedance measurements can also be used for the prediction of the FFM and hence body fat percentage. For those prediction equations, the impedance index was related to measures of FFM, normally obtained by densitometry or DXA as reference methods or the four-compartment model as a gold standard.

Box 5.7

In a simplified model the body consists of a cylinder with a uniform cross-section that is filled with a homogeneous conducting material of a specific resistivity (p). End-to-end impedance of the cylinder is the resistivity times the length (L) divided by the cross-sectional area (A) because impedance increases with increasing length of the conductor (height of the body) and decreases with increasing area ($Z = pL/A$). Multiplying the right side of the equation by L/L gives $Z = pL^2/\text{volume}$. Rearranging this equation gives volume = pL^2/Z. The conductive volume that is total body water is therefore proportional to L^2 that is the square height of the body (Ht^2) and inversely related to the impedance (Z) of the cross-sectional body area ($TBW \sim Ht^2/Z$).

Box 5.8

The current flows through all conducting material in the body in the path between the source and detector electrodes (usually located on the wrist and ankle) and generates voltages between different points in the body volume according to Ohm's law. The voltage (V) is measured and expressed as a ratio, V/I, which is also called impedance (Z). The carriers of the current (I) are predominantly charged ions, such as sodium or potassium ions, which move within the tissue volume. Because the current will flow predominantly through materials with higher conductivities (e.g., blood and muscle), small changes in fluid compartments cause a significant change in the resulting impedance, whereas even larger changes in high-resistance compartments such as bone or fat, will not have a big impact on the BIA-results. In addition, in regions where the conductor has a larger cross-sectional area (i.e., the body trunk or the thigh) there is a lower resistance to current flow, whereas a higher resistance occurs in regions with a smaller cross-sectional area (e.g., the forearm and calf). Finally, impedance is lower in tissues with fewer cells because cell membranes form barriers to charge movement.

Today many different algorithms for BIA calibration exist. All these equations are clearly specific for a certain device (arrangement and conductivity of the electrodes) and also specific for the characteristics of the population that has been investigated to generate that equation. To a large extent the population specificity of a BIA equation is explained by differences in body shape (i.e., the length and volume of arms and legs relative to the trunk) (Bosy-Westphal *et al.*, 2013).

If currents of low frequency (<5kHz) are used, body impedance is a measure of ECW, as a low-frequency current cannot penetrate the cell membrane, which acts, with its layers of protein, lipids, and proteins, as an electrical capacitor. With increasing frequencies the capacitor features of the cell membrane diminish and gradually ICW also participates in the conductance of the current, resulting in lower impedance values at higher frequencies. Hence, at higher frequencies, TBW is measured. TBW and ECW can be predicted from impedance at high and low frequency, respectively, using empirically derived prediction formulae.

BIA-results for body composition depend on the frequency of the current used and on body water distribution between the extracellular and intracellular space and between the different geometrical body compartments (legs, trunk, and arms). As such this calls for extreme caution in the interpretation of calculated body composition values in situations where body water distribution can be disturbed, as is the case, for example, in dialysis patients and in ascites. In these clinical states, TBW, FFM or FM are not the most useful outcome parameters. However, BIA is able to provide some qualitative indices of the quality of lean mass (i.e., hydration and cellularity) that can be obtained from BIA raw data and do not require statistical relationships. For this use it is important to understand that the measured impedance to the current flow is a function of two components (vectors): the resistance (R) of the tissue that is inverse proportional to the electrolyte containing water, and the reactance (Xc) caused by the capacitance of cell membranes, tissue interfaces, and nonionic tissues (Figure 5.6a-c; impedance = $(R^2 + Xc^2)^{1/2}$).

Non-phase sensitive BIA-devices that only measure the absolute value of the impedance (|Z|) do not provide an output for reactance (Xc). Reactance reflects the number of cell membranes and was shown to be important because it is a valuable predictor of muscle mass beyond resistance index (Ht^2/R). In addition, Xc is used to calculate phase angle (phase angle = arctan(Xc/R) x (180/π)) that is a clinically important parameter because it is related to patients prognosis (predictor of survival) in a wide spectrum of diseases. Possible underlying mechanisms are a positive relationship between phase angle and the ICW/ECW-ratio, the number of cells and the integrity of cell membranes.

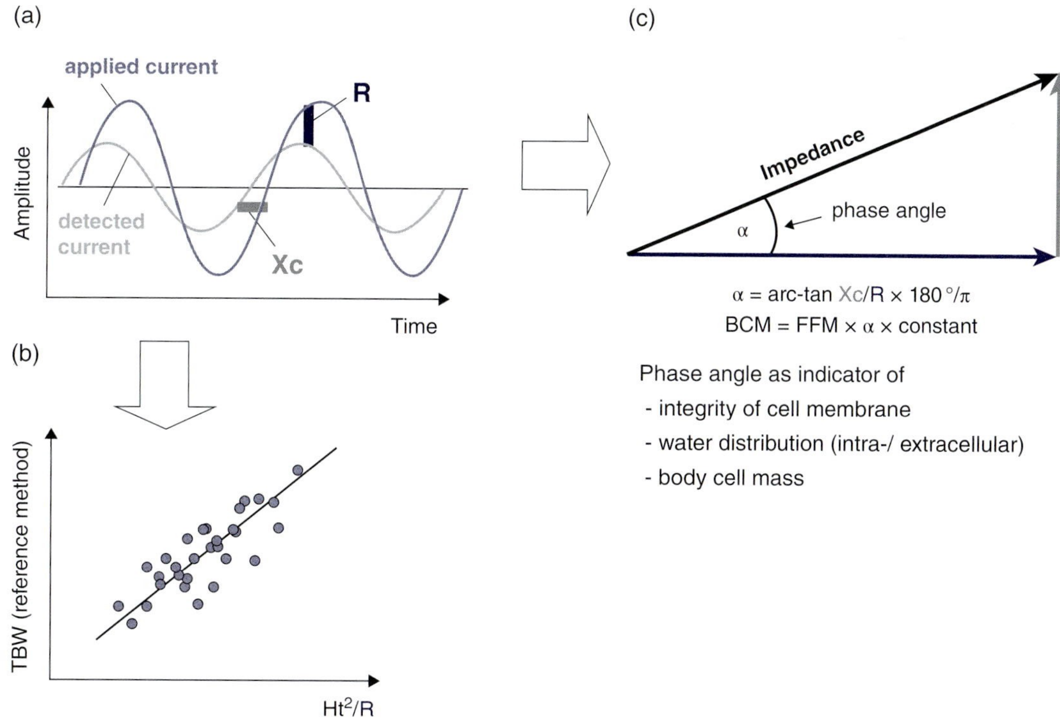

Figure 5.6 Bioelectrical Impedance Analysis (BIA): (a) illustration of BIA resistance R and reactance Xc; (b) relation between resistance index and outcome parameter included in impedance algorithms; (c) phase angle calculated from measured resistance parameters.

Finally, bioelectrical impedance vector analysis (BIVA) can be used to assess hydration status and catabolic states (Box 5.9, Figure 5.7) e.g., in critically ill patients, malnutrition and wasting diseases (Fassini *et al.*, 2016).

Currently available impedance analysers vary in their electrical features and in their principles. Many companies have developed impedance analysers for personal use, anticipating considerable interest among the public in determining their body fat percentage. There are instruments that measure impedance from foot to foot while standing on a weighing scale and provide not only body weight but also body fat percentage. Other instruments measure impedance from hand to hand and allow the reading of body fat percentage, using a built-in software program in which weight, height, age, and gender have to be entered. Combinations of foot-to-foot and hand-to-hand impedance analyzers are also marketed.

Box 5.9

Vector bioelectrical impedance analysis (BIA, RXc-graph method) is a pattern analysis of direct impedance measurements (resistance, *R*, and reactance, *Xc*) plotted as a bivariate vector standardised by height (i.e., expressing *R*/*Ht* and *Xc*/*Ht*). BIVA can be used to monitor hydration status and changes in BCM during cata- and anabolism. In the clinical setting, a great advantage of BIVA is that no algorithms for conversion of impedance raw data into body composition compartments are required. Results are therefore not biased by the choice of regression equation, the accuracy of the criterion method, or the selection criteria of the reference population. Because vector distribution patterns differ between sexes and by race or ethnicity and are dependent on BMI and age, normalised Z-score ellipses are important for the interpretation of BIVA results. This is however of less importance when individual vector migration is interpreted during the course of therapy. Differences in body shape (i.e., the distribution of lean mass) are often overlooked as an important additional confounder of BIVA-results. Because legs have a small diameter relative to their length, when compared with the trunk, they contribute to approximately half the total body resistance, whereas the trunk only contributes 9% (Foster and Lukaski, 1996).

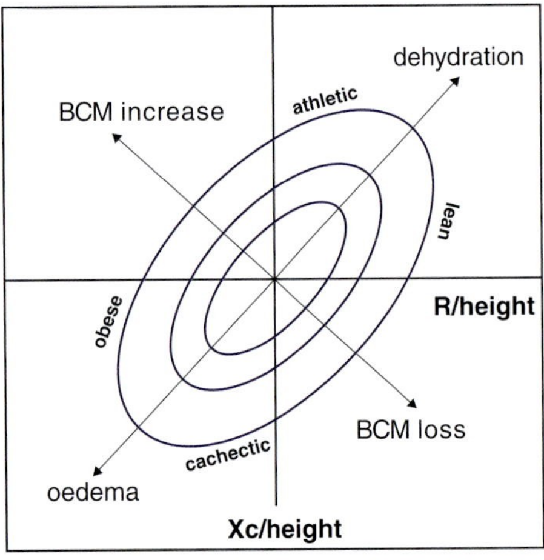

Figure 5.7 Bioelectrical Impedance Vector analysis (BIVA) including z-transformed* vector components (*measured value – mean value / standard deviation).

Recent advances in the technology of multi-frequency BIA facilitated the development of new phase-sensitive impedance analyzers that are innovative in design (e.g., shape and arrangement of electrodes) and technology (high accuracy of electrical reactance measurement) and sold as an approved medical device. This new generation of medical BIA-devices provides a high precision and accuracy due to the use of eight electrodes that allow the assessment of the upper and lower body, as well as the left and right side of the body. This segmental measurement of arms, legs, and the trunk may reduce the assumptions about body shape. In the prediction equations 94-97% of the variance in FFM, TBW, ECW or skeletal muscle mass measured by reference methods (four-compartment model, dilution methods, and whole body MRI) was explained by resistance index (Ht^2/R) only and other variables like weight, sex, and age had only a minor contribution to the prediction of the outcome parameters (Bosy-Westphal *et al.*, 2013, 2017). Limits of agreement of the bias between BIA and whole body MRI as the reference method were calculated as a percentage of the mean reference value: These values revealed that the predictive accuracy of BIA compared to MRI is clinically acceptable when whole body skeletal muscle mass was assessed (between 11% and 12% for different ethnicities), but it becomes limited when small compartments of the body are assessed (e.g., it ranged between 20% and 29% for the arms).

Anthropometry

Body mass index (BMI)

The Quetelet index or body mass index (BMI: weight[kg]/height[m]^2) is the most widely used index today. Its correlation with body fat is high (depending on the age group r = 0.6–0.8). The correlation of BMI with body height is generally low, i.e., the BMI is a stature-independent measure of body weight allowing to compare the body weight of short and tall subjects, an increase in BMI is associated with an increase in mortality risk. The BMI is simple to calculate and applicable to every population.

The World Health Organization (WHO) promotes the BMI as a crude indicator for weight judgement. BMI is used to define overweight and obesity based on the association with cardio-metabolic risk estimates and mortality. In prospective population studies (see GBD, 2015; Obesity Collaborators, 2017; Kivimäki *et al.*, 2017), the lowest mortality is observed in normal and moderately overweight subjects. The nadir of the BMI-all-cause mortality curve is between 24 and 30 kg/m^2. Above the age of 70 years, the lowest mortality was observed in overweight and class I obese subjects, i.e., when compared to young and middle aged adults the BMI-associated risk is shifted upwards. By contrast, in older people, mortality also increased with low body weight, i.e., at a BMI <23 kg/m^2.

In Table 5.1, the cut-off points for underweight, normal weight, overweight, and obesity according to the WHO are given. These cut-off values are based on the relation of BMI with mortality and with risk factors for disease (e.g., biomarkers of insulin resistance) as found in Caucasian populations. For non-Caucasian populations other cut-off values may apply (WHO, 2004).

Indirect estimates of the nutritional status, e.g., BMI and waist circumference, are at best crude indicators of body composition and health; both show a high inter-individual variance and a weak association with detailed body composition (Müller *et al.*, 2016) cannot characterise biological phenotypes to assess (i) tracking of metabolic traits and health risks throughout lifespan; (ii) constitution-dependent metabolic functions and their disturbances (e.g., in obesity, sarcopenia and cachexia); and (iii) models of metabolism and pharmacokinetics.

Cut-off values for BMI and WC as shown in Table 5.1 cannot be used in children. In younger children, weight compared with height is relatively low, and so is the BMI. During growth, the increase in weight is larger than the increase in height and, consequently, the BMI increases with age during the pubertal phase of life. Using a normative approach, there are age-related BMI *cut-off*-values for overweight, obesity as well as for underweight and malnutrition for children as calculated from centiles obtained in reference populations (see Cole *et al.*, 2000). Using a calculation software or respective charts and tables, BMI values above the 90th age- and sex-defined centile are considered as overweight with the 97th centile defining obesity. By contrast BMI values below the 10th age- and sex-related centile are defined as underweight while data below the 3th centile characterise severe malnutrition.

BMI can be used at the population level; it is a measure of general adiposity. As shown in Figure 5.8 there is a linear relationship between BMI and body fat percentage in under-, normal, and overweight subjects within a BMI-rage between 17 to 31kg/m^2. This association is age- and gender- dependent, it is also different among certain ethnic groups (Box 5.10). Including

Table 5.1 Classification of weight status and central obesity in adults according to body mass index and waist circumference in Caucasian populations.

Classification	Body mass index (kg/m^2)	Waist circumference (cm) women	Waist circumference (cm) men
Underweight	<18.5	≥80	≥94
Normal range	18.5–24.9		
Overweight	≥25.0		
Pre-obese	25.0–29.9		
Obese class I	30.0–34.9	≥88	≥102
Obese class II	35.0–39.9		
Obese class III	>40		

Reproduced with permission of the World Health Organization.
In clinical practice these cut-off-values are used as a basis of decision making, e.g., bariatric surgery may be indicated in obese class II and III patients only.

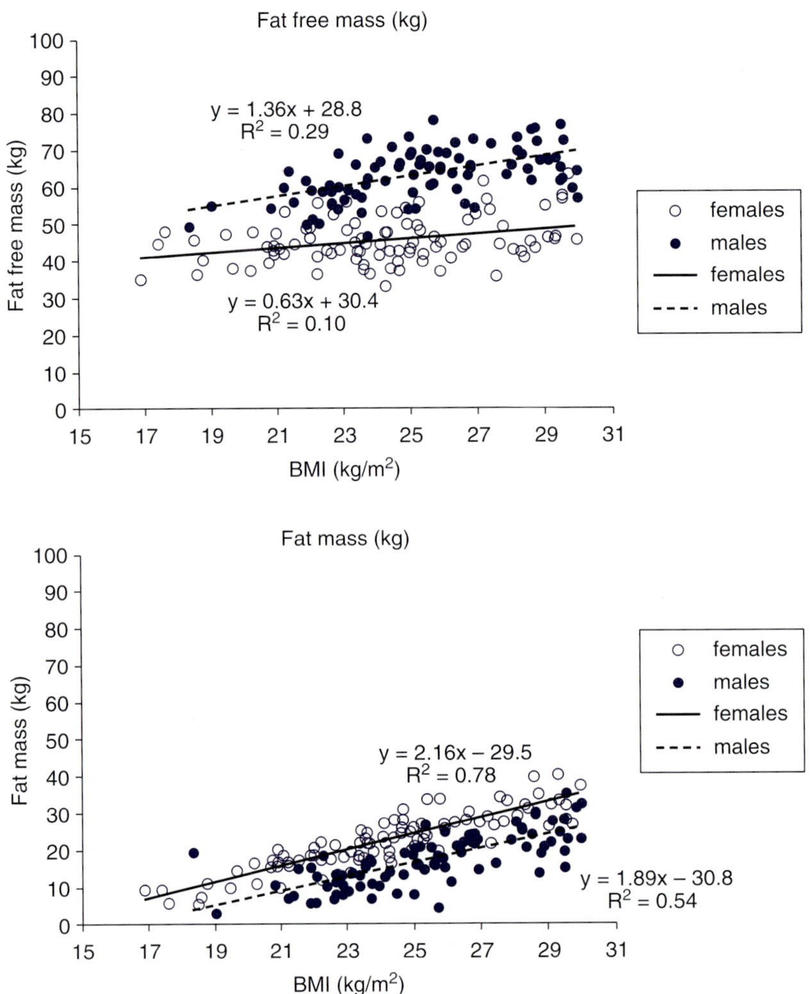

Figure 5.8 Correlation between BMI and fat-free mass (FFM, upper panel) and fat mass (FM, lower panel) in under-, normal- and overweight subjects. Data are taken from the data base of the Kiel Reference Center for Body Composition.

Box 5.10

The relationship between body mass index (BMI) and body fat percentage differs among ethnic groups. For example, compared with Caucasian populations some Asian populations have 3–5% more body fat for the same BMI, age, and gender. The differences can be explained by differences in body build or frame size, subjects with a smaller frame having more body fat at the same BMI.

These differences can have important consequences for the definition of obesity (based on BMI cut-off values) and the prevalence of obesity in a population. In Indonesia, obesity has recently been redefined as BMI ≥ 27 kg/m². At this BMI, Indonesians have a similar body fat to Caucasians with a BMI of 30 kg/m². The lowering of the cut-off point for obesity from 30 to 27 kg/m² increased the prevalence of obesity from less than 5% to over 10%. The World Health Organization (WHO) published new guidelines to redefine "action points" in non-Caucasian populations (WHO, 2004). There are differences in the relationship between BMI and body fat percentage among ethnic groups. Some Aboriginal and Asian people have a higher fat percentage and therefore greater risk for several chronic diseases at a given BMI than Caucasian populations.

obese subjects the association between BMI and body fat percentage becomes curve-linear with a stronger association in the obese compared with the respective association observed in normal- and overweight subjects. However BMI is associated with both major body components, i.e., FM and FFM (see Figure 5.8). BMI has certain limitations at the individual level. At a given BMI, inter-individual variances of FM and FFM are high, for example, FM may vary by more than 100% (Figure 5.8; Müller *et al.*, 2016a). The BMI is inaccurate in subjects with elevated FFM and skeletal muscle mass, such as athletes and body builders, and cannot be generalised among different ethnic groups (Bergman *et al.*, 2011).

WC, hip circumference (HC), Body Adiposity Index (BAI)

WC (as an indirect measure of abdominal fat and VAT), HC and waist-to-hip ratio (WHR) (the ratio of WC to HC as a measure of fat distribution, i.e., the relation between abdominal and gluteal FMs to characterise so-called apple-shaped and pear-shaped body fat distribution) have BMI-independent effects on cardiometabolic risk in overweight and obese subjects (Müller *et al.*, 2016a). For risk assessment, it is recommended to use WC in combination with BMI in overweight and class I obese subjects (see Table 1). BMI, WC, and WHR all have similar correlations to coronary heart disease and ischemic stroke. In addition, BMI, WC, and WHR are inter-correlated with each other (i.e., r = 0.85 between BMI and WC, r = 0.43 between BMI and WHR, and r = 0.70 between WC and WHR) and, thus, they have to be adjusted for each other. Furthermore, WC does not correlate with liver fat. As for BMI, WC is a crude estimate of body composition, metabolic functions, and disease risks associated with individual body components. In daily practice, it is used for risk stratification following the cut-offs given in Table 5.1. *Cut-offs* for defining abdominal obesity were WC-values of 88 cm in women and 102 cm in men (according to the National Cholesterol Education Program Adult Treatment Panel III, 2003 and WHO, 1999) and 80 cm in women and 94 cm in men (according to the International Diabetes Federation; Alberti *et al.*, 2005).

As for WC assessment, different anatomic sites are used. Presently, there are at least eight different protocols and there is no universally accepted protocol for measurement of WC (Bosy-Westphal *et al.*, 2010). Most frequently, WC is measured in the mid-axillar line: (i) below the lowest rib (WC_{rib}, i.e., at the distal border of the lowest rib); (ii) above the iliac crest ($WC_{iliac\ crest}$, i.e., lateral at the superior border of the iliac crest); and (iii) midway between both sites (WC_{middle}, i.e., midway between both measurement sites). Each WC has a stronger correlation with abdominal subcutaneous adipose tissue (aSAT) than with VAT, suggesting that WC is predominantly an index of aSAT, WC cannot differentiate between aSAT and VAT. In men and children, all WC estimates have similar relations with VAT, aSAT, and cardiometabolic risk factors. In women, WCr_{ib} correlates with weight loss-induced decreases in VAT. By contrast, $WC_{iliac\ crest}$ has the lowest associations with VAT and cardiometabolic risk factors in women. In prepubertal and pubertal children, none of the WC measures was consistently better than the other. As far as the association between WC and VAT is concerned the absolute values of the corresponding WC differed among measurement sites. In addition, at both *cut-off* levels (80 or 94 cm and 88 or 102 cm, see Table 5.1), men had ~3.8 times more VAT than women.

Compared with Caucasians of the same WC or BMI, African Americans have a lower VAT and Asians have a higher VAT. Because ethnic differences in body fat distribution may therefore alter the associations between WC sites and VAT, the above-mentioned cut-offs apply to Caucasians only.

The association between WC and VAT is linear with the slopes greater in men compared with women (Bosy-Westphal *et al.*, 2010). Although there are reasonable correlations between all WC and VAT in pre-pubertal and pubertal children, absolute amounts of VAT and the VAT/SAT-ratio are very low in this age group. This observation questions the use of WC, at least in pre-pubertal children.

Today WHR is rarely used only. It is worthwhile mentioning that the authors of the INTERHEART-Study proposed that WHR, rather than WC, is the best adiposity related risk marker to predict myocardial infarction (Yusuf *et al.*, 2005). These data may suggest that while WC (as an index of abdominal fat) is better correlated to risks of metabolic health (e.g., to assess the risk of insulin resistance and hypertriglyceridemia), WHR (as an index of fat distribution) is a better risk marker for cardiovascular health.

For standardisation, WC_{middle} is recommended to assess. In addition to WC, hip circumference (HC) or hip size is measured at the symphysis, i.e., at the level of maximum posterior extension of the buttocks. In the past, HC has been taken as a measure of gluteal fat, it is also correlated with BF%. Measuring HC is rarely done today. It can be used to calculate WHR as a measure of fat distribution. As for WHR, suitable cut-offs are >1.0 and >0.85 in males and females, respectively. HC is also used to calculate the so-called Body Adiposity Index (BAI, i.e.,) ($HC/(height^{1.5})$) - 18 (i.e., BAI can be done without weighing; Bergman *et al.*, 2011). The BAI is in concordance with DXA-derived %body fat with a slope similar to 1.0. However, the relationship between BAI and %FM is not exactly linear. BAI is considered superior BMI in predicting FM and FM-associated health risks (Bergman *et al.*, 2011).

Skinfold thickness measurements (SF), mid-upper arm circumference (MUAC)

Anthropometry applies simple instruments such as low-cost measuring rods and tapes, calipers, and scales that can be safely applied by trained and experienced observers even in remote settings (e.g., during a hunger crisis in Africa).

Body fat is located both internally and subcutaneously, its major component is SAT. If one assumes a constant relationship between subcutaneous fat and total body fat, then total body fat can be estimated by measuring the amount of the SAT. SAT can be assessed as the thickness of the subcutaneous fat layer at different sites of the body using a standardised skinfold caliper (exerting a constant tension of $10 g/mm^2$), infrared inter-actance, or ultrasound measurements. In a given age group, the relation between subcutaneous fat and total fat is indeed relatively constant. However, this relationship is different between males and females, females having relatively more internal fat. Using age- and gender-specific algorithms based on concomitant densitometric and skinfold measurements it is possible to predict the total amount of body fat by measuring skinfolds at different sites of the body.

Skinfolds (SF) can be measured all over the body (see Behnke, 1963; Durnin and Wormersley, 1974; Heymsfield *et al.*, 2005 as references for how to undertake these measurements). The method has a limited precision. SFs for the assessment of total body fat are SFs on the upper arm biceps (biceps SF, BSF) and triceps (triceps SF, TSF) measured at the midpoint of the front or back of the upper arm, under the scapula (subscapular SF, SSF) as measured below and laterally to the left shoulder blade and above the iliac crest (suprailiac SF, SIF). In daily practice, TSF is the most frequently measured SF and it correlates with estimates of total body fat in women and children. SSF is better than TSF as a measure of total body fat in men. SFs should not be used to assess short-term changes in body composition.

The sum of multiple SFs is used to reduce the error in measurement and to correct for possible differences in subcutaneous body fat distribution between subjects within the same age and gender group. In bed-ridden or seriously ill patients the measurement of the trunkal SF (i.e., SSF, SIF) can be difficult. This can be overcome by measuring only the SF at the upper arm. However, the error can be large because the triceps does not necessarily represent the total amount of subcutaneous fat. Assessment of SFs (and mid upper arm circumference, MUAC; see below) may be the only methods of BCA to apply in bed-bound hospitalised patients and when other medical conditions are present that preclude the evaluation of weight, height, and body composition.

With advancing age, the TSF becomes less representative of total body fat. In elderly subjects, the correlation between SFs and total body fat as measured by densitometry is generally lower than in young and middle-aged adults. This is due to an increased amount of internal fat in the elderly. Obese subjects are difficult to measure and the error is large even when measured by trained observers. This is also the case in subjects with oedema, in whom the thickness of SAT is easily overestimated. In patients with human immunodeficiency virus (HIV) and lipodystrophy, peripheral subcutaneous fat may be almost absent, while abdominal fat is increased. In this situation, SFs can be misleading as indicators of total body fat, and should be used only to assess regional fat only.

Various prediction formulae for body fat from SF have been published. For children, in whom the relationship between SF thickness and body fat depends on biological age, separate formulae must be used. The prediction error in BF% is 3–5% compared with densitometry, depending on age, gender, and level of body fatness. Given the possible error in densitometry (3%), this means that in extreme cases body fat may differ from SFs by as much as 10–15%. The calculation of the BF% once the SFs have been measured is very simple. For a given SF, the amount of body fat can be read from a table (see Durnin and Wormersley, 1974; Heymsfield *et al.*, 2005).

Reference values for TSF, BSF, SSF, SIF and the sum of SFs are available by age and sex. Conventional anthropometric data basis are mostly historical and the most frequently used reference charts are those from Durnin and Wormersley (1974). More recent anthropometric reference values have been reported as part of the NHANES study (Freedman *et al.*, 2017; Addo *et al.*, 2017).

Circumferences of arms and legs are used to obtain information on body composition. From the MUAC, in combination with the triceps skinfold thickness, information on muscle mass of the upper arm can be obtained, i.e., mid arm muscle area (MUAMC) as calculated from: MUAC - (π x TSF). Arm muscle area (AMA) can be then calculated from from: $(\text{MUAMC}/4\pi)^2$ - 10 or -6.5 in males and females, respectively. MUAC is measured using a flexible non-stretch tape laid at the midpoint between the acromion process of the shoulder and olecranon process of the ulna, respectively. MUAC is relatively unchanged between the age of six months and five years and it is still used as an age-independent measure of malnutrition in infants and young children (i.e., a MUAC $<$12.5cm). However, MUAC cannot be used as a measure of growth. Most MUAC age-, sex- and also height-related reference data are historical but more recent reference data have been published for US children and adolescents (Addo 2017). In children, malnutrition is defined for a MUAC of less than 80% expected for height.

Rarely available methods

In vivo neutron activation analysis (IVNAA) allows the determination of specific chemical elements in the body. The body is bombarded with fast neutrons of known energy level. The neutrons can be captured by chemical elements (as part of molecules) in the body, resulting in a transition state of higher energy for that element – energy that is finally emitted as gamma rays. For example, capture of neutrons by nitrogen results in the formation of the isotope ^{15}N, which will emit the excess energy as gamma rays:

$$^{14}\text{N} + {}^{1}\text{n} \rightarrow {}^{15}\text{N}^* + \text{gamma rays}$$

where ^{14}N is nitrogen with atomic mass 14, ^{15}N is nitrogen with atomic mass 15, and ^{1}n is a neutron.

With IVNAA, many elements in the body can be determined, including calcium, phosphorus, nitrogen, oxygen, potassium, and chlorine. The information obtained at the atomic level can be converted to more useful information. For example, from total body nitrogen total body protein can be calculated as 6.25 times the total nitrogen, assuming that body protein consists of 16% nitrogen. The disadvantage of IVNAA is not only the price. The subject is irradiated, with the radiation dose used depending on the number and kind of elements to be determined. It is relatively low for nitrogen (0.26mSv) but high for calcium (2.5mSv).

Total body potassium: Chemical carcass analysis has revealed that the amount of potassium in the fat-free body is relatively constant, although the amount of potassium in different tissues varies widely. The determination of total body potassium (TBK) is relatively easy, owing to the natural occurrence of three potassium isotopes (^{39}K, ^{40}K, and ^{41}K), in constant relative amounts, of which ^{40}K is radioactive (gamma emission). Counting the emission of the gamma rays from the body reveals the amount of radioactive potassium, from which TBK and hence FFM and body cell mass (BCM), which contains 98% of TBK, can be calculated. TBK-content of BCM is constant, it is independent of tissue hydration and thus can be used as a risk-free measure of the nutritional status at all stages of life, e.g., during pregnancy, in the first 1000 days of life, during growth and also in disease.

Up until about 50 years ago, there were numerous accessible TBK facilities across the world. However, today this method is rarely used. The chamber in which the subject is scanned has to be carefully shielded to avoid any background radiation (cosmic radiation). The scanning of the body for potassium lasts for 20–30min and the reproducibility is 2–3%.

Several authors have shown that the amount of potassium in the FFM is different between males and females, is lower in obese subjects, and is probably also age dependent. Thus, TBK is much more useful as a measure of body cell mass (BCM) than as a measure of FFM. However, this discrepancy can be used to calculate the "quality" of FFM, defined as the ratio of cellular to extracellular components of FFM, or operationally as BCM/FFM.

Quantitative Magnetic Resonance (QMR) measures FM, lean mass (without solid components that are mainly located in bone) and total body water. QMR technology is based on the modification of spin-patterns of protons in a magnetic field by radiofrequency pulses with each scan producing a series of nuclear magnetic resonance (NMR) responses. The sequence comprises alternating periodic Carr-Purcell-Meiboom-Gill parts and pauses of different duration that are designed to capture all relevant characteristic (relaxation) time scales of the NMR responses (transverse and longitudinal relaxation) typical for fat, lean, and free water. QMR instruments are produced for different sizes ranging from tissue samples >0.3g to small animals, infants and children up to adults <250 kg. In contrast to MRI, QMR requires only a low magnetic field (67 Gauss = 0.0067 Tesla) that can be obtained without complex equipment that entails high maintenance costs. Although QMR has already become a standard of *in vivo* BCA in animals only a few instruments are used worldwide in humans. The QMR instrument is calibrated with canola oil (1 g canola oil at 37°C is assumed to resemble 1 g of human FM). QMR was found to be very accurate and more precise than all conventional body composition methods. The method was predicted to detect >250g changes in FM or >1 kg weight change.

5.4 Applications of body composition methods

Assessment of healthy growth, development and ageing

In children and adolescents, BMI is interpreted by comparison of an individual to age- and sex-specific percentiles from a reference population. In early childhood, the so called adiposity rebound indicates the second rise in the BMI curve that occurs between ages five and seven years. A premature adiposity rebound (e.g., at three to four years) reflects accelerated growth and is often a consequence of low initial BMI that results in increased fat rather than lean body mass after the rebound. An energy deficit early in life may therefore be a risk factor for overweight and obesity. Likewise, infection and malnutrition constrain growth and facilitate subsequent rapid weight gain (upward centile crossing or catch-up growth) that may increase the long-term risk of obesity and non-communicable disease.

Due to the rapid increase in child overweight and obesity worldwide, current BMI-reference percentiles are of limited value for evaluation of weight status. Therefore, cut-off values at childhood percentiles were developed that correspond to the adult values for overweight and obesity 25 and 30 kg/m^2 which are related to morbidity and mortality (Cole *et al.*, 2000). However, BMI is not independent of stature in children and therefore has only low-to-moderate sensitivity in identifying children with excess FM. Changes in body composition during growth determine energy requirement and have a wide range of health implications. During puberty, adolescent growth spurt leads to an increase in FM, FFM and bone mineral content. In girls, FFM increases until the age of 15 years, and remains relatively unchanged thereafter whereas FM increases at a constant rate between 8–16 years, after which the rate of increase slows down. In boys, FFM increases steadily between 8–18 years, with a more rapid increase between 12–15 years whereas FM increases between 8–14 years and decreases again until a plateau is reached at 16 years.

Aging is associated with an increase in FM and a greater relative increase in intra-abdominal fat compared with subcutaneous or total body fat as well as a decrease in muscle and bone mass. In addition, intermuscular, intramuscular and intrahepatic fat are higher in the elderly and associated with insulin resistance. FFM (primarily skeletal muscle) progressively decreases up to 40% from 20 to 70 years of age, whereas FM increases and reaches a maximum at~60–70 years. The increase in lean mass with increasing adiposity is gender-specific but similar between age groups in both genders.

There are various population-based percentiles for FFM and FM (also for FFMI and FMI) e.g., in healthy Caucasian adults (aged 18 to 89 years), children and adolescents (Schutz *et al.*, 2002; Plachta-Danielzik *et al.*, 2012). All these reference data a device- and population-specific.

Assessment of obesity associated cardio-metabolic risk

Although it seems reasonable to recommend that overweight and obesity should be defined based on body composition the use of percentage FM or even FM normalised by height^2 (fat mass index, FMI) is of similar and limited value for cardio-metabolic disease risk prediction at the population level and does not extend beyond the use of BMI or waist circumference. This may be explained by the observation that fat distribution is more important than total FM with respect to the risk of type 2 diabetes and cardiovascular disease. Due to differences in vascularity, adipocyte size, secretome and receptor expression subcutaneous adipose tissue is known to exert less deleterious effects when compared to visceral FM that is prone to inflammatory infiltration and is secreting large quantities of pro-inflammatory, pro-atherogenic cytokines, and free fatty acids. In addition, there is a close correlation between VAT and liver fat that suggests that VAT can be a marker of a high risk body composition phenotype characterised by ectopic fat accumulation in the liver. Importantly, intrahepatic fat is better linked to insulin resistance of the liver, skeletal muscle, and adipose tissue when compared to VAT. Hepatic steatosis is however not necessarily responsible for impaired insulin-stimulated hepatic glycogen synthesis and increased gluconeogenesis. The key is subcellular lipid distribution because hepatic accumulation of diacylglycerol in cytosol but not in the cell membrane was associated with insulin resistance. This finding may also explain the non-association of hepatic steatosis and hepatic insulin resistance in some circumstances of fatty liver that do not involve intracellular diacylglycerol accumulation in hepatocyte. In summary, measurement of fat distribution, ectopic fat and intracellular lipid distribution contribute to our understanding of obesity associated metabolic impairments (see Chapter 9).

Assessment of malnutrition

Malnutrition impairs recovery from disease, trauma and surgery and is associated with increased length of hospital stay, morbidity, and mortality. Screening tools for malnutrition risk assessment used in routine clinical practice are based on anthropometric indices like BMI or MUAC. The European Society for Clinical Nutrition and Metabolism has proposed the following criteria of malnutrition: BMI <18.5 kg/m^2 or weight loss $>10\%$ (indefinite time) or 5% within the last three months, or a BMI <20 or 22 kg/m^2 for patients at age <70 or >70 years, respectively.

In addition, malnutrition has been defined according to detailed body composition data, i.e., a cut-off of FFMI of <17 or <15 kg/m^2 in males and females, respectively (Cederholm *et al.*, 2015). In Caucasian adults, these cut-off data refer to the 10th percentiles of the BIA-reference data obtained in a healthy European population (Schutz *et al.*, 2002). In cancer patients, method specific height squared adjusted cut-offs have been recommended to characterise cancer cachexia, i.e., <32 and <18cm^2 for AMA in males and females, respectively, with corresponding values for appendicular skeletal mass index according to DXA (<7.26 and 5.45 kg/m^2), CT- or MRI-derived muscle area at the height of lumbar vertebra 3 (<55 and 39 cm^2/m^2) and FFMI according to BIA measurements (<14.6 and <11.4 kg/m^2) (Fearon *et al.*, 2013). However, there will be also a problem with different devices (e.g., BIA devices, see box 5.9), but this has not been taken into account by the cut off-values presented by Fearon et la, 2013. These data were calculated from the association between muscularity and the hazard ratio of death where the cut-offs correspond to the threshold of increased health risk (e.g., an increased risk of toxicity related to chemotherapy).

Available bedside tools for BCA are sparse and mainly refined to BIA. Inflammatory diseases enhance catabolism of muscle and loss of FM and contribute to anabolic resistance. The diagnosis of malnutrition therefore ideally includes an evaluation of skeletal muscle and FM. Muscle mass is an important outcome parameter because a low muscle mass is associated with impaired prognosis in patients with chronic disease and reduced life expectancy in healthy subjects, more post-operative complications, increased side effects of medical therapy, impaired quality of life as well as increased health care costs.

The term sarcopenia was originally used to define loss of muscle mass and strength associated with ageing. A low muscle mass also occurs related to an unhealthy lifestyle (inactivity, inadequate diet), diseases and obesity (e.g., insulin resistance, inflammation, oxidative stress), or therapy (e.g., cortisol, operation, chemotherapy). In obese cancer patients, lean mass deficiency is referred to as "hidden cachexia" due to the masking effect of expanded adipose tissue that impedes the clinical identification of lean mass deficiency. The demographic change with an increasing number of elderly people and a concomitant obesity epidemic may increase the prevalence of an overlap between age-related sarcopenia and sarcopenic obesity.

Whole body MRI is the gold standard method for assessment of skeletal muscle mass. Because MRI is laborious and expensive, FFM and LST are often used as a proxy for skeletal muscle mass. However, FFM comprises not only skeletal muscle mass but also organ mass and parts of connective tissue. Because the decrease in muscle mass with age may be compensated by an increase in connective tissue (i.e., an increase in the FFM-component of adipose tissue), FFM is insensitive to age-related changes in muscle mass.

In clinical practice, FFM is mainly measured by DXA (by summing total bone mineral content and LST mass), densitometry (air-displacement plethysmography) or bioelectrical impedance analysis. Percentage of FM (%FM) can be misleading as an indicator of nutritional status in patients with sarcopenia or wasting disease where depletion of lean mass is a crucial factor.

LST can be measured by DXA (total body mass without FM and bone mineral mass) and if derived from arms and legs is a more specific measure for skeletal muscle mass than FFM because most of lean soft tissues from the extremities comes from skeletal muscle mass. This appendicular skeletal muscle mass (ASM) is normalised by height^2 and expressed as skeletal muscle mass index (SMI = ASM [kg] /height [m]^2).

Acute or chronic diseases lead to tissue catabolism and a decrease in BCM with a concomitant increase in FFM-hydration. These changes in the composition of FFM violate the assumptions of two-compartment methods for BCA and also for the determination of skeletal muscle mass by MRI, DXA or BIA. Changes in the quality of lean tissue are however an important determinant of patients′ prognosis and a more valid outcome parameter than an accurate assessment of total FFM. Phase angle by BIA is therefore an established indicator of mortality because it may reflect changes in tissue cellularity, hydration and the integrity of cell membranes. Phase angle is one component of Bioelectrical impedance vector analysis (BIVA). Monitoring an individual patient′s impedance vector in the vector graph (Figure 5.7) extends the information of phase angle (vector angle to the x-axis of the BIVA graph) by information on vector length that is related to fluid shifts). BIVA is therefore increasingly recognised as a promising technique in monitoring the nutritional and hydration status and, thus, the composition or quality of muscle mass or FFM of individual patients with different types of diseases. Therefore, BIVA adds to the information of DXA or MRI data as direct estimates of skeletal muscle mass while BIVA does not replace these techniques.

Assessment of changes in energy balance and energy intake

Long-term changes in energy balance can be estimated from changes in FM and FFM. The energy equivalents (or so-called energy densities) of FM and FFM are lower during weight loss (9,500 kcal/kg or 39·7 MJ/kg FM lost and 1020 kcal/kg or 4·39 MJ/kg FFM lost) when compared with weight gain (13,100 kcal/kg FM gained and 2,200 kcal/kg of FFM gained) because they include the energy cost of tissue synthesis (Hall 2012; Box 5.11).

Box 5.11

Energy-partitioning with weight gain and weight loss can be expressed as protein energy (gained or lost) as a fraction of total tissue energy (protein +fat) gained or lost (= p-ratio). So, the p-ratio for weight loss can be calculated as:

$$\text{p-ratio} = \frac{\Delta FFM}{\Delta FFM + 9.05 \times \Delta FM}$$

where 9·05 is the ratio of energy equivalents for FFM and FM (38.9/4.3 MJ/kg).

People with a higher percentage of FM have a greater proportion of weight loss as FM compared to leaner people. The "Forbes rule" developed by Gilbert Forbes (1987) describes the composition of weight loss as a function of the initial FM and magnitude of weight loss (Δ BW):

$$\Delta FFM / \Delta BW = 10 \cdot 4 / (10 \cdot 4 + FM)$$

Among two people with the same body weight, the person with the higher %FM will therefore have a slower rate of weight loss at the same energy intake because of a higher contribution and energy content of FM to weight loss.

Since assessment of energy intake (EI) by self-report is inaccurate (by a mean of 15-20% of expected values reaching about -50% in obese subjects) there is need of its quantitative assessment. EI can be quantitatively calculated from changes in body composition and a measure of energy expenditure (EE) (i.e., either by doubly labeled water, DLW, or assessment of resting energy expenditure (REE) by indirect calorimetry plus application of a validated activity monitor). This idea is based on mathematical modeling using a 2C-model with changes of FM and FFM during overfeeding and caloric restriction (Hall 2012) given that the estimates of individual body components expenditure are accurate. Then for a given time period (T), EI (in kcal/d) is calculated from:

$$1020 \times \Delta FFM(kg) / \Delta T + 9500 \times \Delta FM(kg) / \Delta T + EE(\text{kcal/d})$$

(Shook 2018). This is called the Intake Balance Method (IBM). Over longer observation periods this method provides an accurate measure of EI (i.e., at the population level it is within agreement of about 40 kcal/d). However, the limited precision of body composition methods at the individual level limits the application of the IBM for short-term measurements in individuals.

Application of BCA in the context of precision and validity of techniques applied

Measurement of changes in FFM and FM with weight loss and weight gain is limited by the systematic and random errors (validity and precision) of methods for body composition analysis

Precision is based on the test–retest reliability of FFM and FM measurements in weight stable persons and can be given as SD, relative SD (SD/mean) or percent relative SD ((SD/mean) x 100). When comparing the precision of different methods as % relative SD the size of the compartment should be considered: a precision of 2% for FM in a lean person with 10 kg FM and 80 kg FFM contributes to a very high precision in the larger FFM compartment whereas a precision of 2% in the measurement of FFM results in a poor precision of 16% in the smaller FM compartment.

The precision determines the minimal detectable change (MDC) in FFM and FM (i.e., the amount by which a patient's FM needs to change to be sure the change is greater than measurement error, Box 5.12).

The **validity** of body composition measurements in the initial phase of weight loss is a challenge to all two-compartment methods because these methods can only distinguish between FM

Box 5.12

The MDC can be interpreted as the magnitude of change below which there is more than a 95% chance that no real change has occurred. MDC is calculated as:

$$MDC_{95} = 1.96 * \sqrt{2} * SEM \quad 1$$

1.96 is the two-sided tabled z-value for the 95% CI of no change; √2 is used to account for the variance of two measurements that are involved in measuring change; SEM (standard error of measurement) links the reliability of the measurement instrument to the standard deviation of the population: SEM = SD√(1-reliability), reliability = Pearson's correlation co-efficient between test and retest values.

The MDC can also be expressed as a percentage, which is defined as:

$$MDC_{95}\% = (MDC_{95} / \text{mean}) \times 100 \quad 2$$

The mean is the mean for all of the measures for test and retest.

The MDC for FM determined in lean subjects lies between 1 and 2 kg for densitometry, DXA, deuterium dilution and bioelectrical impedance analysis. Quantitative magnetic resonance (QMR) has an exceptionally high precision that leads to a MDC >250 g FM.

and FFM by assuming a constant composition of FFM. With weight loss, up to 300 g glycogen are catabolised and about 500 g water and associated electrolytes are lost from intracellular compartments. Additional intracellular water losses come from accelerated protein degradation whereas the decrease in insulin levels contributes to a negative sodium balance and a concomitant loss in extracellular water. A negative water balance and thus a lower hydration of FFM lead to a method-inherent bias using deuterium dilution, densitometry, or dual X-ray absorptiometry. Because of similar densities of fat and water (0.9007 and 0.99371 g/cm^3) a decrease in FFM-hydration leads to an increase body density and thus to an overestimation of the loss in FM by air displacement plethysmography, under water weighing and dual X-ray absorptiometry. By contrast, deuterium dilution overestimates the loss of FFM and thus underestimates FM loss. To overcome these limitations of two-compartment methods, hydration can be measured by a combination of deuterium dilution with DXA or ADP in a three-compartment model. By contrast, long-term changes in body composition that exceed the initial rapid phase of weight loss can be measured without bias using two-compartment methods.

Adjusting metabolic and endocrine functions

There is a high inter-individual variance in metabolic and endocrine data. Therefore a quantitative and predictive framework is needed to normalise these data. If metabolic and endocrine variables are closely related to body weight and individual body components (as is the case e.g., for resting energy expenditure (REE) *vs.* body mass and FFM and plasma leptin levels *vs.* body mass and FM) a suitable adjustment is needed. FFM is the major determinant of REE. Within a "normal" population (characterised by an FFM range between 40 to 80 kg) REE scales linearly with FFM explaining 60-85% of its variance. Since the REE to FFM relationship has a non-zero intercept, thus, simple REE/body weight or REE/FFM-ratios are misleading, i.e., these ratios decrease with increasing body weight suggesting that when compared with normal weight subjects, overweight subjects have a lower metabolic rate per kg of body weight. To avoid erroneous conclusions REE should be expressed in terms of FFM using a multiple regression analysis taking into account the slopes and the intercepts of the REE on body mass (or REE on FFM) relationship (Ravussin *et al.*, 1989). Since FFM has a heterogeneous composition and it's individual organs differ with respect to their specific metabolic rates (e.g., energy expenditure of the heart is about 440 kcal/d compared with that of skeletal muscle of about 13 kcal/d; Müller *et al.*, 2002) a further adjustment of REE for the composition of FFM reduces the non-zero intercept (Müller *et al.*, 2018).

Functional Body Composition (FBC)

Body composition data are mostly about absolute or relative values and normative data are used as a reference for comparison of individual data. To go on, individual body components and their inter-relationships have to be seen in the context of their related functions.

FBC is about interpretation of body functions (e.g., REE or leptin secretion or insulin resistance) and their disturbances by body composition as well as the interpretation of the meaning of individual body components in the context of related functions (Müller, 2013; Müller *et al.*, 2016b). FBC takes into account the relationship between different body components. It thus combines different levels of body composition (e.g., the anatomical and the physical properties of body components). In addition, FBC integrates body components into different regulatory systems (e.g., FFM and FM as determinants of REE which is under control of Sympathetic Nervous System (SNS) thyroid status and leptin) and into substrate metabolism (e.g., muscle mass as a determinant of protein and glucose turnover turnover). Finally, FBC relates to systemic outcomes, e.g., body temperature, heart rate, glomerular filtration and respiration.

To summarise, FBC is about horizontal (i.e., within a level) and vertical (i.e., between levels taking into account neuro-endocrine control and metabolism) relationships between body components and their related functions finally reaching systemic outcomes like heart rate, body temperature etc. (Figure 5.9; Müller *et al.*, 2016b).

"Healthy" body composition is about the relationships between masses of organs, tissues and

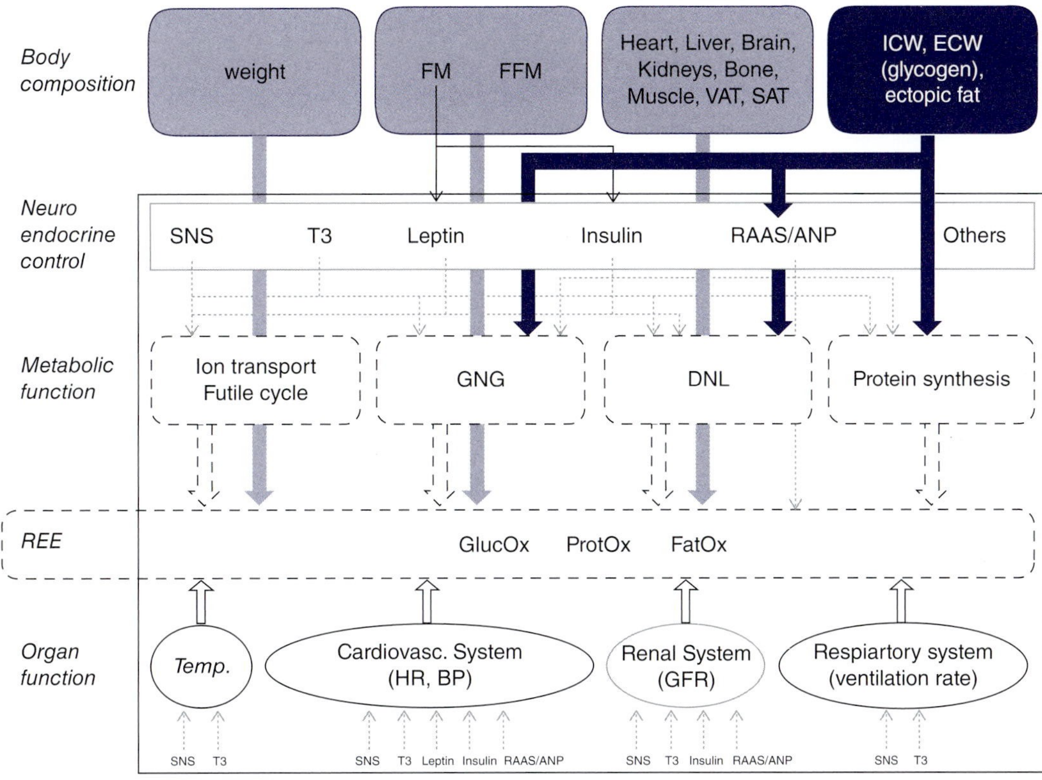

Figure 5.9 Proposed model of metabolism (REE, resting energy expenditure; GluOx, ProtOX and FatOx: substrate oxidation rates) based on its structural and functional determinants (FFM, fat free mass; FM, fat mass; VAT, visceral adipose tissue; SAT, subcutaneous adipose tissue; SNS, sympathetic nervous system activity; T3, 3,5,3′ triiodothyronine; RAAS, rennin angiotensin aldosterone system; ANP, atrial natriuretic peptide; GNG, gluconeogenesis; DNL, de novo lipogenesis; GlucOx; glucose' oxidation; ProtOX, protein oxidation; FatOx, lipid oxidation; HR, heart rate; BP, blood pressure; GFR, glomerular filtration rate; Temp, body temperature) defining healthy body composition (HBC) by hierarchical multi-level-multi-scale analysis. (reproduced from Müller *et al.*, 2016b)

body components and functions in the context of neuroendocrine control adding up to whole body systems. These relationships display mechanisms of biological control (e.g., by hormones as well as by inter-organ/tissue cross talks mediated by substrates and cytokines) and determinants of specific body functions (e.g., REE and glucose metabolism). Using a *multi-level/multi-scale approach* it is possible to integrate and combine data horizontally (i.e., between compartments, organs, and tissues, and at the cellular level) and vertically (from masses to functions taking into account neuroendocrine control, metabolism, and different organ systems).

So-called "Body component units" (BCU) are a further extension of the FBC-concept. A BCU is on the inter-relationship of organs and tissues with a further focus on their interactive associations as well as their metabolic and/or inflammatory impact. BCU are health-related; for example, a "skeletal muscle mass-VAT-CRP-unit" is added to explain the issue of sarcopenia. In addition, a "BMC-SAT-leptin/skeletal muscle mass-muscle strength unit" characterises the issues of frailty and osteoporosis. Similarly, a "liver fat-VAT-epicardial fat/muscle mass-unit" changes with positive or negative energy balance and impacts insulin sensitivity and inflammation. Finally, a "muscle mass-organ mass-SNS activity + T3-unit" explains inter-individual variances in REE. BCUs reflects functional traits, which are worthwhile to study.

A related concept is the so-called "capacity-load-model" integrating two traits, which maintain and challenge homeostasis and thus are related to the risk of Non-communicable Diseases (NCD), e.g., diabetes mellitus (Wells, 2010 and 2017). In this concept "metabolic capacity" (i.e., muscle mass and glucose utilisation, pancreatic ß-cell function and insulin

Table 5.2 A problem-oriented approach to the assessment of the nutritional status. See Figure 5.9 and text for further details.

Anthropometric, two-compartment model	Age (y), sex (m,f), weight (kg), height (cm), BMI (kg/m^2), WC (cm) FFM, FM. first line approach; crude stratification of patients according to overweight, underweight, at cardiometabolic risk.
Composition of FFM (kg)	MM, bone mass, brain, heart, liver, kidneys, spleen, residual mass (i.e., lung, pancreas etc). targeted approach in patients with sarcopenia, osteoporosis, diseases of specific organs etc.
Composition of FM (kg)	TAT, SAT, VAT, liver fat targeted approach in overweight and obese patients at cardio-metabolic risk
Physical characteristic	Density, hydration, phase angle, resistance, reactance targeted approach in patients with fluid imbalances and in cachectic patients
Cardio-metabolic risk factors, systemic correlates	Insulin, HOMA, adiponectin, leptin, thyroid hormones, plasma lipids, CRP, blood pressure, temperature, heart rate, GFR, respiration. assessing neuroendocrine, metabolic and systemic correlates of body composition
Functional body composition units	Relation between: MM ↔ IR; VAT or SAT ↔ IR, Hypertension; MM ↔ BMD; MM ↔ muscle strength; VAT/SAT ↔ CRP, lipid profile; MM/VAT ↔ CRP; Ghrelin/Leptin ↔ BW, FM, FM/FFM; MM,OM. addressing functional body composition (FBC)

FFM, fat free mass; MM, muscle mass; RM, residual mass, FM, fat mass; TAT, total adipose tissue; SAT, subcutaneous adipose tissue; VAT, visceral adipose tissue; GFR, glomerular filtration rate; HOMA,

secretion) promotes glucose homeostasis whereas the "metabolic load" (i.e., as characterized by the sum of liver fat + glycemic load + inactivity) challenges glucose homeostasis. Then, diabetes may result from both, a low "capacity" and a high "load". By contrast to a "low metabolic capacity", a high "metabolic load. The "capacity-load model" is used to define phenotypes worthwhile to study as well as to predict disease risks (Siervo *et al.*, 2015).

A problem-oriented approach to the assessment of nutritional status

Based on the concept of FBC, BCA should follow a systematic and stratified approach based on the question of interest. Today the routine assessment of the nutritional status covers anthropometrics, including the assessments of BMI and waist circumference as well as a 2C-model of body composition. These data serve as a basis for further stratification according to weight status and a crude risk assessment. A deeper phenotyping includes the composition of FFM and FM with special reference to regional differences. To assess the physical properties of the body and its components adds to the understanding of the mass-dependent functions. In a clinical setting, masses and properties of organs and tissues have then to be seen in the context of related risk factors, neuro-endocrine control, metabolism, and systemic outcomes. Finally, functional body component units have to be generated based on a problem-oriented approach. Insulin resistance, for example, is seen in the context of muscle mass, liver fat and VAT. Regional fat depots, and the ratio of muscle mass to VAT have to be characterised in the context of plasma lipids and inflammation, etc. (see Table 5.2). BCA, thus, is an integrated part of assessment; it is a prerequisite for detailed phenotyping of individuals providing a sound basis for in depth biomedical research and clinical decision making.

Acknowledgement

This chapter has been revised and updated by Anja Bosy-Westphal, Manfred J. Müller and Paul Deurenberg, based on the original chapter by Paul Deurenberg and Ronenn Roubenoff. Anja Bosy- Westphal is a consultant for seca Gmbh & Co. KG, Hamburg, Germany.

References

Addo, O., Himes, J.H., Zemel, B.S. (2017). Reference ranges for midupper arm circumference, upper arm muscle area, and upper arm fat area in US children and adolescents aged 1-20 y. *Am J Clin Nutr.* 105:111–120.

Alberti, K.G., Zimmet, P., and Shaw, J. (2005). IDF Epidemiology Task Force Consensus Group. The metabolic syndrome-a new worldwide definition. *Lancet* 366:1059–62.

Baracos, V., Caserotti, P., Earthman, C.P. *et al.* (2012). Advances in the science and application of body composition measurement. *JPEN J Parenteral Enteral Nutr.* 36: 96–107.

Behnke, A.R. (1963). Anthropometric evaluation of body composition throughout life. *Ann New York Acad Sci.* 110: 450–464.

Behnke, A.R. and Royce, J. (1966). Body size, shape, and composition in several types of athletes. *J Sports Med Phys Fitness.* 6: 75–88.

Bergman, R.N., Stefanovski, D., Buchanan, T.A. *et al* (2011). A better index of body adiposity. *Obesity* 19: 1083–1089.

Bosy-Westphal, A., Booke, C.A., Blöcker, T. *et al.* (2010). Measurement site for waist circumference affects its accuracy as an index of visceral and abdominal subcutaneous fat in a Caucasian population. *J Nutr.* 140: 954–961.

Bosy-Westphal, A. and Müller, M.J. (2015). Identification of skeletal muscle mass depletion across age and BMI groups in health and disease--there is need for a unified definition. *Int J Obes (Lond).* 39:379–86.

Bosy-Westphal, A. and Müller, M.J. (2014). Measuring the impact of weight cycling on body composition: a methodological challenge. *Curr Opin Clin Nutr Metab Care.* 17:396–400.

Bosy-Westphal, A., Schautz, B., Later, W. *et al* (2013). What makes a BIA equation unique? Validity of eight-electrode multifrequency BIA to estimate body composition in a healthy adult population. *Eur J Clin Nutr.* 67 Suppl 1: S14–21.

Bosy-Westphal, A., Jensen, B., Braun, W. *et al* (2017). Quantification of whole-body and segmental skeletal muscle mass using phase-sensitive 8-electrode medical bioelectrical impedance devices. *Eur J Clin Nutr.* 71:1061–1067.

Cederholm, T., Bosaeus, I., Barazzoni, R. *et al.* Diagnostic criteria for malnutrition - an ESPEN consensus statement. *Clin Nutr.* 34:335–340.

Cole, T.J., Bellizzi, M.C., Flegal, K.M. *et al.* (2000). Establishing a standard definition for child overweight and obesity worldwide: international survey. *BMJ.* 320(7244):1240–3.

Dixon, W.T. (1984). Simple proton spectroscopic imaging. *Radiology.* 153:189–194.

Durnin, J.V.G.A. and Womersley, J. (1974). Body fat assessed from total body density and its estimation from skinfold thickness: measurements on 481 men and women aged from 17 to 72 years. *Br J Nutr.* 32: 77–97.

Fassini, P.G., Nicoletti, C.F., Pfrimer, K. *et al* (2016). Bioelectrical impedance vector analysis as a useful predictor of nutritional status in patients with short bowel syndrome. *Clin Nutr.* 36: 1117–1121.

Fearon, K., Arends, J., and Baracos, V. (2013). Understanding the mechanisms and treatment options in cancer cachexia. *Nat Rev Clin Oncol.* 10: 90–99.

Forbes, G.B. (1987). *Human Body Composition*. New York: Springer.

Foster, K.R. and Lukaski, H.C. (1996). Whole-body impedance-what does it measure? *Am J Clin Nutr.* 64 (3 Suppl): 388S–396S.

Freedman, D.S., Zemel, B.S., and Ogden, C.L. (2017). Secular trends for skinfolds differ from those of BMI and waist circumference among adults examined in NHANES from 1988-1994 through 2009-2010. *Am J Clin Nutr.* 105:169–176.

Gallagher, D., Belmonte, D., Deurenberg, P. *et al* (1998). Organ-tissue mass measurement by MRI allows accurate in vivo modeling of REE and metabolic active tissue mass. *Am J Physiol.* 275: E249–258.

The GBD 2015 Obesity Collaborators (2017). Health effects of overweight and obesity in 195 countries over 25years. *N Engl J Med* 377: 13–27.

Geisler, C.F., Prado, C.M., and Müller, M.J. (2016). Inadequacy of Body Weight-Based Recommendations for Individual Protein Intake-Lessons from Body Composition Analysis. *Nutrients* 9 (1). pii: E23.

Hall, K. (2012). Modeling metabolic adaptations and energy regulation in humans. *Ann Rev Nutr.* 32:35–54.

Heymsfield, S.B., Lohman, T.G., Wang, Z.W. *et al.* (2005). *Human Body Composition*, 2e. Champaign, IL.: Human Kinetics

Hu, H.H. and Kan, H.E. (2013). Quantitative Proton Magnetic Resonance Techniques for Measuring Fat. *NMR Biomed.* 26: 1609–1629.

Kivimäki, M., Kuosma, E., Ferrie, J.E. *et al* (2017). Overweight, obesity, and risk of cardiometabolic multimorbidity: pooled analysis of indivudual-level data for 120813 adults from 16 cohort studies from the USA and Europe. *Lancet Public Health* 2: e277–e285.

Later, W., Bosy-Westphal, A., Kossel, E. *et al.* (2010). Is the 1975 reference man still a suitable reference? *Eur J Clin Nutr.* 64: 954–961.

Lemos, T. and Gallagher, D. (2017). Current body composition measurement techniques. *Curr Opin Endocrinol Diabetes Obes.* 24:310–314.

Lukaski, H.C., Bolonchuk, W.W., Hall, C.B. *et al.* (1986). Validity of tetrapolar bioelectrical impedance method to assess human body composition. *J Appl Physiol.* 60: 1327–1332.

Lukaski, H.C. (Ed.). (2017). *Body Composition: Health and Performance in Exercise and Sport*. Productivity Press.

McLaughlin, P.D., Chawke, L., Twomey, M. *et al.* (2018). Body composition determinants of radiation dose during abdomino-pelvic CT. *Insights Imaging.* 9:9–16.

Müller, M.J., Bosy-Westphal, A., Kutzner, D. *et al.* (2002). Metabolically active components of fat free mass and resting energy expenditure in humans: Recent lessons from imaging technologies. *Obesity Rev.* 3: 113–122.

Müller, M.J. (2013). From BMI to functional body composition. *Eur J Clin Nutr.* 67: 1119–1121.

Müller, M.J., Baracos, V., Bosy-Westphal, A. *et al.* (2013). Functional body composition and related aspects in research on obesity and cachexia: report on the 12th Stock Conference held on 6 and 7 September 2013 in Hamburg, Germany. *Obes Rev.* 15:640–56.

Müller, M.J., Braun, W., Enderle, J. *et al.* (2016a). Beyond BMI: Conceptual issues related to overweight and obese patients. *Obesity Facts* 9: 193–205.

Müller, M.J., Braun, W., Pourhassan, M. *et al.* (2016b). Application of standards and models in body composition analysis. *Proc Nutr Soc.* 75: 181–187.

Müller, M.J., Geisler, C., Hübers, M. *et al.* (2018). Normalizing resting energy expenditure across life course in humans: challenges and hopes. *Eur J Clin Nutr.* 72 (5 May 2018): in press.

Plachta-Danielzik, S., Gehrke, M.I., Kehden, B. *et al.* (2012). Body fat percentiles for German children and adolescents. *Obes facts.* 5: 77–90.

Prado, C.M., Baracos, V.E., McCargar, L.J. *et al.* (2007). Body composition as an independent determinant of 5-fluorouracil-based chemotherapy toxicity. *Clin Cancer Res.* 13:3264–8.

Prado CM, Baracos VE, McCargar LJ, et al. (2009). Sarcopenia as a determinant of chemotherapy toxicity and time to tumor progression in metastatic breast cancer patients receiving capecitabine treatment. *Clin Cancer Res.* 15:2920–6.

Prado, C.M. and Heymsfield, S.B. (2014). Lean tissue imaging: a new era for nutritional assessment and intervention. *J Par Enter Nutr.* 38: 940–953.

Ravussin, E., Bogardus, C. (1989). Relationship of genetics, age, and physical fitness to daily energy expenditure and fuel utilization. *Am J Clin Nutr.* 49:968–975.

Schutz, Y., Kyle, U.U.G., and Pichard, C. (2002). Fat free mass index and fat mass index percentiles for Caucasians aged 18-24 y. *Int J Obes.* 26:953–960.

Schweitzer, L., Geisler, C., Pourhassan, M. *et al.* What is the best reference site for a single MRI slice to assess whole body skeletal muscle and adipose tissue volumes in healthy adults? *Am J Clin Nutr.* 102:58–65.

Segal, KR, Van Loan M, Fitzgerald PI *et al.* (1988). Lean body mass estimation by bio-electrical impedance analysis: a four site cross-validation study. *Am J Clin Nutr.* 47: 7–14.

Shen W, Chen J, Gantz M *et al.* (2012). A Single MRI Slice Does Not Accurately Predict Visceral and Subcutaneous Adipose Tissue Changes During Weight Loss. Obesity (Silver Spring), 20: 2458–2463.

Shook RB, Hand GA, O'Connor DP *et al.* (2018). Energy intake derived from energy balance equation, validated activity monitors, and Dual X-ray aborptiometry provide acceptable energy intake data among young adults. *J Nutr.* 148: 490–496.

Siervo M, Prado C, Mire E *et al.* (2015). Body composition indices of a low-capacity model: gender- and BMI-specific reference curves. Public Health Nutr. 18: 1245–1254.

Siri, W.E. (1961). Body composition from fluid spaces and density: analysis of methods. In: *Techniques for Measuring Body Composition* (ed. J. Brozek and A. Henschel). Washington, DC: National Academy of Sciences, pp. 223–244.

Teigen, L.M., Kuchnia, A.J., Mourtzakis, M. *et al.* (2017). The Use of Technology for Estimating Body CompositionStrengths and Weaknesses of Common Modalities in a Clinical Setting. Nutr Clin Pract. 32:20–29.

Visser, M., Heuvel, van den E., and Deurenberg, P. (1994). Prediction equations for the estimation of body composition in the elderly using anthropometric data. *Br J Nutr.* 71: 823–833.

Wells, J.C. (2010). *The Evolutionary Biology of Human Body Fat: Thrift And Control.* Cambridge: Cambridge University Press.

Wells, J.C.K. (2017). Body composition and susceptibility to type 2 diabetes: an evolutionary perspective. *Eur J Clin Nutr.* 71:881–889.

WHO (1999). *Definition, diagnosis and classification of diabetes mellitus and its complications: report of a WHO consultation*. Geneva: WHO.

WHO Expert Consultation (2004). Appropriate body-mass index for Asian populations and its implications for policy and intervention strategies. *Lancet* 363: 157–163.

Yusuf, S., Hawken, S., Ounpuu, S. et al (2005). INTERHEART Study Investigators. Obesity and the risk of myocardial infarction in 27,000 participants from 52 countries: a case-control study. *Lancet* 366:1640–9.

6
Energy Metabolism

Gareth A. Wallis

Key messages

- Energy balance in the body is the balance between how much energy is consumed (energy intake) and how much energy is expended (energy expenditure). Individuals who maintain their body weight over a sustained period of time are considered to be in a state of energy balance. A reduction or gain in body weight is attributable to sustained periods of negative or positive energy balance, respectively.
- Energy intake corresponds to the energy content of macronutrients in foods. The metabolisable energy content of the macronutrients within foods is as follows: carbohydrate (16 kJ/g, 3.8 kcal/g), protein (17 kJ/g, 4.0 kcal/g), fat (37 kJ/g, 9.0 kcal/g). In addition, alcohol provides 29 kJ/g (6.9 kcal/g).
- Energy intake is a behaviour governed by appetite sensations, with the overall drive to eat controlled by a complex interplay of biological homeostatic mechanisms and psychological or other non-homeostatic factors.
- Total energy expenditure is generally composed of three components: basal or resting metabolic rate (BMR or RMR), thermic effect of food, and physical activity energy expenditure. BMR or RMR refers to the energy cost of basic physiological functions such as heartbeat, muscle function, and respiration. The thermic effect of food is about 10% of the energy content of consumed food, and is needed to digest, metabolise, and store ingested macronutrients.
- Total energy expenditure and its components can be measured by direct (calorimetry) or indirect (indirect calorimetry) methods; for the latter, measurements of respiratory gas exchange determine rates of oxygen consumption and carbon dioxide production which are used to calculate energy expenditure. The doubly labelled water technique is the gold standard approach for measuring total energy expenditure in free-living environments, typically over 7 to 14 day periods.
- Energy requirement is the amount of food energy needed to balance energy expenditure in order to maintain body size, body composition, and a level of physical activity consistent with long-term good health. This includes the energy needs for optimal growth and development in children, and the needs of pregnancy and lactation (deposition of tissue and milk production, respectively).
- Obesity is the most common form of a disruption in energy balance and now constitutes one of the major and most prevalent disorders related to nutrition. Obesity arises from a sustained period of positive energy balance; that is an overconsumption of energy relative to energy expended. A sustained period of negative energy balance is required to attain a healthy body weight in obese individuals. Negative energy balance can be achieved by reducing energy intake or increasing energy expenditure (particularly physical activity energy expenditure). However, powerful signals exist to resist against negative energy balance, and this may explain the failure of many individuals to achieve and maintain successful body weight loss.

6.1 Introduction

Definition and conceptualisation of energy balance

Energy balance is classically defined as dietary energy intake minus total energy expenditure. It is the amount of dietary energy added to or lost from the body's energy stores after the body's physiological systems have done all their work for the day. Individuals who maintain their body weight over a sustained period of time are considered to be in a state of energy balance. A reduction or gain in body weight is attributable

Introduction to Human Nutrition, Third Edition. Edited on behalf of The Nutrition Society by Susan A. Lanham-New, Thomas R. Hill, Alison M. Gallagher and Hester H. Vorster.

Companion website: www.wiley.com/go/lanham-new/humannutrition

to a sustained period of negative or positive energy balance, respectively. The concept of energy balance follows the principles driven by the first law of thermodynamics, which states that energy can neither be destroyed nor created. While the definition and concept of energy balance may appear straightforward, its regulation is less so. This is because dietary energy intake and energy expenditure are not simply static independent components of energy balance. They are dynamic variables that interact with each other and body weight to influence physiology, behaviour, and ultimately overall energy balance. This chapter will overview the components and determinants of dietary energy intake and total energy expenditure. This will be followed by describing the energy requirements of various populations and sub-groups. Finally, implications of the complexity of energy balance regulation will be considered in the context of obesity, which continues to be a major public health issue.

Components of energy balance

Energy intake

Energy intake is defined as the energy content of food (and drink) ingested as provided by the major sources of dietary energy: carbohydrate, protein, fat, and alcohol. The gross energy content of a food can be measured by bomb calorimetry, which involves combustion of a known weight of food inside a sealed chamber and measuring the amount of heat that is produced during this process. However, not all gross energy in food is available for human metabolism because of losses during food utilisation. Accordingly, the energy available from food is defined as metabolisable energy. In the United Kingdom (UK), metabolisable energy is the value quoted as the energy content of foods on food labels and composition tables. It can be calculated from the amounts of carbohydrate (16 kJ/g, 3.8 kcal/g), protein (17 kJ/g, 4.0 kcal/g), fat (37 kJ/g, 9.0 kcal/g), and alcohol (29 kJ/g, 6.9 kcal/g) in the food, which are determined by chemical analysis (4.184 kJ = 1 kcal). Thus, if the macronutrient gram quantities of any type of food are known, the energy content can be easily calculated. For example, if a protein-rich nutrition snack contains 21 g of carbohydrate, 6 g of fat, and 14 g of protein then the total energy content is $(21 \times 16) + (6 \times 37) + (14 \times 17) =$ 796 kJ (190 kcal). The macronutrient composition is often expressed as the percentage contribution of each macronutrient to the total energy content of a food or diet. If a food has a carbohydrate content of 21 g, which is 336 kJ, and the total energy content is 796 kJ the proportion of energy derived from carbohydrate is 42%; the fat content is 6 g, or 222 kJ, equivalent to 28% of the energy, and the protein contributes 14 g, 238 kJ and 30% of the energy.

Energy expenditure

The energy that is consumed in the form of food is required by the body for metabolic, cellular, and mechanical work such as breathing, heartbeat, and muscular work, all of which require energy and result in heat production. Total energy expenditure is generally composed of three components: basal or resting metabolic rate (BMR or RMR), thermic effect of food, and physical activity energy expenditure. Growth, pregnancy, and lactation are other components that can contribute to energy expenditure and these will be addressed later in this chapter.

BMR or RMR (also called basal or resting energy expenditure) refers to the energy expended by the body to maintain basic physiological functions (e.g., heartbeat, muscle contraction and function, respiration). BMR represents the minimum level of energy expended by the body to sustain life in the awake state. It is measured after a 12 hour fast while the individual is resting physically and mentally, and maintained in a thermoneutral, quiet environment. The BMR is slightly elevated above the metabolic rate during sleep (sleeping metabolic rate) due to the energy cost of arousal. The RMR is often measured due to practical convenience, whereby similar controlled environmental conditions are applied as for the determination of BMR but without the need for adherence to a 12 hour fast. The terms BMR and RMR are often used interchangeably, although energy expenditure will be slightly higher (~3%) when RMR is determined. RMR occurs in a continued manner throughout the 24 hours of a day and remains relatively constant within individuals over time. RMR typically comprises the largest component of energy expenditure, ranging from 40–70% of total energy expenditure, depending on age and lifestyle.

In addition to RMR, there is an increase in energy expenditure in response to food intake. Often referred to as the thermic effect of food (or diet-induced thermogenesis), this increase in energy expenditure reflects the energy that is expended to digest, absorb, and metabolise ingested food and nutrients. The energy cost associated with food ingestion is primarily influenced by the quantity and composition of the food that is consumed, and also is relatively stable within individuals over time. For typical diet compositions, the thermic effect of food constitutes approximately 10% of the energy content of the meal that is consumed. Physical activity energy expenditure is the term used to describe the increase in energy expenditure that occurs during physical activity that is caused primarily by the use of skeletal muscles for any type of physical movement. It is important to note that physical activity energy expenditure encompasses all forms of physical activity, including structured volitional exercise and physical activity related to activities of daily living, often referred to as spontaneous physical activity or non-exercise activity thermogenesis. Physical activity energy expenditure usually accounts for 25–50% of energy expenditure but is the most variable component of daily energy expenditure and can vary greatly within and between individuals due to the volitional and variable nature of physical activity patterns.

Energy balance

Energy balance occurs when metabolisable energy intake is matched to total energy expenditure. It is important to note that energy balance can occur regardless of the levels of energy intake and expenditure. Energy balance can occur in very inactive individuals as well as highly active individuals provided adequate energy sources are available; thus highly active individuals maintain energy balance but at a higher rate of energy turnover than inactive individuals. When energy intake exceeds energy expenditure a state of positive energy balance occurs, and the body increases its energy stores. Examples of this include periods around major festivals when overeating and inactivity generally prevail, and during pregnancy and lactation when the body purposefully increases its stores of energy. When energy intake is lower than expenditure, a state of negative energy balance occurs, for example during periods of starvation. Short-term day to day fluctuations in energy balance are common in free-living weight-stable individuals and are generally accommodated by the storage or mobilisation of body fat (adipose tissue triglycerides) and carbohydrate (glycogen in liver and muscle) stores. Adipose tissue represents the body's largest energy store and in contrast to glycogen which has a limited storage capacity, adipose tissue displays considerable plasticity in its potential to store energy. Accordingly, if energy intake exceeds expenditure for a sustained period of time, weight gain ensues, with the additional energy stored mainly as adipose tissue triglycerides and a small but fixed ratio of lean tissue. Conversely, sustained negative energy balance, which results in weight loss, is associated with mobilisation and utilisation of stored energy from adipose tissue triglyceride and protein from lean tissue. Sustained alterations in energy intake and/or expenditure clearly have the potential to alter energy balance and body weight, although in practice this is not always realised. For example, resistance to or less than expected body weight loss is commonly observed in the context of obesity treatment. In order to understand the complexities of energy balance and body weight regulation it is necessary to consider the determinants of energy intake and expenditure and in particular their intra- and interrelationships.

6.2 Regulation of appetite control and energy intake

Appetite relates to the psychological desire to eat and is generally used to describe overall sensations related to food intake. Overall appetite sensations are sensed by the brain, specifically within the hypothalamus, which determines feeding behaviour. The brain receives neural, metabolic, and endocrine signals that are assimilated and result in an energy intake response. Subjectively, these integrated signals are manifest as feelings of hunger or satiety. Hunger can be described as a nagging, irritating feeling that signifies food deprivation to a degree that the next eating episode should take place. Satiety can be described as the inhibition over eating, for example the cessation of eating within a meal setting (often referred to as satiation) or the time interval between meals. It is important to recognise that the biological signals underpinning feelings of hunger and satiety are influenced by external factors such as environment, learning, and memory. Further, energy intake does not act independently of energy expenditure (and its determinants). As such overall regulation of appetite control and energy intake is a complex phenomenon and best considered within an overall framework of energy balance, as depicted in Figure 6.1.

The major biological signals that stimulate the drive to eat are the metabolic requirements of the body and the hormone ghrelin. As already stated, the body's basic metabolic requirement is largely determined by resting metabolic rate. As resting metabolic rate remains relatively stable it follows that the metabolic requirement can be thought of as exerting a relatively consistent (or tonic) demand on the drive for food intake over time. Ghrelin, the so-called "hunger hormone" is secreted into the bloodstream from specific cells in the stomach and acts on the brain to increase food intake. Ghrelin concentrations in the blood increase during periods of fasting to stimulate hunger, and decrease shortly after meal intake. In this way ghrelin can be thought of an orexigenic hormone (i.e., appetite promoting) that acts in an episodic manner depending on nutrient availability in the gastrointestinal tract.

The biological signals that stimulate food intake are not acting in isolation, and indeed food intake is also subject to modulation by biological factors that suppress appetite (i.e., are anorexigenic). Leptin, sometimes called the "hormone of energy expenditure", is secreted by fat cells in proportion to fat mass and acts primarily within the hypothalamus to reduce food intake and increase energy expenditure. Also, the hormone insulin is secreted by the pancreatic beta cells in response to circulating glucose availability and acts on the hypothalamus to inhibit food intake. Leptin and insulin can be thought of as tonic signals reflecting long-term energy reserves in the body (e.g., availability of fat or carbohydrate). It may seem counterintuitive that obese individuals have

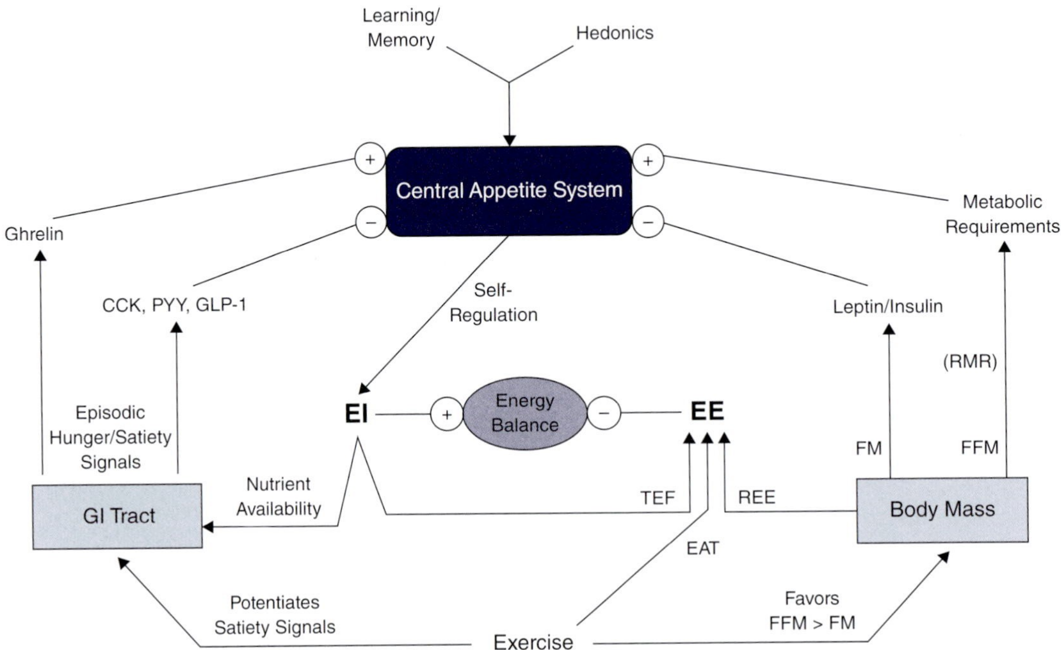

Figure 6.1 Appetite control within an energy balance framework. Energy Intake (EI) is ultimately determined by the balance of stimulatory (+) and inhibitory (–) inputs that include tonic signals related to body mass and episodic signals related to the gastro-intestinal (GI) tract, modified by the influence psychological factors. Further explanation is provided within the text. Reprinted from Maclean *et al.* (2017) with permission.

excessive fat mass and often have high circulating blood leptin and insulin concentrations, which would normally be appetite suppressive. This can be reconciled in that it is likely that the actions of leptin and insulin on appetite regulation are lessened under conditions of chronic energy surplus. Leptin and insulin exert to some extent an ongoing background influence on appetite regulation but other strong satiety signals also exist arising from the gastro-intestinal tract in an episodic manner related to both food and nutrient availability.

The mere presence of food in the gastro-intestinal tract upon consumption of food or drink results in distension and the resulting increased pressure in the stomach and intestine may satisfy feelings of hunger and regulate food intake. As well, the gastro-intestinal tract secretes many so-called "gut-peptides" in response to nutrient exposure following food intake including cholecystokinin (CCK), glucagon-like peptide-1 (GLP-1) and peptide YY (PYY) which stimulate neural and endocrine-mediated appetite suppression. Following absorption, there is an increase in the digested products of nutrients (e.g., glucose, amino acids and fatty acids) in the blood stream and their subsequent metabolism in the liver and other tissues. The metabolism of these substrates particularly in the liver through its neural connection to the brain via the vagus nerve, provides a further level of appetite regulation. Thus, circulating factors provide a link between the digestive system, nutrient metabolism, and the central nervous system for regulating food intake. The episodic biological promoters and suppressors of food intake allow for homeostatic control of appetite, and the integration of these processes have been described within what is known as the Satiety Cascade (see Figure 6.2).

The Satiety Cascade and the model described in Figure 6.1 illustrate the complexity of appetite regulation from a biological perspective but critically they both recognise the importance of psychological and other non-homeostatic factors on appetite regulation. For example, hedonic factors including food liking (i.e., perceived pleasurable sensory properties of food) and motivational "wanting" (i.e., attraction to a specific food over available alternatives) play an

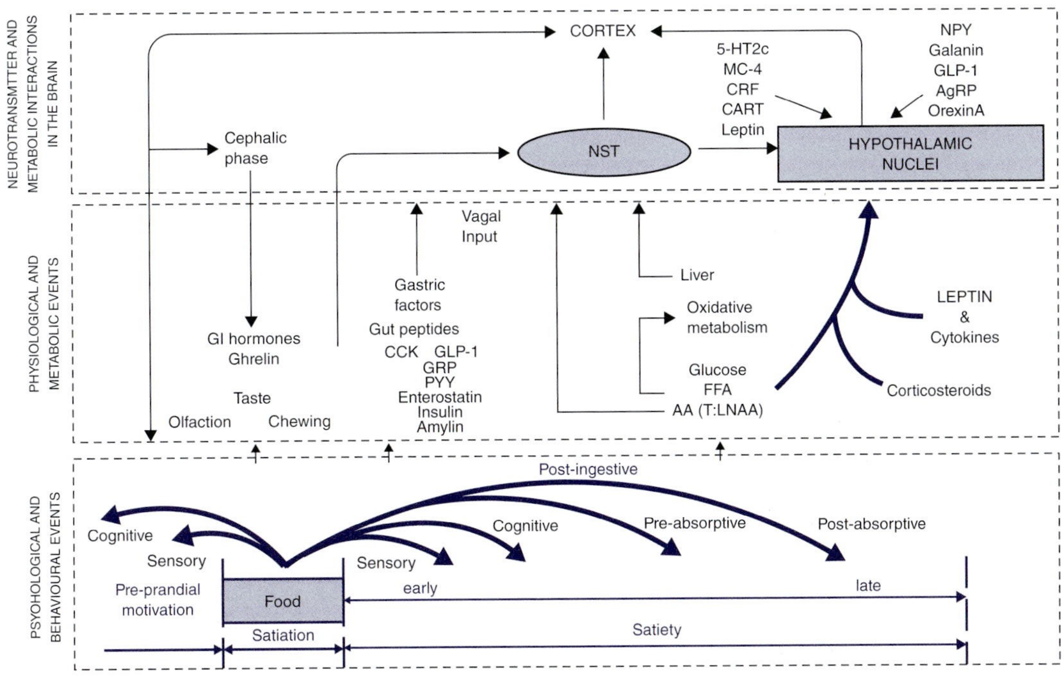

Figure 6.2 The Satiety Cascade. This model describes the complex expression of appetite on three related levels including psychological and behavioural events, physiological and metabolic events and biological actions in the brain. Reprinted from Hopkins and Blundell (2016) with permission.

important role in the control of food intake and in some cases override homeostatic mechanisms of appetite control. Learning and memory play an important role in the establishment of food and taste preference in early life which can continue to influence eating behaviour across the lifespan. Other external factors such as climate, social factors, peer influence, food availability, and cultural practices can play a role in influencing food intake behaviour at any one time. Collectively, the complexities of the regulation of appetite control and energy intake, including compensatory eating behaviours (e.g., in response to exercise or weight loss), mean that a one-size-fits-all solution is unlikely for example in the prevention and treatment of body weight gain.

6.3 Energy expenditure

Energy is expended within the body to support its physiological functions through the oxidation (or combustion) of fuel substrates, principally carbohydrate and fat but also some protein. The fuels oxidised may already be present within the body, for example glucose derived from the breakdown of liver glycogen, or nutrients may be directly oxidised from ingested food. The oxidation of fuel substrates requires the consumption of oxygen (O_2) and results in the formation of adenosine triphosphate (ATP; the energy currency used by cells support metabolic functions) and also the production of carbon dioxide (CO_2), water (H_2O), and heat. As a simple example of how the body uses fuel for energy, consider the combustion of a simple glucose molecule:

$$C_6H_{12}O_6 + 6O_2 \rightarrow 6H_2O + 6CO_2 + \text{Heat}$$

Similar chemical reactions can be described for the oxidation of other sources of energy such as fats and proteins. Knowledge of these types of reactions, which occur continuously in the body and constitute energy expenditure, can be used for the measurement of energy expenditure and its components.

Measurement of energy expenditure

As the oxidation of fuel for energy within the body requires oxygen and results in heat production, it is possible to measure heat production and thus energy expenditure in a manner analogous to the way heat production can be used for determining the energy content of food. This was elegantly demonstrated by the pioneering work of the French chemist Antoine Lavoisier, who demonstrated that living animals breathe (requiring oxygen) and give off heat. Lavoisier created a sealed device (known as a calorimeter) within which a small animal could be placed, surrounded the calorimeter with a sealed pocket of ice and then placed the device and ice layer inside an insulated chamber. The animal's warmth melted the ice and by measuring the volume of melted ice water produced, and knowing the quantity of heat required to melt a given quantity of ice, Lavoisier could accurately calculate the amount of heat produced by the animal. This *direct calorimetry* approach, which directly measures heat production has been developed and used to quantify human energy expenditure. However, the technically demanding nature of these devices means that direct human calorimeter chambers are infrequently used.

A commonly used alternative to direct calorimetry for the assessment of energy expenditure in humans is *indirect calorimetry*. Indirect calorimetry uses determinations of oxygen consumption and carbon dioxide production via respiratory gas analysis, which reflects the oxidation processes of fuel substrate such as glucose, to estimate metabolic rate. Respiratory gas exchange can be measured with relative ease in humans over short durations at rest, after feeding or during physical activity under laboratory conditions using a face mask, mouthpiece, or canopy system for gas collections and over longer periods of 24 h and beyond with individuals living in a whole-room metabolic chamber. Indirect calorimetry has the added advantage that the ratio of carbon dioxide production to oxygen consumption (the respiratory quotient, or RQ) is indicative of the type of fuel substrate being oxidised (i.e., fat versus carbohydrate). For example, carbohydrate oxidation has an RQ of 1.0 and fat oxidation has an RQ close to 0.7 (RQ for protein is ~0.8). In fact, given that the caloric equivalent for oxygen is similar for the three main energy substrates (21 kJ/L O_2 for carbohydrates, 19 kJ/L O_2 for fat, and 17.8 kJ/L O_2 for protein; protein typically contributes only modestly to energy expenditure), energy expenditure can be calculated with reasonable accuracy by simply knowing the rate of oxygen consumption ($\dot{V}O_2$) determined by indirect calorimetry.

$$\text{Energy expenditure}(\text{kJ/min}) = 20\,\text{kJ/L} \times \dot{V}O_2(\text{L/min})$$

Energy expenditure can be calculated with more precision using indirect calorimetry by using measures of $\dot{V}O_2$, rates of carbon dioxide production ($\dot{V}CO_2$), and knowledge of the contribution of protein oxidation by collecting urine during the measurement period to analyse the excreted nitrogen (Box 6.1).

Indirect calorimetry enables the measurement of energy expenditure within laboratory settings. While it is possible to determine total energy expenditure across a whole day or a few days within whole room metabolic chambers, this is a somewhat artificial environment and is not always representative of the normal daily pattern of physical activity. The doubly labelled water (DLW) technique can be used to obtain an integrated measure of total energy expenditure over extended periods while subjects are living in their usual environment. The DLW method requires a person to ingest small amounts of "heavy" water that is isotopically labelled with deuterium and oxygen-18 (^2H_2O and $H_2^{18}O$). These are stable (non-radioactive) isotopes of water that are safe to administer to humans and have the advantage of acting like molecular tags

Box 6.1 Calculation of energy expenditure from indirect calorimetry measurements.

Step 1
First the contribution of protein oxidation to $\dot{V}O_2$ and $\dot{V}CO_2$ is estimated with knowledge that 1 g nitrogen (*n*) corresponds to 6.25 g protein:

$$\dot{V}O_{2(prot)} = n \times 6.25 \times 0.97$$

$$\dot{V}CO_{2(prot)} = n \times 6.25 \times 0.77$$

where $\dot{V}O_{2(prot)}$ and $\dot{V}CO_{2(prot)}$ refer to the rates of O_2 consumption and CO_2 production, respectively, from protein oxidation; 0.97 and 0.77 are the respective volumes (L) of O_2 consume and CO_2 produced by the biological oxidation of 1 g of protein.

Step 2
Next, the contribution of protein oxidation is subtracted from the measured $\dot{V}O_2$ and $\dot{V}CO_2$ to obtain nonprotein $\dot{V}O_2$ ($\dot{V}O_{2(nonprot)}$) and nonprotein $\dot{V}CO_2$ ($\dot{V}CO_{2(nonprot)}$):

$$\dot{V}O_{2(nonprot)} = \dot{V}O_2 - \dot{V}O_{2(prot)}$$

$$\dot{V}CO_{2(nonprot)} = \dot{V}CO_2 - \dot{V}CO_{2(prot)}$$

$$\dot{V}O_{2(nonprot)} = C \times 0.828 + F \times 2.03$$

$$\dot{V}CO_{2(nonprot)} = C \times 0.828 + F \times 1.43$$

where *C* and *F* are grams of oxidised carbohydrate and fat, respectively, and can be found by solving the two equations with two unknowns: O_2 consumed and CO_2 produced by the oxidation of 1 g carbohydrate is 0.828 L while the oxidation of 1 g triglyceride consumes 2.03 L O_2 and produces 1.43 L CO_2.

Step 3
The straightforward output from indirect calorimetry allows the quantitation of RQ as previously described ($\dot{V}CO^2/\dot{V}O_2$), but it is the nonprotein RQ ($RQ_{(nonprot)}$) that is required for calculation of energy expenditure:

$$RQ_{(nonprot)} = \dot{V}CO_{2(nonprot)} / \dot{V}O_{2(nonprot)}$$

Step 4
Energy expenditure can be calculated from:

$$\text{Energy expenditure}(\text{kJ/min}) = [19.63 + 4.59(RQ_{(nonprot)} - 0.707] \times \dot{V}O_{2(nonprot)} + 18.78 \times \dot{V}O_{2(nonprot)}$$

or

$$\text{Energy expenditure}(\text{kJ/min}) = 17 \times P + 17.5 \times C + 38.9 \times F$$

where 17, 17.5, and 38.9 are the heat project (kJ) by the oxidation of 1 g of protein, glycogen and triglyceride, respectively. The protein oxidation (P) is $n \times 6.25$ g.

Step 5
Based on the stoichiometry of the fuel substrates and with measures of urine nitrogen production it is also possible to determine the oxidation of protein, carbohydrate, and fat using indirect calorimetry and the following equations (Frayn, 1983):

$$P(\text{g/min}) = 6.25 \times n$$

$$C(\text{g/min}) = 4.55 \times \dot{V}CO_2 - 3.21 \times \dot{V}O_2 - 2.87 \times n$$

$$F(\text{g/min}) = 1.67 \times \dot{V}O_2 - 1.67 \times \dot{V}CO_2 - 1.92 \times n$$

It is not uncommon to simplify calculations of energy expenditure and fuel substrate oxidation by ignoring the protein component, with the assumption of minimal or constant contribution of protein oxidation to the overall measured responses; in such cases this should be acknowledged as a possible limitation to the accuracy of the values produced.

such that water can be "traced" in the body. After providing a dose of DLW, the deuterium labelled water is washed out of the body as a function of body water turnover; ^{18}O is also lost from the body through water turnover, but is lost via carbon dioxide production as well. The difference between the two "tracer" excretion rates represents the carbon dioxide production rate. Knowledge of the carbon dioxide production rate combined with an estimate of the respiratory quotient (measured by indirect calorimetry or approximated by the food quotient), enables the calculation of energy expenditure.

The main advantages of the DLW water technique are that it is non-invasive and does not interfere with everyday life and therefore free-living energy expenditure can be estimated over extended periods of time (typically 7 to 14 days). As well, in combination with assessments of RMR by indirect calorimetry, it is possible to obtain estimates of physical activity energy expenditure by subtracting RMR and an estimate of the thermic effect of feeding from total energy expenditure. The DLW technique can also provide a measure of energy intake in individuals in energy balance, and in such a state total energy intake must equal total energy expenditure. In this respect the DLW technique has been used to validate other methods such as determination of energy intake by food record or dietary recall or in the prediction of energy expenditure by using accelerometers. For example, it has long been known that obese subjects self-report a lower than expected value for energy intake. At one time it was thought that this was due to low energy requirements in the obese due to low energy expenditure and reduced physical activity. However, using DLW, it was established that obese populations systematically under-report their actual energy intake by 30-40% and actually, have normal energy expenditure relative to their body size.

The main disadvantages of the DLW technique are the expense of the isotopes, their periodic availability, and access to the required equipment and expertise for the analysis of samples (usually urine or saliva) which limits wider adoption. The approach does not inform on the nature of physical activity undertaken during the measurement period (e.g., duration, intensity) although combining DLW with valid accelerometry methods would be one way to address this. No method is without limitation, including the DLW technique, but it has been validated in a number of laboratories, has sufficient accuracy and precision to be considered the "gold standard" measure of free-living total energy expenditure, and has become an integral tool for the determination of energy requirements in a wide-range of populations.

6.4 Factors that influence energy expenditure

Resting metabolic rate

Each of the components that make up total energy expenditure is determined by various factors. RMR is highly variable between individuals (±25%), but is quite consistent within individuals (±5%). In general terms the RMR is higher in individuals of larger body size and in particular body weight due to higher amounts of total tissue mass. In terms of the components of body tissue mass, the RMR is primarily related to the body's fat-free mass (FFM; the total mass of the body that is not fat, i.e., muscle, skin, bone and organs) and thus FFM explains 60-80% of the variation in RMR between individuals. The RMR is dependent on the relative contribution of the different organs that make up the FFM and different tissues have markedly different metabolic rates. For example, skeletal muscle comprises ~43% of total body mass in an adult and contributes between 22-36% of the RMR. In contrast, the brain contributes 20-24% of the RMR despite accounting for only ~2% of total body mass. While FFM is the biggest determinant of RMR, fat mass (FM), age, biological sex, and physical activity make additional contributions to collectively explain 80-90% of the variance in RMR.

Thus, FM is not metabolically inert and can contribute ~5% of RMR and this may be related to changes in sympathetic nervous system activity resulting from changes in FM that affect the metabolism of other tissues. In infants, children, and adolescents, RMR generally increases with age due to growth and increasing body size. RMR seems to decrease in older age which may be related to progressive losses in FFM with aging (for example, loss of muscle mass or sarcopenia is a common feature of the ageing process). RMR differences are apparent as a function of biological sex and largely reflect the fact that men are typically larger than women and have a body composition composed of less FM and more FFM. Physical activity level also seems to influence RMR, with more active people tending to have a higher RMR than inactive individuals. From a practical perspective this can in part be related to the residual effects of the last exercise bout on metabolic rate. The effects of regular exercise training on other determinants of RMR such as skeletal muscle mass may also contribute to increased RMR independent of the last exercise bout. Finally, genetics may play a role in determining RMR directly or indirectly by influencing other factors that determine RMR.

Several equations have been developed to estimate resting energy requirements from simple measures such as age, weight and/or height, and in this case the equations typically predict BMR. These equations are often useful for making estimates in clinical or practice situations when the direct measurement cannot be made, or for making estimates of energy requirements. The classic equations of Harris and Benedict are frequently used for this purpose, although these equations were developed from limited measures performed in the early 1900s. More recent equations such as those developed by Schofield (1985) and those by Henry (2005) appear to offer more accuracy, and have been adopted by the Food and Agriculture Organisation of the United Nations/World Health Organisation/United Nations University (FAO/WHO/UNU) and the UK Scientific Advisory Committee on Nutrition (SACN), respectively, for the purpose of estimating energy requirements in various populations. The equations proposed by Henry based on weight and height are presented in this chapter (Table 6.1), but note that these are just predictive and as such measurements of BMR/RMR should be made wherever possible.

Thermic effect of feeding

The thermic effect of feeding can be measured as the increase in metabolic rate that occurs after feeding and typically occurs over an extended period of at least five hours. The thermic effect of feeding typically corresponds to around 10% of the energy ingested when following a Western diet, that is, if one consumed a mixed meal of 2.1 MJ, the body would require 210 kJ to digest, process, and metabolise the meals contents. Nonetheless, the quantity and macronutrient composition of the ingested calories can modulate the magnitude of the response. Higher energy intakes typically increase the thermic effect of feeding, with recent estimates suggesting 1.1-1.2 kJ/h increases in energy expended for every 100 kJ increase in meal energy intake. Indeed, consuming fewer larger meals would be expected to increase the thermic effect of feeding to a greater extent than more frequent smaller meals. The thermic effect of feeding is generally higher for protein (20-30% of the energy ingested) and carbohydrate (5-10%) than it is for fat (0-3%). This is because the energy storage process is more efficient for fat, while there is an additional energy cost associated with the processing of protein or carbohydrate (i.e., synthesis of

Table 6.1 Simple equations for estimating BMR from body weight and height in men and women according the age category (Henry, 2005).

	BMR (MJ/day)	
Age (years)	Equation for men	Equation for women
<3	{0.118 × wt) + (3.59 × ht) + (−1.55)	(0.127 × wt) + (2.94 × ht) + (−1.2)
3-10	(0.0632 × wt) + (3.59 × ht) + (1.28)	(0.0666 × wt) + (0.878 × ht) + (1.46)
10-18	(0.0651 × wt) + (1.11 × ht) + (1.25)	(0.0393 × wt) + (1.04 × ht) + (1.93)
18-30	(0.0600 × wt) + (1.31 × ht) + (0.473)	(0.0433 × wt) + (2.57 × ht) + (−1.180)
30-60	(0.0476 × wt) + (2.26 × ht) + (−0.574)	(0.0342 × wt) + (2.1 × wt) + (−0.0486)
>60	(0.0478 × wt) + (2.26 × ht) + (−1.070)	(0.0356 × wt) + (1.76 × ht) + (0.0448)

wt, body weight (kg); ht, height (m)

proteins from amino acids, storage of glucose as glycogen). In addition to the obligatory energetic cost of processing and storage of nutrients, a more variable facultative thermogenic component has been described. This component is mainly pertinent to carbohydrates which through increased insulin secretion results in activation of the sympathoadrenal system to increase energy expenditure. Thus, there are a number of factors that can influence the thermic effect of feeding, although the extent to which the thermic effect of feeding can be modified in a clinically meaningful way (e.g., to assist weight loss) remains subject to debate.

Physical activity energy expenditure

The energy expended as a result of physical activity is perhaps the most significant and variable factor of energy expenditure and as such is the component through which large changes in energy expenditure can be achieved. However, as discussed later in this textbook, physical activity levels are generally below those required to attain the health-benefits in large proportions of the general populations of most industrialised societies. Nonetheless, the degree to which energy expenditure is increased by physical activity is determined by the duration of activity, the type of physical activity (e.g., walking, running, cycling) and the intensity at which the particular activity is performed. Thus, physical activity energy expenditure can be accumulated through a number of different ways, including performing lower intensity activities such as standing and walking for longer durations or undertaking higher intensity activities such as running for briefer periods of time. The actual energetic costs of different types of physical activity have been expressed in a variety of ways. For example, the metabolic equivalent (MET) is frequently used to describe the energetic cost of physical activity (Ainsworth *et al.*, 2011), whereby 1 MET is equivalent to the RMR measured during supine rest (defined as 3.5 ml oxygen consumption/kg body weight/min, roughly equivalent to 4.184 kJ/kg body weight/hour). Accordingly, exercise intensity can be expressed as multiples of the MET, and MET values have been assigned to a large range of physical activities (Table 6.2).

Table 6.2 Examples of metabolic equivalent (MET) values for various physical activities.

Activity	MET	Description
Bicycling	6.8	Bicycling, to/from work, self-selected pace
Bicycling	8.0	Bicycling, 19-22 km/h, leisure, moderate effort
Conditioning exercise	3.5	Resistance (weight) training, multiple exercises, 8-15 repetitions at varied resistance
Conditioning exercise	2.5	Stretching, mild
Conditioning exercise	2.5	Yoga, Hatha
Home activities	3.3	Kitchen activity, general (e.g., cooking, washing dishes, cleaning up), moderate effort
Home activities	2.3	Food shopping
Lawn and garden	4.5	Mowing lawn, power mower, light or moderate effort
Lawn and garden	4.0	Raking lawn
Running	9.8	Running (10 min/mile)
Running	11.8	Running (8 min/mile)
Walking	3.5	Walking for pleasure
Sports	7.0	Soccer, casual, general
Sports	7.3	Tennis, general
Sports	4.3	Golf, walking, carrying clubs

MET values assigned to an extensive range of activities can be found at: https://sites.google.com/site/compendiumofphysicalactivities/home

The energetic cost of a physical activity bout can then be approximated with the equation:

$$\text{kilajoules} = (\text{MET value} \times 4.184) \times \text{body weight (kg)} \times \text{duration of activity (hours)}$$

The physical activity ratio (PAR) is another way of presenting the energy cost of physical activity, whereby the PAR is defined in multiples of the BMR. These approaches can be useful in estimating the energy costs of specific activities although they may underestimate true energy costs as they will not account for the short-term elevations in RMR that.can occur in response to exercise (generally termed the excess post-exercise oxygen consumption; EPOC). Thus, in the context of understanding overall dietary energy requirement, estimation of the overall total energy expenditure on a daily basis becomes important.

6.5 Energy requirements

How much energy do we need to sustain life and maintain our body energy stores? Why do some people require more energy and others less? In other words, what are the energy requirements of different types of people? Based on our earlier definition of energy balance, the energy needs or energy requirements of the body to maintain energy balance must be equal to total daily energy expenditure (i.e., the sum of all of the previously described individual components of energy expenditure). From a public health perspective, most recommendations for energy requirements (sometimes called energy reference values) set by authoritative sources (such as the UK SACN) are based on the level of energy intake required to maintain a healthy body weight (i.e., a body mass index [BMI] of 18.5-24.9 kg/m^2) in otherwise healthy people at existing population levels of physical activity. Most approaches rely on the use of DLW studies in appropriate reference populations (e.g., age range, sex) to identify energy expenditures (and thus energy intakes when weight stable) associated with the healthy body weight range. In doing this, it is recognised that the set energy reference values should also support the transition of underweight or overweight individuals to the body weight range consistent with long-term good health.

With knowledge of DLW determined energy expenditures in a reference population, total energy expenditure is divided by the measured or estimated BMR values from that population to determine the physical activity level (PAL). For example, if the total energy expenditure was 12.6 MJ/day and the BMR was 6.3 MJ/day, the PAL value would be 2.0 (i.e., twice the BMR). Thus, it is possible to predict energy requirements for a population of interest by multiplying the estimated BMR by the PAL value (i.e., BMR × PAL). The BMR can be estimated as previously described (Table 6.1). For the PAL value, the most recent UK report by the SACN (SACN, 2011) identified PAL values that reflect the median population physical activity levels (PAL = 1.63) with additional PAL values appropriate to those who are less (PAL = 1.49) or more active (PAL = 1.78). The PAL value associated with the more active category likely reflects a level at which health benefits of regular physical activity are accrued. Regardless, the energy reference values calculated for a given population can be tailored based on sex, age, and physical activity level, with the latter clearly having the potential to strongly affect energy requirements. Biological sex (men typically have higher total energy expenditures and thus energy requirements than women), age and a number of other conditions can also influence energy requirements at various points across the lifespan, and thus require further consideration.

6.6 Energy balance in various conditions

Infancy and childhood

During the first year of life a major contributor to energy requirements is the cost of energy deposited in growing tissues. In this case, energy requirements can be determined based on data from DLW studies plus the energy deposited as growth, assessed by measuring the size of the protein and fat stores in the body. The energy deposited as new tissue is highest in the first three months of life and subsides over the first year of life. For example, energy is deposited in growing tissue at a rate of ~833 kj/day (~199 kcal/day) in the first three months of life in boys and ~749 kj/day (~179 kcal/day) in the same time frame in girls which approximates 36% of the average energy requirement for breast-fed infants of that age. In contrast, by months 10–12 of life, energy deposition falls to ~93 and 78 kj/day (22 and 19 kcal/day) respectively in boys and girls, corresponding to ~3% of the energy requirement. Individual growth rates and early infancy feeding behaviour are at least two known factors that would cause variation in these figures. Nonetheless, from this information and in contrast to requirements for most other healthy population groups, the early infancy period is characterised by an energy requirement that is higher than the total energy expenditure resulting in a positive energy balance to account for growth. For older children and adolescents (e.g., 1 to 18 years), the energy cost associated with growth represents a much smaller overall proportion of total energy needs. Therefore population specific energy requirements can be calculated in a similar manner as for adults (i.e., BMR × PAL) but with a 1% adjustment of the PAL values to account for growth (SACN, 2011).

Ageing

In general the energy requirements of older adults who maintain good general health and mobility are unlikely to differ substantially than those of younger adults. Nonetheless, physical activity levels in the ageing population are often even lower than in younger adult populations and as such the energy requirement in such groups would most likely need to assume a less active PAL to avoid excessive weight gain. However, a careful balance is required in the messages provided to older adults, as some groups inadvertently consume insufficient energy and combined with physical inactivity are at high risk for the development of sarcopenia and related co-morbidities. As well, there is some evidence that being slightly overweight may help to provide resilience in older age but this notion requires further study before altering energy requirements in ageing. It may be that a more individualised approach is required to ensure that older adults meet the energy and nutrient intakes likely to be consistent with good health, especially in those at risk of low energy intake and who exhibit low levels of physical activity. This may be particularly necessary in meeting the energy needs of special conditions associated with the elderly such as Alzheimer's and Parkinson's disease, which frequently can lead to malnourished states and body weight loss due to a reduction in food intake as a result of reduced functionality.

Energy requirements in physically active groups

Some population groups exhibit extremely high levels of physical activity and as such energy requirements will be substantially elevated above those typically accommodated within public health energy reference values. Indeed, a recent DLW study employed at a 24-days professional cycling race (the Giro d'Italia) showed that total daily energy expenditure was on average 32 MJ/day, corresponding to a PAL value of 4.4. Similarly, a recent study undertaken in older adults who performed 2706 km of cycling in Scandinavia over 14 consecutive days showed average energy expenditures of 30 MJ/day, equivalent to 4.0 times the BMR (i.e., a PAL of 4). Clearly, in such extreme situations there can be challenges with balancing energy intake with energy expenditure to ensure the demands of the physical activity can be sustained. Nonetheless, even professional sportspersons rarely maintain extremely high levels of energy expenditure all year round and indeed must alter their energy intakes in accordance with expenditures depending on the specific goals of their training or competition.

There have been suggestions on the basis of low self-reported energy intakes that some endurance athletes may have increased energetic efficiency (i.e., they remain weight stable despite seemingly consuming less energy than is predicted to be required for a particular physical activity level). However, some of this discrepancy may be because food intake has been under-reported, a common issue when measuring dietary intake in most population groups including athletes, rather than the differences between energy intake and expenditure resulting from energy saving metabolic adaptations. Nonetheless, there are some groups of athletes such as endurance athletes or those involved in sports where a low body mass may be advantageous where energy intakes genuinely do fall below requirements. Whilst there may be short-term benefits to aesthetics or sports performance associated with such practices, longer-term health consequences of sustained periods of low energy availability can be severe.

Moving away from professional athletes, it is also likely that recreationally active people within the general population who perform regular sports or exercise have elevated energy requirements. One way to account for this is to use estimates of the likely change in PAL for a given activity, and then to modify the overall PAL value which is ultimately multiplied by BMR to obtain total energy expenditure. For example, 60 minutes of active sport performed five times per week (equivalent to jogging at 10:44 min/miles or 9 km/h) would be expected to increase PAL by 0.3, whereas those involved in an intense daily exercise program associated with training for competitive sports would be expected to increase PAL by 0.6. The assumption here is that there is no compensatory reduction in other activities such that the change in PAL from the activity is additive to overall PAL. Of course, in some cases, for example where weight loss is a goal, a potential increase in energy requirement associated regular exercise may purposely not be met by an increased energy intake in order to create a negative energy balance. Although, as will be discussed later, compensatory mechanisms exist that can work against negative energy balances induced by exercise.

Energy requirements in pregnancy and lactation

Pregnancy and lactation are two other examples in which energy metabolism may be altered. During pregnancy additional energy costs can come from increased body tissue mass (maternal and feto-placental), increased basal metabolic rate, and in the cost of physical activity through losses in movement efficiency. The estimated extra energy cost of pregnancy is approximately 0.3 (85), 1.2 (285) and 2.0 (475) MJ/day (kcal/day) for the first, second and third trimesters, respectively. However, at least in the UK, an additional energy intake of 0.8 MJ/day (191 kcal/day) during the last trimester is the only set recommendation as compensatory reductions in physical activity energy expenditure that typically occur as pregnancy progresses tend to offset the additional energy needs. Lactation increases energy requirements due to the direct energy costs of milk production. Some of the additional energy costs can be met by the mobilisation of energy from tissue (mainly fat) stores accumulated during pregnancy, and this will contribute to weight loss during the post-partum period. An increased energy requirement of 1380 kj/day (330 kcal/day) is generally recommended for the first six months after birth during which exclusive breastfeeding is recommended. Overall, pregnancy and lactation are associated with modest elevations in energy requirement, although such requirements may vary depending on the health status of the mother (e.g., an undernourished mother may require additional energy to ensure both maternal and fetal health is not compromised during pregnancy).

Energy requirements in disease and trauma

Information on the energy requirements during disease and trauma is important because:

- energy expenditure may be altered by disease or injury
- physical activity levels are often reduced
- underfeeding or overfeeding of patients, particularly those who are critically ill, may lead to metabolic complications

Therefore, correct assessment of energy requirements in disease and trauma is an important part of disease management and recovery. However, there is a dearth of well-developed databases documenting total energy expenditures across a wide-range of diseases, which make accurate predictions of energy requirements difficult. In acute and chronic disease BMR is often increased, but total energy expenditure often remains normal or is reduced as a result of reductions in body weight, FFM (e.g., muscle wasting) and physical activity. In contrast, in diseases such as anorexia nervosa or cystic fibrosis some groups of patients will display increased total energy expenditure. It is important to note however that even with knowledge of energy expenditure, the energy requirement for optimal management of disease may be different. For example, measured energy expenditure may be low in undernourished patients, but rather than achieving energy balance, energy requirements might need to be increased in order to provide repletion. Clearly, the energy requirements for specific diseases are likely to be variable between disease states, between patients with a specific type of disease or trauma and even within patients, which makes establishing the appropriate level of energy intake a critical but highly complex task.

6.7 Obesity

Basic metabolic principles

Obesity is the most common form of a disruption in energy balance and now constitutes one of the major and most prevalent disorders related to nutrition. Because of the strong relationship between obesity and health risk, obesity is now generally considered a disease by health professionals.

Although the body continuously consumes a mixed diet of carbohydrate, protein, and fat, and sometimes alcohol, the preferred store of energy is fat. There is a clearly defined hierarchy of energy stores that outlines a preferential storage of excess calories as fat. For alcohol there is no storage capacity in the body. Thus, alcohol that is consumed is immediately oxidised for energy. For protein, there is a very limited storage capacity, and in most situations protein metabolism is very well regulated. For carbohydrate there is only a very limited storage capacity, in the form of glycogen, which can be found in the liver and muscle. Glycogen provides a very small and short-term energy store, and the stores in the liver can easily be low after an overnight fast, with additional reductions in the muscle glycogen store occurring after a bout of exercise. When excess carbohydrates are consumed, the body adapts by preferentially increasing its use of carbohydrate as a fuel. Contrary to popular belief, excess carbohydrates above requirements are unlikely to make any quantitatively meaningful contribution to fat storage.

If excess fat is consumed, the body fails to quickly adjust fuel substrate utilisation to favour fat oxidation, and thus excess fat is accumulated as an energy store in the body. This process occurs at a very low metabolic cost and is therefore and extremely efficient process. Storing excess carbohydrate as glycogen is more metabolically expensive and is therefore a less efficient option. There also appears to be a limit to how much glycogen can be stored in liver and muscle, whereas the body can store excess fat across multiple body sites. There is another reason why the body would prefer to store fat rather than glycogen. Glycogen can only be stored in a hydrated form that requires 3 g water for each gram of glycogen, whereas fat does not require any such process. In other words, for each gram of glycogen that is stored, the body has to store an additional 3 g of water. Thus, for each 4 g of storage tissue, the body only stores 16.8 kJ (4.0 kcal), equivalent to just 4.2 kJ/g (1.0 kcal/g), compared with the benefit of fat which can be stored as 37.8 kJ/g (9.0 kcal/g). Thus, a typical adult with 15 kg of fat carries 567.0 MJ of stored energy. If the adult did not eat and was inactive, he or she might require 8.4 MJ/day for survival, and the energy stores would be sufficient for almost 70 days. This length is about the limit of human survival without food. Given that glycogen stores requires 4 g to store 4.2 kJ (3 g water plus 1 g glycogen = 16.8 kJ), we can calculate that to carry this much energy in the form of glycogen requires 135 kg of weight. It is no wonder therefore that the body's metabolism favours fat as the preferred energy store.

Definition of obesity

Obesity has traditionally been defined as an excess accumulation of body energy, in the form of fat or adipose tissue. Thus, obesity is a disease resulting from sustained positive energy balance, which arises as a result of dysregulation in the energy balance system – a failure of the regulation systems to make appropriate adjustments between energy intake and expenditure. It is now clear that the increased health risks of obesity (e.g., cardiovascular disease, type 2 diabetes) may be conferred by the distribution of body fat. In addition, the influence of altered body fat and/or body fat distribution on health risk may vary across individuals. Thus, obesity is best defined by indices of body fat accumulation, body fat pattern, and alterations in health risk profile.

The BMI is the most widely used crude index of obesity and classifies weight relative to height squared (i.e., weight in kg divided by height squared in meters, and expressed as kg/m^2). In adults, the normal range of BMI is considered 18.5 – 24.9 kg/m^2, while cut-offs for underweight, overweight, and obesity are defined as ≤18.5, ≥25 and ≥30 kg/m^2, respectively. It is important to recognise that there are ethnic differences in the relationship between BMI and health, such that lower BMI cut-off points are used for certain populations (e.g., BMI's of 23 and 27.5 kg/m^2 indicate increased health risk and high health risk, respectively, among South Asian and Chinese populations). In children it is more difficult to classify obesity by BMI because height varies with age during growth; thus age-adjusted BMI percentiles are generally used. Whilst measurement of BMI is a convenient measure, it is not without limitations. For example, BMI does not distinguish between excess muscle weight and excess fat weight. Thus, although BMI is strongly related to body fatness, at any given BMI in a population, there may be large individual differences in the range of body fatness. A classic example of misclassification that may arise from the use of BMI is a body builder with a large muscle mass who may have a BMI ≥30 kg/m^2 but is not obese; rather, this person has a high body weight for his height resulting from increased FFM.

Since the health risks of obesity are related to body fat distribution, and in particular excess abdominal fat, other anthropometric indices of body shape are useful in the definition of obesity. Traditionally, the waist-to-hip ratio has been used as a marker of upper versus lower body-fat distribution. It is however now more common to use the waist circumference alone or in combination with BMI, as waist circumference provides a strong index of central body-fat pattern and increased risk of obesity-related conditions. The risk of obesity-related diseases is increased above a waist circumference of 94 cm in men and above 80 cm in women. Assessment of BMI and waist circumference are convenient practical ways to estimate adiposity, although they do not reveal the extent of fat accumulation on non-traditional sites such as the liver, pancreas, and skeletal muscle, which can also play an important role in the development of metabolic complications associated with obesity.

Etiology of obesity: excess intake or decreased physical activity

Stated simply, obesity is the end-result of positive energy balance, or an increased energy intake relative to expenditure. It is often stated, or assumed that obesity is simply the result of overeating or lack of physical activity. However, the aetiology of obesity is not as simple as this, and many complex interrelated factors are likely to contribute to the development of obesity. It is unlikely that any single factor causes obesity. Many cultural, behavioural, and biological factors drive energy intake and energy expenditure and contribute to the homeostatic regulation of body energy stores. In addition, many of these factors are influenced by individual susceptibility which may be driven by genetic, cultural, or hormonal factors. Despite this complexity, the "obesogenic environment" now present in many societies globally, which influences behaviour to promote energy intake and minimise energy expenditure, undoubtedly plays a key role in the development of weight gain.

While lack of physical activity as a key driver of obesity presents an attractive view, from an energetics perspective a clear relationship between physical activity energy expenditure or sedentary behaviour and long-term weight gain has been difficult to delineate. Similarly, links between diet composition and risk of weight gain have not been consistently shown. It is possible that methodological limitations prevent clear links between physical activity or diet composition and weight gain from being revealed. Also, as obesity may develop gradually over time, the actual energy imbalance is often negligible and undetectable. It could also be that considering energy intake and expenditure in isolation results in failure to appreciate their inter-relationship, and that it is disturbances in this dynamic relationship that underpin the risk for positive energy balance. For example, there is evidence to suggest that energy intake and energy expenditure are more tightly coupled at higher levels of physical activity, and thus the likelihood of remaining in energy balance is stronger. In contrast, at low levels of physical activity the coupling between energy intake and expenditure may be weaker and there may be overconsumption of energy relative to energy expended, thus increasing the risk for positive energy imbalance (Figure 6.3). This type of evidence would support a role for exercise or physical activity in the maintenance of energy balance and prevention of weight gain, by enabling more sensitive appetite regulation and possibly by contributing to higher total daily energy expenditures.

Body weight reduction and energy balance

In order to reduce body weight, for example, in those who are overweight or obese, it is of course necessary to reach a negative energy balance over a sustained period of time. It may therefore seem straightforward, that increasing energy expenditure, reducing energy intake, or some

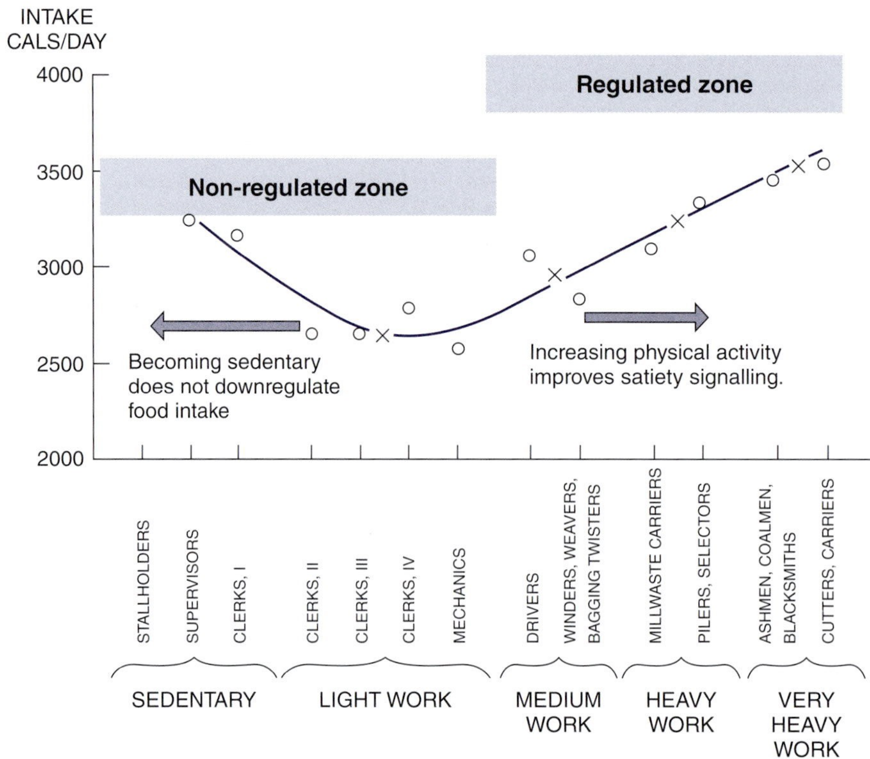

Figure 6.3 Original observations of a J-shaped relationship between energy expended in physical work and food intake for workers in Bengali jute mills (Mayer et al., 1956). More recently, the work of John Blundell (e.g., Hopkins and Blundell, 2016) has confirmed such relationships and introduced the concept of regulated and non-regulated zones to describe higher physical activity levels where energy intake is tightly coupled to energy expenditure or more sedentary activity where there is a disconnect between energy intake and expenditure, promoting overconsumption of energy. Reprinted from Blundell (2011) with permission.

combination of the two should lead to weight loss. However, this assumes that both components of energy balance act independently from one another, and also do not have an influence on their own function. In reality, there is variability in the degree of weight loss achieved regardless of the strategy applied to create a negative energy balance, and it is also clear that weight loss is often much less than expected based on the predicted energy deficit induced. Thus, a more dynamic understanding of the intra- and interrelationships between the components of energy balance are required rather than the simple "calories in, calories out model" of considered for body weight reduction.

Exercise is a good example of the complexities of sustaining a negative energy balance. It is intuitive to think that as regular exercisers tend to be lean and of a healthy body weight, embarking on an exercise program will lead to weight loss. However, overall exercise alone on average does not typically result in substantially body weight loss. Some individuals do experience weight loss on an exercise program, but some may experience less than expected weight loss or none at all. This is because exercise can result in compensatory adjustments to energy intake that serve to resist against negative energy balance. Quite simply, in those people who lose less than expected or no body weight based on the energy expended during exercise training, it is highly likely they adjust their dietary habits to consume more food. As shown in Figure 6.1, the regulation of food intake is complex, and exercise could influence elements of both the homeostatic/biological and non-homeostatic mechanisms of appetite control to ultimately influence energy intake and overall energy balance. Whether less than expected weight loss with exercise training is due to reductions in non-exercise physical activity energy expenditure is less clear, and it seems the major source of energy compensation occurs due to increased energy intake. It is important to recognise that even in the absence of body weight changes with exercise training; there may be favourable alterations to other important aspects of health such as body fat content and distribution, blood lipid profiles, and insulin sensitivity.

Reducing energy intake appears to result in more consistent reductions in body weight in those who have high levels of adherence. It does not appear that one particular method of reducing energy intake for weight loss is any more effective than another (e.g., reducing fat intake or reducing carbohydrate intake). Rather, the energy deficit induced and compliance to the weight reduction strategy are the critical aspects. Nonetheless, even with reduced energy intake it can be difficult to achieve successful and sustained weight loss. Partly this is explained by the fact that restricting food intake tends to lead to increases in hunger and subsequent food intake which would limit the magnitude of negative energy balance achieved. As well, food intake restriction can lead to compensatory reductions in energy expenditure because body weight loss will result in a reduction in fat mass and importantly fat-free mass which will reduce RMR. There may also be metabolic adaptation to reduced energy intake whereby the decrease in energy expenditure observed with food restriction is greater than that predicted from changes in body composition or the thermic effect of food. In this respect it is interestingly to note that exercise can assist more consistently with modest weight loss when combined with reduced energy intake and is particularly effective in preventing weight regain following a period of weight loss; in these situations exercise works by making direct and indirect (e.g., maintenance of RMR) contributions to total energy expenditure.

6.8 Future perspectives

A key development in recent years has been the consideration of energy balance as a dynamic concept whereby the intra- and interrelationships of its component parts (i.e., energy intake and energy expenditure) ultimately determine the likelihood of falling within or outside of energy balance over a sustained period over time. As well, it is clear that there are large individual differences in the susceptibility to weight gain and indeed in the response to weight loss interventions. Understanding the biological (including genetic and epigenetic) and behavioural basis of individual differences in energy balance regulation, within the framework of energy balance as a dynamic construct will represent an important step in the development of personalised approaches for management of body weight. It is also time to move beyond body weight as the only marker of health in respect of energy balance, and to consider how the components of energy balance and their interactions can be modified to improve a broader range of relevant disease risk factors. In this respect, in individuals who appear to be markedly resistant to weight loss interventions, this will bring acceptance that there are still health benefits to be gained from modifying components of energy balance, such as physical activity energy expenditure, independent of weight loss. Importantly, new scientific knowledge needs to be generated in a way that facilitates seamless translation into practice in order to exert efficient and effective impacts upon population health. Along with the strong influence of cultural and environment factors in the regulation of energy balance, clearly more multi- and interdisciplinary working will be required to ensure an integrated and holistic approach to the study of obesity.

Acknowledgement

This chapter has been revised and updated by Gareth Wallis, based on the original chapter by Arne Astrup and Angelo Tremblay.

References

Ainsworth, B.E., Haskell, W.L., Heermann, S.D. *et al.* (2011). Compendium of physical activities: a second update of codes and MET values. *Medicine and Science in Sports and Exercise*, 43(8):1575–1581. doi: 10.1249/MSS.0b013e31821ece12.

Blundell, J.E. (2011). Physical activity and appetite control: can we close the energy gap? *Nutrition Bulletin*, 36:356–366. doi.org/10.1111/j.1467-3010.2011.01911. xFrayn KN. Calculation of substrate oxidation rates in vivo from gaseous exchange. Journal of Applied Physiology, 55(2):628-34, 1983.

Henry, C.J. (2005). Basal metabolic rate studies in humans: measurement and development of new equations. *Public Health Nutrition*, 8:1133–1152.

Hopkins, M., Blundell, J.E. (2016). Energy balance, body composition, sedentariness and appetite regulation: pathways to obesity. *Clinical Science*, 130(18):1615–1628. doi: 10.1042/CS20160006

Maclean, P.S., Blundell, J.E., Mennella, J.A. *et al.* 2017). Biological control of appetite: A daunting complexity. *Obesity*, Suppl 1:S8–S16. doi: 10.1002/oby.21771

Mayer, J., Roy, P., and Mira, K.M. (1956). Relation between caloric intake, body weight and physical work: studies in an industrial male population in West Bengal. *American Journal of Clinical Nutrition*, 4:169–175.

Schofield, W.N., Scholfied, C., and James, W.P.T. (1985). Basal metabolic rate – review and prediction together with an annoted bibliography of source material. *Human Nutrition: Clinical Nutrition*, 39C Suppl1:1–96.

Scientific Advisory Committee of Nurition (2011). *Dietary Reference Values for Energy*. The Stationery Office Limited, London, UK.

Further reading

Hall, K.D. and Guo, J. (2017). Obesity energetics: body weight regulation and the effects of diet composition. *Gastroenterology*, 152(7):1718–1727. DOI: 10.1053/j.gastro.2017.01.052

Lam, Y.Y. and Ravussin, E. (2016). Analysis of energy metabolism in humans: A review of methodologies. *Molecular Metabolism*, 5(11):1057–1071. https://doi.org/10.1016/j.molmet.2016.09.005

Maclean, P.S., Blundell, J.E., Mennella, J.A. *et al.* (2017). Biological control of appetite: A daunting complexity. *Obesity*, Suppl 1:S8–S16. doi: 10.1002/oby.21771

7
Nutrition and Metabolism of Proteins and Amino Acids

D. Joe Millward

Key messages

- Proteins are made up a series of l-α-amino acids (drawn from 21 unique amino acids) linked through peptide bonds with the amino acid side chains conferring protein structure and function, and with their amino acid sequence encoded as triplet sequences of nucleotides in DNA with each gene transcribed and translated into a protein by various RNA molecules.
- All proteins turn over through proteolysis and resynthesis: an energetically expensive dynamic state which serves a number of homeostatic roles.
- Free amino acids serve as precursors to a wide range of compounds, the provision of which drives the obligatory nitrogen losses (ONL) observed in subjects adapted to a protein free diet.
- Amino acid oxidation involves removal of the amino group by transamination and deamination reactions to give ammonia and urea, with the carbon skeleton converted to either glucose or acetyl CoA.
- Many amino acids are nutritionally dispensable and can be synthesised from ammonia and glucose: 9 are nutritionally indispensable (IAAs) with carbon skeletons which cannot be synthesised, while some become indispensable in the absence of other essential precursor amino acids, or when their synthesis is limited under certain conditions. The essentiality of dietary protein is therefore the need for sufficient IAAs and a source of non-essential nitrogen.
- The dietary requirement for protein = metabolic demand/efficiency of utilization and a 2007 WHO report defined the minimum protein requirements (MPR) as: *the lowest level of dietary protein intake that will balance the losses of nitrogen from the body, and thus maintain the body protein mass, in persons at energy balance with modest levels of physical activity, plus, in children or in pregnant or lactating women, the needs associated with the deposition of tissues or the secretion of milk at rates consistent with good health.*
- Part of the demand is obligatory, comprising a) those metabolic pathways that irreversibly consume amino acids giving rise to the ONL and (b) any special needs for growth, pregnancy and lactation.
- Part of the demand is adaptive, involving amino acid oxidation at a particular rate set by the habitual protein intake, enabling the disposal of those potentially toxic IAAs which are maintained in very low concentrations in the free amino acid pool.
- Nitrogen balance (N balance) studies indicate a median MPR value for nitrogen equilibrium from a meta-analysis of multi-level short term balance studies of 0.65g protein/kg/d. Because of the adaptive metabolic demand, the slope of N balance studies markedly underestimates the actual efficiency of protein utilisation so that factorial calculations of the special needs for growth, pregnancy and lactation have been overestimated and need to be revised.
- Dietary protein quality varies with its digestibility and IAA content compared with the IAA content of the demand (the amino acid score). Digestibility is best measured at the terminal ileum, but in practice the available data involves faecal digestibility. IAA requirements for adult maintenance derive from N balance and various stable isotope studies and scoring patterns for protein quality assessment derive from a factorial calculation using the adult pattern and the pattern of tissue protein deposited during growth.
- Although all cereal proteins are limited by lysine with some legumes marginally limited by the sulphur amino acids, most mixed plant-based diets provide sufficient IAAs and are only limited by their digestibility. Many new plant protein sources contain an IAA pattern indistinguishable from animal protein.

Introduction to Human Nutrition, Third Edition. Edited on behalf of The Nutrition Society by Susan A. Lanham-New, Thomas R. Hill, Alison M. Gallagher and Hester H. Vorster.

Companion website: www.wiley.com/go/lanham-new/humannutrition

7.1 Introduction

Proteins, polymers of l-α-amino acids linked through peptide bonds, are by far the most diverse of the large macromolecules which provide structure and enable function of the organism. Diversity reflects the chemistry of the side chains of the 21 unique amino acids occurring in proteins (see Figure 7.1). The human proteome comprises less than 20 000 primary proteins out of an unimaginably large number of different amino acid sequences which could exist for an average protein molecule of about 400 amino acids. Proteins display a unique shape determined by the interactions of the amino acid side chains both within each primary molecule and between different polypeptide chains which form multimeric protein structures. As a result, human proteins comprise a wide range of structures with many different functions (see Table 7.1).

This chapter begins with a brief discussion of the amino acids and the genetic code as determinants of the amino acid content of proteins, followed by a review of protein and amino acid metabolism as the metabolic setting for a consideration of the nutritional requirement for protein and amino acids. This includes a short historical perspective on the nutritional importance of protein and amino acid essentiality, a consideration of the nutritional classification of amino acids, with a brief review of the magnitude of the protein and amino acid requirement in the context of an adaptive metabolic demands model focussing on the implications of this model for current values of protein requirement requirements. Finally, protein quality and the general nutritional properties of plant proteins are reviewed.

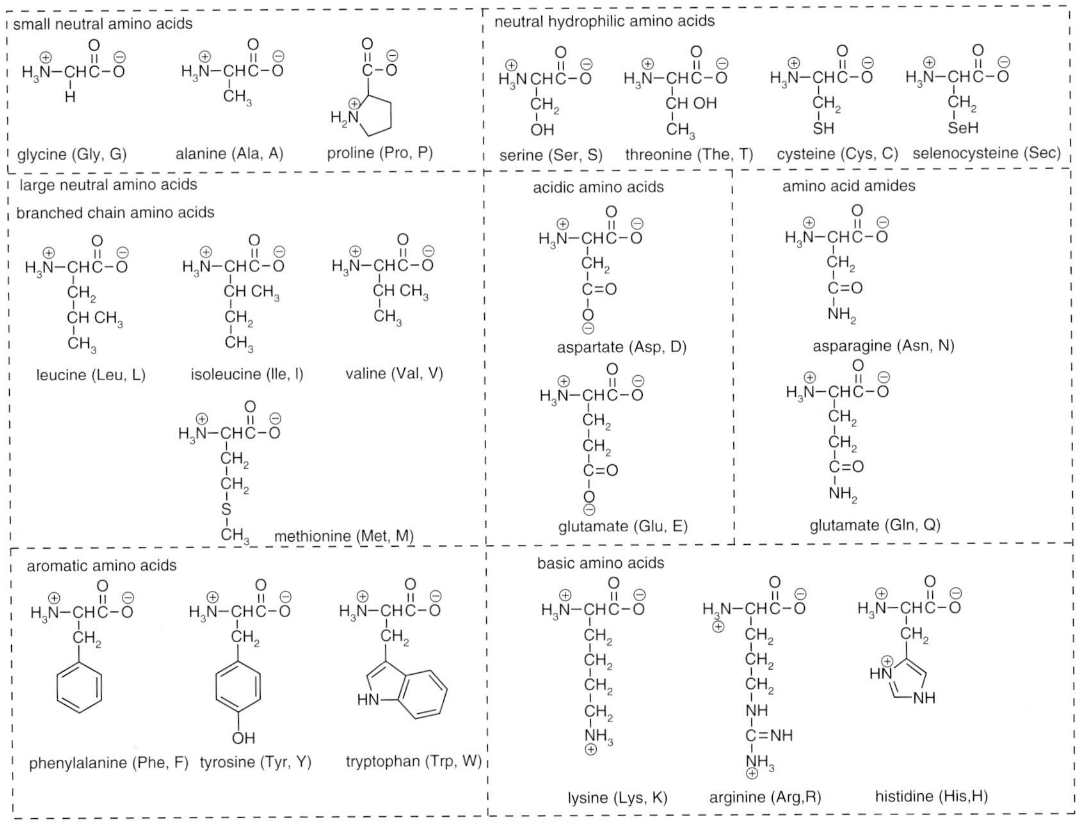

small neutral amino acids
glycine (Gly, G) alanine (Ala, A) proline (Pro, P)

neutral hydrophilic amino acids
serine (Ser, S) threonine (The, T) cysteine (Cys, C) selenocysteine (Sec)

large neutral amino acids
branched chain amino acids
leucine (Leu, L) isoleucine (Ile, I) valine (Val, V)
methionine (Met, M)

acidic amino acids
aspartate (Asp, D)
glutamate (Glu, E)

amino acid amides
asparagine (Asn, N)
glutamate (Gln, Q)

aromatic amino acids
phenylalanine (Phe, F) tyrosine (Tyr, Y) tryptophan (Trp, W)

basic amino acids
lysine (Lys, K) arginine (Arg,R) histidine (His,H)

Figure 7.1 The amino acids, showing three and one letter codes. Those on the left are hydrophobic with those on the right, hydrophilic. Within the protein molecule in general the hydrophobic sequences will tend to avoid water and form the interior of the final structure with the hydrophilic sequences on the outside.

Table 7.1 What do proteins do?

Function	Examples
Muscular contraction	myosin, actin, tropomysin & troponin
Intracellular movement	kinesin;
Structure	collagens, elastin; actin
Enzymatic catalysis	hexokinase, citrate synthetase, glutamate dehydrogenase,
Transport in blood	B_{12} binding proteins; ceruloplasmin; apolipoproteins;
Immunity	antibodies
Plasma oncotic pressure	albumin
Storage/sequestration	ferritin; metallothionein
Peptide hormones	insulin, glucagon, growth hormone, IGF-1
Intercellular signalling molecules	cytokines
Intracellular signalling molecules	tyrosine kinase, mTOR
Regulatory proteins	protein synthesis initiation factors, peptide growth factors;

7.2 The amino acids, the genetic code and protein synthesis

The primary structure of all 20 000 proteins in the organism, the polypeptide amino acid sequence, is encoded as the human genome in the double helix of DNA, mostly in nuclear chromosomes. A few genes (<40) occur in mitochondria which are inherited exclusively from the maternal line because sperm cell mitochondria do not survive fertilisation of the ovum. Remarkably the genome comprises only 1–2% of all DNA, with the importance of the rest of the inter-genic non-coding material not entirely understood. Within the DNA genome each amino acid is coded by a triplet sequence of the four nucleotides from which the DNA helix is made. Because the triplet code involves 64 (4x4x4) triplet combinations, (codons), with only 21 amino acids, this means that there are several codons for each amino acid. The double helix of DNA involves two strands which bind together because of the purine-pyrimidine base pairing, discovered by Watson and Crick, in which the purines adenine (A) and guanine (G) bind to the pyrimidines thymine (T) and cytosine (C). Of these two strands, the "sense" strand contains the genes and the "antisense" strand is a sequence of anti-codons exactly matching the sense strand.

The conversion of the codon sequence of a gene into a protein molecule involves the two phases of protein synthesis. *Transcription* involves the copying of the DNA nucleotide sequence of an individual gene on the sense strand to make an exactly matching ribonucleotide sequence of a messenger (m)RNA molecule, which, after some processing, moves out of the nucleus into the cytoplasm. Thus, RNA contains the same nucleotide sequence as the anti-sense strand of the DNA double helix, apart from the replacement of the thymine in DNA by a uracil in RNA, and the triplet sequences in mRNA are what we identify as the genetic code, (see Table 7.2). *Translation* involves the assembly of the polypeptide sequence as indicated by the mRNA molecule. The translation apparatus involves ribosomes, large protein-RNA complexes, and the smaller amino-acyl transfer RNA (tRNA) molecules which contain a

Table 7.2 The genetic code, showing the codons in mRNA

	second base				
first base	U	C	A	G	third base
U	Phe	Ser	Tyr	Cys	U
U	Phe	Ser	Tyr	Cys	C
U	Leu	Ser	STOP	STOP[1]	A
U	Leu	Ser	STOP	Trp	G
C	Leu	Pro	His	Arg	U
C	Leu	Pro	His	Arg	C
C	Leu	Pro	Gln	Arg	A
C	Leu	Pro	Gln	Arg	G
A	Ile	Thr	Asn	Ser	U
A	Ile	Thr	Asn	Ser	C
A	Ile	Thr	Lys	Arg	A
A	Met	Thr	Lys	Arg	G
G	Val	Ala	Asp	Gly	U
G	Val	Ala	Asp	Gly	C
G	Val	Ala	Glu	Gly	A
G	Val	Ala	Glu	Gly	G

[1] UGA also codes for selenocysteine in a specific context.

binding site for a specific amino acid and a triplet nucleotide sequence associated with the specific amino acid, an anticodon. A specific enzyme, a tRNA ligase, recognises the amino acid and its anticodon on the corresponding tRNA molecule and "charges" the tRNA with its amino acid. The ribosome then enables the anticodon on each tRNA charged with its amino acid, to bind with its appropriate codon on the mRNA and form a peptide bond with the next amino acid in the sequence. What this means is that the faithfulness of translation of the mRNA into a specific protein is determined by the ability of the tRNA ligase enzyme to recognise and join together each tRNA and its amino acid.

Of the 64 possible mRNA codons, three are used to designate the end of a protein chain, (STOP codons), the other 61 code for amino acids (Table 7.2). Thus, the genetic code is degenerate, i.e., there is more than one codon for each amino acid, three on average with methionine and tryptophan having only one codon, and leucine, serine, and arginine having six each. This uneven distribution of codons between amino acids has influenced to some extent the amino acid composition of proteins since, in the database of >0.5-m known protein sequences, the frequency of occurrence of leucine, methionine, and tryptophan is 9.7%, 2.4% and 1.1% respectively, with their frequency in some food proteins shown in Table 7.3.

The average amino acid content of plant and animal source proteins in food differs because of the specific amino acid sequence of the individual proteins most abundant in the food protein source (see Table 7.3). Thus, in muscle proteins, (e.g., beef in Table 7.3), lysine is more abundant than would be expected from its two codons as are the sulphur amino acids (methionine and cysteine) in egg albumin. In cereal grains, the major proteins are the prolamin storage proteins, which contain a high glutamine and proline and low lysine content. These include wheat gluten, barley hordein, rye secalin, maize zein, sorghum kafirin, and as a minor protein, avenin in oats. The unique structure and high content of gluten in wheat enables wheat flour to be made into bread and pasta. Zein in maize is low in tryptophan as well as lysine. The globulin storage proteins in legumes have lower levels of the sulphur amino acids than in cereals or in animal source foods. The implications of these differences in amino acid content for the nutritional quality of food proteins is discussed below.

7.3 Protein and amino acid metabolism

A simplified scheme describing protein and amino acid metabolism in relation to dietary intake and nitrogen excretion is shown in Figure 7.2. The processes shown are turnover, continual degradation, and re-synthesis of tissue proteins: diurnal cycling in which post-absorptive protein losses are replaced by post-prandial net protein synthesis, net protein deposition for special needs, and synthesis of proteins in skin, hair, and various secretions from the body surface. Other useful pathways include amino acids irreversibly transformed to a variety of other compounds. Oxidation is the catabolism of amino acid to urea and ammonia generating ATP and CO_2, while de

Table 7.3 Amino acid composition of food proteins.

	codons	egg	beef	milk	soya	wheat	potato	rice	maize	mean plant	mean animal
					mg/g protein						
Leu	6	83	80	104	76	72	61	86	136	86	89
Thr	4	51	46	44	38	29	38	35	36	35	47
Val	4	75	53	51	50	48	51	61	53	53	60
Ile	3	56	51	38	48	36	42	40	37	41	48
Lys	2	62	91	71	65	26	54	39	26	42	75
Phe + Tyr	2,2	46	42	41	43	40	37	46	48	43	43
Cys + Met	2,1	25	20	18	13	22	14	19	15	17	21
Trp	1	18	13	25	13	12	14	13	7	12	18

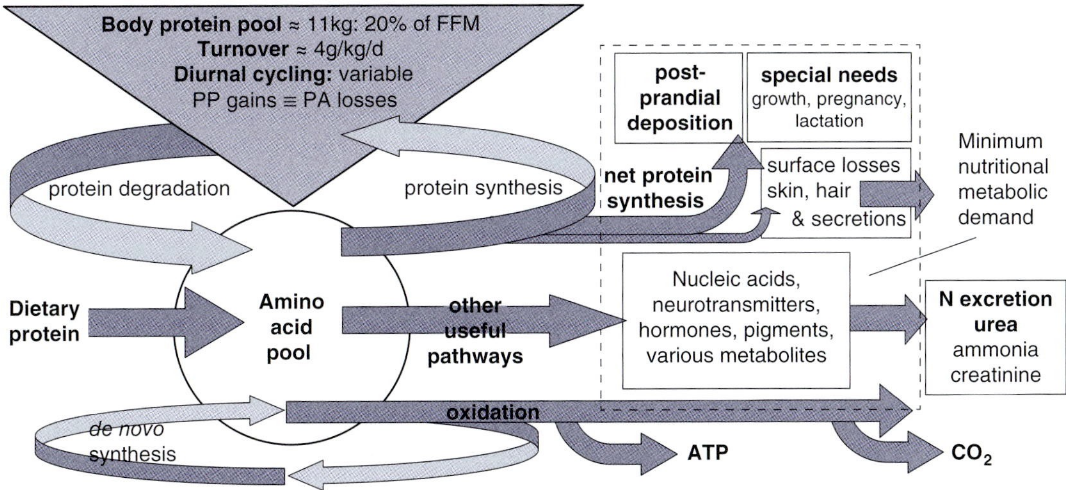

Figure 7.2 Protein metabolism and the metabolic demand for amino acids:-a simplified scheme.

novo formation is the synthesis of amino acids from other amino acids, glucose, and other nitrogen sources (e.g., urea and ammonia). Those pathways within the dotted area identified as the minimum nutritional demand are discussed further below.

The body protein pool

The body protein pool, about 11 kg for a 70 kg adult man, which is 20% of the fat free mass, is distributed between the cellular mass (75%), extra cellular solids (bone, cartilage, tendons, fascia) 23%, and a minor part in the extracellular fluid (2%). Of the cellular mass within the organs, skeletal muscle protein accounts for about 50%.

Protein turnover

All intracellular proteins and many extracellular proteins continually turn over, i.e., they are hydrolyzed to their constituent amino acids by proteolytic enzymes in all cells and replaced by new synthesis, a process which accounts for a significant part of cellular energy expenditure.

The idea that cells undertake continual replacement had been first suggested by the French physiologist Francois Magendie in Paris early in the nineteenth century. However, this was not pursued until a century later when Rudolf Schoenheimer and David Rittenberg in New York, in the late 1930s, early 1940s, developed stable isotope tracer techniques with the newly discovered isotopes [^{2}H] (deuterium) and [^{15}N]. They synthesised isotopically enriched amino acids and gave them to rats observing their incorporation into tissue proteins, identifying what they called metabolic "regeneration," the continual release and uptake of chemical substances by tissues to and from a circulating metabolic "pool." Subsequently, in the 1960s John Waterlow, who was investigating protein metabolism in malnutrition, simplified the methods for measuring whole body and tissue protein turnover and they became widely used with amino acids labelled both with radioactive isotopes (^{3}H and ^{14}C) for animal studies and stable isotopes (^{2}H,^{13}C and ^{15}N) for human studies. These studies have shown that individual proteins in the nucleus and cytosol, as well as in the endoplasmic reticulum (ER) and mitochondria, are degraded at widely differing rates that vary from minutes for some regulatory enzymes to days or weeks for proteins such as actin and myosin in skeletal muscle or months for haemoglobin in the red cell. In the latter case, it is the erythrocyte itself which is "turning over" through its destruction within the spleen. With the development of proteomic techniques for the separation and analysis of all proteins within cells, and with stable isotope labelling, it is now possible to evaluate the turnover rates of proteins within the entire proteome.

Protein degradation

Multiple proteolytic systems in cells enable turnover with complex regulatory mechanisms to ensure that turnover is highly selective and excessive breakdown of cell constituents is prevented. One major proteolytic system is the autophagic–lysosomal pathway which involves a number of acidic proteases within the membrane-bound lysosome which are capable of degrading any protein or even cellar structures to amino acids. Entry into the lysosome involves several different autophagic mechanisms. Another major system is the ubiquitin-proteasome pathway. This involves an initial linkage of a polypeptide co-factor, ubiquitin, onto proteins to mark them for degradation by a very large multicatalytic protease complex, the proteasome. This proteolytic machine degrades ubiquitinated proteins to small peptides, to be subsequently degraded to amino acids by cytosolic peptidases, with the ubiquitin recycled. A third system, the calpain-calpastatin system, comprises two calcium-activated calpain proteinases and their inhibitor calpastatin. This system is present in muscle and many other cell types and is associated primarily with subcellular organelles such as myofibrils in skeletal muscle and the cytoskeleton, vesicles, and the plasma membrane in other cell types. Finally, the caspases are a family of cytosolic proteases which are critical in the destruction of cell constituents during apoptosis, (programmed cell death). Although these four systems are well described as far as the proteinases involved, protein turnover remains a very poorly understood process in terms of how it works and is regulated on a day-to-day basis.

Overall, the rates of cellular protein synthesis and degradation within cells are balanced precisely to avoid a marked growth or loss of mass in the organism. This is achieved through highly complex multiple signalling systems which exert fine control over both protein synthesis and proteolysis, in response to hormones, such as IGF-1 and insulin, cytokines and metabolites, of which amino acids especially some individual amino acids like glutamine and leucine, are the most important. In addition, cell swelling and shrinkage in result to changes in cellular hydration exerts overall anabolic and catabolic influences.

The functional importance of protein turnover

Although most discussion of cellular protein degradation systems relates to tissue wasting in starvation and diseases states, with the four known systems having different specific roles, it is the case that in healthy individuals in the post-absorptive state there is a net loss of protein from muscle and other tissues resulting in amino acid oxidation and urea excretion, because of an excess of protein degradation over protein synthesis. This continues until a meal provides energy and protein to reverse the catabolism and mediate net protein deposition to replace the post-absorptive losses. This diurnal cycling can only occur because of continuing protein degradation and because both protein synthesis and degradation are sensitive to nutrition. Measurements of whole body and tissue protein turnover show that both protein degradation and synthesis are sensitive to feeding which mediates an inhibition of the post-absorptive rate of degradation of up to 50% together with an increase in protein synthesis. The continuing intracellular proteolysis even in the post-prandial state means that the continual removal and replacement of cellular proteins must be absolutely necessary for normal functioning of cellular processes and metabolism.

It is often stated that the reutilisation of amino acids during protein turnover is inefficient, with only 70% of amino acids reutilised, and that this accounts for a major part of the nutritional requirement for protein. In fact, there is no direct evidence about the extent of amino acid recycling and the 70% efficiency figure derives from an inadequate understanding of the regulation of oxidative pathways of amino acids which generates a metabolic demand for their dietary replacement. This is discussed further below in relation to the metabolic basis of the protein requirement.

The free amino acid pool and amino acid metabolism

Free amino acids occur in both extracellular (ecf) and intracellular (icf) pools. The ecf pool present in blood plasma and interstitial fluid is of mainly uniform composition throughout the body because of blood flow. The plasma membrane of cells is impermeable to amino acids, but specific transporters mediate amino acid transport which allows rapid exchange between ecf and icf compartments. The icf pools within individual tissues and organs, differ in their amino acid composition from the ecf pool and vary between organs and tissues. Both ecf and icf amino acid composition bear very little relationship to that of dietary protein. Figure 7.3 shows amino acid concentrations in the human ecf and the largest ICF compartment (skeletal muscle), with many amino acids concentrated within the icf through active transport systems which link the inward transport to that of Na+ influx which is then pumped out in exchange for K+ by the Na+/K+ ATPase pump. Glutamine is the most abundant within muscle and its gradient is used to energise the inward transport of other amino acids such as leucine. Note that the concentrations of the branched chain, aromatic, and sulphur amino acids are maintained at very low levels both in the ecf and icf pools even though they may be very abundant in proteins as with leucine. The implication of this, at first sight, quite surprising difference between the composition of the free amino acid pool from that of dietary and body proteins which replenish it is discussed further below.

Free amino acids not only provide for protein synthesis but also serve as precursors to most nitrogen-containing compounds in the organism, shown as other useful pathways in Figure 7.2. These range from small molecules like nitric oxide (NO), an important signalling molecule within the vascular system, to the nucleotides which make up the nucleic acids. Some important examples are listed in Table 7.4.

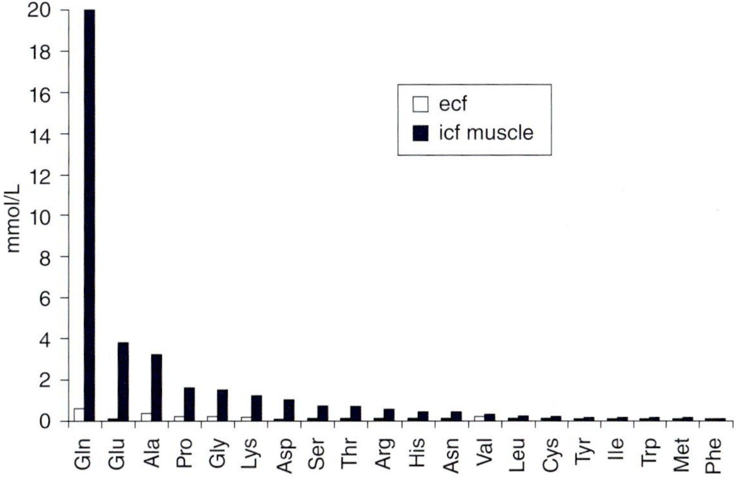

Figure 7.3 Amino acid concentrations in the extracellular fluid (ecf), blood plasma and intracellular fluid (icf), human muscle.

Table 7.4 Useful pathways of amino acid consumption

Amino acid	Molecules synthesised
Arginine	Creatine, nitric oxide, proline, polyamines
Aspartate	Purine and pyrimidine nucleotides
Cysteine	Glutathione, Taurine
Glutamate	Glutathione, N-acetylglutamate, γ-aminobutyrate,
Glutamine	Purine and pyrimidine nucleotides, amino sugars, ammonia transport, cellular fuel
Glycine	Creatine, porphyrins (for haemoglobin and cytochromes), purines, bile acids, glutathione, hippuric acid
Histidine	Histamine, carnosine, anserine
Lysine	Carnitine
Methionine	Creatine, carnitine, choline, acetylcholine, ornithine, putrescine,
Serine	Ethanolamine, choline, sphingosine
Tyrosine	Adrenaline, noradrenaline, dopamine, melanin pigments, thyroxine
Tryptophan	Serotonin (5-hydroxytryptamine), melatonin (N-acetyl-5-methoxy tryptamine), nicotinamide

These include *neurotransmitters*; serotonin, dopamine, glutamate, and acetyl choline, *hormones*; adrenaline, noradrenaline, thyroxine, *inflammatory mediators*; histamine, *cofactor precursors*; nicotinamide, *antioxidants* (glutathione) and numerous other compounds. These are formed in many cases through unidirectional pathways and are either eventually converted to urea after catabolism of the intermediates, or excreted directly (as with creatinine). The amounts involved for some of these pathways may be quite small as with nitric oxide for example. Arginine is the precursor of NO and the total amount of NO synthesised (and degraded) per day may represent less than 1% of the daily arginine intake. In contrast, the synthesis and turnover of glutathione, (GSH), a major intracellular thiol and important antioxidant, formed from glutamate, glycine, and cysteine, that protects cells against damage by reactive oxygen species, accounts for a high rate of cysteine utilisation. This is especially the case in conditions of oxidative stress, where the oxidised form of glutathione (GSSG) may leak out of the tissues and some of it may be transformed into mercapturic acid and excreted. When this occurs, there will be an increased demand for the sulphur amino acids (methionine and/or cysteine) and some suggest they should be supplemented as part of nutritional therapy of trauma patients. This is discussed further below.

Urinary creatinine derives from muscle creatine phosphate, the store of high energy phosphate which can regenerate ATP from ADP. Both creatine and creatine phosphate concentrations are regulated at a specific level but undergo an irreversible spontaneous reaction to form creatinine at a constant rate of about 2% per day. This is no longer useful and leaves muscle to be excreted by the kidneys by very efficient renal clearance. This means that the urinary creatinine excretion rate varies with the skeletal muscle creatine/creatine phosphate pool size, itself a function of skeletal muscle mass. The assumed relationship is 1 g/d of excreted creatinine is equivalent to 18–22 kg of muscle mass. This also means that the amount of creatinine in a single sample of urine can be used to calculate what proportion of the daily urine production the sample represents, enabling the amount of any urinary metabolite in the urine sample, (e.g., sodium or iodine) to be scaled up to a 24 hour equivalent, where 24 hour urine samples cannot be obtained. In the same way a urinary metabolite concentration can be standardised by expressing it as the metabolite/creatinine concentration. However variable dietary creatine intakes (from meat), variation in hepatic creatine synthesis and an influence of physical activity on creatinine formation from creatine, means that the precision of this relationship is low with quite large day to day variations in creatinine excretion (≈20%).

The quantitative importance of amino acid utilisation as precursors for such compounds as those shown in Table 7.4 is poorly understood although we can make some estimates. An upper limit can be estimated from the obligatory nitrogen losses (ONL), the total urinary and faecal nitrogen losses from healthy adults after their adaptation, (usually over two weeks), to a protein-free diet. This is about 50 mg N/kg/d, equivalent to about 0.3 g protein/kg/d lost from the body protein store which is assumed to provide for the basal amino acid needs. However, this net loss of tissue protein releases amino acids in proportion to their occurrence in tissue protein and this pattern is unlikely to be the same as the pattern of basal amino acid consumption with many amino acids present in excess of their basal metabolic requirement. It is possible however, that the requirement of only one amino acid can be identified in this way, i.e., the limiting amino acid, with the highest ratio of metabolic demand for maintenance to tissue protein content. The metabolic consumption of methionine is believed to be the amino acid which in effect "drives" the ONL. This means that the overall metabolic requirements for amino acids in other pathways is considerably less than their content in 0.3 g protein/kg/d.

Oxidation of amino acids The oxidation of amino acids requires the removal of the amino group and its subsequent conversion to urea, and the disposal of the remaining α-oxoacid carbon skeletons in energy-generating pathways. Although urea production occurs in the liver, there is considerable amino acid metabolism and oxidation in extrahepatic tissues including muscle, brain, kidney, adipose tissues, and the intestine.

Transamination reactions and de novo synthesis of amino acids The amino group of most amino acids is very labile and can exchange between amino acids and form new amino acids (de novo synthesis) when the α- oxoacid carbon skeleton can be synthesised from simple metabolic intermediates. The exchange of amino groups with α- oxoacids involves pyridoxal phosphate-dependent transamination reactions. The α- oxoacids include α-ketoglutarate, pyruvate, 3-phosphohydroxypyruvate, and oxaloacetate which form glutamate, alanine, serine (via phosphoserine), and aspartate.

Removal of the amino nitrogen group Some amino acids can be directly oxidised to their corresponding α-oxoacids releasing ammonia—the process of deamination. There is a general amino acid oxidase that catalyses this reaction, but it has a low activity. Four amino acids (glutamate, glycine, serine, and threonine) are deaminated by specific enzymes. Of these glutamate dehydrogenase, a mitochondrial enzyme which is present in most tissues, and especially in the liver, is particularly important, mediating the oxidative deamination of glutamate and releasing ammonia in an NAD/NADH-linked reaction capturing some of the energy of the α-amino group for subsequent ATP production.

$$\text{Glutamate} + H_2O + NAD^+ \rightarrow \alpha\text{-ketoglutarate} + {NH^+}_4 + NADH$$

Glycine is oxidised by the mitochondrial glycine cleavage system generating, tetrahydrofolate, ammonia and NADH, while serine, threonine, and histidine deamination by their dehydratase enzymes liberate ammonia without any NAD/NADH-linked reactions, i.e., no ATP is generated, only heat.

Glutamine also plays an important role in nitrogen transport and amino acid oxidation. It is synthesised from glutamate and ammonia by glutamine synthetase, an ATP requiring enzyme.

$$\text{Glutamate} + {NH^+}_4 + ATP \rightarrow \text{Glutamine} + ADP + P_i + H^+$$

Glutaminase mediates the reverse reaction liberating glutamate and ammonia.

$$\text{Glutamine} + H_2 0 \rightarrow \text{glutamate} + {NH^+}_4$$

Both glutamate and glutamine play an important role in the oxidation of the branched chain amino acids (BCAAs), which can account for 20% of dietary protein. The BCAAs reversibly transaminate with α-ketoglutarate (α-KG) to make glutamate and their α- oxoacids, a reaction mediated by the branched chain amino transferase enzyme (BCAT), which acts on all three BCAAs. Subsequently, the irreversible dehydrogenase enzyme (BCKD), acts on the branched chain α-oxoacids, such as α-oxo isocaproate (OIC), which is the first step in their oxidation. These two enzymes are widespread in peripheral tissues, especially muscle, brain, and adipose tissue, as well as liver, kidney, intestine, and heart. The peripheral location of BCAA metabolism means that they can serve as a source α-amino nitrogen to the periphery.

For example, human brain avidly extracts leucine and releases glutamine, with the entry of leucine exceeding that of any other amino acid. Although not neuroactive, leucine shares the same large neutral amino acid transporter of the aromatic amino acids and can influence their tissue uptake and the synthesis of neurotransmitters deriving from them (dopamine from tyrosine and serotonin from tryptophan). Leucine is especially important for brain glutamate metabolism being "trafficked" between cellular compartments, providing -NH_2 groups for glutamate synthesis in compartments of high glutamate concentration and supplying OIC to act as a sink for -NH_2 groups from glutamate in compartments of low glutamate concentration.

In skeletal muscle, the uptake of BCAA represents ≅ 50% of all amino acids taken up after a meal, with their nitrogen released as alanine and glutamine. Alanine synthesis can occur through the mitochondrial form of alanine amino-transferase, which is expressed in muscle, allowing glutamate produced by BCAT to be recycled back to α-KG through transamination with pyruvate. Glutamine can be synthesised as described above, and is present in skeletal muscle in very high concentrations (see Figure 7.3), its concentration maintained by a secondary, (Na^+ linked), active transporter (SNAT2).

In the liver, alanine and glutamine from peripheral BCAA oxidation make ammonia available for urea synthesis. Glutamine is also taken up by enterocytes in the gastrointestinal tract and in some circumstances by the kidney as discussed below.

Urea synthesis

The ornithine cycle of urea synthesis (see Figure 7.4), was discovered by Krebs and Henseleit in 1932. This is the way in which mammals detoxify ammonia liberated from amino acids and excrete it as urea. In fish, the abundance of water allows ammonia to be removed without the need for urea synthesis, whilst in birds the need to conserve water results in the formation and excretion of the insoluble uric acid, without the formation of urine per se. Whilst the urea cycle is usually discussed solely in these terms, it does serve a second important function as a means of getting rid of bicarbonate, (HCO_3^-). The complete oxidation of amino acids yields HCO_3^- and NH_4^+. Air-breathing animals can excrete volatile CO_2 from their lungs, but not HCO_3^-. The kidney, with its usual range of urine production, cannot remove the daily HCO_3^- production associated with oxidation of amino acids from usual protein intakes. Thus, hepatic urea synthesis, which consumes two moles of HCO_3^- and two moles of NH_4^+ per mole urea formed is the major pathway for disposal of HCO_3^-.

$$\text{i.e., } HCO_3^- + 2NH_4^+ \rightarrow H_2NCONH_2 + H^+ + 2H_20$$

$$\underline{HCO_3^- + H^+ \rightarrow H_2O + CO_2}$$

$$2HCO_3^- + 2NH_4^+ \rightarrow H_2NCONH_2 + CO_2 + 3H_20$$

a. Sources of ammonia The two nitrogen atoms of urea derive from ammonia and aspartate (shown in bold in Figure 7.4). Whereas urea production takes place largely within the liver, much of the ammonia used in urea synthesis is derived, directly or indirectly, from extrahepatic tissues. One source is alanine and glutamine from the peripheral oxidation of the BCAAs as described above, the other is the intestine as described below.

A major source of ammonia for the first step of the urea cycle, the formation of carbamyl phosphate, is glutamate, via the action of mitochondrial glutamate dehydrogenase. The glutamate is derived by transamination from alanine, aspartate and other transaminating amino acids and by the deamidation of glutamine another important source of ammonia. Ammonia is also

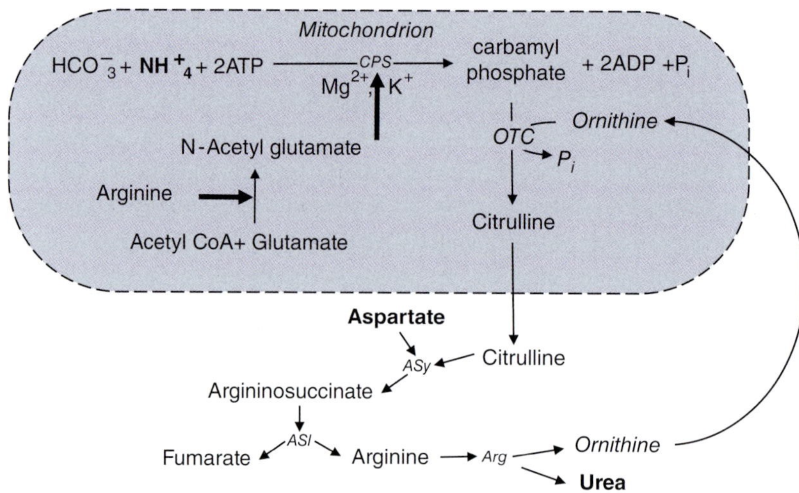

Figure 7.4 The ornithine cycle enzymes and their distribution in the liver. *CPS*, carbamoyl phosphate synthetase; *OTC*, ornithine transcarbamylase; Asy, argininosuccinicsynthetase; ASI, argininosuccinate lyase; Arg, arginase.

generated by the deamidation of asparagine and the deamination of glycine, serine, threonine, and histidine.

The aspartate which provides the second nitrogen molecule in urea derives from the citric acid cycle intermediate oxaloacetate by transamination from alanine or other transaminating amino acids by the abundant aspartate aminotransferase. Aspartate is always present in excess and as fast as it is used up in the formation of argininosuccinate, it is replenished.

25% of the ammonia utilised in urea synthesis reaches the liver via the portal vein, because the intestine is a major site of ammonia production by two important pathways. Firstly, the intestinal mucosa produces a significant quantity of ammonia, which comes from the metabolism of glutamine removed from arterial blood, and from oxidation of some intraluminal amino acids from food (e.g., alanine, glutamate, and aspartate). A second source of ammonia is from salvage of 15–30% of the urea synthesised by the liver, which enters the intestinal lumen where it is degraded by bacterial ureases mainly in the mucosa or the juxtamucosal area of the colon, and to a lesser extent in the small intestine, with the liberation of ammonia (and carbon dioxide). This ammonia from the intestine enters the portal circulation, where the ammonia concentration in the portal vein is up to 10-fold greater than elsewhere in the circulation, and it is converted back to urea in the liver.

b. Ammonia detoxication by glutamine synthesis Apart from urea synthesis the other major pathway for ammonia detoxication in liver is glutamine synthesis by glutamine synthetase, which is anatomically separate from the urea cycle enzymes. Portal blood from the GIT to the liver first encounters the urea cycle system in periportal hepatocytes which will remove intestinal ammonia. However, after this at the perivenous end of the liver functional unit a small hepatocyte subpopulation, perivenous scavenger cells, contains no urea-cycle enzymes but do contain glutamine synthetase which can eliminate with high affinity any ammonia that was not used by the upstream urea-synthesising compartment. These cells are of crucial importance for the maintenance of non-toxic ammonia levels in the hepatic vein and throughout the body. Up to 25% of the ammonia delivered via the portal vein escapes periportal urea synthesis and is used for glutamine synthesis in these cells which exhibit high-affinity uptake of carbon precursors for glutamine synthesis, mainly α – ketoglutarate. Perivenous glutamine synthesis allows excess NH_4^+ to be transported via the bloodstream to the kidney as glutamine, to be degraded by renal glutaminase with NH_4^+ excreted via the tubules. By intricate intercellular compartmentation in the liver of a more periportal localisation of urea synthesis and glutaminase, the regulation of hepatic glutaminase provides a major point of pH control in the organism. In acidosis, both these processes are shut off, decreasing bicarbonate removal, favouring hepatic glutamine formation by the perivenously located glutamine synthetase, and causing increased renal excretion of NH_4^+ instead of urea. The converse holds in alkalosis. Thus, a hepatic intercellular glutamine cycle between periportal and perivenous cells of the lobule serves a regulatory function in the pH homeostasis of the organism. While such a scheme is clear from animal studies, the relationship between pH homeostasis and ureagenesis in human metabolism is a controversial issue.

c. Regulation of the urea cycle Experimental in vitro studies indicate that the operation of the urea cycle is automatic, controlled entirely by kinetic and thermodynamic factors. The activity of the first enzyme, CPS-1, is irreversible and appears to control the rate of urea production. However, CPS-1 is inactive without a co-factor, N-acetyl glutamate (N-AG), which is an allosteric activator (see Figure 7.4). Because the synthesis of N-AG is stimulated by glutamate, through a substrate effect, and also by arginine, many believe N-AG to be a regulator or even overall controller of the urea cycle especially since the amount of N-AG in the liver increases when the amino acid supply and the production of urea is increased: i.e., glutamate stimulates the formation of N-AG which then exerts control over CPS-1. However, others believe that although N-AG activates CPS-1, substrate availability (free NH_3 and ornithine) exerts immediate control. Clearly this is a complex subject.

The metabolism of amino acid carbon skeletons

The various pathways by which the carbon skeletons of amino acids are converted into useful energy result in one of two end products. Most amino acids are glucogenic (glucose-forming), after conversion to pyruvate, oxaloacetate, α-keto glutarate, propionyl CoA, succinyl CoA, or fumarate. The ketogenic amino acids, leucine and lysine, are converted into acetyl CoA which feeds into the tricarboxylic acid cycle and is converted to CO_2 and ATP, or into fatty acid synthesis. Tryptophan, isoleucine, phenylalanine, and tyrosine are both ketogenic and glucogenic.

7.4 Protein and amino acid requirements

The historical background

The nutritional importance of dietary protein

Following the identification of nitrogen by Rutherford in the late nineteenth century our understanding of the nutritional importance of protein began in Paris in the early nineteenth century where the indispensability of dietary N was established by the feeding trials on dogs by Magendie and the balance studies on herbivores of Boussingault. These studies, together with the chemical identification of protein by Mulder, established protein as the determinant of food "quality" and the food constituent which dominated nutritional science for the rest of the nineteenth century.

The first discussions of how much protein was needed in the diet were those of Carl Voit in Germany in the 1880s. Although he reported nitrogen balance studies on dogs and humans, his recommended intake derived simply from observations of what working people choose to eat: i.e., 118 g protein/d. In America, Wilbur Atwater thought that American workmen worked harder and ate more, so his recommendation was 125 g/d. Some disagreed, notably John Harvey Kellogg, a physician and Seventh-day Adventist who promoted a much lower protein vegetarian diet, inventing breakfast cereals including Kelloggs corn flakes. The most prominent low protein advocate was Russell Chittenden, Professor of Physiological Chemistry at Yale in the early twentieth century, who had deliberately reduced his own meat and protein intake (to about 40g/d) and claimed he felt the benefit. With five month trials of low meat diets involving his scientific colleagues, soldiers and then some elite athletes, he demonstrated not only maintenance of fitness on about 0.75 g protein per d, but also an increased strength (by 35% in the athletes), a fall in perceived fatigue with increased wellbeing. He concluded that "man can profitably maintain nitrogen equilibrium and body weight upon a much smaller amount of protein food than he is accustomed to consume." He defined an optimal requirement of about 0.75 g/kg, close to the current safe allowance of 0.83 g/kg/d, with most of this coming from plant protein sources. Chittenden's views were controversial at the time and have been given less prominence than they deserve, although it is likely that his athletes improved their performance because of a higher carbohydrate intake after swopping meat for potatoes. However, the data on protein intakes speak for themselves.

The next important event in attitudes towards protein was inadvertently triggered by articles on kwashiorkor published by Cecily D. Williams in the 1930s. She described the condition of kwashiorkor in Ghana and suggested it was due to protein deficiency, a view which was consonant with reports at the time suggesting, quite incorrectly, that the protein:energy (P:E) ratio of the protein requirement was highest at the age of 2y, falling markedly into adult life. An early FAO/WHO report on kwashiorkor in Africa in 1951 identified it as protein-deficiency after which protein supplies and deficiency became far and away the most important issue for international nutrition. Indeed, the United Nations published in 1968 a call for "International Action to Avert the Impending Protein Crisis". In consequence, the green revolution was initiated involving new seeds, fertilisers and pesticides to allow monoculture, the intensification of livestock production and a massive investment in soya production.

We now know that Kwashiorkor is caused by a combination of infection and multiple micronutrient deficiency, especially the antioxidant micronutrients, not by protein deficiency. Also, even though the protein requirements of infants and young children (per kg) are greater than adults, the P:E ratio of their protein requirement is low, as indicated by the composition of breast milk, (P:E = 6–7%), because their energy requirements (per kg) are much higher than adults. Because of this protein deficiency is much less common than had been believed. Nevertheless the idea of "Protein, the only true nutrient", proposed by Liebig in 1842, on the basis of his incorrect view that it was the fuel for muscular work, still influences attitudes to the importance of protein, as does the view that protein deficiency is widespread in children.

Development of the concept of amino acid essentiality

Recognition of the concept of dietary amino acid essentiality as the determinant of dietary protein quality arose early in the nineteenth century through feeding trials with collagen extracted from bones. This showed that collagen protein was demonstrably nutritionally inferior to proteins such as albumin extracted from serum. The advances in chemical analysis of protein in the latter part of the nineteenth century resulted in the identification of many individual amino acids by the early twentieth century with Hopkins isolating tryptophan (1901) which in turn enabled the unusual composition of collagen and especially its lack of any tryptophan to be demonstrated. Thus, Kaufman showed that gelatin + tryptophan + cystine + tyrosine maintained N balance in dogs and man. The other protein which aroused interest through its inability to allow growth of animals was zein, the principal protein extract from maize. In 1906, Hopkins had shown that mice fed on zein (which contains very low levels of tryptophan) lived longer if they also received a supplement of tryptophan. This established the concept of dietary protein quality determined by its amino acid content. N balance studies with adults with different foods, rapidly established the importance of protein quality in human nutrition. The final refinements of the basic principles of the nutritional quality of protein were the experiments of Osborne and Mendel (1915). As shown in Figure 7.5, they showed that rats fed zein lost weight and died without tryptophan, but maintained weight when supplemented with tryptophan and then grew with additional lysine (i.e., zein was limited by tryptophan for maintenance and by lysine for growth). The implication of these famous experiments is that the pattern of amino acids required for maintenance is different from that for growth as subsequently confirmed in animal studies. After this, in pioneering work, Rose completed the identification of all 20 amino acids by discovering threonine in 1935, and then identified and quantified the 8 indispensable amino acids (IAAs) needed to maintain N balance in adult humans. Although Rose had failed to show that lack of histidine influenced N balance in adults, because of the detrimental effects of histidine-free diets on haemoglobin concentrations in individuals fed such a diet, histidine eventually became the ninth IAA. Rose's N

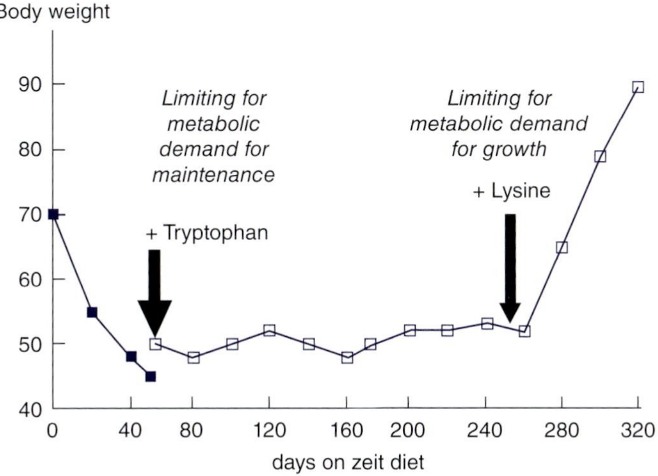

Figure 7.5 Rat growth with zeinprotein. Source: Osborne & Mendel 1915.

balance work was followed up by further N balance studies, some on women, to establish the requirement of individual amino acids like lysine, and many to establish the overall protein requirement of men and women in the 1960s and 70s.

These balance studies also showed that the need for dietary IAAs depends upon the total amount and type of nitrogen in the diet. Thus, the higher the total N, the lower the amount of IAA needed for N balance. The most effective "non-essential nitrogen" for maintenance was a mixture of dispensable amino acids, which was better than one single dispensable amino acid such as glycine, which was better than ammonia and/or urea. The clear implication of this was that the minimum N intake for N balance is determined by the intake of dispensable amino acids (DAA), and this was confirmed with the demonstration that at any given level of N intake with egg protein, partial replacement of the protein with DAA improved N balance.

Subsequently, stable isotope studies in the 1980s and 90s quantified the magnitude of amino acid requirements in adult men and women and these values are used today.

Current nutritional classification of amino acids

After these early studies it became apparent that classification of amino acids into just two categories was insufficient, with a third category introduced to accommodate amino acids which could become essential under certain circumstances when their synthesis in the tissues could become limited. Table 7.5 shows the 21 amino acids found in proteins listed in terms of their currently accepted nutritional dispensability, i.e., whether they can be synthesised in the body.

In many ways, with the exception of histidine, the classification of the 9 IAAs is the most straightforward: they cannot be synthesised in human tissues and therefore must be provided in the diet. Strictly speaking, it is the carbon skeletons which are indispensable, but in no case do these occur naturally in the diet. However, in renal patients when nitrogen excretion becomes compromised, the branched chain α-oxo acids have been used to formulate special diets which would maintain the branched chain amino acid pool through transamination.

Table 7.5 Amino acid essentiality/dispensability of the 21 coded amino acids

	Essential/ indispensable	Conditionally essential/ indispensable	Nonessential/ dispensable
Group	*no synthesis*	*limited synthesis at times*	*unlimited synthesis*
Branched chain	Leucine Isoleucine Valine		
Aromatic	Phenylalanine Tryptophan	→ Tyrosine	
Sulphur/ selenium	Methionine	→ Cysteine	Selenocysteine (from inorganic Se)
Basic	Lysine Histidine	Arginine	
Acidic and amides		Glutamine	Glutamate Aspartate Asparagine
Neutral	Threonine	Glycine Proline	Alanine Serine

Identifying the dispensable group, which exhibit unlimited synthesis in the tissues from a source of transaminating nitrogen, is relatively straightforward. Indeed, because the enterocytes oxidise glutamate, aspartate (and probably asparagine), and glutamine, only a small fraction of these amino acids in food appears in the portal blood after a meal. Their nitrogen is absorbed in the form of ammonia and alanine which enables their resynthesis in the liver and other tissues. Selenocysteine *per se* is not required in the diet since for the few selenoproteins which contain this amino acid, (54 proteins in 2016) it is made from serine and inorganic selenium on a specific tRNA species which directs the selenocysteine to a specific stop codon (UGA) in mRNA by means of a specific elongation factor.

The conditionally IAAs are those for which their synthesis may be limited under specific circumstances so that a dietary requirement has been suggested. Clearly under normal circumstances of protein feeding of healthy subjects they will be provided, and it has never been suggested that their dietary protein content could be limiting, influencing protein quality, comparable to the IAAs. However, in the clinical environment, conditionality may become important when metabolic demands for specific amino acids are increased, when special feeds and feeding modalities differ from usual healthy eating, and when there is an inborn error of metabolism preventing synthesis of an amino acid. One obvious example of the latter situation is phenylketonuria (PKU) when there are very low levels of phenylalanine hydroxylase which converts phenylalanine to tyrosine. For such patients, tyrosine is indispensable. Another example is parenteral nutrition (PN) when a solution of free amino acids is fed intravenously. Glutamine is not normally present in PN solutions because of concern for its instability during heat sterilisation. So, the clinical question is, should efforts be made to ensure glutamine is provided? Similarly, in enterally fed patients when special feeds are formulated, should additional amino acids be added to such feeds? Whilst for tyrosine, with the exception of PKU, it is not thought likely that its supply from phenylalanine is ever limited, the conditionality of cysteine, arginine, proline, glycine, and glutamine has been widely discussed but after several decades of research, in each case a consensus has yet to be reached about the special provision of these amino acids in the various circumstances where they may have benefit. Here the salient issues are reviewed.

Cysteine is formed on the catabolic pathway of methionine although only the sulphur (thiol) group of cysteine actually derives from methionine with the rest of the molecule coming from serine which might limit conversion of methionine to cysteine. In addition, methionine conversion to cysteine is limited or compromised by poor B-vitamin status in infancy and by alcohol consumption. As indicated in Table 7.4, cysteine is part of glutathione a tripeptide (γ-glutamyl-cysteinyl glycine, GSH). GSH is a key part of the cellular antioxidant system found in all cells existing predominantly in its reduced state, GSH with much lower concentrations of its oxidation product, GSSG. The GSH/GSSG redox system maintains an overall reducing environment in the cell. Cysteine availability has been considered limiting for the synthesis of GSH in pathological situations, such as malnutrition or HIV infection, since providing cysteine has been shown to stimulate GSH synthesis and restore GSH stores. Also, immaturity in preterm infants has been suggested as a reason that cysteine is indispensable, so it is added to some but not all PN solutions. Whether cysteine provision for preterm infants should be part of their feeding guidelines is under discussion.

Arginine is an example of an amino acid which may become essential under conditions of stress and catabolic states when the capacity of endogenous amino acid synthesis is exceeded. It as an important amino acid for several reasons but its metabolism is quite complex varying between tissues and is incompletely understood. As the immediate precursor of urea in the urea cycle it is synthesised from ornithine, but its cleavage to urea by arginase in the liver poses a problem for the supply of arginine to extrahepatic tissues. Furthermore, a second arginase enzyme (type II arginase) occurs in enterocytes so that only a small fraction of arginine from dietary protein is absorbed. However, there is cooperation between the intestine and the kidney to supply extrahepatic tissues arginine. This involves the synthesis of citrulline in enterocytes from glutamine and proline which is released into the portal blood and appears to bypass the liver to be extracted by the kidney where it is converted to arginine. This renal arginine is the source of about 60% of the circulating arginine.

As already indicated in Table 7.4, arginine is the precursor of nitric oxide (NO) the endothelium-derived molecule involved in vasodilation, immune responses, neurotransmission, and platelet adhesion, a reaction which occurs in many cell types and which is of great importance. In NO producing cells, this reaction generates citrulline which can be reconverted to arginine from aspartate in an arginine/citrulline cycle. This means there should be no limitation on arginine supply for NO production. However, it appears that under conditions of stress, and the catabolic states of critical illness with catabolism of arginine by arginase, the capacity for endogenous arginine synthesis may become inadequate with arginine limiting for NO production. This will contribute to endothelial dysfunction and/or T-cell dysfunction, depending on the clinical scenario and disease state. Certainly, during wound healing, the citrulline formed from NO production may be converted to proline for collagen synthesis (see below) and under these circumstances, arginine may become limited. This is also why it has been identified as conditionally dispensable.

The metabolism of proline, another conditionally essential amino acid, is closely related to that of arginine and like arginine its metabolism is poorly understood. While proline is widely distributed in protein, it is abundant in collagen accounting for almost a quarter of all amino acid residues (although some of the proline is modified post translationally to hydroxyproline). Since collagen is an important part of scar tissue in wound healing, and in the skin, the provision of proline may become important after injury and burns. Although proline can be synthesised from glutamate, it is likely that its main source in tissues is from ornithine in a reversible reaction which means that it can be formed from arginine and can contribute to arginine synthesis. However, much of dietary proline is consumed in the enterocyte together with glutamine to make ornithine and then citrulline which as discussed above is how arginine reaches peripheral tissues. Some of this arginine in peripheral tissues is converted to citrulline and ornithine which can then be used to synthesise proline. This is particularly important in the mammary gland in which much of the proline in milk derives from arginine. The complicating factor in understanding proline metabolism and its conditional indispensability is that developmental changes occur especially in the intestine where in the neonate proline synthesis is limited suggesting its indispensability.

Glycine is the simplest amino acid in nature and is widespread in all proteins but especially collagen in which it comprises a third of all residues. Furthermore, it is metabolically important in a number of pathways as shown in Table 7.4 and this importance may increase in some circumstances such as oxidative stress where oxidised glutathione is lost from cells and excreted as mercapturic acid. Although glycine synthesis can occur by several pathways (from serine, threonine, choline, glyoxalate, and hyroxyproline) it is nevertheless usually classified as a conditionally indispensable AA. The reason for this is evidence that the amount of glycine synthesised in vivo is insufficient to meet metabolic demands during neonatal development especially in preterm infants for whom supplemental glycine improved growth and in catch-up growth of malnourished infants.

As indicated above, glutamine is central to inter-organ N metabolism and is by far the most abundant free amino acid in the body, so it might be considered to be surprising to find it is classified as conditionally indispensable. Clinical interest in glutamine arose following the discovery of its very high concentration in muscle, its potential importance in the regulation of protein balance in muscle and its role as a major fuel for immune cells and enterocytes. Because the muscle and plasma glutamine pool falls markedly in catabolic situations, this raised the possibility that its provision might be of benefit in terms of maintaining muscle mass and the immune system and reducing risk of intestinal bacterial translocation in critically ill patients by maintaining a healthy population of enterocytes. This was of particular importance during the intravenous nutrition of patients with amino acids because as indicated above glutamine is not normally present in such solutions. This has resulted in many clinical trials of its supplementation both intravenously and enterally as the amino acid or as a dipeptide which is more effective in raising plasma glutamine when given enterally than glutamine. However, although early intravenous and enteral trials indicated benefit (e.g., reduced mortality in critical illness), many subsequent trials failed to confirm this so that its benefit is uncertain. Indeed, some recent large trials have suggested harm with an increase in mortality among critically ill patients with multiorgan failure and this has divided opinion amongst experts.

In summary, although the concept of conditional indispensability is most important and has resulted in a great deal of research, a consensus on generally agreed guidelines for nutritional practice has yet to be agreed.

The magnitude of the protein and amino acid requirement

The amount of dietary protein in an otherwise nutritionally adequate diet, necessary for the desired structure and function of the human organism is the requirement, usually identified as maintenance and any special needs for growth, reproduction, and lactation. It was defined in a 2007 WHO report as: "*the lowest level of dietary protein intake that will balance the losses of nitrogen from the body, and thus maintain the body protein mass, in persons at energy balance with modest levels of physical activity, plus, in children or in pregnant or lactating women, the needs associated with the deposition of tissues or the secretion of milk at rates consistent with good health.*" This has the benefit of being conceptually straightforward with N balance as its main focus. Whilst several stable isotopic approaches based on different paradigms have been described, no consensus has been reached on any specific alternative approach, with some identified as deeply flawed. Nevertheless, N balance studies are very difficult to conduct, and especially to interpret as discussed below.

The requirement as defined above can be described by a generic model which defines the protein requirement in terms of the needs of the organism, i.e., the metabolic demand, and the dietary amount which will satisfy those needs, a function of the efficiency of protein utilisation. Thus:

Dietary requirement = metabolic demand/ efficiency of utilisation

For planning and public health purposes and to minimise risk of deficiency, individual requirements are expressed as dietary allowances, which take into account between-individual variation and are set in the upper range of observed individual requirements so that such intakes will be associated with a low risk of deficiency for any individual.

The metabolic demand is determined by the nature and extent of those pathways which irreversibly consume amino acids as shown in Figure 7.2. The efficiency of protein utilisation to satisfy the metabolic demand and achieve N equilibrium will be determined by those factors associated with digestion and absorption of dietary protein. Thus net protein utilisation may be less than 100% if *digestibility* is incomplete, with a consequent loss of dietary N in the faeces, and if the cellular bioavailability of the absorbed amino acids does not entirely match the amino acid pattern of the demand, reducing the *biological value* of the absorbed amino acids.

One estimate of the metabolic demand for maintenance has traditionally been based on the obligatory nitrogen losses (ONL). These are all nitrogen losses from healthy subjects fed a protein-free but otherwise adequate diet. Such a diet induces initially a marked negative N balance which gradually decreases until it becomes constant as the ONL usually after a period of one to two weeks. The constant ongoing loss of N is assumed to reflect the special circumstances where the metabolic demands are met by protein mobilised from body tissues. In healthy adults the ONL nitrogen is equivalent to about 0.3 g protein/kg/d.

When protein is added to the protein free diet to meet the demand, an intake can be reached which exactly matches the losses, so that N equilibrium is achieved, intake = loss, and this intake will represent the minimum protein requirement (MPR). The 2007 WHO protein report was based on a meta-analysis of all N balance studies in healthy adults. 235 individuals were each studied at three or more test protein intakes for between 10 and 14 days with the urinary and faecal nitrogen excretion data from the last few days used to represent the response to that intake. A linear regression of the N balance data points at each intake (N intake minus N loss), was used to identify the N-equilibrium intake:

i.e., N intake for equilibrium = intercept/slope.

Median slopes, intercept and requirements were identified as 0.47, –48.1 mg N/kg/d and 104.6 mg N/kg/d: i.e., 0.65g protein/kg/d (as protein=Nx6.25). The intercept is similar to the directly determined ONL (equivalent to 0.30g protein/kg/d). The distribution of individual values of the MPR are shown in Figure 7.6. The range was from <0.4 to >1.1g/kg/d and no between study factors, age, gender or type of diet (animal or vegetable proteins), could be identified to explain such wide variation. Between individual variation was determined statistically, enabling the *safe individual intake* to be identified as 0.83g/kg/d. The report also identified a *safe population intake*, (based on variability of both requirement and intake) which is higher than safe individual requirement at 1.05 g/kg/d. One cause of variability is that N-equilibrium can be influenced by energy intakes and ensuring that subjects are at exact energy balance at each protein intake in the studies is difficult. Excess energy intake leads to some weight and lean tissue gain, with a less negative or even a

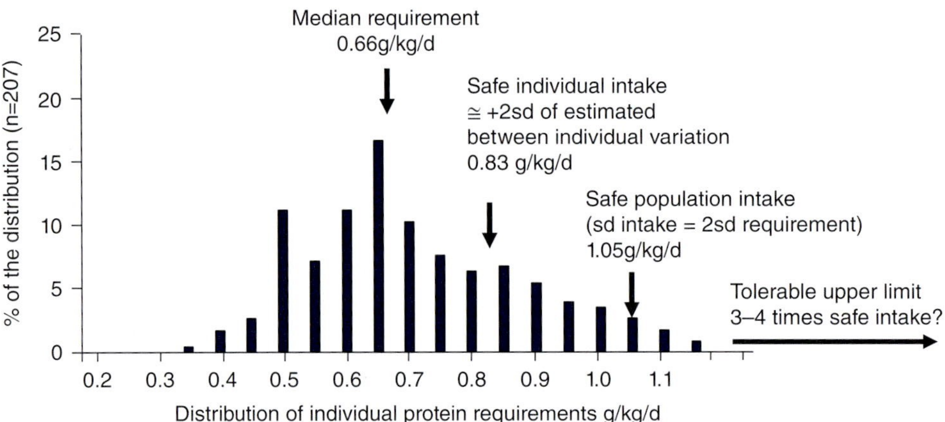

Figure 7.6 Adult protein requirements as indicated by meta analysis of all acceptable published studies on adults.

positive N balance, thus underestimating the requirement. With too little energy intake, protein is oxidised as an energy source resulting in a more negative N balance thus overestimating the requirement. This means that the MPR is a function of the state of energy balance with an error of only ±10% in estimating energy needs equivalent to about 85% of the estimated true between-individual variance in the studies shown in Figure 7.6.

Nevertheless, the observed MPR was much greater than the ONL (in terms of protein nitrogen) because the apparent efficiency of utilisation of dietary proteins in the N balance studies was on average only 47%. In the WHO report, as with previous reports, no explanation was given for this low efficiency of utilisation. However metabolic studies of amino acid oxidation, post-prandial protein utilisation, and nitrogen excretion during the diurnal cycle of feeding and fasting have explained why the MPR is substantially greater than the ONL; this work has established a different model of the protein requirement based on the concept of an adaptive metabolic demand.

Metabolic demand: obligatory and adaptive

The metabolic demand for amino acids comprises two components; namely, obligatory and adaptive demands. The obligatory demands are conceptually straightforward. They comprise the irreversible conversion of some individual amino acids into important metabolites which maintain the structure and function of the body and which are subsequently further transformed into nitrogenous end products, mainly urea and other compounds in urine, faeces or sweat. Net synthesis of proteins lost from the body as skin, hair, and any other secretions is also included. It is this obligatory demand which gives rise to the ONL.

The adaptive metabolic demand

This represents simple oxidative losses of amino acids. The rate is set by the habitual protein intake, which in turn sets the activity levels of pathways of oxidative catabolism. It can be identified as a demand because it occurs continuously, day and night, and changes only slowly, over several weeks, when the habitual protein intake changes. This adaptive and therefore variable demand is one reason why protein requirements have proved so difficult to determine. This aspect of amino acid metabolism is not entirely understood and may have evolved as a consequence of the slow growth and weight maintenance of humans consuming diets which provide protein, which is often considerably in excess of minimum needs. Four aspects of human protein and amino acid metabolism and behaviour explain the adaptive metabolic demand.

Some amino acids are potentially toxic The branched chain, aromatic, and sulphur amino acids, are toxic at high concentrations in the blood and tissues. In-born errors of metabolism in children associated with the oxidative disposal of these amino acids result in severe pathologies. Figure 7.3 shows their very low concentrations in blood and muscle tissue even though for three of them, leucine, valine, and isoleucine, they are the most abundant amino acids in tissue and food proteins (see Table 7.3). This is not a general feature of amino acids since Figure 7.3 shows that some, especially glutamine, are present in very much higher (100 fold), concentrations. This means that after a meal, the potentially toxic amino acids must be rapidly disposed of by high capacity oxidative pathways or by deposition as tissue protein.

There are no protein stores Although there is a small capacity for the liver protein mass to increase, generally it is not possible to simply deposit protein from food in tissues. The largest tissue protein mass is skeletal muscle. Muscle differs from many other tissues in that its cells, the myofibres are encased in an inelastic connective tissue framework, through which the transmission of the force of muscle contraction occurs and which defines myofibre volume. During growth, remodelling of muscle connective tissue occurs in response to the passive stretch of bone lengthening which allows myofibre mass to increase so that a proportionality between strength and body weight is maintained. In the adult, after epiphyseal fusion of the long bones, height growth stops with muscle mass fixed at its phenotypical size which is a function of height. No further growth can occur unless muscle is subject to passive stretch through resistance exercise. This means that after a meal of protein in excess of the minimum demands, the excess protein cannot be simply stored as larger muscles.

Humans are usually day-time meal-eaters Human eating behaviour solves the problem of meal protein disposal. The diurnal cycle of feeding and fasting with long periods between meals especially during sleep involves a substantial post-absorptive state during each 24 hours when there is a net loss of tissue protein, with amino acid oxidation and urea production. These losses of protein from muscle and other tissues in effect, create a space into which excess protein can be deposited after a meal, repleting post-absorptive losses until the regulated size of the muscle mass is reached.

The rate limiting steps in the oxidative catabolism of the essential amino acids appear to adapt to the habitual protein intake This is the least understood feature. In effect the capacity or Vmax for the oxidative amino acid catabolism of the potentially toxic amino acids adapts to the habitual protein intake at a level which appears to be maintained throughout the diurnal cycle of feeding and fasting and does not change until a sustained period of a higher or lower protein intake occurs. Furthermore, the acute regulation of amino acid oxidation appears to be less sensitive to food intake than indicated by studies of the rate-controlling enzymes so that the adapted rate does not appear to change markedly throughout the diurnal cycle. This ensures that after adaptation to a particular level of protein intake, disposal of dietary amino acids can occur by protein deposition which replaces the tissue protein lost in the post-absorptive state and by amino acid oxidation throughout each daily cycle.

The consequences of these features of protein and amino acid metabolism are shown in Figure 7.7 in terms of body protein balance regulation during the diurnal cycle. Figure 7.7a shows the two components of amino acid oxidative losses which comprise the metabolic demand occurring continuously throughout each 24 hours of the diurnal cycle. This is measurable as the hourly rate of post absorptive losses as leucine oxidation or nitrogen excretion, scaled up to 24 hours. In the post-absorptive state, the demand is met from tissue protein resulting in a negative balance as tissue protein is lost. In response to a protein meal the metabolic demand is met by the dietary protein which also repletes the tissue protein pool and this allows the essential amino acids to be disposed of without excessive increases in the free amino acid pool. Arbitrary responses to three meals are shown with very brief between meal periods of negative balance which might occur. Any dietary protein in excess of the demand or amino acids not matching the amino acid pattern of the demand will be oxidised and these are shown as meal dependent amino acid losses, i.e.. an increase in amino acid oxidation above the post-absorptive

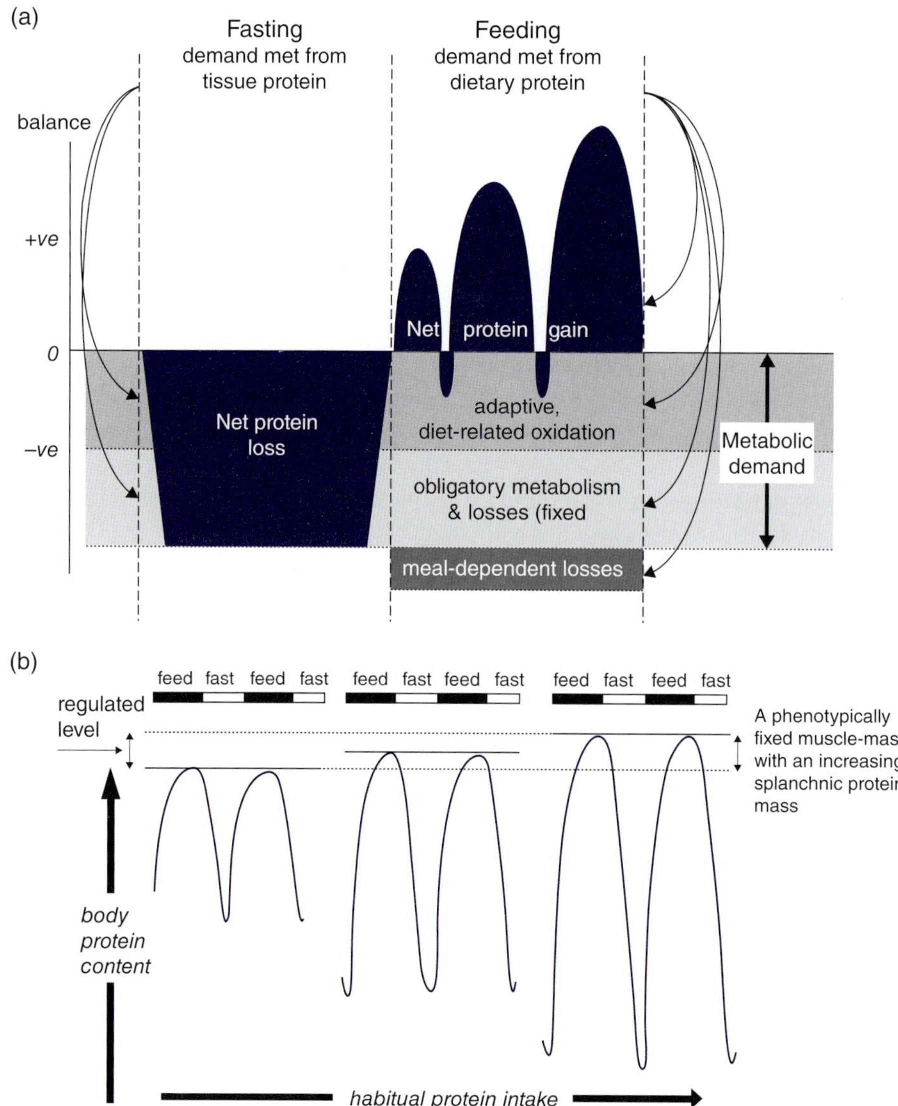

Figure 7.7 Body protein balance regulation during the diurnal cycle (a) (Top). Gains and losses in relation to the metabolic demand over 24h (b) (Bottom). Influence of adaptation to increasing protein intakes on diurnal gains and losses of protein in relation to the regulated size of the skeletal muscle mass.

rate. The extent of this increase will determine the true efficiency of protein utilisation. Clearly because protein intake varies from day to day, so will overall 24 hour nitrogen balance but for any particular habitual dietary pattern of protein intake above the minimal level, the adaptive metabolic demand will ensure overall balance.

Figure 7.7b shows how the body protein content, mainly a function of muscle mass, is regulated at its phenotypical level, throughout the diurnal cycle with two days indicated at each of three levels of habitual protein intake. With an increased habitual protein intake level after complete adaptation, the amplitude of the post-absorptive losses and repletion increases. Although there is a phenotypically fixed muscle mass there may be a small increasing splanchnic protein mass associated with digestion absorption and metabolism of the increasing protein intakes. The increasing post-absorptive losses resulting from the adaptive increases in the capacity of the amino acid oxidation pathways with increasing habitual dietary protein intakes, mean that to maintain muscle at its phenotypic regulated mass, increasing deposition of muscle protein will be observed in the post-prandial state to replete the increased post-absorptive losses.

When protein intake changes to a lower habitual intake, mobilisation of tissue protein occurs with a negative N balance for as long as it takes oxidative losses to adapt to the lower intake. This was previously identified as the labile protein reserves, but no specific protein stores were ever identified, and it is now believed to originate from both skeletal muscle and the splanchnic organs. Change to a new higher intake poses a problem for the immediate disposal of dietary amino acids in excess of the adapted metabolic demand. This is partially solved by the appetite mechanism in which protein is the most satiating nutrient, especially when eaten in excess of habitual intakes.

Implications of the adaptive metabolic demand model of the protein requirement

By definition, the adaptive metabolic demand model sets the protein requirement at the habitual intake within an adaptive range. The practical problem involves both the limits of that range and the timescale of adaptation. Long term balance studies in the 1960s indicated a time scale greatly in excess of one to two weeks (the time in most of the multilevel balance studies analysed in the WHO 2007 report), was necessary for N-losses to match very low intakes. This would suggest that some of the observed MPR variability between studies shown in Figure 7.6 reflects incomplete adaptation to the test diets, and that the true MPR may be in the lower range of observed values between 0.3 g/kg/d the ONL and 0.65 g/kg/d the median value of all studies. However, protein intakes as low as this are rare and probably not possible from otherwise nutritionally complete diets. For example, a 70 kg young adult male consuming either cereal or starchy roots, tubers or fruit staples as sole sources of energy at the rate of 1·75 x BMR (183 kJ or 43·7 kcal)/kg), would consume digestible protein intakes of 0·82 g/kg/d from potatoes, between 0.76 and 1·80 g/kg/d from cereals, with only a few non-cereal staples providing intakes substantially less than 0·50 g/kg/d; e.g., Ethiopian banana (Ensete) 0·36, plantain 0·35 or cassava 0·23g/kg/d. Furthermore, such diets are seldom consumed as sole sources of energy with other constituents providing protein and even if they were, they would almost certainly be nutritionally limiting in several key micronutrients that would impact on most indicators of nutritional status. This means that the actual value of the true MPR becomes of academic rather than practical interest with no reason not to continue with the currently accepted EAR of 0.65 g/kg/d. However, there are other important consequences of this metabolic model that are of practical importance.

The slope of the N balance regression line markedly underestimates the efficiency of protein utilisation This is a quite complicated conceptual issue. It is the case that many N balance studies have involved proteins of high digestibility and biological value, so that such a low efficiency of utilisation (median value = 0.47), is not biologically plausible. However, it is of great importance because the protein requirements for children and for pregnancy and lactation in the 2007 WHO report are derived with a factorial model in which the efficiency of utilisation of dietary protein from N balance studies is used to calculate the extra dietary requirements for these special needs. For children (see Figure 7.8) the dietary intake to meet the demands for growth is experimentally determined lean-tissue gain adjusted by an efficiency factor 0.58, the slope of N balance studies in children. In practical terms the overestimation of the growth component in children is probably not of great importance. For pregnancy and lactation (see Table 7.6), the extra protein intakes derive from calculations in which the protein deposition during gestational weight gain, for which there is a consensus, is adjusted by an efficiency factor of only 0.42, deriving from N balance studies in pregnant women. These values in Table 7.6 are almost double previous reports in which much higher efficiency values were used. In view of the literature indicating an increase in neonatal death with supplements that are very high in protein, the report recommended that the higher intake during pregnancy should consist of normal food, rather than commercially prepared

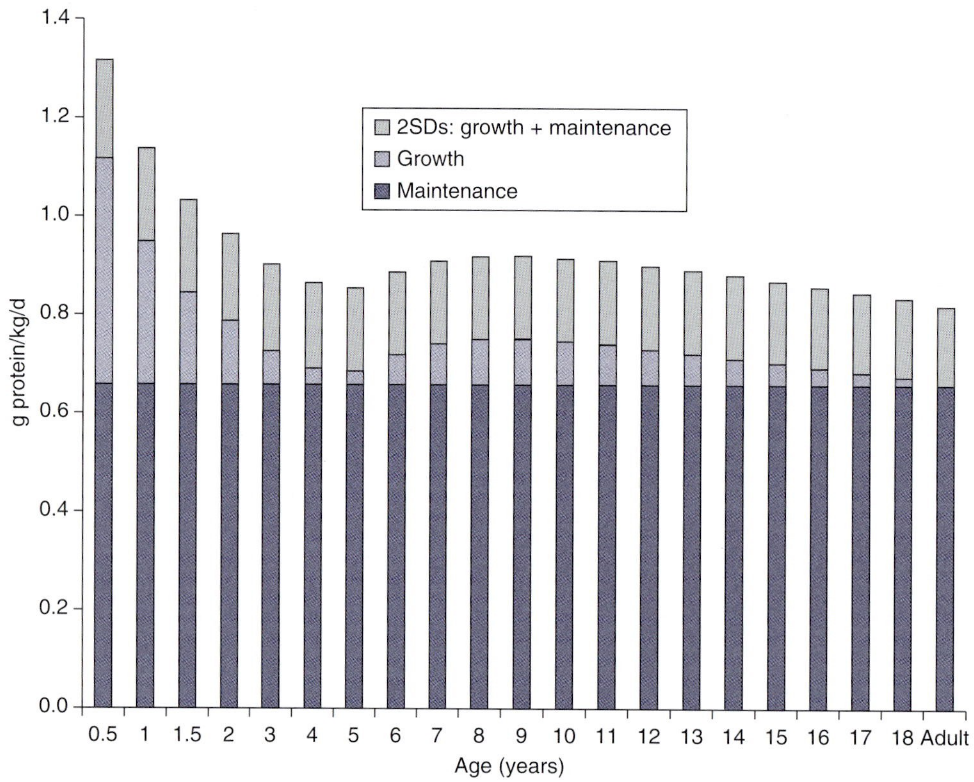

Figure 7.8 The safe allowances for infants children adolescents and adults showing components of the factorial model used to derive them. Growth is experimentally determined lean tissue gain adjusted by an efficiency factor 0.58 to determine the dietary intake to meet the demands for growth.

Table 7.6 Extra protein requirements for pregnancy and lactation.

	Safe intake (g/day)	Additional energy requirement (kJ/day)	Protein:energy ratio
Pregnancy			
trimester			
1	1	375	0.04
2	10	1200	0.11
3	31	1950	0.23
Lactation			
First 6 months	19	2800	0.11
After 6 months	13	1925	0.11

high-protein supplements. However, in the authors' view the overestimation of the values for pregnancy is unsafe because it is doubtful if the usual intakes could be increased sufficiently to provide such extra intakes without the mothers becoming obese.

We now know that post-prandial protein utilisation as depicted in Figure 7.7a does occur with an efficiency similar to what would be expected, i.e., close to 100% with milk proteins for example. This has been observed in studies in which an experimental approach involving [$^{13}C_1$]-leucine oxidation and balance has been used to assess post-prandial protein utilisation (PPU) from the slope of leucine balance studies in subjects in the post-absorptive state fed protein intakes first low and then equivalent to their habitual intake during a single 9 h leucine infusion. In contrast the shallow slope in N balance studies is explained because at each intake the demand has increased above that indicated by the ONL but such changes cannot be identified from the analysis of the balance studies. Thus although 24 h N balance studies, at least as usually implemented, will indicate the intake which allows N-equilibrium, (the requirement) and the obligatory demand, (the intercept) they cannot identify the adaptive component of the demand at each intake so the slope is not an indication of the true efficiency of utilisation. If it is interpreted as such it will markedly overestimate factorial calculations of special needs. Clearly this is an unsatisfactory situation.

Qualitative Aspects of the Metabolic Demand

Given the extensive amino acid interconversions between the dispensable amino acids as discussed above, the dietary protein amino acid pattern need not exactly match the amino acid pattern of the demand. However, intakes must meet the requirement for the IAAs and those which become indispensable under specific physiological or pathological conditions (the conditionally indispensable amino acids) and sufficient total amino acid N or sources of nonessential N such as ammonium compounds (see *Development of the concept of amino acid essentiality* above). In practice, discussion of protein quality is usually limited to the extent to which dietary protein provides enough IAAs.

7.5 Protein quality evaluation

Protein quality in animals

Studies of protein quality evaluation in animal growth assays resulted in the widespread view that there are marked differences in the relative nutritional value (quality) of plant compared with animal protein sources in human nutrition because of deficiencies of some IAAs. As shown in Table 7.3 there are important differences in the IAA content of the main classes of proteins. Cereals have low levels of lysine and in some cases tryptophan and legumes have lower levels of the sulphur amino acids compared with animal source proteins. Thus cereals, and to a lesser extent, legumes, performed poorly in animal growth assays, but when combined, maximal growth occurred. This gave rise to the concept of "complementation" in which the appropriate balance of IAAs is provided from combinations of plant proteins. However, it is now recognised that in human nutrition, with the rapid growth of the newborn infant slowing markedly after weaning, the nutritional demand for IAAs for tissue growth becomes a minor component of the total metabolic demand after the first year of life. Thus, animal growth assays of protein quality have little relevance for protein-quality evaluation in human nutrition.

Protein quality evaluation in human nutrition

Protein quality is influenced by *digestibility*, the amount of the protein which is absorbed from the intestine, and *biological value*, the extent to which the amino acid pattern of the absorbed amino acid mixture matches that of the cellular demand.

Digestibility can vary through limitation by plant-cell walls and by anti-nutritional factors in plant foods. Values range from 60 to 80% in legumes and cereals with tough cell walls such as millet and sorghum to 97% for egg. Anti-nutritional factors in legumes and seeds include amylase and trypsin inhibitors, tannins in most legumes and cyanogens in lima beans.

Biological value (BV) varies according to the cross match between the composition of the absorbed amino acid mixture and the pattern of the metabolic demand for maintenance and net protein deposition. During human growth and development, after the second year of life metabolic demands for growth are quite low, so that amino acid needs are mainly for maintenance. We know from extensive work in farm animals and rats that the amino acid pattern for maintenance is quite different from that for growth, with a much lower proportion of IAAs. N balance studies in adults indicate very small differences when comparisons are made between single proteins, and no differences in the apparent MPR were observed between plant based or animal source diets in the meta-analysis of all N balance studies in adults in the 2007 WHO report. Because of these difficulties in assessing protein quality directly in human nutrition, current approaches attempt to predict quality from digestibility and amino acid scoring.

Predicting protein quality: PDCAAS and DIAAS methods

If the IAA pattern of the protein requirement is known as mg IAA/g protein, then the measured BV of a dietary protein should be predictable from its composition relative to that of the requirement pattern. If the digestibility and the amino acid score are both known, then overall protein quality in terms of digestibility and amino acid score can be predicted as

$$\text{Protein quality} = \text{digestibility} \times \text{amino acid score}$$

This was formalised by FAO as the protein digestibility corrected amino acid score (PDCAAS).

Digestibility Digestibility, the proportion of food protein which is absorbed has been defined from measurements of the N content of the foods and N loss in faeces, with "true" digestibility adjusted for endogenous N loss: i.e., faecal N loss on a protein-free diet. Concern has been expressed over correction for faecal as opposed to ileal protein digestibility in the calculation of PDCAAS. Ileal digestibility of dietary proteins is a specific measure of amino acid absorption in the small intestine and is measured at the terminal ileum. In contrast faecal digestibility indicates how much of the N in food has been absorbed by the organism. Thus, digestibility is more complex than usually assumed. On the one hand ileal digestibility is a measure of residual amino acids from both dietary and endogenous sources. Faecal digestibility is a measure of residual nitrogen, much of which is bacterial protein, to some extent a function of the bacterial biomass in the colon. This is related to dietary non-starch polysaccharide (NSP) intake which supports bacterial growth after its fermentation, together with N deriving largely from urea salvage. Taken together this means that for human diets containing large amounts of non-digestible carbohydrate, faecal N may not be a reliable measure of digestibility. Thus, the concepts of both ileal digestibility and faecal digestibility are subject to important limitations.

The FAO has suggested that conceptually, ileal digestibility of individual amino acids was the appropriate measure from which to develop a digestibility-corrected amino acid score, proposing a new term the Digestible Indispensable Amino acid Score (DIAAS): i.e.,

$$\text{DIAAS} = \frac{\text{digestible dietary indispensable amino acid in the dietary protein}}{\text{dietary indispensable amino acid in the reference amino acid scoring pattern.}}$$

However, because ileal digestibility studies are difficult to conduct, only a very few human studies have been undertaken and the currently available data is insufficient to recommend adoption of this new approach until sufficient data has accumulated. Thus, in the meantime, FAO has suggested that faecal digestibility (in effect PDCAAS) should continue to be used.

Amino acid scoring

To score a protein, the single limiting amino acid is identified from the ratios of each individual amino acid in the protein with that in a reference pattern. Values <1 indicate potential deficiency, with the limiting amino acid indicated by the lowest ratio. This is the extent of the limitation: the score. Thus, if the lysine score for wheat gluten is only 0.5, to achieve the required intake of lysine and all IAAs, the digestible intake of the gluten will have to be increased by 1/0.5 = 2 times the reference protein intake.

The reference pattern is that of an ideal protein which would provide requirement levels of all amino acids when fed at the protein requirement level. So that:

$$\text{reference IAA pattern}\left(\text{as mg / g protein}\right) = \frac{\text{amino acid requirement / kg / d}}{\text{protein requirement / kg / d}}$$

Defining amino acid requirement levels and a reference protein scoring pattern

The definition of amino acid requirement values has been challenging and remains subject to considerable controversy. Current values for the adult maintenance requirement pattern are derived from both N balance studies in adults and stable-isotope studies which include various types of amino acid oxidation balance studies with ^{13}C-labelled amino acids, none of which have been judged entirely satisfactory. The requirement for the sulphur amino acids has been predicted from the obligatory oxidative loss. The "best estimate" of different values is often chosen from a wide range, e.g., for lysine, 30 mg/kg/d chosen from a range of values from 12-45 mg/kg/d. No suitable values exist for infants, children or other population groups so that a factorial model has been developed. This is based on the amino acid requirements for maintenance, assumed to be the same for all

Table 7.7 Recommended amino acid scoring patterns for infants, children and older children, adolescents and adults

	His	Ile	Leu	Lys	SAA	AAA	Thr	Trp	Val
Tissue amino acid pattern (mg/g protein)[1]	27	35	75	73	35	73	42	12	49
Maintenance (adult) amino acid pattern (mg/g protein)[2]	15	30	59	45	22	38	23	6	39
Age group		scoring pattern mg/g protein requirement							
Infant (birth to 6 months)[3]	21	55	96	69	33	94	44	17	55
Child (6 months to 3 years)[4]	20	32	66	57	27	52	31	8.5	43
Older child, adolescent, adult[5]	16	30	61	48	23	41	25	6.6	40

[1] Composition of mixed tissue proteins
[2] Adult amino acid requirement pattern
[3] Based on the gross amino acid content of human milk.
[4] The 6-month (0.5 y) requirement pattern
[5] The 3-10 year requirement pattern.
The adaptive metabolic demand and amino acid scoring.

ages, and for growth assumed to be the same as the composition of mixed tissue proteins. The final age-related pattern was calculated as a weighted mean of the growth and maintenance patterns. These values are shown in Table 7.7.

The inherent difficulty in defining amino acid requirements for growth and maintenance is that the distinction becomes difficult when the metabolic response of humans to varying protein intakes shown in Figure 7.7 is taken into account. As the habitual protein intake increases, the consequence of the increasing post-absorptive losses and post-prandial gains is that the pattern of the amino acid requirement will increasingly reflect the pattern of tissue and decreasingly that of the obligatory demands of maintenance. Furthermore, predicting the impact of the increased losses and gains of body protein throughout the day on the overall requirement pattern is not straight forward because of the potential recycling of some IAAs such as lysine and threonine. These have larger free amino acid pools (see Figure 7.3) and are less likely to be immediately oxidised in the post-absorptive state when released from tissue protein. Nevertheless within the normal range of protein intakes which occur, the pattern of the demand will to some extent be that of growth, especially for those amino acids which are immediately oxidised on release from tissue protein in the post-absorptive state, such as the branched chain, aromatic and sulphur amino acids. This means that only at very low protein intakes is it likely that the pattern of the requirement will reflect that of the obligatory demand as has been identified in animal studies. At usual protein takes it will include a component reflecting the needs for post-prandial net protein gain, but the actual overall pattern will be difficult to predict. However, since the main food sources which result in higher than average protein intakes are animal source foods, a shift with higher intakes towards the growth requirement pattern should not present a problem.

7.6 Sources and general nutritional properties of plant proteins

The relative quality of plant protein sources is an issue of great current importance given the increasing demand to feed a growing global population and to develop food sources which have a low footprint in terms of both water and other resources for their production and their damaging influence on the environment in terms of both nitrification by waste products and greenhouse gas production. Thus, a wide range of novel plant and single cell foods are appearing. Plant foods are chemically diverse often containing secondary metabolites which may be either beneficial phytoprotectants or anti-nutritional, adversely influencing digestibility, having allergenic properties or generally undesirable such as oxalates.

Major current sources of plant proteins in the human diet are cereals, especially wheat, rice and maize, starchy roots such as cassava and potato and legumes including peas and various beans, especially soya, (although only 2-3% of soya production is consumed as human food directly). Cereals represent globally the most important protein source, which is limited by low levels of lysine and, for maize, by tryptophan in the major protein fraction, i.e., the prolamin storage protein.

As to the significance of the low lysine, it is the case that there is considerable uncertainty in the current adult lysine value so that the deficiency may be more apparent than real. In the case of zein, it is also low in tryptophan, one contributing factor to pellagra given that the bioavailability of niacin from maize is low (unless treated with lime), and the insufficient tryptophan limits its conversion to nicotinamide. Another important factor in the provision of tryptophan is its supply compared with that of the other large neutral amino acids (LNAAs). These are all transported into cells by the same large neutral amino acid transporter. When levels of these other LNAAs are high this will prevent the uptake of tryptophan into tissues. In fact, the ratio of tryptophan to LNAA is particularly low in maize and in sorghum, and both cereals have been implicated in pellagra.

In practice, the protein quality and quantity in cereals can be quite variable. The relative amounts of storage as opposed to cytoplasmic proteins (as in the germ) influences the IAA profile so that that the profile of whole grain is better than that of gluten. Thus, the amino acid quality worsens as the germ and bran are removed in flour production. Also, the relative amounts of storage and cytoplasmic protein can be altered with plant breeding as with varieties of maize developed from opaque-2(o2), sugary-2(su2) hybrids with higher cytoplasmic protein:zein ratios. These are now in use under the name Quality Protein Maize. As shown in Table 7.8 these new maize strains have higher levels of all the IAA. Field trials in Ethiopia and elsewhere have shown better rates of weight gain and height growth in children where these hybrid strains are farmed.

Protein sources currently under investigation as alternative human food protein include oilseeds such as rapeseed (canola), marine microalgae (e.g., chlorella), aquatic plants such as duckweed, and the cyanobacterium (blue-green algae) spirulina. The single-cell fungal mycoprotein (sold as "Quorn") has been widely available at least in the UK and Europe for some time. In fact, all green leafy vegetables such as spinach are sources of high-quality protein.

When the amino acid profile (biological value) of these various plant source proteins (PSPs) is judged against an animal source protein (ASP) such as beef and the scoring pattern for school children adolescents and adults (Figure 7.9) the most obvious features are that:

- All PSPs contain all IAA: often not appreciated.
- Most PSPs contain more IAA than in the requirement pattern although relative proportions of some key amino acids like lysine, tryptophan, and the sulphur amino acids vary.
- Some (but by no means all) are indistinguishable from ASPs in terms of total amount and pattern of IAAs.

Table 7.8 Protein and amino acid content and quality of animal and plant food protein sources.

		Lysine	Threonine	Sulphur AAs	Tryptophan					
	P:E ratio		mg/g protein			SCORE	Limiting AA	Digestibility	PDCAAS	Adjusted P:E ratios
Requirement pattern		48	25	23	6.6					
Beef	0.66	91	47	40	13	100		100	100	0.660
Egg	0.34	70	47	57	17	100		100	100	0.340
Cow's milk	0.19	78	44	33	14	100		100	100	0.194
Breast milk	0.060	69	44	33	17	100		100	100	0.060
Soya	0.388	65	38	25	13	100		90	90	0.349
Wheat	0.160	26	29	45	12	54	Lysine	95	51	0.082
Maize	0.130	29	36	29	5	60	Lysine	82	50	0.064
Improved maize	0.135	40	44	48	7	83	Lysine	80	67	0.090
Potatoes	0.100	54	38	29	14	100		82	82	0.082
Rice	0.072	36	37	40	11	75	Lysine	82	62	0.044
Yam	0.061	42	34	28	13	88	Lysine	80	70	0.043
Cassava	0.034	32	21	29	14	67	Lysine	80	53	0.018

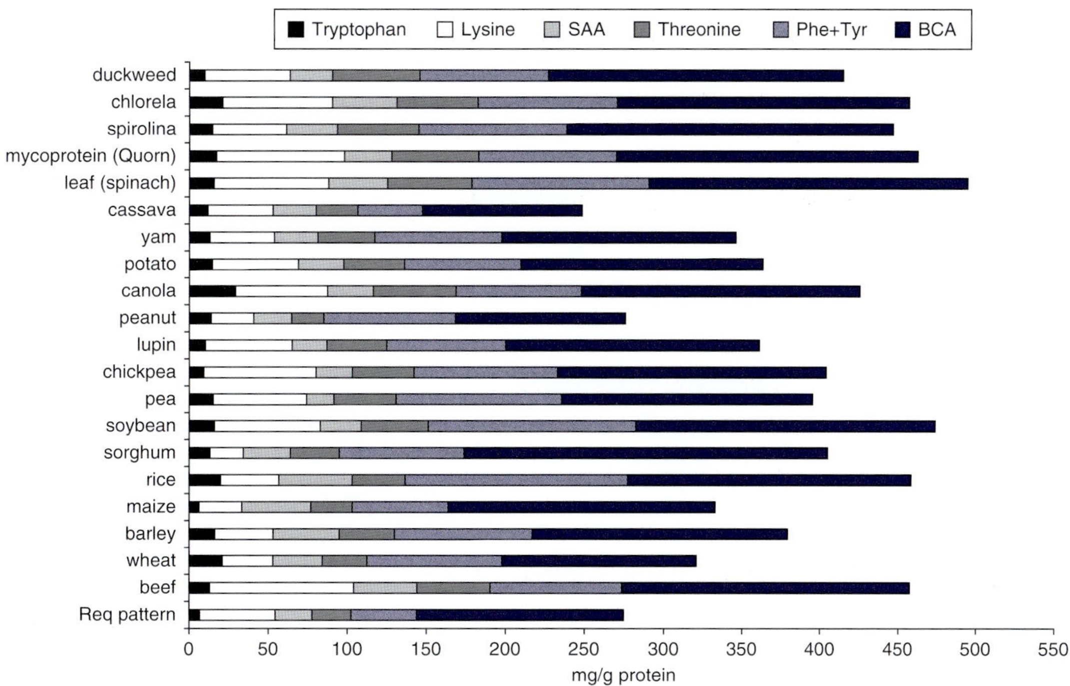

Figure 7.9 Amino-acid profile of various plant source proteins PSPs) is judged against beef and the requirement pattern, ((FAO 2013 scoring pattern for older child, adolescent and adult: see table 7).

It is clear that duckweed, chlorella, spirolena, mycoprotein and leaf protein (of which spinach is typical of the food group) have similar levels of all the IAAs as meat and these have protein contents ranging from 25 to 50% of the energy. Clearly with leaves in the human diet accounting for minor fractions of energy, leaves represent usually a minor part of total protein. Nevertheless, as consumed in some countries such as Greece as *Horta* (Steamed Greens), in a serving of up to 500 g, this would amount to 10 g of very high-quality protein which would complement protein from bread to provide a balanced intake. The starchy roots exemplified by cassava, yam, and potato, are quite variable in terms of both amino acid profile and protein content, with cassava quite poor in both respects and potato a much better protein source. The IAA profile of potato exceeds the requirement for every IAA and at ≈11% energy has been the major source of protein in many traditional diets.

Oilseeds, (canola) are used in the developed world mainly in animal feed, but have an IAA profile which exceeds the requirement for every IAA being especially rich in the sulphur amino acids (SAA).

Legumes are traditionally viewed as protein-rich foods limited by their SAA but in the examples shown (lupin, chickpea, pea, and soybean), only pea protein has less of the SAA compared with the reference pattern (about 70%).They are all rich in lysine and tryptophan especially soybean and pea and in many diets are consumed with cereals such as rice to complement the low lysine levels.

Figure 7.10 shows the adequacy of the amino acid levels of the various PSPs as a percentage of that in the requirement pattern for older children and adults for the main current food protein groups, starchy roots, legumes, cereals and animal source proteins. Thus, some starchy root proteins like cassava and yam are marginally deficient in lysine, some legume proteins like pea are deficient in the SAA, while all cereals are deficient in lysine.

Taken together these data show that in terms of their amino acid content there are many sources of PSPs which can be considered as alternatives to ASPs, and it is clear that currently available food sources make it relatively easy to construct nutritionally adequate vegetarian or vegan diets in terms of the quality of the protein

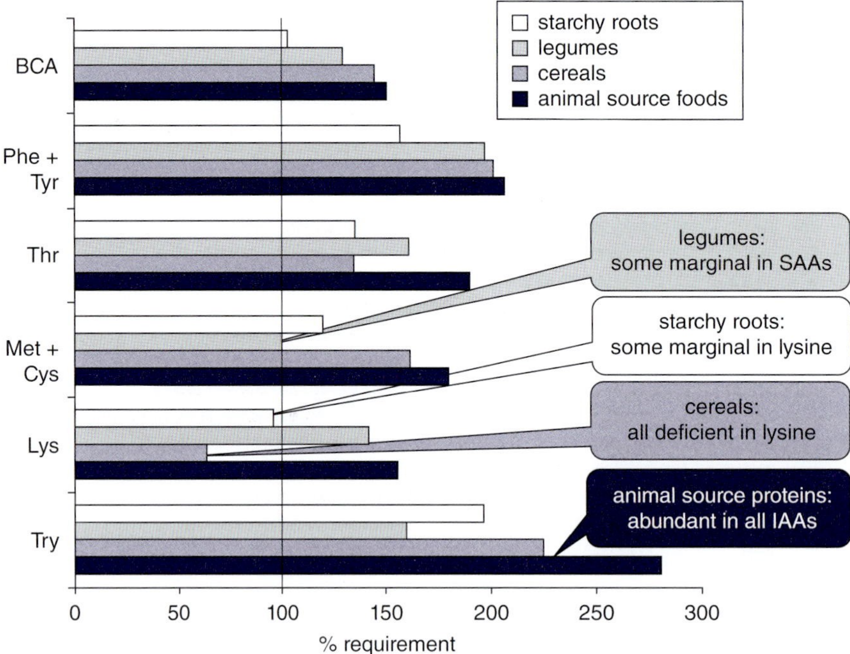

Figure 7.10 Amino-acid profile of the main food protein sources as judged against the requirement pattern, ((FAO 2013 scoring pattern for older child, adolescent and adult: see table 7).

content. Thus, their protein quality in terms of food sources may well only be limited by their digestibility.

Table 7.8 shows PDCAAS values of dietary protein sources, based on the scoring pattern for the older child, adolescent and adult shown in Table 7.7 and digestibility, and the PDCAAS-adjusted P:E ratios. The adjusted P:E ratio is the important measure: i.e., available protein in foods determined by both protein content and quality.

Animal foods generally perform well on both counts. Lysine is the limiting amino acid for cereal proteins, yam and cassava. Maize also contains less than the reference tryptophan level, but at 83% of reference, compared with lysine at 60%, lysine is limiting, and adjusting intake to supply lysine needs will supply more than enough tryptophan. The improved maize variety, opaque maize has adequate tryptophan and 83% of the reference lysine. Soya, in common with all legumes, has low levels of sulphur amino acids, but with this scoring pattern, this is just sufficient.

Potatoes provide sufficient supply of all amino acids and after correcting for digestibility the adjusted P:E ratio of potato at 8.2%, which is higher than that of breast milk. However, even though the protein density of potato is adequate, the growth of a newborn could not be supported on mashed potato because its energy density is insufficient with mashed potato being too bulky to allow the newborn to eat enough to satisfy energy needs. Breast milk is high-fat and therefore energy-dense. For a young adult however energy requirements per kg are only half that of infants so the potato could supply all of the energy needs. The high protein level in wheat together with its high digestibility means that it provides a much higher level of utilisable protein (PDCAAS-adjusted P:E ratio) than rice, yam, or cassava, even though wheat has the lowest lysine level of any staple at 54% of the reference. Clearly cassava does badly mainly due to its low protein content so that only 1.8% of its energy is utilisable protein.

7.7 Conclusions and perspectives on the future

This introductory review has attempted to identify the core knowledge of the nutrition and metabolism of proteins and amino acids. There is a large literature with considerable work published in the decade since the 2007 WHO report on human protein and amino acid nutrition, and that report was comprehensive. This means that in this review only brief references have been made to many of the outstanding issues and uncertainties. Nevertheless, it should be clear that after two centuries of study, protein remains a controversial and "difficult" nutrient. Our knowledge of amino acid metabolism is inadequate so that questions about the clinical relevance of the conditionally indispensable amino acids remain. The protein requirement, considered here only as defined by WHO, with no consideration of optimal intakes for long term health, is often identified as the best understood of any nutrient but remains controversial with current values inadequate and potentially unsafe in some cases. Uncertainties exist for the magnitude of the requirements for the indispensable amino acids, for amino acid scoring patterns which derive from them and even whether we should adopt the newly recommended DIAAS approach to judge protein quality or continue with the simpler PDCAAS approach. What has not been discussed is the debate about the need for animal source protein in the human diet in the context of both climate change and concern for the role of livestock in greenhouse gas emissions, and potentially adverse influences of the major source of dietary protein, red meat, for human health. The brief review of plant protein amino acid quality presented above should make it clear that there are several alternative potential plant sources, although their incorporation into acceptable food sources remains to be demonstrated. Clearly much remains to be done.

Acknowledgement

The author declares no conflicts of interest.

References

FAO/WHO (1991). Protein quality evaluation: report of the Joint FAO/WHO Expert Consultation. *FAO Food and Nutrition Paper 51*. Rome: FAO.

FAO (2013). Dietary protein quality evaluation in human nutrition: report of an FAO Expert Consultation. *FAO Food and Nutrition Paper 92*. Rome: FAO.

FAO (2014). *Research approaches and methods for evaluating the protein quality of human foods: report of a FAO Expert Working Group*. Rome: FAO.

Millward, D.J. (1995). A protein-stat mechanism for the regulation of growth and maintenance of the lean-body mass. *Nutrition Research Reviews* **8**: 93–120.

Millward, D.J. (2003). An adaptive metabolic demand model for protein and amino acid requirements. *British Journal of Nutrition* **90**: 249–260

Millward, D.J. (2012). Identifying recommended dietary allowances for protein and amino acids: a critique of the 2007 WHO report. *British Journal of Nutrition* **108**(Suppl. 2): S3–S21 doi: 10.1017/S0007114512002450. PubMed PMID: 23107542.

Millward, D.J. (2012). Amino acid scoring patterns for protein quality assessment. *British Journal of Nutrition.* **108** (Suppl. 2): S31–S43. doi: 10.1017/S0007114512002462. PubMed PMID:23107544.

Osborne, T.B. and Mendel, L.B. (1915). The comparative nutritive value of proteins in growth, and the problem of the protein minimum. *J. Biol. Chem.* **20**:351–378.

Rand, W.M., Pellett, P.L., and Young, V.R. (2003). Meta-analysis of nitrogen balance studies for estimating protein requirements in healthy adults. *American Journal of Clinical Nutrition* **77**:109–127

WHO (2007). Protein and amino acid requirements in human nutrition. Report of a joint WHO/FAO/UNU expert consultation. *WHO Tech Rep Ser* 935 Geneva: WHO.

Further reading

Darling, A.L., Millward, D.J., Torgerson, D.J. *et al.* (2009). Dietary protein and bone health: a systematic review and meta-analysis. *Am J Clin Nutr.* **90**(6):1674–92. doi: 10.3945/ajcn.2009.27799. Epub 2009 Nov 4. Review. PubMed PMID: 19889822.

Haussinger, D. (1983). Hepatocyte heterogeneity in glutamine and ammonia metabolism and the role of an intracellular glutamine cycle during ureogenesis in perfused rat liver. *European Journal of Biochemistry* **133**, 269 ± 275.

Haussinger, D.D., Gerok, W., and Sies, H. (1984). Hepatic role in pH regulation: role of the intercellular glutamine cycle. *Trends in Biochemical Sciences* **9**, 300 ± 302.

Millward, D.J. (2008). Sufficient protein for our elders? *American Journal of Clinical Nutrition.* **88**(5):1187–8. PubMed PMID: 18996850.

Millward, D.J. (2013). The use of protein:energy ratios for defining protein requirements, allowances and dietary protein contents. *Public Health Nutrition* **16**(5):763–8. doi:10.1017/S1368980013000396. PubMed PMID: 23570877.

Millward, D.J., Fereday, A., Gibson, N.R. *et al.* (2000). Human adult protein and amino acid requirements: $[^{13}C_{-1}]$ leucine balance evaluation of the efficiency of utilization and apparent requirements for wheat protein and lysine compared with milk protein in healthy adults. *American Journal of Clinical Nutrition.* **72**:112–21.

Millward, D.J. and Garnett, T. (2010). Food and the planet: nutritional dilemmas of greenhouse gas emission reductions through reduced intakes of meat and dairy foods. *Proc Nutr Soc.* **69**(1):103–18. doi: 10.1017/S0029665109991868. Epub 2009 Dec 15. PubMed PMID: 20003639.

Millward, D.J. and Jackson, A.A. (2003). Reference protein: energy ratios of diets in relation to current diets in developed and developing countries: Implications of proposed protein and amino acid requirements values. *Public Health Nutrition*, **7** (2003), pp. 387–405

Millward, D.J. and Jackson, A.A. (2012). Protein requirements and the indicator amino acid oxidation method. *Am J Clin Nutr*. Jun; **95**(6):1498–501; author reply 1501-2. doi: 10.3945/ajcn.112.036830. PubMed PMID: 22611079.

Millward, D.J. and Pacy, P.J. (1995). Postprandial protein utilisation and protein quality assessment in man. *Clinical Science*. **88**: 597–606.

Reeds, P.J. (2000). Dispensable and indispensable amino acids for humans. *J Nutr.* 2000; **130**: 1835S–1840S.

Waterlow, J.C. (1999). The mysteries of nitrogen balance. *Nutrition Research Reviews*. **12**: 25–54.

8
Digestion and Metabolism of Carbohydrates

John C. Mathers

Key messages

- Carbohydrates are the single most abundant source of food energy in the human diet, providing 40–80% of total energy intake in different populations.
- Carbohydrates are classified according to their degree of polymerisation into sugars, oligosaccharides, and polysaccharides. The latter include starches (mostly digested in the small intestine) and dietary fibre which is not digested in the small intestine.
- Glycaemic carbohydrates are digested (hydrolysed by enzymes) to sugars (monosaccharides) in the small bowel and absorbed via specific transporter proteins. Absorbed sugars are metabolised to produce energy and used for structural purposes e.g., in the synthesis of glycoproteins and glycolipids.
- Dietary fibre flows to the large bowel where it is fermented to a greater or lesser extent leading to the production of short-chain fatty acids (SCFAs), carbon dioxide, hydrogen, and methane. Absorbed SCFAs are metabolised in the colonic epithelial, hepatic, and muscle cells.
- For optimum function of the nervous system and other cells, blood glucose concentration is controlled within a narrow range by a consortium of hormones (insulin in the absorptive phase; glucagon, adrenaline, and cortisol in the postabsorptive phase),
- Current public health advice recommends low intakes of sugars (not more that 5% of dietary energy) and higher intakes of dietary fibre (at least 30 g/d) to reduce the risk of obesity and of multiple non-communicable diseases.

8.1 Introduction: carbohydrates in foods

Carbohydrates are one of the four major classes of biomolecules and play several important roles in all life forms, including as:

- sources of metabolic fuels and energy stores;
- structural components of cell walls in plants and of the exoskeleton of arthropods;
- parts of RNA and DNA in which ribose and deoxyribose, respectively, are linked by N-glycosidic bonds to purine and pyrimidine bases;
- integral features of many proteins and lipids (glycoproteins and glycolipids, respectively), especially in cell membranes where they are essential for cell–cell recognition and molecular targeting.

Carbohydrates are very diverse molecules that can be classified by their molecular size (degree of polymerisation or DP) into sugars (DP 1–2), oligosaccharides (DP 3–9), and polysaccharides (DP > 9). The physicochemical properties of carbohydrates and their fates within the body are influenced by their monosaccharide composition and by the type of linkage between sugar residues. Examples of food carbohydrates and an overview of their digestive fates are given in Table 8.1.

Introduction to Human Nutrition, Third Edition. Edited on behalf of The Nutrition Society by Susan A. Lanham-New, Thomas R. Hill, Alison M. Gallagher and Hester H. Vorster.

Companion website: www.wiley.com/go/lanham-new/humannutrition

Table 8.1 Classes of food carbohydrates and their likely fates in the human gut

Class	DP	Example	Site of digestion	Absorbed molecules
Monosaccharides	1	Glucose	Small bowel	Glucose
	1	Fructose	Small bowel[a]	Fructose
	2	Sucrose	Small bowel	Glucose + fructose
	2	Lactose	Small bowel[b]	Glucose + galactose
	2	Trehalose	Small bowel	Glucose
Oligosaccharides	3	Raffinose	Large bowel	SCFA
	3–9	Inulin	Large bowel	SCFA
	3–8	Galacto-oligosaccharides	Large bowel	SCFA
Polysaccharides	>9	Starches	Predominantly small bowel[c]	Glucose
	>9	Non-starch polysaccharides	Large bowel	SCFA

[a] Except where very large doses are consumed in a single meal.
[b] Except in lactose-intolerant individuals, in whom lactose flows to the large bowel.
[c] Some starch escapes small bowel digestion (resistant starch) and becomes a substrate for bacterial fermentation to short-chain fatty acids (SCFAs) in the large bowel.
DP, degree of polymerisation.

From birth, carbohydrate provides a large part of the energy in human diets, with approximately 40% of the energy in mature breast milk being provided as lactose. After weaning, carbohydrates are the largest source (40–80%) of the energy in many human diets, with most of this derived from plant material except when substantial amounts of milk or milk products containing lactose are consumed.

8.2 Digestive fate of dietary carbohydrates

As with other food components, the digestive fate of each individual carbohydrate depends on its inherent chemical nature and on the supramolecular structures within foods of which they are a part. To be absorbed from the gut, carbohydrates must be broken down to their constituent monosaccharide units, and a battery of hydrolytic (digestive) enzymes capable of splitting the bonds between sugar residues is secreted within the mouth, from the pancreas, and on the apical membrane of enterocytes. While these carbohydrases ensure that about 95% of the carbohydrate in most human diets is digested and absorbed within the small intestine, there is considerable variation in bioavailability between different carbohydrate classes and between different foods. Carbohydrates that are digested to sugars and absorbed as such in the small bowel are called "glycaemic" carbohydrates because they have the potential to raise blood glucose concentration.

Hydrolysis in the mouth and small bowel

The salivary glands and the acinar cells of the pancreas secrete the endoglycosidase α-amylase (EC 3.2.1.1] which hydrolyses internal α-1,4-linkages in amylose and amylopectin molecules to yield maltose, maltotriose, and dextrins. These oligosaccharides, together with the food disaccharides sucrose, lactose (from milk), and trehalose (from fungi, insects and other invertebrates), are hydrolyzed by specific oligosaccharidases expressed on the apical membrane of the epithelial cells that populate the small intestinal villi. Each of these oligosaccharidases is a glycoprotein anchored via its amino-terminal domain in the apical membrane and with the hydrolytic portion of the molecule protruding into the gut lumen. Sucrase–isomaltase [EC 3.2.1.10] hydrolyzes all of the sucrose and most of the maltose and isomaltose, lactase [EC 3.2.1.108] hydrolyses lactose, whilst trehalase [EC 3.2.1.28] hydrolyses trehalose and the resulting monomeric sugars are then available for transport into the enterocytes. These disaccharidases are expressed early during foetal development in humans and are active at birth. After weaning, lactase [EC 3.2.1.108] activity usually declines. However, lactase [EC 3.2.1.108] continues to be expressed throughout life in about 35% of the world's population mainly those of Northern European descent, some residents of the Middle East and Northern India and among traditionally pastoralist populations in sub-Saharan Africa where lactose intolerance is usually <5%. This lactase [EC 3.2.1.108] persistence is due to relevantly recently acquired mutations in an intron (non-coding region) in the *MCM6* gene (located close to the lactase *LCT* gene) that is important for the control of lactase expression. Evolutionary evidence suggests that the acquisition of lactase persistence-associated alleles occurred around the time of animal domestication and the development of dairying.

Absorption and malabsorption in the small bowel

Glucose and galactose are transported across the apical membrane by the sodium–glucose transport protein-1 (SGLT1), a process that is powered by Na^+/ K^+-ATPase on the basolateral membrane (Figure 8.1). In contrast, fructose is absorbed by facilitated transport via the membrane-spanning GLUT5 protein. A member of the same family of transporter proteins, GLUT2, is the facilitated transporter on the basolateral membrane which shuttles all three monosaccharides from the enterocyte towards the blood vessels linking with the portal vein for onward transport to the liver.

The capacity of the human intestine for transport of glucose, galactose, and fructose is enormous – estimated to be about 10 kg per day – so that this does not limit absorption in healthy individuals. Carbohydrate malabsorption is usually

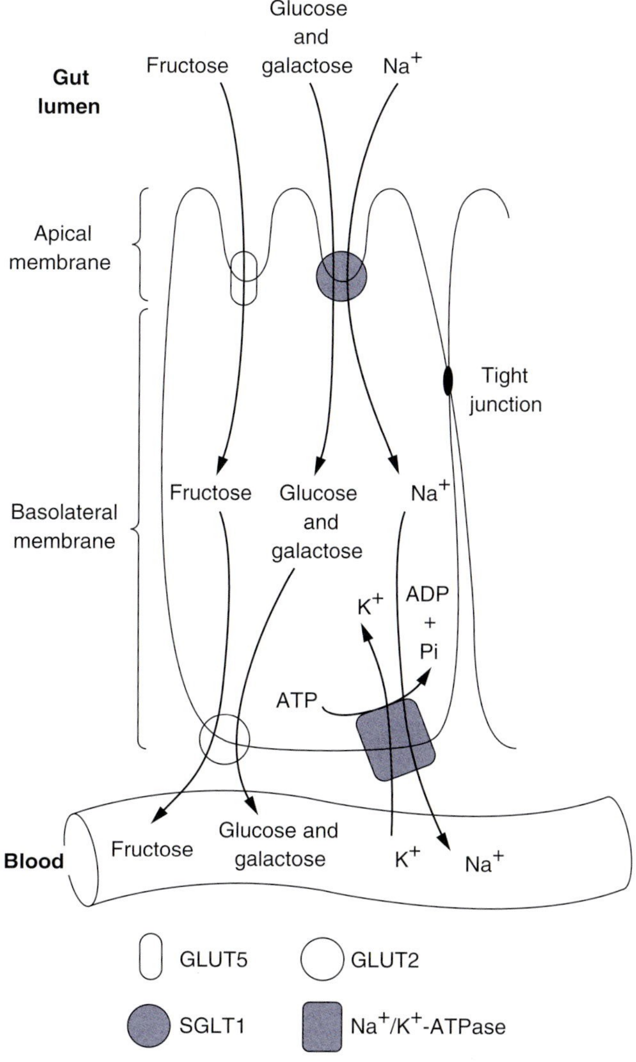

Figure 8.1 Sugar transporters on enterocytes, showing the transport of glucose and galactose across the apical membrane.

caused by an inherited or acquired defect in the brush border oligosaccharides. In the majority (about 65%) of humans, intestinal expression of lactase [EC 3.2.1.108] falls to very low levels after weaning. As a consequence, ingestion of more than small amounts of lactose by such individuals leads to the flow of the sugar to the large bowel, where it is fermented to produce short-chain fatty acids (SCFAs) and gases as end-products. The appearance of hydrogen in the breath (>12ppm hydrogen above baseline) after ingestion of lactose is the basis for diagnosis of malabsorption of this carbohydrate. Failure to see an increase in blood glucose concentration after a test drink containing lactose is an alternative approach for diagnosing lactose intolerance. Diseases of the intestinal tract, such as protein-energy malnutrition, intestinal infections, inflammatory bowel disease and coeliac disease, and gastrointestinal surgery, which reduce the expression of lactase [EC 3.2.1.108] on the enterocyte apical membrane, can result in secondary lactase insufficiency. Sucrase–isomaltase [EC 3.2.1.10] activity, which rises rapidly from the pylorus towards the jejunum and then declines, is inducible by sucrose feeding. About 10% of Greenland Eskimos and 0.2% of North Americans have sucrase–isomaltase [EC 3.2.1.10] deficiency whereas congenital sucrose-isomaltase deficiency is relatively rare (one in 5000) among those of European descent. A mis-sense mutation in the *SGLT1* gene on chromosome 22 (22q13.1) is responsible for the very rare autosomal recessive disorder known as glucose–galactose malabsorption (GGM) in which, shortly after birth and initiation of milk consumption, patients present with severe watery diarrhoea and dehydration. This can be fatal unless lactose, glucose, and galactose are excluded from the diet. Most patients with GGM can absorb fructose so this sugar can be used in the management of the condition.

Carbohydrate malabsorption in Irritable Bowel Syndrome

Irritable Bowel Syndrome (IBS) is a common condition affecting the gastrointestinal tract in which sufferers experience cramps, bloating, diarrhoea, and constipation. Many people with IBS experience symptom relief when they reduce or exclude fermentable oligosaccharides, dissaccharides, monosaccharides, and polyols, e.g., sorbitol and mannitol (collectively known as FODMAPS) from their diet. When tested by ingestion of challenge doses of lactose and fructose and measurement of breath hydrogen, about one third of adults with IBS-like symptoms were shown to malabsorb lactose and nearly two thirds malabsorbed fructose.

8.3 Glycaemic carbohydrates

The rate of uptake of glucose (and other sugars) from the gut is determined by the rate of hydrolysis of oligosaccharides and polysaccharides that are susceptible to pancreatic and brush border enzymes. In addition to the primary structure of the polymers, many factors intrinsic to the ingested foods and to the consumer influence these rates, including:

- food factors
  - particle size
  - macrostructure and microstructure of food, especially whether plant cell walls are intact
  - amylose–amylopectin ratio of starches
  - lipid content of food
  - presence (or otherwise) of enzyme inhibitors including e.g., polyphenols
- consumer factors
  - degree of comminution in the mouth
  - rate of gastric emptying
  - small bowel transit time.

All three main sugars absorbed from the gut (glucose, galactose, and fructose) are transported via the portal vein to the liver (glucose concentrations in the portal vein after a meal can rise to almost 10 mM), but only glucose appears in significant concentrations in the peripheral circulation. Most absorbed galactose and fructose is removed during the first pass through the liver via specific receptors on hepatocytes, so that the blood concentration of these sugars rarely exceeds 1 mM. Within the hepatocytes, galactose is converted to galactose-1-phosphate by the enzyme galactokinase (EC 2.7.1.6] and then to glucose-1-phosphate in three further steps. Fructose is also phosphorylated in hepatocytes (by fructokinase [EC 2.7.1.4]) to fructose-1-phosphate, which is subsequently split by fructose-1,6-bisphosphate aldolase [EC 4.1.2.13] to yield one molecule of each of the glycolytic intermediates, dihydroxyacetone phosphate and glyceraldehyde. Although the liver removes some glucose, using the bidirectional transporter GLUT2, most is transported in the peripheral circulation for utilisation by muscle, adipose, and other tissues.

Metabolic utilisation of glucose

Peripheral organs and tissues including brain, muscle, and adipose tissue remove glucose from the bloodstream via tissue-specific GLUT, or SLC2A family, transporters that are located on the cell's plasma membrane (see Table 8.2).

Once inside the cells, glucose is metabolised in the cytoplasm via glycolysis, a sequence of reactions in which the 6-carbon molecule glucose is converted to the 3-carbon molecule pyruvate, with concomitant production of a small amount of ATP. This is the prelude to the citric acid (Krebs) cycle and the electron transport chain in the mitochondria which, together, release the majority of the energy contained in glucose. Under aerobic conditions, pyruvate enters the mitochondria where it is oxidised completely to carbon dioxide and water. The overall reaction can be summarised stoichiometrically as:

$$C_6H_{12}O_6 + 6O_2 \rightarrow 6CO_2 + 6H_2O$$

Approximately 40% of the free energy (ΔG) released by this transformation is captured by the production of ATP (38 moles of ATP per mole of glucose oxidised), which is used for almost all energy-requiring purposes, including powering muscle contraction, transporting substances across membranes against a concentration gradient, and synthesis of cell macromolecules. The remainder of the free energy in glucose is released as heat.

When the demand for oxygen exceeds supply, as in muscle during intense exercise, and tissues become anaerobic, glycolysis produces lactic acid as a major end-product. The relative lack of oxygen means that oxidative phosphorylation cannot keep up with the supply of reduced dinucleotides and, for glycolysis to proceed, NADH must be recycled back to NAD^+. This is achieved by the reaction:

$$\text{Pyruvate} + \text{NADH} + H^+ \rightarrow \text{Lactate} + \text{NAD}^+$$

which is catalysed by the enzyme lactate dehydrogenase [EC 1.1.1.27]. Anaerobic glycolysis provides ATP for some cells and tissues including erythrocytes, white blood cells, lymphocytes, the kidney medulla, and eye tissues. The lactate released from tissues undergoing anaerobic glycolysis is taken up by other tissues that have a high density of mitochondria in their cells, such as heart muscle, in which the lactate is converted back to pyruvate (a process known as the lactate shuttle). Pyruvate in the cell cytoplasm is transported into the mitochondria and metabolised to acetyl coenzyme A by a consortium of three enzymes known as the pyruvate dehydrogenase complex. Acetyl CoA can then enter the Krebs cycle to generate ATP. In addition, muscle-derived lactate that is taken up by the liver can be converted back to glucose via gluconeogenesis (an energy expensive process) and returned to muscle in a circular pathway known as the Cori cycle.

In hepatic and muscle cells, some glucose is converted to glycogen (a highly branched

Table 8.2 Tissue distribution of glucose transporters

Transporter name	Tissue distribution	Comments
GLUT1	Almost all tissues including red blood cells and, especially, endothelial cells of blood-brain barrier	Also transports the oxidised form of vitamin C i.e., dehydroascorbic acid.
GLUT2	Multiple cell types including enterocytes, renal tubular cells, hepatocytes and pancreatic beta cells	Bi-directional transporter
GLUT3	Neurons and placenta	In placenta, may be of greater importance in early pregnancy
GLUT4	Adipose tissue and striated (skeletal and cardiac) muscle	Insulin-regulated glucose transporter

polymer of $\alpha(1\rightarrow4)$ glycosidic bonds in the straight chains and $\alpha(1\rightarrow6)$ glycosidic bonds at branch points) via the glycogenesis pathway. Human liver can contain up to 6% glycogen whereas muscle cells rarely contain more than 1–2% glycogen so that total body glycogen is about 400 g in a 70 kg adult. In healthy young women, muscle glycogen concentrations are lower in the luteal compared with the follicular phase of the menstrual cycle. However, liver glycogen concentrations are similar in both genders and not significantly different between menstrual cycle phases in young females (Price and Sanders, 2017). Glycogen is a readily mobilised storage form of glucose especially for strenuous muscle activity and its synthesis and degradation are important for the regulation of blood glucose concentration.

Regulation of blood glucose concentration

The exocrine pancreas (and other tissues) is primed to expect a rise in blood glucose concentration by peptide hormones (incretins) including gastric inhibitory peptide (GIP) and glucagon-like peptide-1 (GLP-1) that are secreted from enteroendocrine cells (GIP and GLP1 from K and L cells, respectively) within the mucosa of the small bowel. Following carbohydrate ingestion, digestion and absorption of sugars, blood glucose concentration rises above 5 mM, and these peptide hormones amplify the response of the β-cells of the endocrine pancreas. Incretins are members of the G protein-coupled receptor (GPCR) family and binding of the incretin to its receptor on the plasma membrane of the β-cell leads to increased intracellular concentration of cyclic adenosine monophosphate (cyclic AMP) – an important second messenger. This results in the discharge of the hormone insulin from secretory granules which fuse with the cell membrane. Insulin has several effects on metabolism, including facilitating the transport, by GLUT4, of glucose into adipocytes and into muscle cells.

In healthy people, blood glucose concentration (glycaemia) is homeostatically controlled within a fairly narrow range. It seldom falls below 5 mM, even after a prolonged fast, rises to 7–8 mM after consumption of a carbohydrate-containing meal and returns to this concentration two to three hours later. However, glucose continues to be absorbed from the gut for up to five to six hours after a meal and in this later post-prandial phase there is little or no change in blood glucose concentration because the rate of glucose removal from the blood by liver and peripheral tissues matches the rate of uptake from the gut.

In the absence of uptake from the gut (the postabsorptive state), about 8 g glucose per hour is provided for those tissues with an obligatory demand for glucose – namely, the brain, red blood cells, mammary gland, and testis – by breakdown of stores of glycogen in the liver and muscle and by gluconeogenesis. An adult human brain is about 2% of total body mass but uses approximately 20% of whole-body glucose-derived energy. A typical brain weighs approximately 1350 g, requires approximately 5.6 mg glucose per 100g brain tissue per minute or about 110 g/day. Glycogen breakdown can supply the required glucose for one to two days but, in longer periods of fasting and starvation, the requirement for glucose is met from non-carbohydrate sources by a process known as gluconeogenesis which occurs in the liver (responsible for about 90% of gluconeogenesis) and kidney. Gluconeogenesis is the synthesis of glucose from a range of substrates including pyruvate, lactate, glycerol, and amino acids. Body proteins are turned over (catabolised and re-synthesised) continuously and the amino acids required for gluconeogenesis are derived by this catabolism. All amino acids, with the exceptions of lysine and leucine, are glucogenic. Triacylglycerols (from adipose tissue) are catabolised to release glycerol, which is also glucogenic. These gluconeogenic processes are triggered by a fall in blood glucose concentration below about 5 mM and are signalled to the tissues by the secretion of glucagon and the glucocorticoid hormones.

Diabetes and its consequences

Symptoms of diabetes include the presence of glucose in urine, passage of large volumes of urine, body weight loss, and, in extreme cases, ketosis (excess production of acetone, acetoacetate, and β-hydroxybutyrate). Diabetes is characterised by higher than usual fasting blood glucose concentration and an exaggerated response in blood glucose concentration following ingestion of a fixed amount of glucose (a glucose tolerance test). When blood glucose concentrations are higher than normal for prolonged periods, weeks and months, this leads to a form of damage to the body's proteins called glycation. In glycation, glucose binds non-enzymatically to the amino group of amino acid residues (usually lysine) in proteins and, eventually forms a stable ketoamine. This process is exploited in the diagnosis and management of diabetes through the measurement of glycated haemoglobin (HbA1c) which provides an integrated index of blood glucose concentration over the previous two to three months. An HbA1c concentration greater than 48 mM (6.5%) is used in the diagnosis of diabetes.

The most common forms of diabetes are type 1 diabetes (T1DM) and type 2 diabetes (T2DM). T1DM results from the autoimmune destruction of the β-cells of the endocrine pancreas (possibly following viral exposure) which results in insulin insufficiency. Control of blood glucose concentrations in T1DM requires the exogenous supply of insulin by injection, or increasingly often, by implanted insulin mini-pumps. There has been rapid progress in research on use of implanted pancreatic β-cells which is likely to offer a more physiological form of treatment in the future.

Although more than 100 genetic variants are associated with risk of T2DM, expression of the disease is due mainly to adverse lifestyle choices (excess energy intake and low physical activity) that result in obesity, especially when the extra fat is accumulated on the trunk. The early stages of T2DM are characterised by insulin insensitivity/resistance, i.e., failure of the tissues to produce a normal response to insulin release that can be seen as relatively wide swings (excursions) in blood glucose concentrations following a carbohydrate-containing meal. Raised blood glucose concentration sustained for several years is causal for the spectrum of complications, including macrovascular (atherosclerosis) and microvascular diseases and problems with the kidneys (nephropathy), nerves (neuropathy), and eyes (retinopathy and cataract) experienced by diabetics. Until recently, it had been assumed that T2DM was a permanent, life-long condition. However, studies of weight loss induced by bariatric surgery or low energy diet have shown clearly that significant weight loss leads to diabetes remission. In the DiRECT Study, carried out in primary care in the UK, 86% of participants who had maintained at least 15 kg weight loss after one year achieved remission of their T2DM (Lean *et al.* 2018). Rapid and substantial weight loss leading to removal of fat from the pancreas (and liver) seems to be important in enabling β-cell recovery and diabetes remission (Taylor *et al.* 2018).

Dietary management of blood glucose concentration

Glycaemic index

GD Campbell appears to have been the first to attempt to quantify and rank carbohydrate-rich foods according to the change in blood glucose concentration (glycaemia) that they induced after a standard amount of carbohydrate (50 g) was ingested (Cummings and Engineer, 2018). This idea was developed further by Crapo *et al.* (1971) and by Jenkins and colleagues (1981) who introduced the concept of the glycaemic index (GI). GI provides a means of comparing quantitatively the blood glucose responses (determined directly by *in vivo* experiments) following ingestion of equivalent amounts of digestible carbohydrate from different foods. In practice, GI is calculated as the ratio of incremental area under the curve for blood glucose (iAUC) after ingestion of 50g of available carbohydrate from the test food compared with the iAUC after ingestion of 50g of glucose (Brouns F *et al.*, 2005). When a range of carbohydrate-containing foods was ranked according to their GI values, there was a strong linear relationship with the rapidly available glucose (RAG) from similar foods determined *in vitro* as the sum of free glucose, glucose from sucrose, and glucose released from starches over a 20 minute period of hydrolysis with a battery of enzymes under strictly controlled conditions (Englyst *et al.* 1999). This offers the possibility of assaying foods *in vitro* for their RAG content, which is faster and less expensive than the approach based on GI measurements *in vivo*.

Studies with glucose and starches enriched with the stable isotope carbon-13 have demonstrated that glucose absorption from the gut following a meal continues for several hours after blood concentrations have returned to fasting levels. In this later postprandial period, insulin secretion is sufficient to ensure that the rate of glucose absorption is matched by the rate of glucose removal from the circulation. ^{13}C-labelled substrates are valuable tools for investigating the kinetics of digestion, absorption, and metabolic disposal of glucose and other sugars from a range of foods. Such kinetic studies are likely to be helpful in identifying foods with slower rates of intestinal hydrolysis – information that can be used in public health advice or in counselling individuals. Recent studies suggest that multiple factors, including the activity of the gut microbiome (more details below), determine individual blood glucose responses to consumption of specific foods (Zeevi *et al.*, 2015). This concept is being used to develop personalised approaches to food choice that are intended to avoid unnecessarily large excursions in blood glucose concentration. However, this approach has been criticised (Wolever, 2016) and its utility remains to be demonstrated.

Fructose

When glucose and fructose are available simultaneously after a meal containing sucrose, how does the body select which fuel to use first for oxidative purposes? This question has been resolved by experiments in which volunteers consumed, on two separate occasions, high-sucrose test meals which were identical except that one or other of the constituent monomeric sugars was ^{13}C-labelled in each meal (Daly *et al.*, 2000). The volunteers blew into tubes at intervals after the meals to provide breath samples for measurement of the enrichment of expired carbon dioxide with ^{13}C. The results showed that, after the high sucrose meal, fructose was oxidised much more rapidly and extensively than was glucose (Figure 8.2). This rapid oxidation of fructose may be explained by the fact that, because it is phosphorylated in hepatocytes, it bypasses 6-phosphofructokinase [EC 2.7.1.11], one of the key regulatory enzymes in glycolysis.

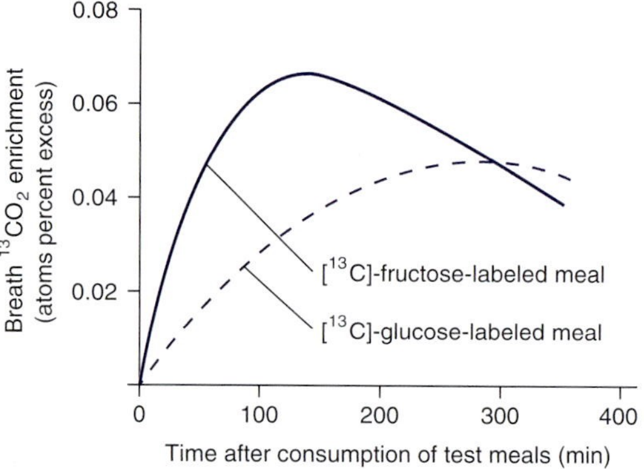

Figure 8.2 Enrichment of breath $^{13}CO_2$ following ingestion of high-sucrose test meals labelled with [^{13}C]-fructose and [^{13}C]-glucose. Source: Redrawn from Daly *et al.*, 2000, with permission of the American Society for Nutrition.

8.4 Dietary fibre

Carbohydrates that are not absorbed in the small intestine enter the large bowel, where they are partially or completely catabolised by bacteria in the colon by a process called fermentation (discussed below). McCance and Lawrence in 1929 were the first to classify carbohydrates as "available" and "unavailable" when they realised that not all food carbohydrates provide "carbohydrates for metabolism" to the body. They called these carbohydrates "unavailable." This was a useful concept because it drew attention to the fact that some carbohydrate is not digested and absorbed in the small intestine. However, it is misleading to consider this carbohydrate as "unavailable" because some so-called non-digestible carbohydrate can provide the body with energy through fermentation in the colon (discussed further below). The potential importance of plant cell wall material (which makes up the bulk of unavailable carbohydrate in most human diets) in promoting human health was identified in the late 1960s and early 1970s though pioneering research by Denis Burkitt using ideas from and, sometimes in collaboration with, a small group of clinicians and biochemists including Campbell, Cleave, Painter, Trowell, and Walker. Whilst working in East Africa, Burkitt had made his scientific reputation by discovering that swellings in the jaws of children were due to an aggressive form of non-Hodgkin's lymphoma (now known as Burkitt's lymphoma) that is rare in most parts of the world but common in children living in sub-Saharan Africa. His second major scientific contribution was in recognising the potential importance of (dietary) "fibre" in preventing coronary heart disease, obesity, diabetes, dental caries, various vascular disorders, and large bowel conditions such as cancer, appendicitis, and diverticulosis (now classified as non-communicable diseases (NCDs)) (Burkitt and Trowell, 1975). Burkitt's idea of grouping these diseases together as having a common cause was ground-breaking (Cummings & Engineer, 2018) and the hypothesis that these NCDs were caused by a relative lack of non-digestible carbohydrates (dietary fibre) was met with much scepticism. However, epidemiological and experimental research over the last 40+ years has shown that Burkitt and his colleagues were broadly correct. Plant-based diets rich in dietary fibre are now recognised as a key component of healthier eating patterns that make a significant contribution to lowering NCD risk.

Several names, definitions, and methods for assaying these so-called non-digestible carbohydrates have been used by different authorities and have led to problems in food labelling and in the conduct and interpretation of nutritional epidemiological studies. In an attempt to rationalise this complex field, the Food and Agriculture Organization (FAO 1998) of the United Nations and World Health Organization suggested that the term "non-glycaemic carbohydrates" is more appropriate. This proposal was not adopted widely by either relevant scientists and clinicians or by the food industry because the term "dietary fibre" was already in widespread use. In 2010, the European Food Safety Authority (EFSA) proposed that the term "dietary fibre" should be used to describe the sum of all non-digestible (or non-glycaemic) carbohydrates plus lignin. This is in accord with the definition of dietary fibre approved by the Codex Alimentarius Committee in 2009 (Lupton *et al.*, 2009). The amounts of dietary fibre in foods that meet the Codex and EFSA definitions can be quantified using an enzyme-based method, i.e., AOAC Method 2009.01 (McCleary *et al.*, 2013).

Nature of carbohydrates that enter the colon

Carbohydrates that enter the colon can be classified either physiologically or chemically. Neither of these classifications is entirely satisfactory because it is difficult to measure the physiologically indigestible carbohydrates, and this varies in different people. Further, the chemical structure of carbohydrates does not always predict their physiological behaviour in the gut.

Physiological classification of carbohydrates entering the colon

Carbohydrates enter the colon because (i) monosaccharide transporters do not exist in the intestinal mucosa or do not function at a high enough rate; (ii) the enzymes needed to digest the carbohydrates are not present in the small intestine; (iii) the enzymes are present but cannot gain access to the carbohydrates, e.g., because of food structure; or (iv) the enzymes do not digest the carbohydrates sufficiently rapidly for them to be completely absorbed. In addition, a small amount of carbohydrate enters the colon as carbohydrate residues occurring on mucopolysaccharides (mucus) secreted by the small and large intestinal mucosal cells.

Although some carbohydrates (e.g., cellulose found in plant cell walls) are always non-glycaemic because humans do not express the enzymes necessary for their digestion, a significant proportion (perhaps up to half) of all carbohydrates that escape digestion in the small intestine have a chemical structure which means that they could potentially be digested or absorbed in the small intestine. However, for various reasons, digestion in this part of the gut is incomplete.

Some monosaccharides and sugar alcohols are only partially absorbed because of low affinity for intestinal transporters. Xylose is taken up by the glucose transporter SGLT1, but is only partly absorbed because of low affinity for the transporter. On its own, fructose is poorly absorbed, but it is readily absorbed in the presence of glucose (most rapid absorption with 1:1 molar ratio). In addition, GLUT5, the transporter responsible for fructose absorption across the enterocyte, is inducible and sustained exposure to higher intakes of fructose leads to higher GLUT5 expression. The surface area of the small intestine available for absorption is reduced by diseases that cause atrophy of the intestinal mucosa, such as tropical sprue or coeliac disease, or surgical resection of a portion of the intestine (e.g., for Crohn's disease or in some types of bariatric (weight loss) surgery). An increased rate of intestinal transit (e.g., high osmotic load in the small intestinal lumen from undigested sugars) reduces the time available for absorption to occur.

As discussed above, most adult humans (except for those of European descent or other groups with a long tradition of dairying) have low or absent intestinal lactase [EC 3.2.1.108] activity leading to partial or complete lactose non-absorption. Starch hydrolysis is dependent on the supply of amylase [EC 3.2.1.1] from the pancreas and inadequate pancreatic amylase will result in starch escaping small bowel digestion (resistant start – see below). Amylase [EC 3.2.1.1] supply may be reduced in those with exocrine pancreatic insufficiency which occurs in cystic fibrosis, in individuals who have undergone surgical removal of all or part of the pancreas (pancreatectomy) and in those with chronic pancreatitis. Such individuals may be treated with pancreatic enzyme replacement therapy.

All amylopectin and amylose which make up the starch complex is potentially digested in the small intestine but if it is trapped inside intact plant cell walls or other plant cell structures, pancreatic amylase [EC 3.2.1.1] may be unable to gain access to it, and so it remains undigested. The digestibility of the carbohydrates in banana depends on the degree of ripeness of the fruit. The starch in green banana is very indigestible but, as the banana ripens, the starch is converted to sugars including sucrose (>70%), glucose and fructose.

For carbohydrates that are digested and/or absorbed slowly, the time that the food residues spend in the small intestine (transit time; typically, about four hours) influences the amount of it that escapes to flow to the large bowel. Some forms of retrograded or resistant starch, or foods with a large particle size, are digested so slowly that the time spent in the small intestine is too short for their complete digestion. Digestion of these carbohydrates can be altered by factors that affect transit time including other components of the meal, ageing and intestinal diseases For example, gastroparesis (reduced gastric function and slowing of digesta release from the stomach) occurs in some people with T1DM and in some of those treated with opioid pain relievers, with certain antidepressants and with some allergy medications.

Chemical classification of carbohydrates entering the colon

The chemical classification of carbohydrates entering the colon is as follows:

- *Monosaccharides:* all except for glucose, fructose, and galactose are partly or completely unabsorbed in the small intestine. Fructose in the absence of a source of glucose (mono-, di-, or polysaccharide) is partly unabsorbed.
- *Sugar alcohols:* all are partly or completely unabsorbed in the small intestine.
- *Disaccharides:* all except for maltose, sucrose, and lactose are unabsorbed in the small intestine. Lactose is completely or partly unabsorbed in individuals with low intestinal lactase [EC 3.2.1.108] activity.
- *Oligosaccharides:* all are unabsorbed in the small intestine except for maltodextrins.
- *Non-starch polysaccharides:* all non-starch polysaccharides, e.g., cellulose, xylans, and pectin are not hydrolysed by human pancreatic enzymes.
- *Resistant starch:* by definition, starch that escapes digestion in the small intestine and enters the colon (discussed below).

Amount of carbohydrate entering the colon

It is difficult to measure the amount of carbohydrate entering the human colon. However, it has been estimated that at least 30 g of carbohydrate is required to support the growth of the bacterial population in the colon of an individual on a typical Western diet producing about 100 g stool per day. About half of that amount comes from non-starch polysaccharide (NSP), 1–2 g from indigestible oligosaccharides, and probably about 1–2 g from intestinal mucopolysaccharides. The other 10–12 g is believed to come from starch that has escaped digestion in the small bowel (resistant starch; see below). The amount of carbohydrate entering the colon, however, can be increased several-fold, up to 100 g/day or more, by changes in diet such as increased intake of dietary fibre-rich foods such as wholegrain cereals, pulses (e.g., peas, beans and lentils), vegetables and slowly digested, low-GI foods.

Resistant starch

Resistant starch is starch that escapes digestion in the small intestine and enters the colon (Asp *et al.,* 1996). In the 1970s and early 1980s it first became apparent that appreciable amounts of starch are not digested in the small bowel, from experiments showing that breath hydrogen increased after eating normal starchy foods. Hydrogen gas is a product of the anaerobic fermentation of carbohydrates by colonic bacteria (see below). Subsequently, other ways of measuring carbohydrate entering the colon were developed. In one technique, study participants swallowed a tube that was passed through the stomach and along to the end of the small intestine so that the material leaving the small intestine and about to enter the colon could be sampled directly and quantified. Another method was to study people who have had their colons removed surgically and in whom the end of the ileum was sutured to a stoma in the body wall (an ileostomy). In this way, the material leaving their small intestine could be collected quantitatively. With these methods, the amount of carbohydrate leaving the small intestine can be measured directly and all methods confirmed that a substantial amount of starch enters the colon (Englyst *et al.,* 1996).

The main forms of resistant starch (RS) are physically enclosed starch, for example within intact cell structures (known at RS_1); raw starch granules (RS_2); and retrograded amylose (RS_3). In addition, chemically modified starches (RS_4; etherised, esterified or cross-linked starches) are used for technical purposes by the food industry. These kinds of starch can be quantified using methods developed by Englyst and colleagues (Englyst *et al.,* 1996).

Dietary fibre

Originally, Burkitt and Trowell (1975) defined dietary fibre as the components of plant cell walls that are indigestible in the human small intestine. Later, the definition was expanded to include storage polysaccharides within plant cells (e.g., the gums in some legumes). Over time, the definition has evolved in an attempt to be holistic in assessing all carbohydrates that escape digestion in the small intestine and now most authorities accept the Codex (2009) or EFSA (2010) definitions. However, readers of the scientific literature should be aware that several different methods for assessing dietary fibre have been used over the past 40+ years which were more or less restrictive in the components measured, and that quite different analytical approaches were adopted. The methods that have been used in Europe and their potential implications for health are reviewed in detail by Stephen and colleagues (Stephen AM *et al.,* 2017). Since different analytical methods can yield quite different estimates of the dietary fibre content of specific foods, readers are advised to take note of the specific method used when reading, and interpreting, earlier publications.

The gut microbiome: what it is and what it does

Burkitt, and the other pioneers who laid the foundation for understanding the physiological actions of dietary fibre, recognised that gut bacteria may play a role human health but, 40 years ago, the scientific tools for investigating this complex issue were limited. However, in the last 15 years, the development of genetic and bioinformatics tools has facilitated a revolution in research on complex ecosystems such as the human large bowel. We can now characterise the composition and function of microbiomes in considerable detail. In addition to a very high density of multiple bacterial species (there are at least as many bacterial cells in the colon as eukaryotic cells in the human body), other key microorganisms in the human large bowel include archeae (a class of prokaryotes distinct from bacteria), viruses, phages, yeast, and fungi (Ohland & Jobin, 2015). To date, most research has focused on the gut bacteria, but it is becoming clear that the other members of this highly integrated ecosystem may also be important for human nutrition and health. For example, there are ten times more phage than bacteria and these phages may play a role in maintaining the balance between those gut microbes that live in symbiosis with their human host (symbionts) and those normal gut inhabitants that could potentially cause diseases (pathobionts). In addition to the rapid progress in characterising the gut microbiota and in describing their complex interactions, the other major recent advance has been in understanding the intimate interactions between these gut residents and their human host (Figure 8.3). As discussed above, the gut epithelial cells have a primary function in digestion and absorption of nutrients, but they also play a major role in defence by acting as a barrier to infective organisms and other damaging particles. Epithelial cells also transfer key information from gut bacteria to the immune cells located in the lamina propria – the thin layer of loose areolar connective tissue located below the epithelium. The lamina propria contains many types of immune cell including activated T cells, plasma cells, mast cells, dendritic cells, and macrophages, and the gut also contains the organised lymphoid tissues known as Peyer's patches and mesenteric lymph nodes. Chemical "crosstalk" between the microbiota, epithelial cells, and immune cells is essential to maintain gut (and, perhaps, whole body) homeostasis. Therefore, since the gut provides the home for the vast majority of the body's microbes, it is not a surprise that the gut also harbours most of the immune cells that are present in the human body.

Although the colonic lumen is largely devoid of oxygen (anaerobic), the bacteria in the human large bowel are metabolically very active and ferment a wide range of substrates including food residues, host cells and other endogenous constituents flowing into the distal gut from the small intestine. This microbial metabolism results in multiple end-products which can influence host nutrition and metabolism such as folate, indoles,

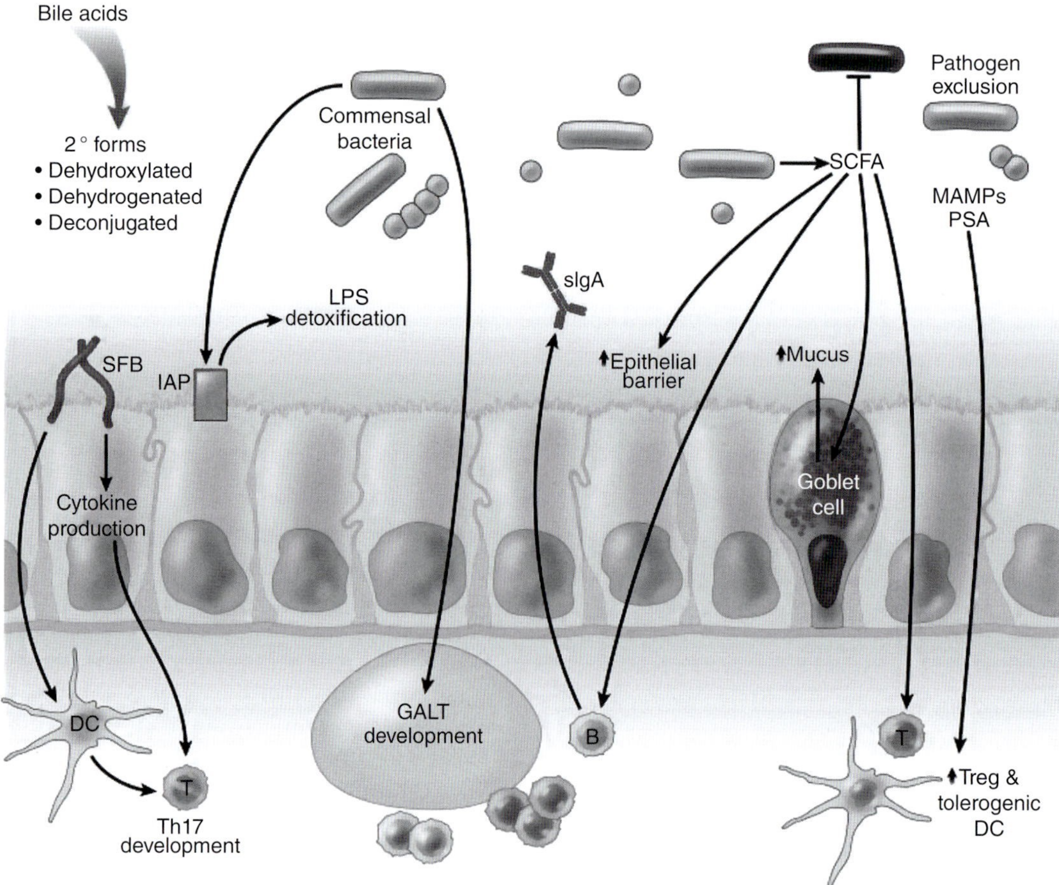

Figure 8.3 Overview of the crosstalk between the human gut microbes and the host immune system. MAMP (microbe-associated molecular pattern); SCFA (short-chain fatty acids); IAP (intestinal alkaline phosphatase); LPS (lipopolysaccharides); SFB (segmented filamentous bacteria); DC (dendritic cells); GALT (gut-associated lymphoid tissue) including Peyer's patches and mesenteric lymph nodes. (Reproduced from Ohland and Jobin, 2015)

secondary bile acids, trimethylamine-N-oxide (TMAO), and neurotransmitters. However, from the perspective of carbohydrate digestion, the most important end-products are short-chain fatty acids (SCFAs). Fermentation is the process by which the gut microorganisms catabolise monosaccharides to derive energy for their own metabolism. Because they are operating in an essentially anaerobic environment, gut bacteria cannot use molecular oxygen as a terminal electron acceptor and, therefore, they cannot use the Krebs cycle and oxidative phosphorylation to complete oxidation of sugars to CO_2 and water. The first part of this anaerobic catabolism is accomplished using glycolysis which yields pyruvate and the reduced dinucleotide NADH. To allow glycolysis to continue, NAD+ is regenerated by conversion of the glycolytic intermediate pyruvate to SCFAs. These are saturated aliphatic carboxylic acids containing one to six carbons of which acetate (C2), propionate (C3), and butyrate (C4) are the most abundant (Figure 8.4). In addition, fermentation results in the production of CO_2, H_2 and in some cases methane (CH_4) which are lost from the body through breath and flatus (Figure 8.5). There is good evidence that the proportions of individual SCFA produced are influenced by the types of carbohydrate reaching

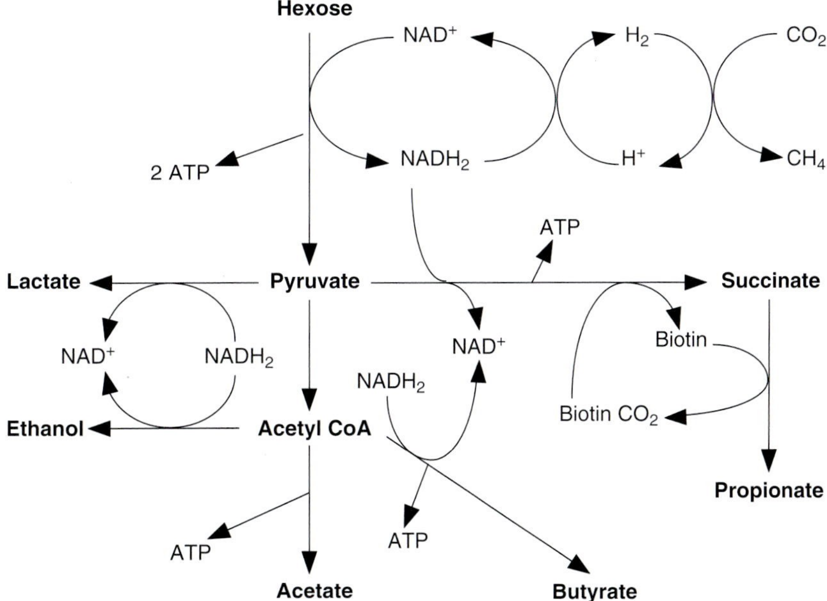

Figure 8.4 Summary of biochemical pathways used by the anaerobic bacteria in the human colon. Acetyl CoA, acetyl coenzyme A.

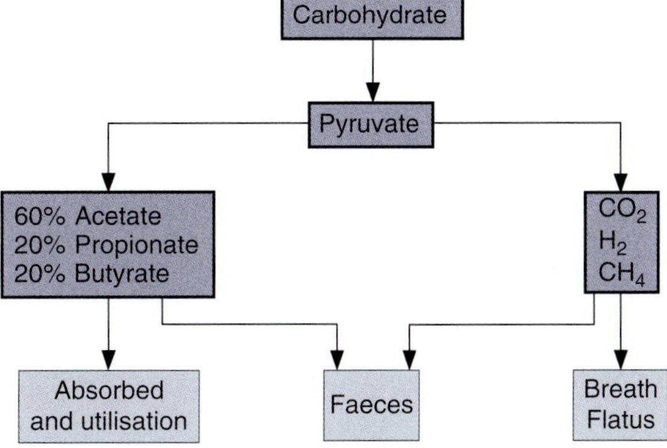

Figure 8.5 Overview of carbohydrate fermentation in the human colon.

the large bowel but, as yet, there is insufficient understanding to allow manipulation of SCFA patterns through dietary choices.

Fate of short-chain fatty acids

SCFA are absorbed readily (Cummings *et al.*, 1987) and used as sources of energy by host tissues. This salvaging of energy with the aid of commensal gut bacteria is probably the primary driver for the evolution of the complex symbiotic relationship between the host human and the gut microbiome. The amount of energy recovered via large bowel fermentation depends mainly on the quantity and fermentability (which can range from 0% to 100%) of the carbohydrate entering the large bowel. On a typical Western diet, about half of the energy in carbohydrate that enters the colon is available to the human host as SCFAs. Some of the butyrate is metabolised by the colonocytes (the epithelial cells lining the large bowel) and the rest, together with the other SCFA, is transported to the liver via the portal vein. Propionate and butyrate are removed in first pass through the liver, but increased concentrations of acetate can be observed in peripheral blood several hours after consumption of indigestible, but fermentable, carbohydrates. Most of the absorbed SCFAs are oxidised and contribute modestly (up to 10%) to the body's energy supply.

SCFA as signalling molecules and potential impact on health

Butyrate, and to a lesser extent propionate, are inhibitors of enzymes known as histone deacetylases [EC 3.5.1.98; HDAC] that remove acetyl groups from histones, the globular proteins around which DNA is wrapped in the cell nucleus. The acetylation status of histones is part of the constellation of epigenetic marks and molecules that regulate access to the genome and control, in part, gene expression (Mathers, 2015). Therefore, through its action as an HDAC inhibitor, butyrate plays a critical role in information transfer from the gut microbiota to multiple cells and tissues in the host including the gut epithelium and immune cells. At physiological concentrations, butyrate alters the expression of many genes with diverse functions, including those involved in cell kinetics (cell proliferation and apoptosis – programmed cell death) and differentiation. Butyrate may help to reduce the risk of cancer in the large bowel (and elsewhere in the body) by inducing differentiation and apoptosis of cancer cells. The antineoplastic effects of the additional SCFA, including butyrate, that are produced in the large bowel with higher intakes of dietary fibre may provide part of the explanation for the lower CRC risk among those with higher intakes of dietary fibre-rich foods.

In addition, SCFA are ligands for G protein-coupled receptors (GPCRs), a large family of receptors that are located on the plasma membrane of the cell, detect molecules outside the cell and activate internal signal transduction pathways which regulate cellular responses. Acetate and propionate are the most potent activators of GPR43 (also known as free fatty acid receptor 2; FFAR2). GPR43 is expressed in specialised enteroendocrine cells known as L cells that are present at high densities in the epithelium of the ileum and colon. When the relevant SCFA bind to their receptors on L cells, the signalling cascade that is initiated leads to secretion of glucagon-like peptide-1 (GLP1), an incretin, and other regulatory peptides including pancreatic peptide YY3-36, oxyntomodulin, and glucagon-like peptide-2. GLP1 has multiple effects on metabolism and also regulates gut movements. For example, through both peripheral and central nervous mechanisms, GLP1 decreases gastric emptying and intestinal motility and contributes to the ileal break, an inhibitory feedback mechanism that slows gastric emptying to provide sufficient time within the small intestine to optimise nutrient digestion and absorption. Such effects may contribute to the better regulation of appetite (reduce likelihood of over-eating) observed with higher fibre intakes and, therefore, greater SCFA production. Since some colon-derived acetate enters the peripheral circulation (not all acetate is cleared during first pass through the liver), acetate may influence metabolism elsewhere in the body through binding to GPR43 on adipocytes and other extra-intestinal tissues. In this way, higher intakes of dietary fibre may influence a wide range of health outcomes including obesity, asthma and cancer.

8.5 Carbohydrates and dental caries

There is a dynamic relationship between dietary carbohydrates and oral health. Starches that can be hydrolysed rapidly by salivary amylase [EC 3.2.1.1] yield mono- and oligo-saccharides which, together with ingested free sugars, become substrates for fermentation by the bacteria in the mouth. The mouth plays host to the second most diverse microbial community in the human body (the most diverse is in the colon), with more than 700 species of bacteria colonising both the teeth and the soft tissues of the oral mucosa. The resident bacteria in the mouth ferment carbohydrates to yield acidic end-products (mainly lactic acid but also some formic, acetic, and propionic acids), which result in a drop in dental plaque pH. When the pH falls below 5.5, the dental enamel dissolves in the plaque fluid and repeated exposure to periods of very low pH can lead to caries. With higher frequency of sugar intake, or reduced saliva production (as a result of diseases such as diabetes mellitus, radiation therapy to the head and neck; or some medications), plaque biofilms on teeth are exposed to lower pH for longer which increases caries risk. In addition, more regular periods of lower pH select for bacteria that produce acids themselves and/or are more tolerant of an acidic environment which exacerbates the situation.

Not all carbohydrates are equally cariogenic. Dietary fibre-rich foods have the potential to reduce caries risk through increased saliva production during chewing, but most such foods are processed and cooked to minimise the need for chewing. Many widely-consumed sugars, including sucrose, fructose, glucose, and maltose, are readily fermented by bacteria in the mouth and are strongly cariogenic when consumed frequently. Lactose, galactose, and starches are less cariogenic, while sugar alcohols such as xylitol (used as a sweetener in some confectionery and chewing gums) are non-cariogenic. Eating sugars with meals reduces the risk of caries, as does the consumption of cheese, which provides phosphates to prevent demineralisation and to encourage demineralisation of the enamel. Fluoride ingestion in foods and drinking water and via toothpastes and mouth rinses prevents dental caries. At a public health level, the strength of the evidence for links between sugar intake and poor oral health was a major factor in the decisions by both the WHO (2015) and the Scientific Advisory Committee on Nutrition (SACN, 2015) in the UK to recommend that the intake of free sugars should not exceed 5% of daily energy intake to improve and protect health.

8.6 Current perspectives and the future for dietary carbohydrates

Carbohydrates provide the largest component of dietary energy intake for most people worldwide and have done so for millennia. However, at present, there is a strong anti-carbohydrate fashion that promotes so-called "low carbohydrate" diets in which intake of sugary foods, pasta, potatoes, rice, and bread is greatly restricted in favour of foods rich in proteins and fats together with "healthy" vegetables. Although the restriction of free sugars is likely to be beneficial for health, there is no good evidence that excluding starchy staple foods is beneficial and, indeed, such diets may be disadvantageous because they are likely to be low in dietary fibre. One reason often advanced by the advocates of "low carbohydrate" diets is that they help with body weight management. However, the recent DIETFITS study in which 609 overweight and obese adults aged 18 to 50 years, without diabetes, were randomised to either a healthy "low carbohydrate" or a healthy "low fat" diet found no difference in weight loss after 12 months intervention (Gardner *et al.*, 2018). In addition, a recent systematic review and meta-analysis of both prospective studies and clinical trials has confirmed that there is a strong dose-response relationship between higher intakes of dietary fibre and lower body weight and lower risk of multiple common non-communicable diseases (Reynolds *et al.*, 2019).

Primary food production, processing, transport, and retail have major impacts on the global environment through the production of greenhouse gases (which drive climate change), demand for farm land use, depletion of freshwater resources, and pollution of aquatic and terrestrial ecosystems by (i) fertilisers and other chemical inputs into agriculture and (ii) excreta from farmed animals. Options for reducing the adverse environmental impact of the food system include dietary changes towards a healthier, more plant-based diet (Springmann *et al.*, 2018), which is likely to mean more emphasis on carbohydrate-rich foods, including starchy staples, pulses, vegetables and fruits, and substantially lower consumption of animal-derived foods.

Acknowledgement

This chapter has been revised and updated by John Mathers, based on the original chapter by John Mathers and Thomas M.S. Wolever.

References

Asp, N.-G., van Amelsvoort, J.M.M., and Hautvast, J.G.A.J. (1996). Nutritional implications of resistant starch. *Nutr. Res. Rev.* **9**: 1–13.

Brouns, F., Bjorck, I., Frayn, K.N. *et al.* (2005). Glycaemic index methodology. *Nutr Res Rev.* **18**, 145–171.

Burkitt, D.P. and Trowell, H.C. (1975). *Refined Carbohydrate Foods and Disease*. London: Academic Press.

Crapo, P.A., Reaven, G., Olefsky, J. (1976). Plasma glucose and insulin responses to orally administered simple and complex carbohydrates. *Diabetes* **25**: 741–747.

Cummings, J.H. and Engineer, A. (2018). Denis Burkitt and the origins of the dietary fibre hypothesis. *Nutr. Res. Rev.* **31**: 1–15.

Cummings, J.H., Pomare, E.W., Branch, W.J. *et al.* (1987). Short chain fatty acids in human large intestine, portal, hepatic and venous blood. *Gut* **28**: 1221–1227.

Daly, M.E., Vale, C., Walker, M. *et al.* (2000). Acute fuel selection in response to high-sucrose and high-starch meals in healthy men. *Am J Clin Nutr* **71**: 1516–1524.

European Food Safety Authority. (2010). *Scientific Opinion on Dietary Reference Values for Carbohydrates and Dietary Fibre by EFSA Panel on Dietetic Products, Nutrition, and Allergies (NDA)*. Parma, Italy: European Food Safety Authority (EFSA).

Englyst, K.N., Englyst, H.N., Hudson, G.L. *et al.* (1999). Rapidly available glucose in foods: an in vitro measurement that reflects the glycemic response. *Amer J Clin Nutr.* **69**: 448–454.

Englyst, H.N., Kingman, S.M., Hudson, G.J. *et al.* (1996). Measurement of resistant starch in vitro and in vivo. *Br J Nutr.* **75**: 749–755.

Joint FAO/WHO Food Standards Programme, Secretariat of the CODEX Alimentarius Commission (2010). *CODEX Alimentarius (CODEX) Guidelines on Nutrition Labeling CAC/GL 2-1985 as Last Amended 2010*. Rome: FAO

Food and Agriculture Organization of the United Nations. (1998). FAO food and nutrition paper 66. *Carbohydrates in human nutrition*. Report of an FAO/WHO Expert Consultation on Carbohydrates, 14–18 April 1997, Rome, Italy. Rome: FAO.

Gardner, C.D., Trepanowski, J.F., Del Gobbo, L.C. *et al.* (2018). Effect of Low-Fat vs Low-Carbohydrate Diet on 12-Month Weight Loss in Overweight Adults and the Association With Genotype Pattern or Insulin Secretion: The DIETFITS Randomized Clinical Trial. *JAMA.* **319**: 667–679.

Jenkins, D.J.A., Wolever, T.M.S., Taylor, R.H. *et al.* (1981). Glycemic index of foods: a physiological basis for carbohydrate exchange. *Am J Clin Nutr.* **34**:362–366.

Lean, M.E., Leslie, W.S., Barnes, A.C. *et al.* (2018). Primary care-led weight management for remission of type 2 diabetes (DiRECT): an open-label, cluster-randomised trial. *Lancet.* **391**:541–551.

Lupton, J.R., Betteridge, V.A., and Pijls, L.T.J. Codex final definition of dietary fibre: issues of implementation. *Crops & Food.* **1**: 206–212.

Mathers, J.C. (2015). Epigenetics. In *Nutrition Research Methodologies*. (ed. J.A. Lovegrove, L. Hodgson, S. Sharma *et al.*). John Wiley & Sons

McCance, R.A. and Lawrence, R.D. (1929). The carbohydrate content of foods. *MRC Special Report Series*, No. 135.

McCleary, B.V., Sloane, N., Draga, A. *et al.* (2013). Measurement of Total Dietary Fiber Using AOAC Method 2009.01 (AACC International Approved Method 32-45.01): Evaluation and Updates. *Cereal Chem.* **90**: 396–414.

Ohland, C.L. and Jobin, C. Microbial Activities and Intestinal Homeostasis: A Delicate Balance Between Health and Disease. *Cell Mol Gastroenterol Hepatol*, **1**(1) 28 - 40

Price, T.B. and Sanders, K. (2017). Muscle and liver glycogen utilization during prolonged lift and carry exercise: male and female responses. *Physiol. Reports* **5**(4): e13113.

Reynolds, A., Mann, J., Cummings, J. *et al.* (2019). *The Lancet* Pub. Online, 10 January 2019.

Scientific Advisory Committee on Nutrition. (2015). *Carbohydrates and Health*. The Stationery Office.

Springmann, M., Clark, M., Mason-D'Croz, D. *et al.* (2018). Options for keeping the food system within environmental limits. *Nature*. Oct 10. doi: 10.1038/s41586-018-0594-0. [Epub ahead of print]

Stephen, A.M., Champ, M.M.-J., Cloran, S.J. *et al.* (2017). Dietary fibre in Europe: current state of knowledge on definitions, sources, recommendations, intakes and relationships to health. *Nutr Res Rev* **30**, 149–190.

Taylor, R., Al-Mrabeh, A., Zhyzhneuskaya, S. *et al.* (2018). Remission of Human Type 2 Diabetes Requires Decrease in Liver and Pancreas Fat Content but Is Dependent upon Capacity for β Cell Recovery. *Cell Metab.* **28**: 547–556.

Wolever, T.M. (2016). Personalized nutrition by prediction of glycaemic responses: fact or fantasy? *Eur J Clin Nutr.* **70**:411–413.

World Health Organisation. (2015). Sugars intake for adults and children.

Zeevi, D., Korem, T., Zmora, N. *et al.* (2015). Personalized Nutrition by Prediction of Glycemic Responses. *Cell.* **163**:1079–1094.

Further reading

Asp, N.-G. (2001). Development of dietary fibre methodology. In: (ed. B.V. McCleary and L. Prosky) *Advanced Dietary Fibre Technology*. Oxford: Blackwell Science 77–88.

Cani, P.D. (2018). Human gut microbiome: hopes, threats and promises. *Gut.* **67**:1716–1725.

Johnson, L.R. (2013). *Gastrointestinal Physiology*, 8e. St Louis, MO: Mosby.

Lanham-New, S., MacDonald, I., and Roche, H. (Eds). (2010) *Nutrition and Metabolism*, 2e. Wiley Blackwell.

Rugg-Gunn, A.J. (1993). *Nutrition and Dental Health*. Oxford: Oxford University Press.

Wolever, T.M.S. (2006). *The Glycaemic Index: A Physiological Classification of Dietary Carbohydrate*. Wallingford: CABI.

9 Nutrition and Metabolism of Lipids

Bruce A. Griffin and Stephen C. Cunnane

Key messages

- Lipids (another word for "fats") are organic compounds composed of a carbon skeleton with hydrogen and oxygen substitutions, which are soluble in non-polar organic solvents, and with a few exceptions, are usually insoluble in water. Lipids, in combination with proteins and carbohydrates, are principal constituents of living cells, e.g., fats, waxes, phosphatides, cerebrosides, and related compounds
- Lipids can be classified as simple (e.g., fatty acids esterified with alcohols like glycerol (triacylglycerol), or cholesterol esters, vitamin A and D), complex (fatty acids esterified with alcohols plus other groups, e.g., phospholipids or lipids attached to proteins e.g., serum lipoproteins), derived (e.g., fatty acids) or miscellaneous (e.g., carotenoids and vitamins E and K).
- Fatty acids are the densest dietary source of energy, but lipids also have important structural roles in membranes. The processes controlling the synthesis, modification, and degradation of fatty acids contribute to the fatty acid profile of cell membranes and storage lipids in the body.
- Linoleate and α-linolenate are polyunsaturated fatty acids that cannot be synthesised by the body *(de novo)* and are termed "essential" and must be obtained in the diet.
- Dietary lipids (fats) contribute to weight gain and obesity, and share associations with chronic, degenerative diseases like cardiovascular disease (CVD) that influence human morbidity and mortality.
- Dietary lipids (fats) are emulsified, lipolyzed (hydrolyzed), and solubilised in the upper small gut before they are absorbed in the ileum, entering enterocytes with the help of fatty acid-binding proteins.
- Cholesterol and fatty acids are precursors of hormones such as steroids and eicosanoids, respectively, while dietary lipids (fats) carry and facilitate the absorption of fat-soluble vitamins.
- Dietary lipids (fats) and lipids synthesised in the body are rendered soluble for transport in an aqueous medium like blood serum by combining with specialised proteins and phospholipids to make large macromolecular complexes called "lipoproteins" e.g., chylomicrons, very low-density, low-density, and high-density lipoproteins. The concentration of serum lipoproteins are strongly influenced by diet and lifestyle factors. They are also associated with the development and protection against CVD, and used in clinical practice as biomarkers of CVD risk.

9.1 Introduction: the history of lipids in human nutrition

The term "lipid" was introduced by Bloor in 1943, by which time the existence of cholesterol had been known for nearly 200 years, and individual fats for 130 years. Cholesterol was named "cholesterine" (Greek for bile-solid) by Chevreul in 1816, although he did not discover it. The earliest association of cholesterol with cardiovascular atherosclerosis dates back to Vogel's work in 1843. Chevreul isolated a mixture of 16- to 18-carbon saturated fatty acids in 1813 that was called margarine because he believed it to be a single 17-carbon fatty acid, margarate. The mixed triacylglycerol (TAG) of palmitate (16:0) and stearate (18:0) was also called margarine, whereas the triacylglycerol of oleate, stearate, and palmitate became known as oleomargarine. Phospholipids were discovered by Thudicum, who isolated and named sphingosine in 1884, and also lecithin (phosphatidylcholine) and kephalin

Introduction to Human Nutrition, Third Edition. Edited on behalf of The Nutrition Society by Susan A. Lanham-New, Thomas R. Hill, Alison M. Gallagher and Hester H. Vorster.

Companion website: www.wiley.com/go/lanham-new/humannutrition

(phosphatidylethanolamine). The difference in polarity across phospholipids is a key attribute of these molecules, enabling them to associate with aqueous and non-aqueous environments, which was termed "amphipathic" by Hartley in 1936 and renamed "amphiphilic" by Winsor in 1948.

The first understanding of how fat was absorbed emerged in 1879 when Munk studied fat emulsions and showed that lymph contained TAG after a fatty meal, and even after a meal not containing TAG. In 1905, Knoop deduced that fatty acid β-oxidation probably occurred by the stepwise removal of two carbons from the fatty acid. The probable role of two carbon units as building blocks in the synthesis of fatty acids was first recognised by Raper in 1907, and confirmed in the 1940s by Schoenheimer, Rittenberg, Bloch, using tracers such as deuterated water and carbon-13. The late 1940s was a seminal period in our understanding of how fatty acid oxidation occurs. Green and colleagues discovered that ketones were fatty acid oxidation products, and Lehninger demonstrated the role of mitochondria as the cellular site of fatty acid oxidation. Microsomal desaturases were shown to introduce an unsaturated bond into long-chain fatty acids by Bloomfield and Bloch in 1960.

In 1929, Mildred and George Burr discovered that the absence of fat in a diet, otherwise believed to contain all essential nutrients, impaired growth, and caused hair loss and scaling of the skin of rats. This led to the isolation of the two primary "essential" polyunsaturated fatty acids, linoleate (18:2n-6) and α-linolenate (18:3n-3). The prostaglandins are a subclass of eicosanoids that were discovered in the early 1930s by Von Euler, who mistakenly believed that they originated from the prostate gland. The link between the eicosanoids and polyunsaturates, principally arachidonate, was established in the 1960s.

9.2 Terminology of dietary fats

Lipids

Like other organic compounds, all lipids are composed of a carbon skeleton with hydrogen and oxygen substitutions. Nitrogen, sulphur, and phosphorus are also present in some lipids. Water insolubility is a key, but not an absolute characteristic distinguishing most lipids from proteins and carbohydrates. There are some exceptions to this general rule, since short- to medium-chain fatty acids, soaps, and some complex lipids are soluble in water. Hence, solubility in a "lipid solvent" such as ether, chloroform, benzene, or acetone is a common, but circular definition of lipids.

There are four categories of lipids, as classified by Bloor: simple, compound (complex), derived, and miscellaneous (Table 9.1). Simple lipids are esters of fatty acids with various alcohols such as glycerol or cholesterol. They include triacylglycerols (TAG = neutral fats and oils), waxes, cholesteryl esters, and vitamin A and D esters. Compound lipids are esters of fatty acids in combination with both alcohols and other groups. They include phospholipids, glycolipids, cerebrosides, sulfolipids, lipoproteins, and lipopolysaccharides. Derived

Table 9.1 Classification of lipids

Simple lipids (fatty acids esterified with alcohols)	Fats (fatty acids esterified with glycerol)
	Waxes (true waxes, sterol esters, vitamin A and D esters)
Complex lipids (fatty acids esterified with alcohols plus other groups)	Phospholipids (contain phosphoric acid and, usually, a nitrogenous base)
	Glycolipids (lipids containing a carbohydrate and nitrogen but no phosphate and no glycerol)
	Sulfolipids (lipids containing a sulfur group)
	Lipoproteins (lipids attached to plasma or other proteins)
	Lipopolysaccharides (lipids attached to polysaccharides)
Derived lipids (obtained by hydrolysis of simple or complex lipids)	Fatty acids (saturated, monounsaturated, or polyunsaturated)
	Monoacylglycerols and diacylglycerols
	Alcohols (include sterols, steroids, vitamin D, vitamin A)
Miscellaneous lipids	Straight-chain hydrocarbons
	Carotenoids
	Squalene
	Vitamins E and K

lipids are hydrolysis products of simple or compound lipids, including fatty acids, monoacylglycerols and diacylglycerols, straight-chain and ring-containing alcohols, sterols, and steroids. Miscellaneous lipids include some wax lipids, carotenoids, squalene, and vitamins E and K.

Saturated and unsaturated fatty acids

The main components of dietary fat or lipids are fatty acids varying in length from one to more than 30 carbons. They are carboxylic acids with the structure RCOOH, where R is hydrogen in formic acid, CH_3 in acetic acid, or else a chain of one to over 30 CH_2 groups terminated by a CH_3 group. The various names for individual fatty acids (common, official) and their abbreviations are complicated, and the use of one or other form is somewhat arbitrary. The basic rule for the abbreviations is that there are three parts: number of carbons, number of double bonds, and position of the first double bond. Thus, the common dietary saturated fatty acid palmitate is 16:0 because it has 16 carbons and no double bonds. The common dietary polyunsaturated fatty acid linoleate is 18:2n-6 because it has 18 carbons, two double bonds, and the first double bond is at the sixth carbon from the methyl-terminal (n-6). Beyond six carbons in length, most fatty acids have an even number of carbons (Table 9.2). Older fatty acid terminology referring to saturated or unsaturated carbons in lipids that still occasionally appears includes: aliphatic (a saturated carbon), olefinic (an unsaturated carbon), allylic (a saturated carbon adjacent to an unsaturated carbon), and doubly allylic carbon (a saturated carbon situated between two unsaturated carbons).

Lengthening of the chain and the introduction of additional double bonds beyond the first one occur from the carboxyl-terminal. The presence of one or more double bonds in a fatty acid defines it as "unsaturated," compared with a saturated fatty acid which contains no double bonds. A saturated fatty acid generally occupies less space than an equivalent chain length unsaturated fatty acid (Figure 9.1). Double bonds allow for isomerisation or different orientation (*cis* or *trans*) of the adjoining carbons across the double bond (Figure 9.2). In longer chain fatty acids, double bonds can also be at different positions in the molecule. Hence, unsaturation introduces a large amount of structural variety in fatty acids and the resulting lipids. Further details about the features of the different families of fatty acids are given in Sections 9.6 and 9.8.

Short- and medium-chain fatty acids

Short-chain fatty acids (less than eight carbons) are water soluble. Except in milk lipids, they are not commonly esterified into body lipids. Short-chain fatty acids are found primarily in dietary products containing ruminant milk fat. Hence, although they are produced in relatively large quantities from the fermentation of undigested carbohydrate in the colon, as such, they do not

Table 9.2 Nomenclature of common fatty acids

Saturated	Monounsaturated	Polyunsaturated
Formic (1:0)	Lauroleic (12:1n-3)	Linoleic (18:2n-6)
Acetic (2:0)	Myristoleic (14:1n-5)	γ-Linolenic (18:3n-6)
Propionic (3:0)	Palmitoleic (16:1n-7)	Dihomo-γ-linolenic (20:3n-6)
Butyric (4:0)	Oleic (18:1n-9)	Arachidonic (20:4n-6)
Valeric (5:0)	Elaidic (trans-18:1n-9)	Adrenic (22:4n-6)
Caproic (6:0)	Vaccenic (18:1n-7)	n-6 Docosapentaenoic (22:5n1-6)
Caprylic (8:0)	Petroselinic (18:1n-12)	α-Linolenic (18:3n-3)
Capric (10:0)	Gadoleic (20:1n-11)	Stearidonic (18:4n-3)
Lauric (12:0)	Gondoic (20:1n-9)	Eicosapentaenoic (20:5n-3)
Myristic (14:0)	Euricic (22:1n-9)	n-3 Docosapentaenoic (22:5n-3)
Palmitic (16:0)	Nervonic (24:1n-9)	Docosahexaenoic (22:6n-3)
Margeric (17:0)		
Stearic (18:0)		
Arachidic (20:0)		
Behenic (22:0)		
Lignoceric (24:0)		

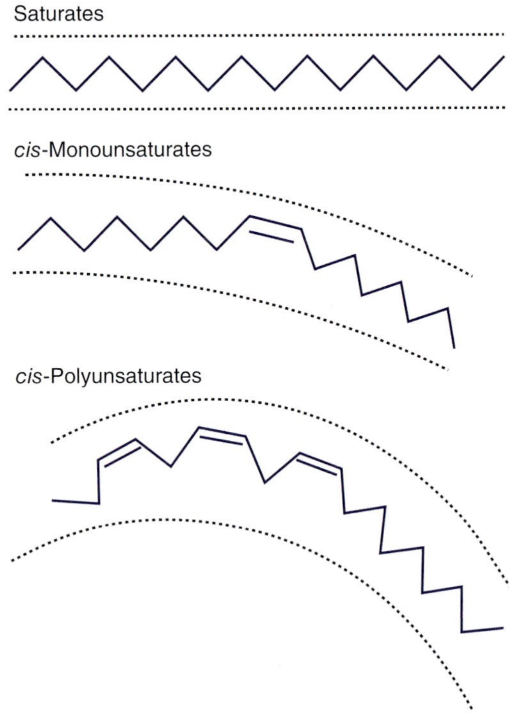

Figure 9.1 Stick models illustrating the basic structural differences between saturated, *cis*-monounsaturated, and *cis*-polyunsaturated fatty acids. As shown in two dimensions, the increasing curvature caused by inserting one or more double bonds increases the area occupied by the fatty acid. The physical area occupied by unsaturated fatty acids is further accentuated in three dimensions because esterified fatty acids rotate around the anchored terminal.

become part of the body lipid pools. Medium-chain fatty acids (8–14 carbons) arise as intermediates in the synthesis of long-chain fatty acids or by the consumption of coconut oil or medium-chain TAG derived from it. Like short-chain fatty acids, medium-chain fatty acids are present in milk, but they are also rarely esterified into body lipids, except when consumed in large amounts in clinical situations requiring alternative energy sources. Medium-chain fatty acids are rare in the diet except for coconut and milk fat.

Long-chain saturated and monounsaturated fatty acids

Long-chain fatty acids (>14 carbons) are the main constituents of dietary fat. The most common saturated fatty acids in the body are palmitate and stearate. They originate from three sources: directly from the diet, by complete synthesis from acetyl-coenzyme A (CoA), or by lengthening (chain elongation) of a pre-existing shorter-chain fatty acid. Hence, dietary or newly synthesised palmitate can be elongated within the body to form stearate and on to arachidate (20:0), behenate (22:0), and lignocerate (24:0). In practice, little stearate present in the human body appears to be derived by chain elongation of pre-existing palmitate. In humans, saturates longer than

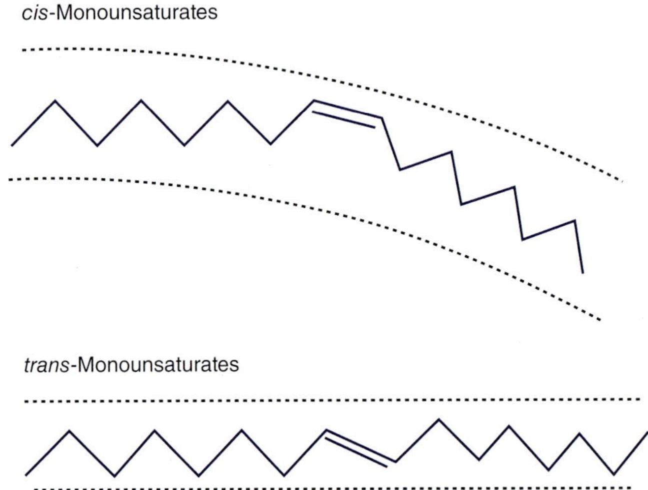

Figure 9.2 Stick models comparing a *cis*- with a *trans*-unsaturated fatty acid. A *cis*-unsaturated double bond creates a U-shaped space and confers curvature to the molecule because, relative to the longitudinal axis of the fatty acid, the two hydrogens at the double bond are on the same side of the molecule. A *trans*-unsaturated double bond does not confer curvature to the molecule because the hydrogens are on opposite sides of the double bond. A *trans*-double bond therefore tends to give the fatty acid physicochemical properties more like that of a saturated fatty acid.

24 carbons do exist, but usually arise only during genetic defects in fatty acid oxidation, as will be discussed later.

Palmitate and stearate are important membrane constituents, being found in most tissue phospholipids at 20–40% of the total fatty acid profile. Brain membranes contain 20- to 24-carbon saturates that, like palmitate and stearate, are synthesised within the brain and have little or no access to the brain from the circulation. The normal membrane content of long-chain saturates can probably be sustained without a dietary source of these fatty acids. In comparison to all other classes of dietary fatty acid, especially monounsaturated or polyunsaturated fatty acids, an excess intake, and possibly synthesis, of some medium and long-chain saturates (with 12-16 carbons) is associated with an increased risk of cardiovascular disease (CVD).

The most common long-chain *cis*-monounsaturated fatty acids in the diet and in the body are oleate (18:1n-9) and palmitoleate (16:1n-7), with the former predominating by far in both the body's storage and membrane lipids. As with stearate, most oleate in the human body appears to be of dietary origin. Hence, although humans have the capacity to desaturate stearate to oleate, dietary oleate is probably the dominant source of oleate in the body. Only plants can further desaturate oleate to linoleate and again to α-linolenate. As with saturates of >18 carbons in length, 20-, 22-, and 24-carbon monounsaturates derived from oleate are present in specialised membranes such as myelin.

Polyunsaturated fatty acids (PUFAs)

Linoleate and α-linolenate are the primary dietary *cis*-polyunsaturated fatty acids in most diets. Neither can be synthesised *de novo* (from acetate) in animals so are "essential" fatty acids. They can be made by chain elongation from the two respective 16-carbon precursors, hexadecadienoate (16:2n-6) and hexadecatrienoate (16:3n-3), which are found in common edible green plants at up to 13% of total fatty acids. Hence, significant consumption of green vegetables will provide 16-carbon polyunsaturates that contribute to the total available linoleate and α-linolenate.

Linoleate is the predominant polyunsaturated fatty acid in the body, commonly accounting for 12–15% of adipose tissue fatty acids. In the body's lean tissues there are at least three polyunsaturates present in amounts >5% of the fatty acid profile (linoleate, arachidonate, docosahexaenoate). In addition, at least two other biologically active polyunsaturates are present in body lipids [dihomo-γ-linolenate (20:3n-6) and eicosapentaenoate (20:5n-3)], although usually in amounts between 1% and 3% of total fatty acids. Marine fish are the richest source of 20- to 22-carbon polyunsaturates. α-Linolenate and its precursor, hexadecatrienoate (16:3n-3), are the only n-3 polyunsaturates in common terrestrial plants.

Hydrogenated and conjugated fatty acid isomers

The introduction of unsaturation with one double bond creates the possibility of both positional and geometric isomers in fatty acids. Among long-chain unsaturated fatty acids, positional isomers exist because the double bond can be introduced into several different locations, i.e., 18:1n-7, 18:1n-9, 18:1n-11, etc. Geometric isomers exist because the two remaining hydrogens at each double bond can be opposite each other (*trans*) or on the same side of the molecule (*cis*; Figure 9.2). Thus, there is *cis*-18:1n-9 (oleate) and *trans*-18:1n-9 (elaidate), and so on for all unsaturated fatty acids, with the combinations mounting exponentially as the number of double bonds increases.

Trans isomers of monounsaturated or polyunsaturated fatty acids occur naturally in ruminants, but can also be produced by partial hydrogenation, a process that was used extensively in the past in the food processing of oils. However, *trans* fatty acids have been shown to raise serum low-density lipoprotein (LDL) cholesterol and lower HDL cholesterol, and have been associated with CVD. For this reason, the industrial partial hydrogenation of oils has been greatly reduced in most countries to reduce the intake of *trans fatty* acids in foods. The number of *trans* isomers increases with the number of double bonds, so there is only one *trans* isomer of oleate, but three *trans* isomers of linoleate and seven of α-linolenate. Virtually all naturally occurring polyunsaturated fatty acids have double bonds that are methylene interrupted, i.e., have a CH_2 group between the two double bonds. However, methylene interruption between double bonds can be lost, again, through food processing, and the bonds moved one carbon closer together, becoming conjugated. Thus, the double bonds in linoleate are at the 9-10 and 11-12 carbons, but in conjugated linoleate, the main conjugated fatty acid, these occur at the 9-10 carbons and the 11-12 carbons. Some degree of further desaturation and chain elongation can occur in conjugated fatty acids, but much less than with methylene-interrupted polyunsaturates.

Fats and oils

Fats are esters of fatty acids with glycerol (Table 9.1). They usually occur as triesters or triacylglycerols (TAGs Figure 9.3), although monoacylglycerols and diacylglycerols occur during fat digestion and are used in food processing. Most common dietary fats contain a mixture of 16- to 18-carbon saturated and unsaturated fatty acids. By convention, fats that are liquid at room temperature are called oils, a feature arising from their lower proportion of saturated (straight-chain) and higher proportion of unsaturated (bent-chain) fatty acids. Unsaturated fatty acids usually have a lower melting point; this facilitates liquefaction of the fats of which they are a component. TAGs of animal origin are commonly fats, whereas those of fish or plant origin are usually oils. Animal fats and fish oils frequently contain cholesterol, whereas plant oils do not contain cholesterol, but usually contain other "phyto" sterols.

TAGs are primarily used as fuels, so dietary fats (mostly TAGs) are commonly associated with energy metabolism rather than with structural lipids found in membranes. However, membrane lipids as well as TAGs are extracted with lipid solvents used to determine the fat content of foods, tissues, or plant material. Hence, because organs such as brain are rich in membrane phospholipids, when the total lipids are extracted to determine the organ's chemical composition, these organs are said to have a certain fat content. On a chemical basis this is true, but this description often misconstrues the nature of the lipid because the brain in particular contains virtually no TAG.

Phospholipids

Phospholipids contain two nonpolar, hydrophobic acyl tail groups and a single functional head group that is polar and hydrophilic. Hence, they are relatively balanced amphiphilic lipids and, in this capacity, are crucial components of biological membranes. The head groups contain phosphorus and amino acids (choline, serine, ethanolamine), sugars (inositol), or an alcohol (glycerol). Phosphatidylcholine (lecithin) is the most abundant phospholipid in animal tissues but phosphatidylglycerols (glycosides) predominate in plant lipids. Phospholipids containing a fatty acid amide are sphingolipids. Various phospholipases can hydrolyze the acyl groups or head group during digestion or metabolism.

One of the outstanding characteristics that make phospholipids suitable as major constituents of biological membranes is their "amphipathicity". In water, they naturally aggregate into spherical or rod-like liposomes or vesicles, with the hydrophilic portion facing outwards and the hydrophobic portion facing inwards (Figure 9.4). Changing the constituent acyl groups from saturated to polyunsaturated changes the fluidity of these aggregates because of the greater amount of space occupied by more unsaturated fatty acids. At interfaces between non-miscible polar and non-polar solvents, phospholipids also form a film or monolayer.

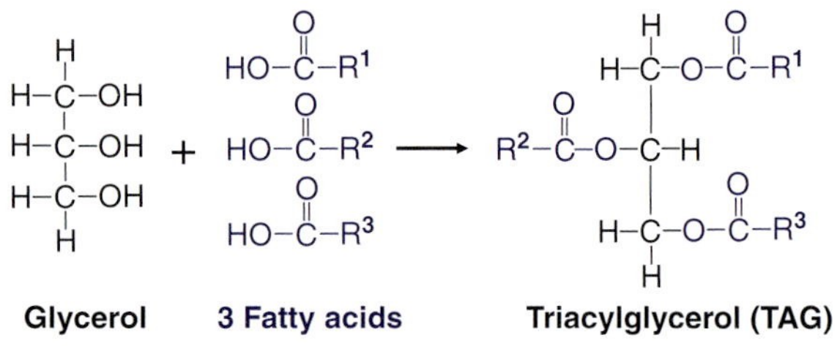

Glycerol + 3 Fatty acids → Triacylglycerol (TAG)

Figure 9.3 General structure of a triaclyglycerol as derived from glycerol and three fatty acids (R′, R″, R‴ = fatty acids).

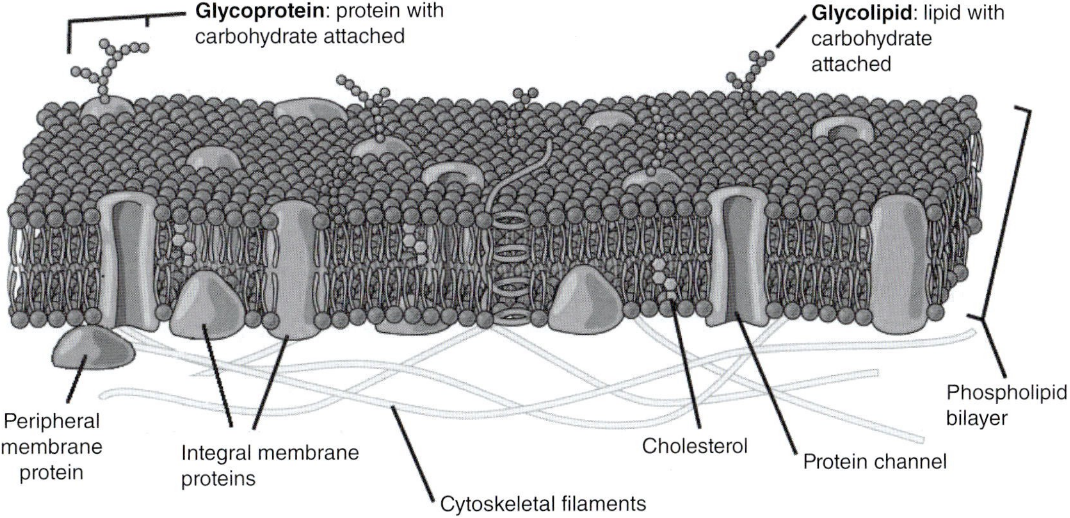

Figure 9.4 Simplified schematic view of a membrane bilayer. The main components are proteins, free cholesterol, phospholipids, and carbohydrates. There are many different proteins with a myriad of shapes, membrane distribution, and functions, of which three are illustrated. Membrane phospholipids principally help to create the bilayer. They have four types of "head groups" (choline, ethanolamine, serine, and inositol) that are located at or near the membrane's two surfaces. The two fatty acids in phospholipids are mixtures of 16- to 22-carbon saturates, monounsaturates, and polyunsaturates in all combinations, with those rich in unsaturated fatty acids occupying more space; hence, their trapezoid shape compared with the narrower, rectangular shape of the more saturated phospholipids. Free cholesterol represents 30–40% of the lipid in most membranes. The many different carbohydrates are on the membrane's surfaces and are bound to lipids and/or proteins in the membrane. Reproduced with thanks to Khan Academy. All Khan Academy content is available for free at www.khanacademy.org.

Sterols

The main sterol of importance in human nutrition is cholesterol. It has multiple roles including being:

- a vital component of biological membranes;
- a precursor to bile salts used in fat digestion;
- a precursor to steroid hormones.

Sterols are secondary alcohols belonging to the polyisoprenoids or terpinoids (terpenes), which have a common precursor, isopentenyl diphosphate. Other members of the terpinoids include squalene, carotenoids, and dolichols. Bacteria appear to be the only life forms not containing cholesterol. Sterols have a common cyclopentano(a)- perhydrophenanthrene skeleton, with different substitutions giving rise to the multiple sterols and steroids.

9.3 Lipids as components of the diet

Dietary sources of lipids are listed in Table 9.3. Cholesterol is found only in animal lipids, while a variety of other phytosterols occur in plants. Soyabeans, leafy plants, and lean animal meat are rich in dietary phospholipids. Animal fat and plant oils from seeds or nuts are rich in TAG.

The leafy and fruit components of plants contain phospholipids and sterols, whereas seeds contain TAG. With rare exceptions such as flaxseed (linseed), edible green leaves are proportionally much richer in α-linolenate than are seeds. Seed oils are usually rich in either linoleate or oleate. Common plant sterols include β-sitosterol, β-sitostanol, and campesterol. Foods enriched with esters of plant sterols are used widely to lower blood cholesterol via the inhibition of cholesterol absorption in the gut.

Phospholipids and cholesterol constitute the majority of lipids in tissues (gut, kidney, brain, skeletal muscle, etc.) of lean, undomesticated animals. By contrast, in domesticated animals, TAGs or non-membrane lipids present in subcutaneous and intramuscular adipose tissue deposits are the dominant form of lipid on a weight basis. This is because domestication usually involves rearing animals with minimal exercise and on higher energy intakes, leading to more subcutaneous and visceral TAG obtained through both fat synthesis and

Table 9.3 Common food sources of lipids

Cholesterol	Eggs, shellfish, organ meats
Phytosterols	Soya products, olive oil
Short-chain fatty acids (1–6 carbons)	Milk fat
Medium-chain fatty acids (8–14 carbons)	Milk fat, coconut fat
Long-chain fatty acids (16–20 carbons)	Saturates: animal fat, shortening, butter, palm oil, peanuts
	Monounsaturates: olive, canola oils
	Linoleate: sunflower, safflower, corn oils, soyabean
	α-Linolenate: flaxseed oil, canola, soyabean oil, walnuts
	γ-Linolenate: evening primrose oil, borage oil, blackcurrant seed oil
	Stearidonate: blackcurrant seed oil
	Arachidonate: lean meat and organ lipids
	Eicosapentaenoate: marine cold-water fish, shellfish, some seaweeds
	Docosahexaenoate: marine cold-water fish, shellfish
	Trans fatty acids: partially hydrogenated fats and oils

deposition of dietary fat. Animal meat lipids are the main dietary source of arachidonate (20:4n-6), although it can also be obtained from tropical marine fish.

Lipoproteins represent the main form of lipid in the blood (see Section 9.5). Like serum lipoproteins, milk lipids also occur as globules consisting of a combination of a mainly TAG core surrounded by a membrane containing proteins, cholesterol, and phospholipids, called the Milk Fat Globule Membrane (MFGM). However, while MFGMs have been ascribed various biological roles associated with health and disease, it is important to appreciate (chiefly to avoid confusion between serum lipoproteins circulating in blood with MFGMs in food!) that serum lipoproteins are entirely distinct from MFGMs in having well defined metabolic origins, structure, composition, physiological roles, and associations with human health and CVD.

Phospholipids and cholesterol constitute the main lipids of undomesticated edible fish, which usually have low amounts of TAG or stored body fat. As in domesticated animals, it is likely that subcutaneous and intramuscular fat deposits of TAG will increase in commercially farmed fish. Cold-water marine fish ("oily" or "pelagic" fish living higher up in the water column, as opposed to "demersal" white fish living nearer the sea bed) are the main dietary source of the long-chain n-3 (omega-3) polyunsaturates eicosapentaenoate (20:5n-3), and docosahexaenoate (22:6n-3), which oily fish accumulate in their flesh by consuming photosynthesising marine algae and phytoplankton. These long-chain n-3 fatty acids are also abundant in certain shell fish, e.g., prawns and shrimp, and in several types of edible seaweed.

9.4 Digestion, absorption, and transport of dietary fat

The average daily intake of fat in a Western diet ranges between 50 and 100 g, and provides between 35% and 40% of total energy. It consists mainly of TAG, which forms the principal component of visible oils and fats, and minor quantities of phospholipids and cholesterol esters (CEs). The physical properties of dietary fat, such as their hardness at room temperature (melting point) and subsequent metabolic properties once in the body, are determined by the number of double bonds in their constituent fatty acids (degree of saturation or unsaturation) and length of the fatty acid carbon chain (see Tables 9.2 and 9.3). As mentioned in Section 9.2, fats that are solid at room temperature tend to consist of long-chain saturated fats (>14 carbons, no double bonds), whereas oils consist of long-chain unsaturated fats with several double bonds. While the terms "lipids" and "fats" are often used synonymously, it's become convention to refer to lipids in foods that we eat as "dietary fats", but as "lipids" once they have been absorbed into the body via the small intestine.

Reception, emulsification, lipolysis, solubilisation, and absorption

The digestion of dietary fat takes place in three phases, known as the gastric, duodenal, and ilial phases. These involve crude emulsification in the stomach, lipolytic breakdown by lipases and solubilisation with bile salts in the duodenum and, finally, absorption into the epithelial cells or enterocytes lining the walls of the small intestine or ileum. Digestion may actually be initiated in the mouth under the influence of a lingual lipase secreted by the palate, although its contribution to lipolysis in adults is questionable and thought to be more important in young suckling infants, in which its release is stimulated by suckling and the presence of milk. It is possible that this lingual lipase is carried into the stomach, where it acts as a human gastric lipase (HGL) that has been shown to degrade up to 10% of ingested fat. Although these early products of fat digestion, fatty acids and monoacylglycerols, represent a relatively minor component of fat digested, their entry into the duodenum is believed to supply a major stimulus for the production of the hormone cholecystokinin (CCK), which inhibits gut motility.

The stomach serves mainly as an organ of mechanical digestion, churning its contents to produce a coarse creamy emulsion known as chyme. The circular pyloric sphincter muscle that separates the stomach from the duodenum regulates the rate of gastric emptying, opening twice a minute to release approximately 3 ml of chyme. Since emulsified fat in chyme is less dense than the aqueous material, the two fractions separate with the fat collecting above the aqueous layer. As a result, the entry of emulsified fat into the duodenum is delayed, allowing sufficient time for the minor breakdown products to act on CCK.

The duodenal phase involves the breakdown of the emulsified fat by a process known as lipolysis and the solubilisation of the products of lipolysis. The entry of chyme containing minor lipolytic products into the duodenum stimulates the:

- release of CCK, which inhibits gut motility;
- secretion of bile acids from the gall bladder; and
- release of pancreatic juice containing a battery of lipases.

Lipolysis is an enzyme-catalyzed hydrolysis that releases fatty acids from lipids (TAGs, phospholipids, and CEs). It involves the hydrolytic cleavage of bonds between a fatty acid and the glycerol backbone of TAGs and phospholipids, and cholesterol in CEs, and occurs not only in the digestive tract but also in circulating and intracellular lipids (Figure 9.5). The lipolysis of emulsified dietary fat entering the duodenum is catalysed by a battery of pancreatic enzymes including a pancreatic lipase that acts chiefly on TAG and phospholipase A_2 and a cholesterol ester hydrolase acting on phospholipids and CEs. The hydrolysis of TAG by pancreatic lipase occurs in a sequential fashion with the initial removal of a fatty acid from position 1 and then position 3 from the glycerol backbone, generating a 2,3-diacylglycerol, followed by a 2-monoacylglycerol (2-MAG).

Solubilisation of emulsified fat

With the notable exceptions mentioned previously (Section 9.2), fats are insoluble in water and must be rendered soluble before they can be absorbed in the gut and transported within cells and in the circulation. In each of these situations, this is achieved by the hydrophobic fat or lipid associating with molecules that are capable of interfacing with both hydrophobic and hydrophilic environments. Molecules with these characteristics are called amphipathic molecules, examples of which are phospholipids, bile salts, and specialised proteins known as apoproteins (Figure 9.6). In the small intestine emulsified fats are solubilised by associating with bile salts produced in the liver and stored and released from the gallbladder, and phospholipids to form complex aggregates known as mixed micelles. Lipids within cells and the circulation are solubilised by combining with specific proteins known as fatty acid-binding proteins (FABPs) and apolipoproteins (ApoA, B, C, E), respectively. Further details of the structure and function of these specialised proteins are given in Section 9.5.

The action of pancreatic lipase on TAG yields free fatty acids and 2-MAG. Fatty acids of short- and medium-chain length (≤14 carbons) tend to be absorbed directly into the portal circulation with free glycerol and transported bound to albumin to the liver, where they are rapidly oxidised. This catabolic pathway provides the principle for the use of medium chain triacylglycerols (MCTs) in parenteral feeds, and less well established claims of MCTs helping to promote weight loss. In contrast, long-chain fatty acids (LCFAs;

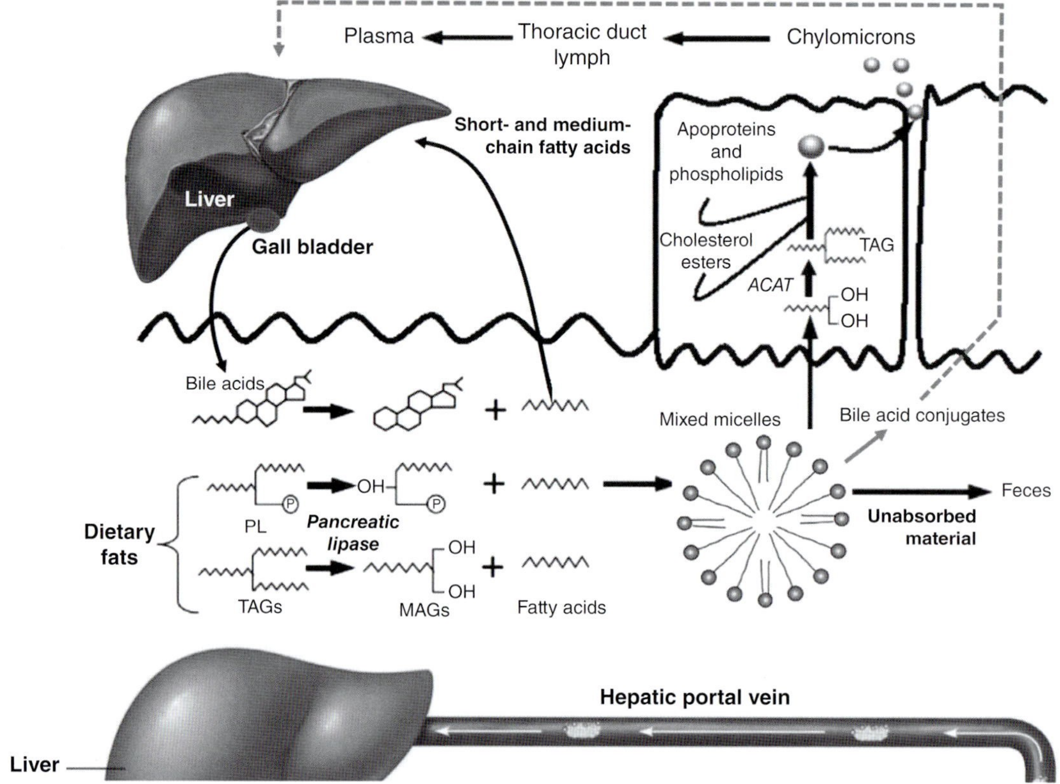

Figure 9.5 Reception, emulsification, lipolysis, solubilization, and absorption of fats. ACAT, acyl-CoA-cholesterol acyltransferase; MAG, monoacylglycerol; TAG, triacylglycerol; PL phospholipid; P, phosphate.

>14 carbons) tend to associate with bile salts in bile juice from the gallbladder, and are absorbed into the enterocyte for further processing and packaging into transport lipoproteins. However, the subdivision of the fates of fatty acids on the basis of their carbon chain length is by no means absolute, since fatty acids with 12 (lauric) and 14 (myristic) carbons are also absorbed and transported in serum lipoproteins.

The primary bile salts, cholic and chenodeoxycholic acids, are produced from cholesterol in the liver under the action of the rate-limiting enzyme 7-α-hydroxylase. These bile salts act as effective detergents, solubilising dietary fat through the formation of mixed micelles. These are spherical associations of amphipathic molecules (with hydrophobic and hydrophilic regions) with a hydrophilic surface of bile salts and phospholipids that encapsulates a hydrophobic core of more insoluble LCFAs and 2-MAG (see Figure 9.6). The core of micelles also contain some lipid-soluble vitamins including tocopherols and carotenoids. The formation of mixed micelles increases the solubility of fat by 100- to 1000-fold, and creates an acidic microenvironment for the lipid core which facilitates the dissociation of LCFAs and 2-MAG from the micelle and diffusion into the enterocyte.

Absorption of solubilised fat

The ilial or absorptive phase of fat digestion involves the transit of dietary fats from mixed micelles into the enterocyte. Although originally believed to be a purely passive process, dependent on factors such as the rate of gastric emptying, extent of mixing, and gut motility, the translocation of LCFAs and 2-MAG from the micelle into the enterocyte is now known to be assisted by the presence of FABPs within the cell membrane and the cell. FABPs maintain a diffusion gradient down which LCFAs and MAGs can flow into the cell, have numerous roles within cells and specificity for different types

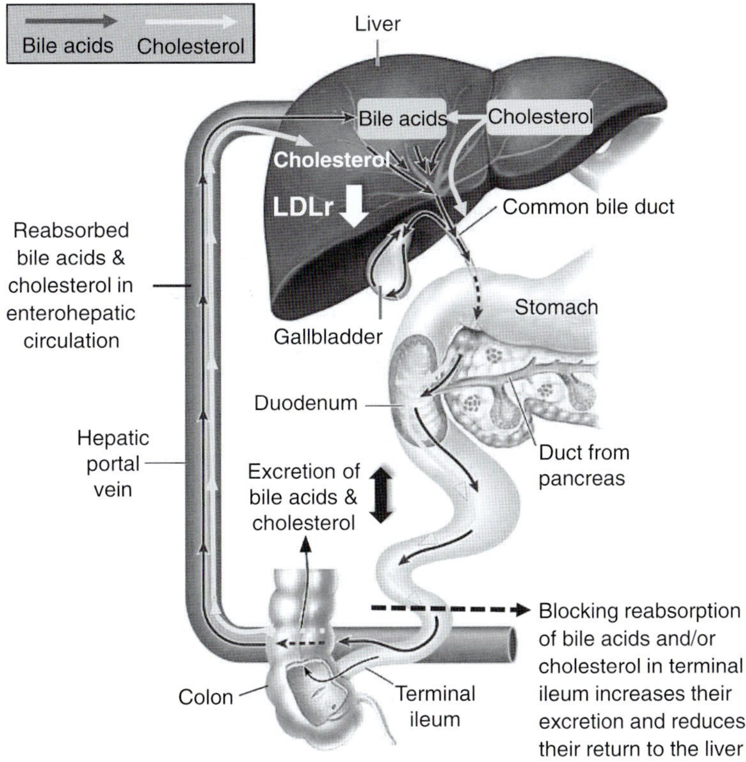

Figure 9.6 Entero-hepatic circulation of bile acids and cholesterol (dietary & biliary). After being secreted by the liver and participating in fat digestion and absorption, the majority (95%) of bile acids are reabsorbed by active transport in the terminal ileum. Between 35–57% of cholesterol in the intestine, mainly from bile (approximately 800–1200mg/day) and the diet (approximately 300–500mg/day), is reabsorbed, mostly in the upper small intestine. This enterohepatic circulation of bile acids and cholesterol effectively repletes the pool of free cholesterol in the liver, reducing the requirement for LDL receptors (LDLr). Blocking the reabsorption of bile acids and/or cholesterol produces the opposite effect by increasing their excretion, which lowers free cholesterol in the liver and stimulates the expression of LDLr.

of LCFAs. Thus, the absorption of LCFAs and 2-MAG derived from dietary TAGs occurs by facilitated diffusion via FABP, which increases membrane permeation and promotes cellular uptake of LCFAs and MAGs. An additional factor that drives the diffusion gradient is the rapid re-esterification of LCFAs into 2-MAG and 2-MAG into TAGs within the enterocyte, by the enzyme acyl-CoA-cholesterol acyltransferase (ACAT). The absorption of dietary TAGs in the small intestine is extremely efficient, with up to 90% being absorbed. Dietary cholesterol also associates within mixed micelles and is absorbed in a similar manner by specific sterol-carrying proteins resident in the enterocyte membrane. Thus, cholesterol is also absorbed by a protein-facilitated mechanism, but in contrast to dietary TAGs, only about 40% of dietary cholesterol is absorbed directly.

Enterohepatic circulation

The absorption of fat in the small intestine is dependent on the availability of bile acids from biliary secretions, which also contain free cholesterol. Dietary and biliary cholesterol, and bile acids are salvaged by an energy-dependent process in the terminal ileum. This active process of resorption via the enterohepatic circulation is tightly controlled by a feedback mechanism that is sensitive to hepatic levels of free cholesterol.

The resorption of cholesterol and bile acids increases their return to the liver, raises intra-hepatocellular cholesterol which suppresses

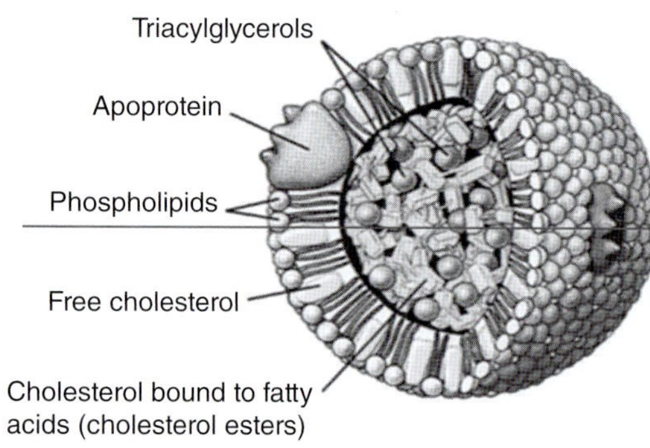

Figure 9.7 General lipoprotein structure. Source: Griffin, 2013.

LDL-receptor production and activity and in the case of bile acids, also suppresses the activity of 7-α-hydroxylase, a rate-limiting enzyme for the production of bile acids. Interruption of this enterohepatic circulation, by substances in the lumen of the gut that are capable of either competing for uptake of cholesterol into mixed micelles (e.g., plant sterols and stanols) or bind bile acids (e.g., dietary soluble fibres such as β-glucan), prevent the resorption of cholesterol and bile acid. This restricts the supply of cholesterol returning to the liver and accelerates the production of bile acids, depleting the liver of cholesterol (Figure 9.7). To replenish this loss, liver cells respond by increasing the LDL-receptor mediated uptake of cholesterol from circulating lipoproteins in the blood, chiefly LDL, resulting in decreased serum cholesterol. For further details of the control mechanism (see Section 9.5).

Re-esterification of triacylglycerols in the enterocyte

Once LCFAs have entered the cell they are activated by acyl-CoA and are re-esterified with glycerol back into TAG and phospholipids by two distinct biochemical pathways, the 2-MAG and glycerol-3-phosphate (G-3-P) pathways. The difference between these two pathways lies in:

- their substrates of activation;
- the former using 2-MAG and the latter α-glycero-3-phosphate;
- their location within different cellular organelles: the 2-MAGs reside in the smooth endoplasmic reticulum and the G-3-P in the rough endoplasmic reticulum; and
- the periods during which they are most active.

The 2-MAG pathway is of greater quantitative importance in the enterocyte of the intestine, and thus predominates in the postprandial period, whereas the G-3-P pathway is more active in the post-absorptive phase in tissues such as liver, muscle, and adipose tissue. Following the absorption of a fatty meal and uptake of 2-MAG into the enterocyte, up to 90% of these molecules are rapidly acylated back to 1, 2-dia-cylglycerol and finally into TAGs by the sequential actions of three enzymes: CoA ligase, mono-glycerol acyltransferase, and diacylglycerol acyltransferase. In a similar fashion, lysophosphatidylcholine, produced by the action of pancreatic phospholipase "A" on dietary phospholipids, is absorbed by the enterocyte and re-esterified back to phosphatidylcholine in the enterocyte by direct acetylation. The bulk of free cholesterol absorbed from the intestinal lumen is also re-esterified in the enterocyte by the enzyme ACAT.

Lipoprotein assembly and secretion

Serum lipoproteins are a family of spherical, macromolecular complexes of lipid and protein (Figure 9.7), the principal function of which is to transport endogenous lipids (synthesised in the liver) and exogenous lipids (synthesised in the gut from dietary fats) from these sites of production and absorption to peripheral sites of utilisation (e.g., oxidation in muscle, incorporation in membranes, or as precursors of biologically active metabolites) and storage (e.g., adipose tissue) (Figure 9.8). In the small intestine, the newly re-esterified TAGs and CEs associate with specific amphipathic proteins and phospholipids in the enterocyte to form the largest and most TAG-rich lipoproteins, known as chylomicrons. The enterocyte is capable of synthesising at least three different apoproteins (apo): apoA-I, apoAIVs and apo B (B-48). The last apoprotein is a smaller isoform (48%) of its larger arbitrarily named relative apoB-100, which is synthesised in the liver. While both apoproteins are products of the same gene, in the enterocyte the mRNA undergoes post-transcriptional editing to produce a truncated polypeptide. ApoB-48 is produced in the rough endoplasmic reticulum and transferred to the smooth endoplasmic reticulum, where it combines with a lipid droplet, or nascent chylomicron, and then migrates to the Golgi apparatus. Here, the apoproteins (A-I, A-IV, and B-48) are glycosylated before the chylomicrons eventually leave the enterocyte by exocytosis through the basement membrane, across the intracellular space between the enterocyte and the lacteal, and are finally discharged into the lymphatic vessels.

Postprandial lipemia

The turbid, milky appearance of serum after the ingestion of dietary fat, marks the arrival of fat (TAG) into the blood in the form of TAG-rich chylomicrons from the intestine. The turbidity of serum arises from the chylomicrons, which are of a sufficient particle size to physically scatter light. The size and composition of the chylomicrons produced after a fatty meal are determined by the fat content of the meal. Hence, the nature of fatty acids in chylomicron TAG reflects the nature of fatty acid in the meal. Each chylomicron particle carries a single molecule of apoB-48 which, unlike its other smaller counterparts A-I and A-IV, remains with the chylomicron throughout its life in the circulation. There is little evidence to suggest that the production of apoB-48, and thus the number of particles, increases in response to an increased flux of dietary fat. Instead, the enterocyte incorporates more TAG into each chylomicron and expands the size of each chylomicron to facilitate the transport of larger amounts of absorbed dietary fat. There is evidence to suggest that chylomicrons containing lipids enriched with polyunsaturated fatty acids (PUFAs) are larger than chylomicrons enriched with saturated fat, since the former occupy more space when packaged into a lipoprotein. This has implications for the subsequent metabolism and fate of these lipoproteins in the circulation, since TAGs associated with larger chylomicrons are known to be hydrolysed more rapidly. ApoB-48 may be produced continuously throughout the post-absorptive phase, as evidenced by the enterocyte-forming pools of apoB-48 in readiness for the sudden reception of dietary fat and production of chylomicrons.

The onset, duration, and magnitude of postprandial lipemia can be monitored in the laboratory after a standard fat-containing meal by making serial measurements of serum TAG or more specifically TAG associated with TAG-rich lipoproteins over a postprandial period of up to eight or nine hours (remnants of chylomicrons can be detected 12 hours after a meal). Alternatively, the levels of apoB-48 or retinyl esters in serum act as useful markers or tracer molecules for following the metabolism of chylomicrons in the postprandial period. In normal subjects postprandial lipemia peaks between three and four hours and subsides to baseline concentration after five to six hours. In some cases, postprandial TAG (mainly in chylomicrons) can appear in the blood within 30 min and peak as early as one hour after the ingestion of fat. So rapid is this rise in TAG that it is believed to represent preformed lipid in the enterocyte from the previous meal that is being shunted into the circulation by the incoming fat load. Note that, in addition to the time taken to emulsify, hydrolyse, and absorb dietary fat, re-esterification of TAG in the enterocyte and lipoprotein assembly alone takes about 15 min, although shunting means that the first TAG can appear well within 30 min, with the first peak after one hour. This shunting phenomenon is particularly noticeable during the day and gives rise to two or even more TAG peaks, whereas postprandial peaks after an overnight fast are usually monophasic.

While chylomicrons clearly contribute significantly to the extent and time course of postprandial lipemia, they are not the only TAG-rich lipoproteins in the postprandial phase. The TAGs in circulating chylomicrons are hydrolysed by a rate-limiting lipase known as lipoprotein lipase (LPL). LPL is tethered to the endothelial lining of blood vessels in peripheral tissues, most notably muscle and adipose tissue, by proteoglycan fibers, and as such is known as an endothelial lipase. Several molecules of LPL can interact and hydrolyse the TAG from a single chylomicron particle to generate a chylomicron remnant, which is removed by specific cell membrane receptors in the liver. The situation is complicated by the fact that TAG-rich lipoproteins from the liver, known as very low-density lipoprotein (VLDL), also contribute to this postprandial lipemia to variable extents in health and disease states. These VLDLs, containing

Table 9.4 Plasma lipoproteins: classes, composition, and distribution

	Chylomicrons	VLDL	LDL	HDL
Mass (10^6 Da)	0.4–3.0	10–100	2–3.5	0.2–0.3
Density (g/ml)	>0.95	<1.006	1.02–1.063	1.063–1.210
Particle diameter (nm)	>90	30–90	22–28	5–12
Apoproteins	B-48, A-I, C-I, C-II, C-III, E	B-100, E	B-100	A-I, A-II
Lipids % mass (molecules/particle)				
Cholesterol	8 (60 000)	22 (10 000)	48 (2000)	20 (100)
Triacylglycerols	83 (500 000)	50 (24 000)	10 (300)	8 (20)
Ratio of particles				
Postabsorptive	1	40	1000	10 000
Postprandial	1	25	250	250 000

VLDL, very low-density lipoprotein; LDL, low-density lipoprotein; HDL, high-density lipoprotein.

endogenously produced TAG, are similar in lipid composition to chylomicrons, but considerably smaller (Table 9.4). Chylomicrons carry up to 80% of measurable plasma TAG during the postprandial period, but VLDL particles can carry up to 80% of the measurable protein (mainly as apo-B), and significantly outnumber chylomicrons at all times. VLDL-TAG are also metabolised by LPL, which creates competition for the clearance of endogenously and dietary derived TAG carried by VLDLs and chylomicrons respectively, by what is known as the "Common saturable pathway".

Postprandial lipemia: relevance to atherosclerosis

In 1979, Donald Zilversmit, an American lipid biochemist, stated that "*Atherosclerosis was a postprandial phenomenon*". This idea was based on the finding that patients either with or at high risk of developing coronary heart disease (CHD) showed an impaired capacity to remove TAG-rich lipoproteins from the circulation after a meal, resulting in enhanced postprandial lipemia, which also became known as the TAG intolerance hypothesis. At about the same time, evidence emerged that TAG-rich lipoproteins, and especially the partially hydrolysed remnants of chylomicrons, were directly atherogenic, meaning that they can damage the endothelial lining of arteries and promote the deposition of cholesterol in coronary arteries. For this reason, there is considerable research interest in the role of excess postprandial lipemia as both a causal factor and therapeutic target for CHD. This interest includes the mechanisms that underlie the production and removal of TAG-rich lipoproteins, not only in the intestine but also in the liver, since the production and removal of VLDL can clearly influence postprandial events. The quality and, to a lesser extent, quantity of dietary fat are extremely important as determinants of the duration and magnitude of postprandial lipemia, and have a major role to play in preventing cardio-metabolic disease.

9.5 Circulating lipids: lipoprotein structures and metabolism

Circulating blood lipids are insoluble in water and must be solubilised for transportation in the extracellular fluid by combining with bipolar molecules with charged and uncharged regions (apoproteins and phospholipids). This makes them perfect for enveloping insoluble lipids, chiefly TAG and CE, in macromolecular lipid-protein complexes called serum lipoproteins. It is worth remembering that, in the absence of lipoproteins, TAG would exist in aqueous blood as immiscible oil droplets, while free fatty acids liberated from TAG and phospholipids in the absence of the blood protein albumin would act as detergents and dissolve cell membranes.

Lipoprotein structure: a "shopping bag and groceries"

The general structure of a lipoprotein consists of a central core of hydrophobic, neutral lipid (TAG and CE) surrounded by a hydrophilic coat of phospholipids, free cholesterol, and apoproteins. A useful analogy for this arrangement of molecules is that of a "shopping bag and groceries," with the lipid core representing the groceries and the outer coat the fabric of the bag. The apoproteins weave in and out of the lipid core and outer surface layer and form the thread of the fabric which holds the bag together (see Figure 9.7). This arrangement of molecules renders the hydrophobic lipids soluble for the purpose of transport in blood. In addition to conferring structural integrity on the lipoprotein particle, apoproteins have a vital role in regulating the metabolism of lipoproteins by acting as ligands for cell membrane receptors and cofactors for key enzymes.

Serum lipoproteins can be subdivided into distinct classes on the basis of their physical properties and/or composition, both of which reflect the physiological role in the transport of lipids from sites of synthesis (endogenous lipids) and absorption (exogenous lipids, absorbed in the gut) to sites of storage (adipose tissue) and utilisation (skeletal muscle) (Figure 9.8). Serum lipoproteins were traditionally classified according to their hydrated density, a property which is determined by the ratio of lipid to protein in the lipoprotein particle. Since lipids tend to occupy a greater molecular volume than proteins, they are lighter and less dense. Thus, particles with high lipid content are larger and less dense (carry more lipid groceries) than lipoproteins enriched with protein. This property relates directly to the transport function and metabolic interrelationships between lipoprotein classes in blood. It can also be used to separate lipoproteins of different densities, because lipoproteins of different density have different flotation characteristics in the ultracentrifuge (note that plasma lipoproteins will float when subjected to centrifugal force, whereas pure proteins sink). Other classification schemes for plasma lipoproteins have exploited differences in their net electrical charge (electrophoretic mobility), particle size (exclusion chromatography, gradient gel electrophoresis), and immunological characteristics conferred upon the lipoprotein by the types of apoproteins in each lipoprotein subclass (see Table 9.4). Some of these techniques permit the further resolution of VLDL, low-density lipoproteins (LDLs), and high-density lipoproteins (HDLs) into discrete subclasses, the distribution of which relates to cardiovascular risk and is determined by genetic, and diet and lifestyle factors.

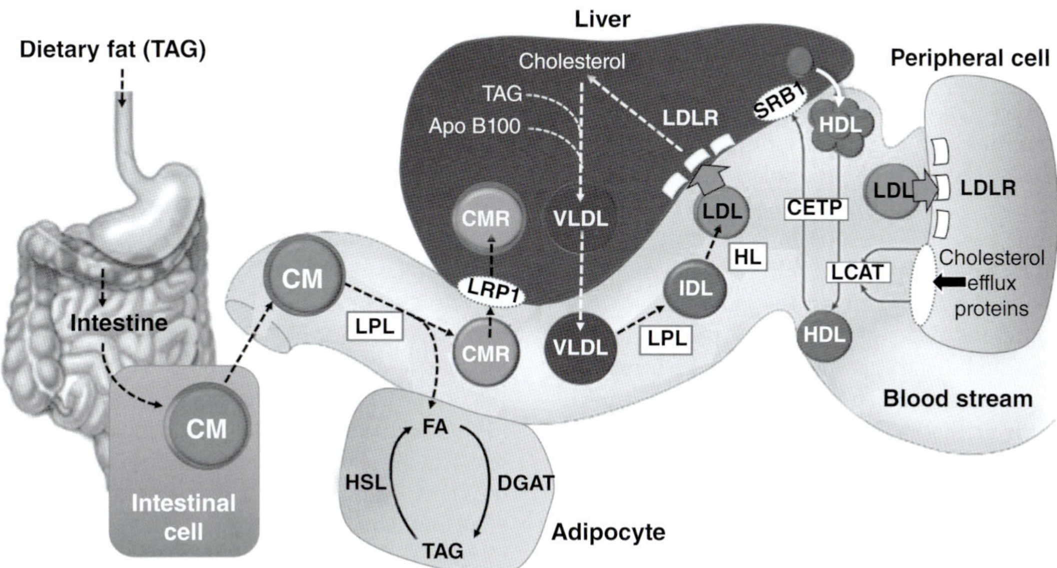

Figure 9.8 Lipoprotein exogenous and endogenous pathways. CM chylomicron; CMR chylomicron remnant, FA fatty acid; IDL, intermediate-density lipoprotein; LDL, low-density lipoprotein; TAG, triacylycerol; VLDL, very low-density lipoprotein, HDL, high-density lipoprotein, LPL, lipoprotein lipase.

Lipoprotein transport pathways

Lipoprotein transport can be described in terms of the production, transport, and removal of cholesterol or TAG from the circulation. In reality, these two processes are inseparable because both TAG and cholesterol are transported together in lipoproteins. Lipoproteins are in a constant state of flux, with lipids and apoproteins constantly shuttling between different lipoproteins that interrelate through integrated metabolic pathways. A useful analogy here is to think of serum lipoproteins as railway carriages, transporting passengers that represent lipids and apoproteins within a complex rail network. The trains and passengers are in a constant state of change within and between stations. Lipoprotein metabolism is controlled by the activity of functional proteins (enzymes, cell surface receptors, receptor ligands in lipoproteins) that determine the rate at which lipoproteins enter and leave the system, and by the physicochemical properties of the lipoprotein themselves. These functional proteins can be viewed as the rate-limiting determinants of a train journey, which control the timetable and type of passengers.

All lipoproteins, with the notable exception of HDL, begin life as TAG-rich particles. The principal transport function of these lipoproteins in the first instance is to deliver fatty acids liberated from the TAG to tissues. The enterocytes in the gut are the producers of lipoproteins called chylomicrons (transport exogenous, dietary TAG), whereas the liver is the central terminus for the production of VLDL and removal of their cholesterol-rich end-product, LDL. VLDLs, although smaller than chylomicrons, resemble the latter in many ways and are often referred to as the liver's chylomicrons. While the rate at which the gut produces chylomicrons depends largely on the amount of absorbed dietary fat, the rate of VLDL production is determined by the supply of fatty acids in the liver that can be re-esterified back to TAG for incorporation into VLDL. These fatty acids are derived chiefly from the systemic circulation in the form of non-esterified fatty acids (NEFAs), and to a lesser extent from the uptake of circulating lipoprotein remnants. It is noteworthy that, although the liver has the capacity to synthesise fatty acids, the amount synthesised by *de novo* lipogenesis is relatively small in humans on a mixed Western diet. However, the contribution of fatty acids from this source may increase in conditions associated with an overproduction of VLDLs, and has been shown to occur on low-fat, high-carbohydrate diets, and in metabolic disease.

Metabolic determinants of lipoprotein metabolism

The metabolism of serum lipoproteins and fate of their transport lipids is controlled by:

- the physical and chemical characteristics of the lipoprotein, such as its size and lipid and apoprotein content;
- the activity of the endothelial LPL and hepatic lipase (HL), so called because they are attached to the surface of endothelial cells lining blood vessels in peripheral tissues, such as adipose tissue and skeletal muscle, and the liver, respectively;
- lipid transfer proteins; cholesteryl ester and phospholipid transfer proteins, (CETP and PLTP, respectively);
- apoproteins that act as activators of enzymes and ligands for specific lipoprotein receptors on the surfaces of cells (apoB-100 and apoE as ligands for the LDLs and remnant receptors in the liver, respectively);
- the activity of specific lipoprotein receptors on cell surfaces.

Lipoprotein transport pathways have been previously described in terms of the forward and reverse transport of cholesterol. Forward transport encompasses the transport of exogenous (dietary) and endogenous (liver) TAG, in chylomicrons and VLDL, respectively, the arrival of cholesterol in the blood from either the gut or the liver and its carriage back to the liver for processing (Figure 9.8). Note, the liver has the unique capacity to secrete cholesterol either as free cholesterol or as bile acids. Conversely, reverse transport describes the "HDL pathway" and the process of cholesterol efflux out of peripheral tissues back to the liver for ultimate excretion in the form of free cholesterol or bile acids via the gut. This "forward" and "reverse" directionality can be misleading, since each pathway directs cholesterol back to the liver. Both the exogenous and endogenous pathways share a common saturable lipolytic pathway that consists of a delipidation cascade in which the TAG-rich lipoproteins (chylomicrons and VLDLs), after receiving apo-C (C-II) from HDL, an essential cofactor for the activation of LPL, are progressively depleted of their TAG in a stepwise fashion by LPL to become cholesterol-rich remnants that are removed by specific, high affinity, cell-surface receptors, found chiefly in the liver. Several molecules of LPL can bind to a single chylomicron or VLDL particle, although LPL shows greater affinity for chylomicrons in preference to VLDL. This situation leads to competition between these TAG-rich lipoproteins for LPL, and provides a mechanism to explain how VLDL can influence the clearance of TAG in the postprandial period.

The hydrolysis of TAG in chylomicrons, generates chylomicron remnants which, during passage through the liver, bind to specific receptors on the surface of hepatocytes that recognise apoE, an apoprotein that is also acquired at an early stage from HDL. The activity of remnant receptors is maintained at a very high level and is not down-regulated through a feedback mechanism (see LDL receptor pathway below). This is fortunate, since lipoprotein remnants can deposit their cholesterol in artery walls, thus promoting coronary atherosclerosis. The secretion of VLDL from the liver is again followed by the sequential lipolysis of TAG by LPL and generation of VLDL remnants or, in this case, the further lipolysis of these remnants into LDL. The remnants and LDLs bind to another receptor in the liver that recognises both apoE exclusively in VLDL remnants and apoB-100 in LDLs, namely the LDL receptor. Approximately 60% of LDL is removed by LDL receptors. The remainder is internalised into cells via scavenger receptors. This latter route has been associated with the development of atherosclerotic disease.

Whether a VLDL particle is removed as a remnant or transcends to LDL largely depends on its pedigree, i.e., its size and lipid composition. Experiments with radioactively labelled VLDL have shown that larger, TAG-rich VLDL particles are less likely to be converted into LDL and are removed as partially delipidated VLDL remnants, whereas smaller VLDLs are precursors of LDL.

The low-density lipoprotein (LDL) receptor pathway

The incontrovertible link between raised serum LDL cholesterol and CHD is directly responsible for the rapid growth, and quantum leaps, in our understanding of cholesterol homeostasis in relation to diet and disease, the most prolific of which was the discovery of the LDL receptor pathway, which won Joseph Goldstein and Michael Brown the Nobel Prize for Medicine or Physiology in 1985. All cells, most notably those in the liver, have a highly developed and sensitive mechanism for regulating intracellular and intravascular levels of cholesterol. The liver synthesises approximately 500 mg of cholesterol a day and while this could be provided by the import of cholesterol from the blood in the form of LDL, in the complete absence of LDL, the cells could theoretically manufacture sufficient cholesterol to meet their metabolic needs. However, cells import cholesterol as LDL in preference to synthesising it for themselves, as the former process requires less energy. Cells acquire cholesterol from the blood by the uptake and degradation of LDL particles. As the requirement for free cholesterol increases within the cell, it increases its production and thus activity of LDL receptors, so that more LDL is extracted from the blood, lowering blood cholesterol. Conversely, if the cell becomes overloaded with cholesterol, it senses that it requires less cholesterol and produces fewer LDL receptors, causing blood cholesterol to increase. Since the production of LDL receptors is regulated by the intracellular level of free cholesterol, anything that increases free cholesterol within the cell will inadvertently lower blood LDL cholesterol. Intracellular free cholesterol represses the activity of a sterol regulatory element binding protein (SREBP), a positive nuclear transcription factor that promotes the transcription of the LDL receptor gene when free cholesterol levels fall (see figure 9.18 for further explanation). Homeostatic interplay between these processes and the enterohepatic circulation of bile acids and cholesterol, maintains a reciprocal relationship between cholesterol biosynthesis and absorption, so the more cholesterol that is synthesised the less will be absorbed in the gut and vice versa. Unfortunately, these processes are not always in complete harmony which upsets cholesterol homeostasis.

The metabolic effects increased of intracellular free cholesterol are:

- it decreases the production of LDL receptors via SREBP;
- it inhibits the synthesis of cholesterol by the enzyme 3-hydroxy-3-methylglutaryl (HMG)-CoA reductase;
- it increases the re-esterification of cholesterol for storage as cholesterol esters.

Goldstein and Brown were aided in their discovery of the LDL receptor by studying a condition known as familial hypercholesterolemia, a genetic abnormality in the LDL receptor gene that produces defects in the LDL receptor pathway and extreme elevation of serum LDL cholesterol (15-20 mmol/l) and premature CVD in early life. Their findings also helped to promote studies on the influence of dietary fats on the activity of the LDL receptor pathway, which led to a credible explanation for the differential effects of dietary fatty acids on serum LDL-cholesterol (see page 210).

Reverse cholesterol transport (high-density lipoprotein pathway)

The removal of cholesterol from tissues back to the liver via HDL represents the only route for the elimination of cholesterol from the body. This physiological role of HDL explains, in part, the cardio-protective effects of these lipoproteins, as indicated by a strong inverse relationship between serum HDL cholesterol and CHD risk in prospective cohort studies. The activity of the HDL pathway is influenced by genetic and environmental factors that can interact to either increase or reduce the efficiency of cholesterol removal. This, in turn, may be reflected in changes in the concentration of serum HDL and their functional properties.

HDL is synthesised in the liver and gut, and transformed from nascent particles into mature spherical HDL particles in serum through the acquisition of cholesterol and apoproteins from two principal sources:

i surface material released from TAG-rich lipoproteins during lipolysis and
ii peripheral tissues. The particles, which are responsible for removing cholesterol from cells, are very small pre-HDLs and are disk-shaped particles composed of phospholipid and apoA-I (ApoA-I is capable of this function on its own). The molecular mechanism for the efflux of free cholesterol from tissue sites, including deposits of cholesterol in the walls of arteries, is understood in detail that lies beyond the scope of this chapter. Efflux is facilitated by the formation of a free cholesterol gradient from the cell across the cell membrane to pre-HDLs. The gradient is generated by the re-esterification of free cholesterol by the enzyme lecithin–cholesterol acyltransferase (LCAT) and via the migration of these newly formed cholesterol esters into the hydrophobic core of what becomes mature, spherical HDL. The newly acquired cholesterol is transported back to the liver, either directly by HDL docking with scavenger receptors on hepatocytes or indirectly by transfer of its cholesterol to apo B-containing lipoproteins VLDL and LDL via the action of cholesteryl ester transfer protein (CETP). The microcirculation of the liver contains a close relative of LPL (hepatic lipase (HL)), which acts on smaller lipoproteins, and especially the surface phospholipids of HDL, where it effectively punches a hole in the surface layer of phospholipids to facilitate access to the lipid core and delivery of CE to the hepatocyte (Figure 9.9).

Inter-relationships among serum TAG and low- and high-density lipoproteins

Lipids and apoproteins are constantly moving between lipoprotein particles. This movement is not totally random but influenced by the relative lipid composition of the lipoproteins and by specific lipid transfer proteins (LTPs) that act as lipid shuttles. In a normal, healthy individual, TAG-rich lipoproteins transfer TAG to LDL and HDL in equimolar exchange for CE. This is mediated through an LTP called CETP. In this way, CEs are transferred from HDL to VLDL for passage back to the liver. Conversely, when the concentration of serum TAG and thus TAG-rich lipoproteins is increased, for example by either the overproduction of TAG in the liver or the impaired removal of TAG by LPL, the result is a net transfer of TAG into LDL and HDL. As LDL

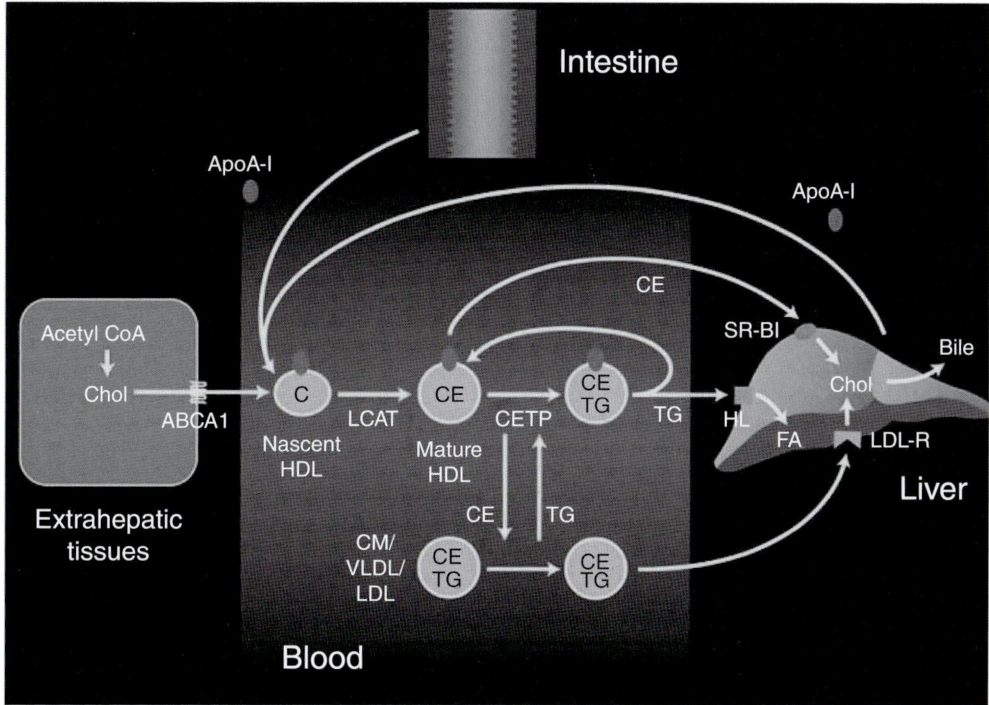

Figure 9.9 Reverse cholesterol transport. CE, cholesterol ester; CETP, cholesterol ester transfer protein; HDL, high-density lipoprotein; LCAT, lecithin–cholesterol acyltransferase; LDL, low-density lipoprotein; LPL, lipoprotein lipase; VLDL, very low-density lipoprotein.

and HDL are overloaded with TAG they become favored substrates for the action of HL and are remodeled into smaller and denser particles. While small, dense HDL is catabolised rapidly in the liver and other tissues, lowering serum HDL and impairing reverse cholesterol transport, small, dense LDLs are removed less effectively by LDL receptors and accumulate in serum. Small, dense LDL, by virtue of its size, has a much greater potential to infiltrate the artery wall and deposit its cholesterol. Even a moderately raised concentration of serum TAG (>1.5 mmol/l) may be inversely associated with reduced HDL cholesterol (<1 mmol/l) and a predominance of small, dense LDL. This collection of findings is known as the atherogenic lipoprotein phenotype (ALP) and is a very common, but modifiable source of increased CHD risk in free-living populations.

Endocrine control of lipoprotein metabolism

Many hormones with endocrine effects exert an influence on lipoprotein metabolism. However, with respect to diet and the control of postprandial lipid metabolism, insulin has by far the greatest impact. Although classically associated with carbohydrate metabolism and the uptake of glucose into cells, the actions of insulin are critical to the control of postprandial lipid metabolism. Insulin is secreted in response to the reception of food in the gut, reaching a peak in serum three to five hours after the consumption of a meal. Insulin coordinates the hydrolysis of TAG of dietary origin in chylomicrons with the uptake of NEFA into adipose tissue by the following actions:

- stimulates lipoprotein lipase (LPL) in adipose tissue capillaries;
- suppresses the intracellular lipolysis of stored TAG in adipose tissue by inhibiting the activity of hormone-sensitive lipase (HSL), reducing serum NEFA;
- increases the esterification of fatty acids in adipose tissue;
- suppresses the release of VLDL from the liver.

Insulin also suppresses the activity of LPL in the capillaries of skeletal muscle after a meal, though this effect is relatively minor in comparison to its effect on HSL in adipose tissue. The sensitivity of the target tissues to insulin, such as the liver, adipose tissue, and to a lesser extent skeletal muscle, is critical to the maintenance of these effects. Failure of insulin action or "insulin resistance", in conditions such as obesity and diabetes results in impaired capacity of LPL to hydrolyse TAG-rich lipoproteins and accumulation of their partially hydrolyzed breakdown products or lipoproteins remnants in the postprandial circulation. This effect is compounded by the failure of insulin to suppress the mobilisation of NEFA from adipose tissue TAG, which increases the flux of NEFA to the liver and stimulates the overproduction of VLDL. The insulin-induced suppression of VLDL secretion is also relieved, so that VLDL is not only overproduced, but also released into the postprandial circulation, where it competes with chylomicrons for LPL, augmenting the magnitude and duration of postprandial lipemia still further. In the long term, this impaired capacity to remove TAG and repeated bouts of enhanced postprandial lipemia, produce abnormalities in serum low and HDL as part of a dyslipidemia that is a characteristic of insulin-resistant conditions (central obesity, metabolic syndrome, type-2 diabetes) known collectively as an ALP. Insulin may also stimulate the synthesis of cholesterol by activating HMG-CoA reductase, and LDL receptors. However, while increased body weight has been linked to elevated serum LDL-cholesterol, the overall impact of insulin resistance on the concentration of serum LDL-cholesterol must be small, since serum LDL-cholesterol levels are often unremarkable in individuals with an ALP.

Effects of sex hormones on serum lipoproteins

The strongest evidence for the effects of sex hormones on serum lipoproteins is provided by the pronounced differences in lipid and lipoprotein profiles between adult men and premenopausal women. Men present with higher total serum and LDL cholesterol, higher serum TAG, and lower HDL cholesterol concentrations than premenopausal women. This difference in lipid profiles confers a relative protection against CHD on premenopausal women, making their CHD risk lag behind that of men of the same age by approximately 10 years. This applies until oestrogen failure at the menopause, when CHD risk in women increases above that of men. Oestrogen was the first compound shown to stimulate LDL receptor activity in cell culture. In the body, this effect not only accounts for lower LDL levels in women, but also the sharp increase in serum LDL cholesterol after the menopause, to levels above those of men. Oestrogens also stimulate the production of TAG and VLDL, but any detriment to the cardiovascular health of women may be outweighed by the efficiency of TAG removal mechanisms that maintain lower serum TAG levels in women than men until the menopause. In addition to these effects, oestrogen selectively inhibits the activity of HL, which contributes to the relatively higher serum HDL-cholesterol in women over men. In direct contrast, the androgenic male hormone, testosterone, suppresses LDL receptor activity, and is a powerful stimulant of HL activity, effects which contribute to elevating serum LDL and lowering HDL cholesterol, respectively, in men. The latter effect can be observed in male body builders taking androgen "anabolic" steroids, in whom serum HDL cholesterol can be almost absent.

Diet, CVD and relative importance of serum cholesterol and TAG as a cardio-metabolic risk factor

Elevated serum LDL cholesterol is a causal risk factor for the development of CVD, which increases the absolute risk of dying from a heart attack or stroke. However, the high prevalence of only moderately elevated levels of serum LDL cholesterol in populations make it difficult to discriminate between those who will succumb to premature CVD from those who will not, on the basis of this single risk factor. Other risk factors with a higher prevalence, and thus higher attributable risk in populations, such as the common cardio-metabolic, co-morbidities of obesity and type-2 diabetes, must be taken into account. In a similar respect, the effects of diet on serum LDL cholesterol provide a relatively small contribution to explaining the impact of diet on CVD risk relative to the effects of diet on CVD risk that arise through the development of obesity and diabetes. While it is imperative to target elevated serum LDL cholesterol with the portfolio of dietary recommendations to lower this risk factor, correction of cardio-metabolic risk factors, including impaired postprandial lipaemia, is a priority that will inadvertently lower serum LDL.

The ability of humans to protect themselves against an over accumulation of cholesterol in their vascular system through nutritional changes depends to a much greater extent on increasing the functional capacity of the HDL pathway, and the efficiency of the utilisation of TAG-rich lipoproteins. The latter represent the precursors of potentially harmful cholesterol-rich remnants and LDLs that contribute to cardiovascular atherosclerosis. The effects of diet, and in particular dietary fats and carbohydrates, in modulating the clearance of TAG-rich lipoproteins in the postprandial period is of paramount importance in preventing the accumulation of atherogenic remnants and development of proatherogenic abnormalities in LDL and HDL. The actions of insulin in co-ordinating the metabolism of TAG-rich lipoproteins, can become defective through energy imbalance, weight gain, and accumulation of central (visceral) and ectopic fat. As a consequence, the most common abnormalities in lipoproteins to increase CVD risk in populations arise from defects in the metabolic handling of TAG (production and catabolism), and not serum cholesterol *per se*. Equally important is the fact that these metabolic defects that increase CVD risk, originate to a large extent through long term exposure to an inappropriate diet and lifestyle, and are thus highly amenable to therapeutic diet and lifestyle changes.

9.6 Body lipid pools

Lipids in the human body exist in two major pools: structural lipids in membranes and storage lipids in body fat. The lipid composition and metabolic fate of these two pools are quite distinct, although many of the fatty acids occupying both pools are the same. The main components of both membrane and storage lipids are the long-chain (16-24 carbons) saturated, monounsaturated, and polyunsaturated fatty acids. Although several of the major long-chain fatty acids in the body are common to both membrane and storage lipids, namely palmitate, stearate, oleate, and linoleate, three important distinctions exist between membrane and storage lipids.

- membrane lipids are not usually hydrolyzed to release free fatty acids for energy metabolism;
- membrane lipids contain a much higher proportion of long-chain PUFAs;
- membrane lipids are more diverse and rarely include TAGs, which are the main component of storage lipids.

Structural lipid pool

Biological membranes surrounding cells and subcellular organelles exist primarily as lipid bilayers (Figure 9.4). The lipids in both the inner and outer surfaces of membranes are composed mainly of phospholipids and free cholesterol, which interface with a myriad of proteins functioning as receptors, transporters, enzymes, ion channels, etc. Some lipids, i.e., PUFAs, confer the feature of "fluidity" to membranes, whereas others, i.e., cholesterol and saturated fatty acids, have the opposite rigidifying effect. Membranes have extraordinarily diverse fatty acid profiles and phospholipid composition depending on their tissue and subcellular location. They are also the body's reservoir of both fat-soluble vitamins and eicosanoid precursors such as arachidonate.

Most of the body's cholesterol is present in the unesterified form in membranes, where it represents 35–45% of total lipids. Skin, plasma, and adrenal cortex contain 55–75% of cholesterol in the esterified form. Bile also contains free cholesterol and bile salts derived from cholesterol.

Storage lipid pool

TAGs are the main energy storage form of lipids and they are the principal component of body fat. TAG-containing fatty acids destined for oxidation are also present in measurable, but much lower amounts in all tissues that can oxidise long-chain fatty acids, i.e., muscle and heart. TAG is synthesised by the intestine and liver, where it is subsequently incorporated into lipoproteins (see Section 9.4) for the transport of lipids to and from other tissues.

The main fatty acids in the TAG of adult human body fat are palmitate (20–30%), stearate (10–20%), oleate (45–55%), and linoleate (10–15%). The fatty acid profile of adult body fat always reflects the profile of dietary fat. Only rarely would this result in other fatty acids being more prevalent in body fat than the four listed here. At birth, the fatty acid profile of body fat is unusual in having very low linoleate (<3%) and α-linolenate (<1%), but a higher proportion of long-chain polyunsaturates than later in life. Body fat occupies several discrete sites that expand and contract as needed. Body fat is about 82% by weight TAG, making it by far the main body pool of palmitate, stearate, oleate, and linoleate.

The main sites of body fat are subcutaneous adipose tissue (SAT) and intra-visceral or visceral adipose tissue (VAT), and they have different rates of response to stimuli for accumulation or release of fatty acids. Within a given site, growing evidence suggests that PUFAs are more easily released from adipose tissue TAG than are saturated fatty acids, especially during fasting or longer term energy deficit. Body fat may also accumulate in sites other than SAT and VAT. This body fat is referred to as ectopic fat, and can be found in organs like the liver, pancreas, heart and skeletal muscle, where it has been associated with metabolic dysfunction.

Plasma and milk lipids

In a way, serum and milk lipids are an exception to the general rule that distinguishes membrane and storage lipids. Serum and milk lipids are present mostly as lipoproteins and fat globules, respectively, comprising mostly phospholipids and cholesterol in the surrounding membrane and TAG in the core (see Section 9.5). The milk fat globule membrane (MFGM) surrounding the fat (TAG) droplets in milk, consists of a complex system of integral and peripheral proteins, enzymes, and lipids, that may have an important role in various cellular processes and defense mechanisms in the newborn. The MFGM may also provide a physical barrier that contributes to the food matrix effects of certain dairy products.

Plasma lipids contain the only significant pool of free fatty acids or non-esterified fatty acids (NEFA) in the body. NEFA are not components of lipoproteins, but are transported in serum bound to albumin. They are liberated mostly from adipose tissue when plasma glucose and insulin are low. Plasma also contains proportionally more fatty acids esterified to cholesterol (cholesteryl esters) than are found in tissues.

Whole body content and organ profile of fatty acids

An estimate of the whole body content of lipids in a healthy adult human is given in Table 9.5. Additional body fat is deposited during pregnancy, but the fatty acid composition remains similar to that of non-pregnant adults and reflects dietary fat intake. The total lipid content of serum rises in the third trimester, with a proportionally greater increase in saturated fatty acids than PUFAs. This downward trend in the percentage of PUFA towards term has led to some concern about the possible adverse consequences for the fetus of deficiency of PUFA. However, the actual amount of PUFA in blood lipids rises but less so than for saturated fatty acids; resulting in a proportional decrease in PUFA.

Soon after birth, body lipid composition starts to change. Brain cholesterol rises moderately from under 40% to nearly 50% of brain lipids. Docosahexaenoate also rises rapidly in brain lipids, followed a little later by an increasing content of long-chain saturates and monounsaturates as myelin develops. Adipose tissue contains very little linoleate or α-linolenate at birth, but its content increases rapidly with milk feeding. Serum cholesterol is relatively low at birth and in infancy, but increases by more than two-fold by adulthood.

In general, regardless of the profile of dietary fatty acids, saturated and monounsaturated fatty

Table 9.5 Body fat content of major fatty acids in humans

Fatty acid	Content (g)
Palmitic acid	3320
Stearic acid	550
Oleic acid	6640
Linoleic acid	1560
Arachidonic acid	80
α-Linolenic acid	130
Eicosapentaenoic acid	<10
Docosahexaenoic acid	<10
Total	12 300

Data are based on a 70 kg adult human with 20% (14 kg) body fat. Fat tissue contains about 88% actual fatty acids by weight, yielding about 12.3 kg fatty acids in this example.

acids predominate in adipose tissue, whereas there is a closer balance between saturates, monounsaturates, and polyunsaturates in structural lipids. Long-chain PUFAs such as docosahexaenoate are present in high concentrations in specialised membranes, including those of the retina photoreceptor, in synapses of the brain, and in sperm.

9.7 Long-chain fatty acid metabolism

Synthesis

Synthesis of fatty acids occurs in the cytosol. It begins with acetyl-CoA being converted to malonyl-CoA by acetyl-CoA carboxylase, an enzyme dependent on biotin. Malonyl-CoA and a second acetyl-CoA then condense via β-ketothiolase. This is subsequently reduced, dehydrated, and then hydrogenated to yield a four-carbon product that recycles through the same series of steps until the most common long-chain fatty acid product, palmitate, is produced (Figure 9.10). Acetyl-CoA is primarily an intra-mitochondrial product. Thus, the transfer of acetyl-CoA to the cytosol for fatty acid synthesis appears to require its conversion to citrate to exit the mitochondria before being reconverted to acetyl-CoA in the cytosol.

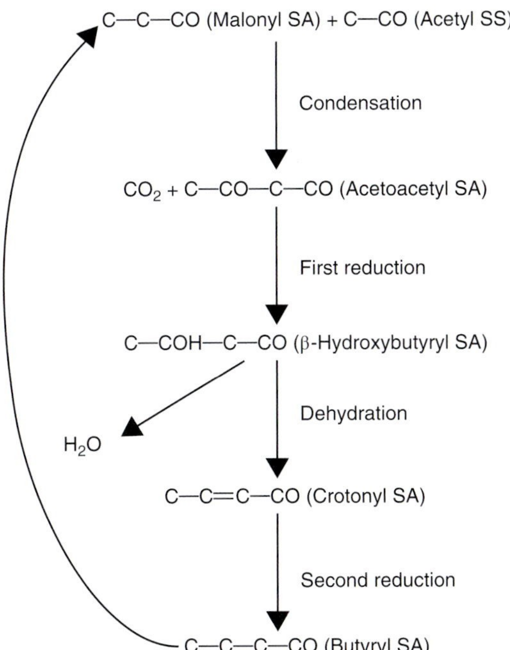

Figure 9.10 Principal steps in fatty acid synthesis. The individual steps occur with the substrate being anchored to the acyl carrier protein. SA, *S*-acyl carrier protein; SS, *S*-synthase.

There are three main features of long-chain fatty acid synthesis in mammals:

- inhibition by starvation;
- stimulation by feeding carbohydrate after fasting;
- general inhibition by dietary fat.

Carbohydrate is an important source of carbon for generating acetyl-CoA and citrate used in fatty acid synthesis. Enzymes of carbohydrate metabolism also help to generate the NADPH needed in fatty acid synthesis. Acetyl-CoA carboxylase is a key control point in the pathway, and is both activated and induced to polymerise by citrate. Acetyl-CoA carboxylase is inhibited by long-chain fatty acids, especially PUFAs such as linoleate. This is probably one important negative feedback mechanism by which both starvation and dietary fat decrease fatty acid synthesis. High amounts of free long-chain fatty acids would also compete for CoA, leading to their β-oxidation. Elongation of palmitate to stearate, etc., can occur in mitochondria using acetyl-CoA, but is more commonly associated with the endoplasmic reticulum where malonyl-CoA is the substrate.

Humans consuming >25% energy as dietary fat, synthesise relatively low amounts of fat (<2 g/day). Compared with other animals, humans also appear to have a relatively low capacity to convert stearate to oleate and linoleate or α-linolenate to the respective longer chain PUFAs. Hence, the fatty acid profiles of most human tissues generally reflect the intake of dietary fatty acids; when long-chain n-3 PUFAs are present in the diet, this is evident in both free-living humans as well as in experimental animals. Nevertheless, fatty acid synthesis is stimulated by fasting/refeeding or weight cycling, so these perturbations in normal food intake can markedly alter tissue fatty acid profiles.

Fatty acid oxidation

β-Oxidation is the process by which fatty acids are utilised for energy. Saturated fatty acids destined for β-oxidation are transported as CoA esters to the outer leaflet of mitochondria by

FABP. They are then translocated inside the mitochondria by carnitine acyl-transferases. The β-oxidation process involves repeated dehydrogenation at sequential two-carbon steps and reduction of the associated flavoproteins (Figure 9.11). Five ATP molecules are produced during production of each acetyl-CoA. A further 12 ATP molecules are produced after the acetyl-CoA condenses with oxaloacetate to form citrate and goes through the tricarboxylic acid cycle.

The efficiency of fatty acid oxidation depends on the availability of oxaloacetate and, hence, concurrent carbohydrate oxidation. β-Oxidation of saturated fatty acids appears to be simpler than oxidation of unsaturated fatty acids because, before the acetyl-CoA cleavage, it involves the formation of a *trans* double bond two carbons from the CoA. In contrast, β-oxidation of unsaturated fatty acids yields a double bond in a different position that then requires further isomerisation or hydrogenation. From a biochemical perspective, this extra step appears to make the oxidation of unsaturated fatty acids less efficient than that of saturated fatty acids. However, evidence from *in vivo* and *in vitro* studies in both humans and animals clearly shows that long-chain *cis*-unsaturated fatty acids with one to three double bonds (oleate, linoleate, α-linolenate) are more readily β-oxidised than saturated fatty acids of equivalent chain length, such as palmitate and stearate.

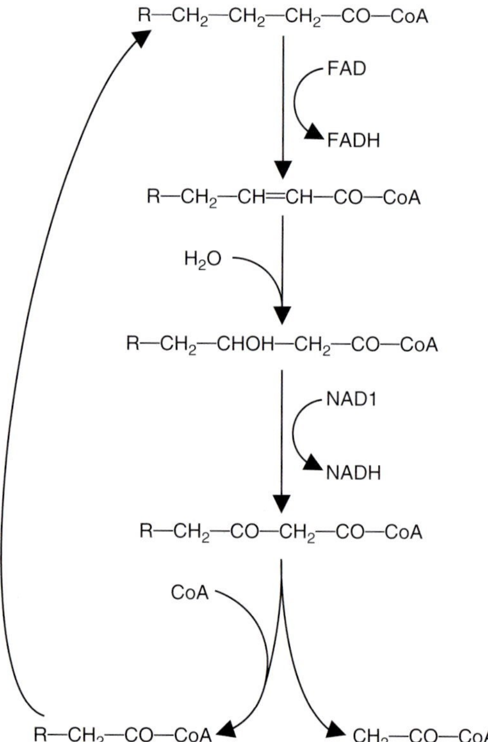

Figure 9.11 Principal steps in β-oxidation of a saturated fatty acid. The steps shown follow fatty acid "activation" (binding to coenzyme A) and carnitine-dependent transport to the inner surface of the mitochondria. Unsaturated fatty acids require additional steps to remove the double bonds before continuing with the pathway shown. FAD, flavin adenine dinucleotide; FADH reduced flavin adenine dinucleotide; R, 12 carbons.

Ketogenesis and ketosis

Large amounts of free fatty acids inhibit glycolysis and the enzymes of the tricarboxylic acid cycle, thereby impairing production of oxaloacetate. When insufficient oxaloacetate is available to support the continued oxidation of acetyl-CoA, two acetyl-CoA molecules condense to form a ketone, acetoacetate. Acetoacetate can be spontaneously decarboxylated to form acetone, a volatile ketone, or converted to a third ketone, β-hydroxybutyrate. When glucose is limiting, ketones are an alternative source of energy for certain organs, particularly the brain. They are also efficient substrates for lipid synthesis during early postnatal development. Conditions favoring ketogenesis include starvation, diabetes, and a very high-fat, low-carbohydrate "ketogenic" diet. There is evidence to suggest that mild ketosis (0.5-3mmol/L) induced through prolonged fasting or very low carbohydrate diets, may exert physiological effects that assist weight loss through decreased appetite and hunger.

Fatty acid peroxidation

Peroxidation (auto-oxidation) is the non-enzyme-catalyzed reaction of molecular oxygen with organic compounds to form peroxides and related breakdown products. PUFAs are particularly vulnerable to peroxidation at the double bonds. Initiating agents such as pre-existing peroxides, transition metals, or ultraviolet or ionising radiation produce singlet oxygen. Singlet oxygen can then abstract hydrogen at the double bonds of polyunsaturates to produce free (peroxy) radicals, which abstract further hydrogens from the same or different fatty acids and propagate the peroxidation process. Eventually, this leads to termination by the formation of stable degradation products or hydroperoxides (Figure 9.12). *Trans* isomers are frequently formed during the process. Hydroperoxides can form further hydroperoxy radicals or can be reduced by antioxidants, which contain thiol groups, i.e., glutathione and cysteine. Peroxidation of dietary fats gives rise to aldehydes, i.e., 2-undecenal, 2-decenal, nonanal, or octanal, which have a particular odor commonly known as rancidity.

Since peroxidation is a feature of PUFA, it is a potential hazard facing most membranes and dietary lipids. Antioxidants such as vitamin E are usually present in sufficient amounts to prevent or block peroxidation in living tissues. Humans and animals readily detect peroxidised fats in foods by their disagreeable odor and avoid them. However, modeling the effects of peroxides produced *in vivo* and *in vitro* is particularly challenging because lipid peroxidation undoubtedly is an important part of several necessary biological processes such as activation of the immune response.

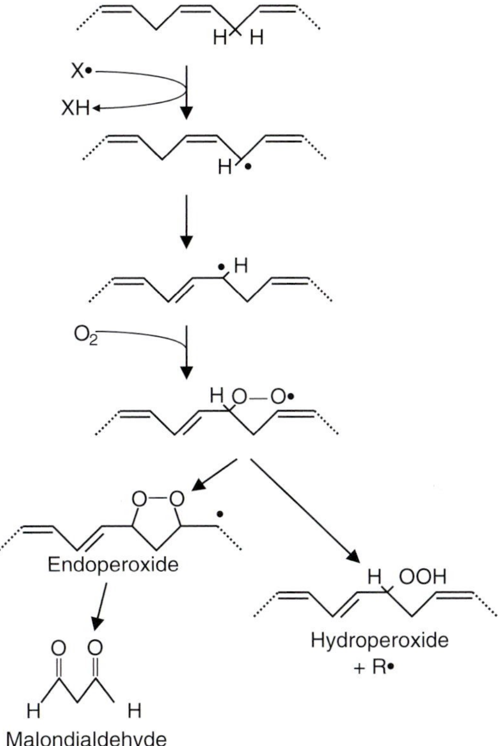

Figure 9.12 Principal steps in peroxidation of a polyunsaturated fatty acid.

Fatty acid desaturation, chain elongation, and chain shortening

One important characteristic of long-chain fatty acid metabolism in both plants and animals is the capacity to convert one to another via the processes of desaturation, chain elongation, and chain shortening.

Plants and animals use desaturases to insert a double bond into long-chain fatty acids. There are several desaturases, depending on the position in the acyl chain into which the double bond is inserted. Although myristate (14:0) and palmitate can be converted to their monounsaturated derivatives, myristoleate (14:1n-5) and palmitoleate (16:1n-7) respectively, commonly it is only the fatty acids of 18 or more carbons that undergo desaturation. The Δ^9desaturases in all organisms, except for anaerobic bacteria, use oxygen and NADPH to introduce a *cis* double bond at carbons 9 and 10 of stearate. This is accomplished by an enzyme complex consisting of a series of two cytochromes and the terminal desaturase itself. The acyl-CoA form of fatty acids is the usual substrate for the desaturases, but fatty acids esterified to phospholipids can also be desaturated *in situ*.

All mammals so far studied, can convert stearate to oleate via Δ^9 desaturase. However, in the absence of dietary oleate, young rats may have insufficient capacity to sustain normal tissue oleate levels. Normal values depend on the reference, which can vary widely depending on the source and amount of oleate in the diet. Nevertheless, it is important to distinguish between the existence of a given desaturase and the capacity of that pathway to make sufficient of the necessary product fatty acid. Hence, as with the long-chain polyunsaturates and, indeed, with other nutrients such as amino acids (see Chapter 4), it is important to keep in mind that the existence of a pathway to make a particular fatty acid or amino acid does not guarantee sufficient capacity of that pathway to make that product. This is the origin of the concept of "conditional essentiality" or "indispensability." Both plants and animals are capable of desaturating at the 9–10 carbon (Δ^9 desaturase) of stearate, resulting in oleate. However, only plants are capable of desaturating oleate to linoleate and then to α-linolenate. Once linoleate and α-linolenate are consumed by animals, their conversion to the longer chain PUFAs of their respective families proceeds, primarily by an alternating series of desaturation (Δ^6 and Δ^5 desaturases) and chain-elongation steps (Figure 9.13). Sequential desaturations or chain elongations are also a possibility, resulting in a large variety, though low abundance, of other PUFAs.

During dietary deficiency of linoleate or α-linolenate, oleate can also be desaturated and chain elongated to the PUFA eicosatrienoate (20:3n-9). Hence, most but not all PUFAs are derived from linoleate or α-linolenate.

Chain elongation of saturated and unsaturated fatty acids occurs primarily in the endoplasmic reticulum, although it has also been demonstrated to occur in mitochondria. Unlike the desaturation steps immediately before and after, the elongation steps do not appear to be rate limiting in the metabolism of linoleate or α-linolenate.

Despite the capacity to insert at least three double bonds in both n-3 and n-6 PUFA, there is no proof that a Δ^4 desaturase exists to insert the final double bond in docosapentaenoate (22:5n-6) or docosahexaenoate (Figure 9.13). Rather, it appears that the precursors of these two fatty acids undergo a second elongation, repeated Δ^6 desaturation followed by chain shortening in peroxisomes. This unexpectedly convoluted series of steps is corroborated by the docosahexaenoate deficiency observed in disorders of peroxisomal biogenesis such as Zellweger's syndrome.

Hydrogenation

Opposite to the desaturation process is hydrogenation or removal of unsaturated bonds in

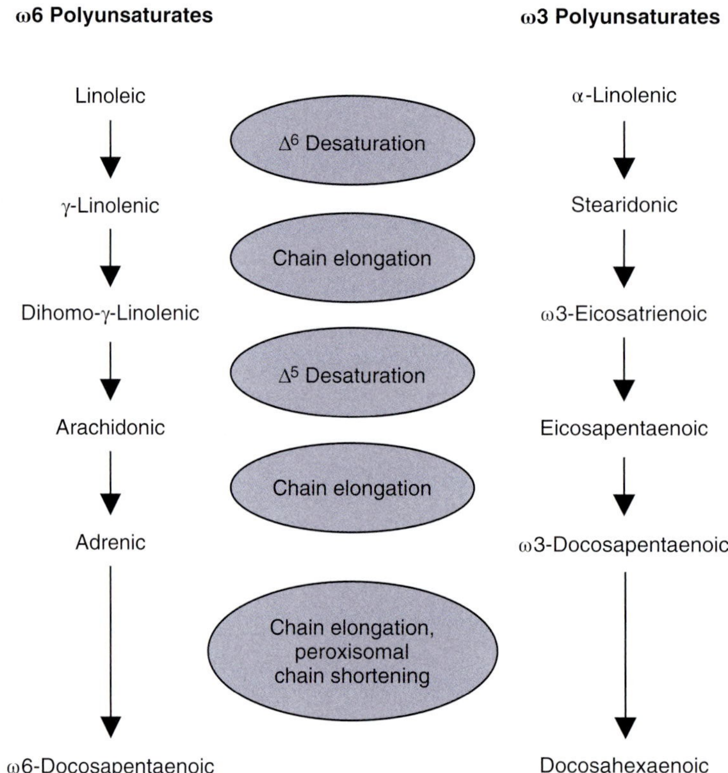

Figure 9.13 Conversion of linoleic (18:2n-6) and α-linolenic (18:3n-3) acids to their respective longer chain, more unsaturated PUFA. In membranes, linoleic and arachidonic acids are the principal n-6 PUFA, while docosahexaenoic acid is the principal n-3 PUFA. Hence, these two families of fatty acids have different affinities for the desaturation and chain-elongation enzymes. This pathway is principally based in the endoplasmic reticulum but appears to depend on peroxisomes for the final chain shortening, which involves 24 carbon intermediates that are not illustrated.

lipids. Rumen bacteria are the only organisms known to have this capability. As in chemical hydrogenation practiced by the food industry, bio-hydrogenation in the rumen can be incomplete, resulting in the formation of small amounts of *trans* isomers, particularly of oleate, linoleate, and α-linolenate, which are found in milk fat.

Eicosanoids

Eicosanoids are 20-carbon, oxygen-substituted cyclised metabolites of cell membrane phospholipid fatty acids, such as dihomo-γ-linolenate, arachidonate, or eicosapentaenoate. They are produced via a cascade of steps starting with the cyclooxygenase or lipoxygenase enzymes present in microsomes. The main cyclooxygenase products comprise the classical prostaglandins, prostacyclin and the thromboxanes. The main lipoxygenase products are the leukotrienes (slow-reacting substances of anaphylaxis) and the noncyclised hydroperoxy derivatives of arachidonate that give rise to the hepoxylins and lipoxins (Figure 9.14).

Eicosanoids are considered to be fast-acting local hormones, the presence of which in the plasma and urine is largely a spillover from localised production, usually in response to an injury or a stimulus that releases the free precursor, most commonly arachidonate. The site of highest eicosanoid concentration appears to be the seminal fluid, although some species have no detectable eicosanoids in semen. Eicosanoids are second messengers modulating, among other pathways, protein phosphorylation. The lung is a major site of eicosanoid inactivation.

Four important characteristics of eicosanoid action should be noted. First, individual eicosanoids often have biphasic actions as one moves from very low through to higher, often pharmacological, concentrations. Thus, effects can vary dramatically depending not only on the experimental system, but also on the eicosanoid concentration used. Second, several of the more abundant eicosanoids arising from the same precursor fatty acid have opposite actions to each other. For instance, prostacyclin and thromboxane A_2 are both derived from arachidonate, but the former originates primarily from the endothelium and inhibits platelet aggregation, while the latter originates primarily from platelets and is a potent platelet-aggregating agent. Third, competing eicosanoids derived from dihomo-γ-linolenate (1 series) and from eicosapentaenoate (3 series) often have effects that oppose those derived from arachidonate (2 series) (Figure 9.14). Thus, unlike prostaglandin E_2, prostaglandin E_1 has anti-inflammatory actions, reduces vascular tone, and inhibits platelet aggregation. Fourth, varying the ratio of the precursor fatty acids in the diet is an effective way to modify eicosanoid production. Thus, eicosapentaenoate and dihomo-γ-linolenate inhibit the

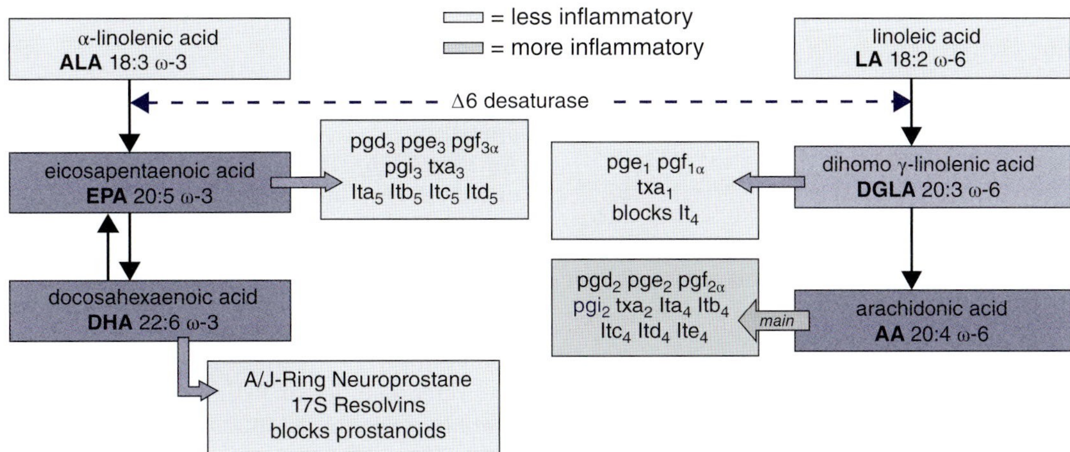

Figure 9.14 Production of eiscosanoids from linoleic and α-linolenic acid in membrane bound phospholipids. Thromboxanes (txa) e.g derived from platelets; prostaglandins (pgi), e.g., derived from the blood vessel wall. Interleukines (lta, ltb). Source: Reproduced under a cc license. Created by David R Throop.

synthesis of 2 series eicosanoids derived from arachidonate. This occurs by inhibiting arachidonate release from membranes by phospholipase A_2 and its cascade through the cyclooxygenases and lipoxygenases. The overproduction of 2 series eicosanoids is associated with higher blood pressure, increased platelet aggregation, and inflammatory processes, and can be effectively inhibited by dietary approaches using oils rich in eicosapentaenoate and γ-linolenate (18:3n-6), the precursor to dihomo-γ-linolenate.

Stable analogues of some classical prostaglandins have specialised medical applications, including the termination of pregnancy and the closing of a patent ductus arteriosus shortly after birth. Many anti-inflammatory and anti-pyretic drugs are inhibitors of eicosanoid synthesis. One potentially dangerous side-effect of inhibiting eicosanoid synthesis is gastric erosion and bleeding. Receptor antagonists of leukotrienes are effective in reducing the symptoms of asthma.

9.8 Nutritional regulation of long-chain fatty acid profiles and metabolism

Phospholipids of all cellular and subcellular membranes contain a diverse range of long-chain fatty acids, the profile of which is subject to both dietary influence and endogenous control. A few organs, notably the brain, maintain extraordinarily strict control of their membrane composition. However, the fatty acid profile of most organs is usually responsive to the influence of changes in dietary fatty acid composition and other nutritional variables, yet maintains the vital "gatekeeper" functions of all membranes. Hence, when changes in dietary fat intake alter membrane fatty acid profiles, appropriate membrane fluidity can be maintained by the addition or removal of other lipids such as cholesterol. Insufficient energy intake and the presence of disease have important consequences for fatty acid synthesis, desaturation, and chain elongation and, consequently, tissue fatty acid profiles.

Saturates and monounsaturates

Inadequate energy intake increases macronutrient oxidation, including fatty acids. Short-term fasting followed by refeeding a carbohydrate-rich meal is the classic way to stimulate fatty acid synthesis. Insulin is implicated in this process. When repeated, fasting/refeeding or weight cycling induces a gradual increase in the proportion of saturated and monounsaturated compared with PUFAs in tissues, especially body fat. This shift occurs because of the increase in fatty acid synthesis, easier oxidation of PUFAs, and the inhibition of desaturation and chain elongation by fasting. The implications of such an alteration in tissue fatty acid profiles have not yet been extensively studied, but may involve changes in insulin sensitivity and other hormone effects. Protein deficiency also inhibits desaturation and chain elongation of PUFAs.

Copper supplementation increases Δ^9 desaturase activity in animals, resulting in higher oleate levels. This effect was first observed when copper was used to reduce gastrointestinal infection in pigs, but also led to softer back fat. Opposite to the effects of copper supplementation, copper deficiency inhibits synthesis of both oleate and docosahexaenoate.

Polyunsaturated fatty acids

There are four key features of the nutritional regulation of the profiles and metabolism of PUFAs. These attributes govern the effects of deficiency or excess of one or more of these families of fatty acids almost as much as their level in the diet. These key features are:

- specificity within families;
- competition between families;
- substrate and end-product inhibition;
- co-factor nutrients.

Specificity

An n-6 PUFA cannot be converted to an n-3 or n-9 PUFA. Thus, deficiency of one family of PUFA cannot be corrected by excess of those in a different family and, indeed, is exacerbated by excess intake of the other families.

Competition

The three families of PUFAs appear to use a common series of desaturases and chain elongases. The preference of these enzymes is for the more unsaturated fatty acids so, everything else being equal, more α-linolenate will be desaturated than linoleate or oleate. However, in practice, more linoleate is consumed than α-linolenate and, as a result, more arachidonate is produced endogenously than eicosapentaenoate. Furthermore, this competition for desaturation and chain elongation between linoleate and α-linolenate can lead to exacerbation of symptoms of deficiency of one or other fatty acid family. Thus, as has been demonstrated both clinically and experimentally, excess linoleate intake using sunflower oil is a common way to accelerate deficiency of n-3 PUFA.

Inhibition

Excess linoleate or α-linolenate intake appears to inhibit production of the respective long-chain products in the same fatty acid family, i.e., high α-linolenate intake inhibits synthesis of docosahexaenoate. Likewise, the main end-products of desaturation and chain elongation tend to inhibit further metabolism through this pathway, so arachidonate inhibits its own synthesis. Similarly, dietary deficiency of linoleate increases activity of the Δ^6 and Δ^5 desaturases, presumably to restore depleted levels of long-chain n-6 polyunsaturates such as arachidonate.

Co-factors

The co-factor requirements of the desaturation chain-elongation enzymes are not yet well understood, but a few relationships are known. The desaturases are metalloenzymes containing iron, and iron deficiency therefore inhibits desaturase activity. Magnesium is needed for microsomal desaturase activity *in vitro*. Zinc deficiency inhibits Δ^6 and Δ^5 desaturation, apparently by interrupting the flow of electrons from NADH. This effect is severe enough that inherited forms of zinc deficiency such as acrodermatitis enteropathica cause a precipitous decline in plasma arachidonate, greater than usually observed with dietary deficiency of n-6 polyunsaturates.

9.9 Nutritional and metabolic effects of dietary fatty acids

Two types of issue exist in relation to the nutritional and health implications of individual dietary lipids.

- Whether synthesised endogenously or only obtained from the diet, what are the specific membrane, precursor, or metabolic effects of dietary fats beyond that of providing energy?
- Whether synthesised endogenously or obtained from the diet, does an excess amount of a dietary fat have beneficial or deleterious implications for health?

Short- and medium-chain fatty acids

Short-chain fatty acids (1–6 carbons) are mostly derived from carbohydrate fermentation in the large bowel and appear to be mainly used for energy, although they are also substrates in several pathways. Butyrate may have an important role as an energy substrate for enterocytes. Medium-chain fatty acids (8–14 carbons) naturally appear in mammalian milk and are almost exclusively used as energy substrates. They may also be chain elongated to palmitate.

Saturated fatty acids

Palmitate and stearate constitute a major proportion of the acyl groups of membrane phospholipids and all mammals have the capacity to synthesise them. Hence, empirically, they presumably have an important function in energy metabolism, cell structure, normal development, and growth. The 20- to 24-carbon saturates are also important constituents of myelin. However, in any of these functions, it is unlikely that a dietary source of saturates is necessary. In fact, the brain is unable to acquire saturated fatty acids from the circulation and relies on its own endogenous synthesis for these fatty acids. Furthermore, chronic excess intake and/or synthesis of palmitate is associated with an increased risk of diabetes and CVD.

Monounsaturated fatty acids

Little is known about the nutritional or health implications of palmitoleate (16:1n-7), but there is a burgeoning interest in the main dietary monounsaturated fatty acid, oleate, and the health implications of olive oil. In the context of the same total fat intake, the main benefit of higher oleate intake seems to be that this reduces intake of palmitate and stearate and that this helps to lower serum cholesterol.

Unlike saturates and MUFA, a dietary source of n-6 and n-3 PUFA is a necessity for normal growth and development. As with other essential nutrients, this has given rise to assessment of the dietary requirements for PUFA and the implications of inadequate dietary intake of them.

It has been accepted for over 50 years that n-6 PUFA, particularly linoleate, are required in the diet of all mammals, including humans. Official dietary guidelines generally recommend a dietary source of linoleate at 1-2% of energy intake. It has taken much longer to demonstrate that n-3 PUFAs are required by humans, although this now seems widely accepted among nutrition researchers. As with other nutrients, the requirement for PUFA varies according to the stage of the life cycle, with pregnancy, lactation, and infancy being the most vulnerable. Symptoms of linoleate deficiency are virtually impossible to induce in healthy adult humans, so the concept of "conditional indispensability or dispensability" of PUFAs was devised to replace the older, but ambiguous term "essential fatty acid." Linoleate appears to be conditionally dispensable in healthy non-pregnant adults, but is not in pregnancy, lactation, or infancy.

Because of the competition between the two families of PUFAs, deficiency of n-3 PUFA is commonly induced by an excess of dietary linoleate. Hence, discussion of the requirements for linoleate and α-linolenate has focused on their ratio in the diet. The ratio of n-6 to n-3 PUFA in human milk (5:1 to 10:1) has been widely viewed as a suitable reference for this ratio in the general diet. In most affluent countries, this ratio remains much higher, at about 20:1, and has been implicated in subclinical deficiency of n-3 PUFA. There is recent evidence to suggest that it is the absolute amounts of long-chain n-3 and n-6 fatty acids that are important in predicting health outcomes, and not the dietary ratio of these PUFA.

Essential fatty acid deficiency

The first experimental model of deficiency of PUFA was total fat deficiency. The elimination of dietary fat had to be extreme because the traces of fat found in starch and dietary proteins were sufficient to prevent reproducible symptoms of fat deficiency. The deficiency symptoms are now well known and involve dry, scaly skin, growth retardation, and reproductive failure. Most of these gross symptoms are relieved by linoleate and arachidonate. Although α-linolenate cannot be synthesised *de novo*, it has little effect on these gross symptoms. However, careful studies using a diet that is extremely deficient in n-3 PUFA and contains an excess of n-6 PUFA led to deficiency of n-3 PUFA, characterised by delayed and impaired neuronal development and impaired vision. These symptoms have been traced in many species to the inadequate accumulation of docosahexaenoate in the brain and eye. Hence, the main function of n-3 PUFA appears to hinge on synthesis of docosahexaenoate. In contrast, the function of n-6 PUFA involves independent roles of at least linoleate and arachidonate.

Human cases of deficiency of PUFAs, usually involve a clinical disorder, often involving weight loss, trauma such as surgery, or a disease requiring parenteral nutrition. However, reports of these cases are uncommon and describe dissimilar characteristics, leading one to question whether the same deficiency exists. Recent investigations into the amount of PUFA in the whole body and the rate at which they can be oxidised suggest that traumatic or disease-related processes leading to weight loss affect metabolism of PUFA more severely than simple dietary deficiency in a weight-stable, healthy individual. For example, deficiency of linoleate has been long suspected, but has been difficult to demonstrate in cystic fibrosis. Despite poor fat digestion, intake levels of linoleate may not be inadequate, but its β-oxidation could well be abnormally high owing to the chronic infectious challenge.

Clinical importance of polyunsaturates

Infant brain and visual development is dependent on adequate accumulation of docosahexaenoate. Several clinical studies and extensive use of formulae containing docosahexaenoate and arachidonate have shown that they are safe. Many, but not all such studies show an improvement in visual and cognitive scores compared with matched formulae containing no docosahexaenoate or arachidonate. The infant brain and body as a whole clearly acquire less docosahexaenoate when only α-linolenate is given. As a whole, these data suggest that docosahexaenoate is a conditionally indispensable fatty acid.

Aside from questionable deficiency of PUFA in cystic fibrosis (see above), one of the most graphic examples of their deficiency being caused by an inherited disease is Zellweger's syndrome. This condition causes severe mental retardation and early death. It is a disorder of peroxisomal biogenesis and one outcome is markedly impaired synthesis of docosahexaenoate. Dietary supplementation with docosahexaenoate appears to partially restore neurological development.

Epidemiological evidence shows that chronic degenerative diseases of affluence are directly associated with the deficiency of n-3 PUFAs. Indeed, countries with relatively high rates of these diseases usually have an adequate to perhaps unnecessarily higher intake of linoleate. High intakes of linoleate have been implicated in death from CVD and several types of cancer because these diseases are associated with low intakes of n-3 PUFA. Mental illnesses such as schizophrenia may also be associated with low intake of n-3 PUFA and respond to supplements of n-3 PUFA. A more balanced ratio of intake of n-6 and n-3 PUFA might achieve a reduction in the rate of these degenerative diseases, but has not yet been widely investigated.

Diets in Paleolithic times contained no processed food and probably balanced amounts of n-3 to n-6 PUFA and a lower level of saturates. Such diets would be predicted to lead to a lower incidence of degenerative disease. Since the brain has a very high energy requirement, it has also been speculated that human brain evolution beyond that of other primates was dependent on a reliable and rich source of dietary energy, and a direct source of long-chain PUFA, particularly docosahexaenoate.

9.10 Cholesterol synthesis and regulation

Cholesterol and the brain

Mammalian brain function is dependent on specialised membranes designed for signal transmission. Greater cognitive sophistication in humans appears to depend on a much greater number of connections and, consequently, greater potential for signal processing. Like the membrane lipids of most other mammalian organs, brain lipids contain a relatively high proportion of cholesterol, which increases from about 40% of the lipid content in neonates to nearly 50% in adults.

Unlike other organs, the mammalian brain is probably unique in being unable to acquire appreciable amounts of cholesterol from the circulation, i.e., from the diet or from synthesis outside the brain. This has been extensively studied in the young rat and supporting, although inconclusive, evidence is also available for the pig. The brain has sufficient capacity to synthesise cholesterol from acetyl-CoA derived primarily from either glucose or ketones. Hence, it achieves the required level of cholesterol apparently entirely by endogenous synthesis. In neonates, ketones appear to play a greater role as substrates for brain cholesterol than in adults, in whom their main function seems to be as an alternative fuel to glucose. Among the common dietary long-chain fatty acids that would give rise to ketones during fat oxidation, PUFAs, particularly linoleate and α-linolenate, appear to be the best substrates for ketogenesis, since carbon from these fatty acids readily appears in brain cholesterol in suckling rats.

9.11 Evidence for the complex relationship between diet and CVD

Definitive evidence for a direct causal relationship between diet and CVD, and more specifically the link between dietary macronutrients (fatty acids, carbohydrates and protein) and cardiovascular atherosclerosis in the large coronary arteries of the heart (coronary heart disease) is lacking, and will always fall short of the stronger evidence for the clinical efficacy of drugs. It comes as no surprise that nutrients, as consumed in foods and whole diets, do not exert the same biological effects as drugs because of the chemical complexity of foods, whole diets and variation in the lifestyles and biological response of humans to diet. This level of complexity confounds the strength of association between diet and disease, and diminishes the role of nutrition in the management of public health. Degenerative diseases like CVD and cancer develop under the influence of multiple genetic and environmental (diet and lifestyle) factors, and critically interactions between the two, giving these diseases multi-factorial origins. Statistical correlations that underlie associations between single nutrients and endpoints of CVD as for example, between SFA, non-fatal myocardial infarction (MI), stroke, and CVD death in observational studies (cross-sectional population and prospective cohorts studies), seldom translate into evidence for causality when particular nutrients are fed to humans in randomly controlled intervention trials, or meta-analyses of the same. While there are some notable exceptions where there is evidence for a direct effect of diet on CVD, this is rarely related to the effects of single nutrients, but a balanced mixture of nutrients consumed in whole foods within a dietary pattern, the best example of which is the benefit of the Mediterranean diet in reducing CVD mortality/risk. There is much stronger and consistent evidence for a relationship between diet and CVD (morbidity) and mortality, when the impact of diet is mediated indirectly through its effects on a factor that has been causally related to the development of CVD. Good examples include the indirect effects of dietary sodium in salt on blood pressure, and serum cholesterol-raising properties of dietary saturated fatty acids (SFA).

Diet, serum cholesterol, and CHD

Macronutrients, especially dietary fatty acids and carbohydrates, exert significant effects on the concentration, composition and metabolism of human serum lipids and lipoproteins, and as such, should always be a major component of dietary intervention strategies for the primary prevention of CHD in those at increased risk, and for secondary prevention in those with existing CHD. In 1953, Ancel Keys proposed that CHD was not simply a natural consequence of ageing, but that diet may contribute to its development, making it a preventable disease. Keys demonstrated a significant positive association between the level of serum cholesterol and risk of CHD death, and believed initially that this could be explained by the intake of total dietary fat. Sugar intake also showed a positive, but slightly weaker association with CHD risk. Some years later, after the initiation of his landmark Seven Countries study in 1958, Keys advanced his theory by linking the association between raised serum cholesterol and increased CHD mortality to the amount of energy derived from dietary SFA, stating in 1959; "*…saturated fats in ordinary foods raise the serum cholesterol level, those of polyunsaturated fats (mainly linoleic acid) lower it*". The cholesterol-raising effect of SFA was first described in terms of total serum cholesterol, since serum LDL and HDL, as discovered by an atomic physicist John Gofman in 1949, were still in their infancy. Counter-intuitively, dietary SFA with a chain length of 12-16 carbons, also raise the concentration of serum HDL-cholesterol, a phenomenon that may occur as compensation, to counter effect the increase in serum LDL. From his findings, Keys was able to formulate equations to predict the quantitative impact of SFA and PUFA fat on serum cholesterol, modified versions of which are still used in clinical practice today. With hindsight, we can appreciate that Ancel Keys was correct to move away from the idea that it was important to lower all types of dietary fat to prevent CHD, and to support the restriction of SFA, chiefly from animal sources in favour of unsaturated fatty from plants. He was also an early advocate of the health benefits of the Mediterranean diet, and in 1959 co-authored one of the first Mediterranean cook books.

Dietary Guidelines to reduce intake of saturated fat: controversy and confirmation

Advice to reduce intake of SFA has been the mainstay of dietary guidelines to decrease CVD risk since the early 1980s, largely on the grounds that this advice will reduce CVD risk by lowering serum LDL-cholesterol. Nevertheless, despite evidence for associations between diet, serum cholesterol, and CVD across a range of study types, several meta-analyses have failed to establish a direct relationship between the intake of dietary SFA and premature death from CVD. These studies cast a shadow of doubt over the validity of this dietary guideline, and were followed by accusations that Ancel Keys had manipulated his data to produce a positive relationship between the intake of SFA and CHD mortality. These accusations were later dismissed in a White Paper that examined Keys' original data and helped to restore confidence in his original findings (Pett *et al.*, 2017). Soon after, the World Health Organization and Scientific Advisory Committee on Nutrition in the UK published independent reports that re-examined the evidence for the relationship between dietary SFA and CHD/CVD mortality. The outcome of these independent reports were unanimous in concluding that the existing recommendation to reduce intake of dietary saturated fat to no more than 10% of total energy intake (11% food energy) was scientifically valid in reducing CVD risk in children and adults, and thus relevant to public health. The reports advised that SFA should be replaced by dietary unsaturated fatty acids (n-6 PUFA, WHO; PUFA and MUFA, SACN), but not carbohydrate. The controversy over SFA and CVD revealed that the relationship between dietary fats (SFA) and serum LDL cholesterol is complex, and depends on many factors, including the variable effects of different types of fatty acids (SFA, PUFA, MUFA) on LDL-cholesterol (Figure 9.15).

Note, the nature of the substituting macronutrient for SFA is also important in translating to positive and negative effects on CHD risk (Figure 9.16).

Additional factors to consider when replacing dietary SFA are that not all SFA exert the same effect on serum LDL-cholesterol, as for example stearic acid, a fatty acid that is widely abundant in our diet having relatively little effect in raising serum LDL cholesterol in comparison to its main counterparts, palmitic, myristic and lauric acids (Figure 9.17). The effects of SFA are also strongly influenced by the type of food containing the SFA, through the so called "food matrix" effect, a good example of which is the lesser LDL-cholesterol raising effect of SFA in cheese in comparison to the same amount and type of SFA in butter.

Lastly, the response of serum LDL-cholesterol to dietary SFA is also highly variable between individuals. While this phenomenon will have confounded attempts to study the inter-relationships between SFA, LDL and CVD, it creates the opportunity for the tailoring of dietary guidelines on SFA reduction to the needs of groups of individuals who show either a hyper of hypo LDL-cholesterol response to reductions in SFA. The identification of the metabolic traits or phenotypes that underlie variable LDL responsiveness to SFA, provides a good example of the study of what is called "personalised" or "precision" nutrition.

Saturated fatty acids and low-density lipoprotein cholesterol

The most well established mechanism to explain how different dietary fats produce variable effects on serum LDL-cholesterol is through the LDL receptor pathway, the control of which has been described in Section 9.5. The ability of the cell to regulate its pool of free cholesterol depends to a large extent on the nature of the fatty acids available for esterification by the enzyme ACAT, an intracellular relative of LCAT. ACAT favors

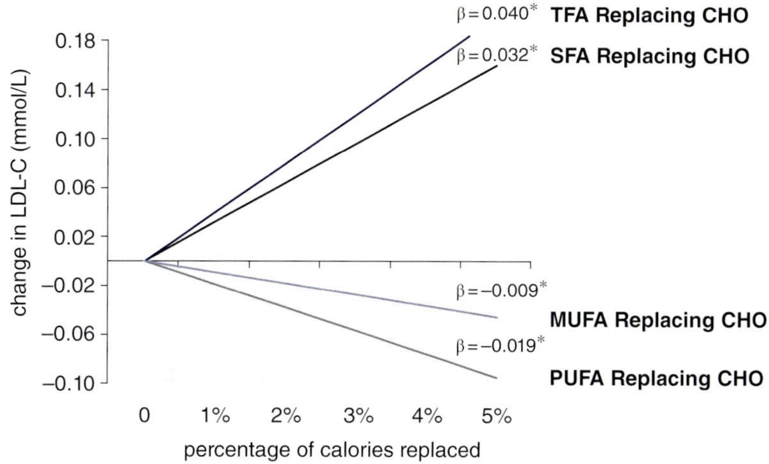

Figure 9.15 Effects of iso-energetic substitution of carbohydrate with different fatty acids on serum LDL-cholesterol. Source: Figure taken from: Micha & Mozaffarian (2010) *Lipids* 45, 893–905.

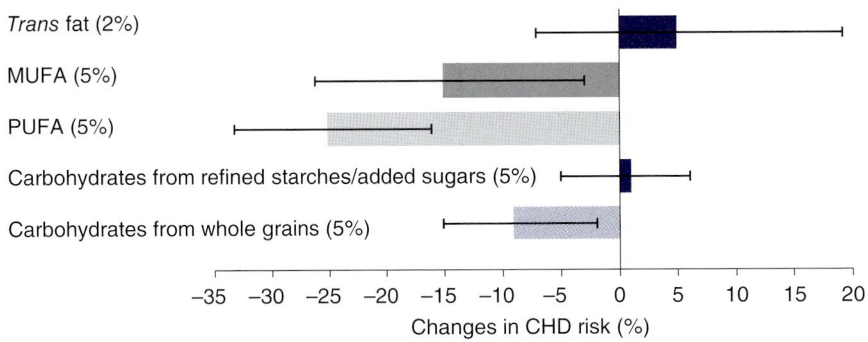

Figure 9.16 Effects of iso-energetic substitution of SFA with different fatty acids and types of carbohydrate on CHD risk. Source: Figure taken from Yanping Li *et al.* (2015) *J Am Coll Cardiol* 66, 1538–47.

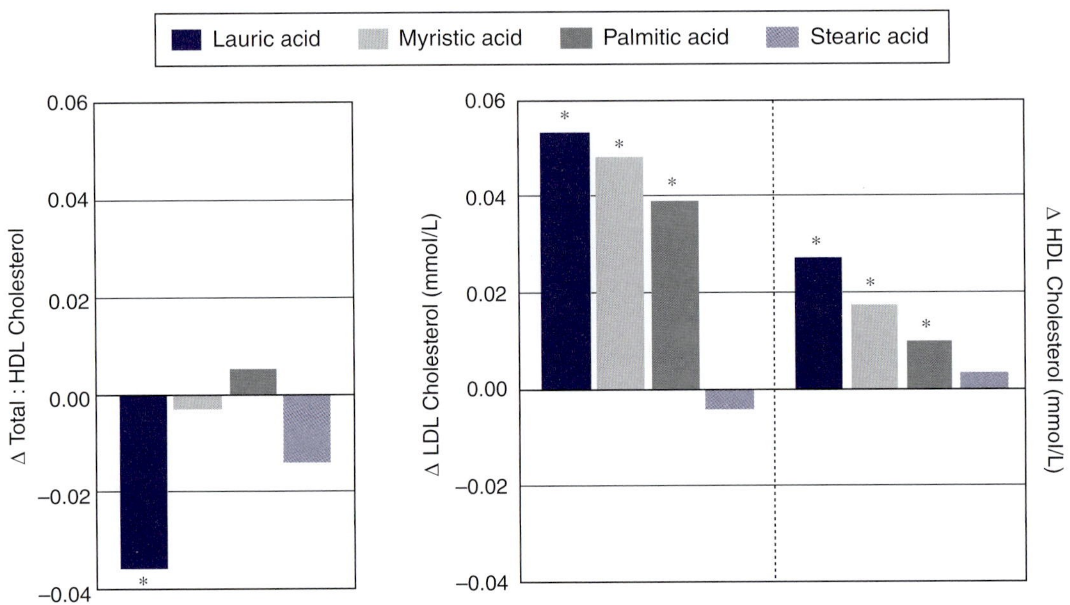

Figure 9.17 Differential effects of dietary saturated fatty acids on serum LDL-cholesterol and HDL-cholesterol. Source: Adapted from Mensink RP *et al.* (2003) *Am J Clin Nutr* 77, 1146–55.

unsaturated fatty acids (MUFAs and PUFAs) as substrates for esterification, which utilises free cholesterol within the cell. The resulting reduction in intracellular free cholesterol stimulates the transcription of the LDL receptor gene and production of new LDL receptors through the SREBP mechanism, and fall in circulating LDL as already described. Conversely, SFAs are poor substrates for ACAT, and their presence in the cell exerts the opposite effect on free cholesterol levels, thus increasing circulating LDL cholesterol and total serum cholesterol (Figure 9.18). Fatty acids may also exert direct effects on the activity of LDL receptors by altering the composition of membrane phospholipids and thus membrane fluidity. Alternatively, there is evidence to suggest that dietary PUFA could upregulate LDL receptors indirectly, by increasing the cholesterol content (lithogenicity) of bile and in this way accelerate the excretion of cholesterol.

Fat oxidation; a flawed theory for the development of CVD: Important difference between the oxidation of fatty acids in food and the body

There are two established chemical phenomena which involve the oxidation of fatty acids, which are frequently linked to provide an

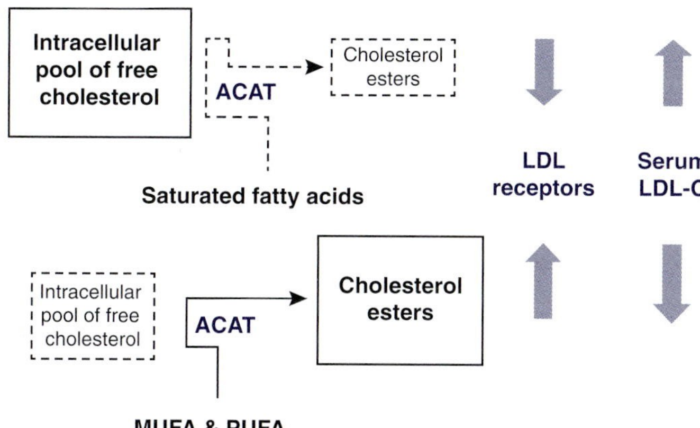

Figure 9.18 Influence of dietary fatty acids on serum LDL-cholesterol; through differential effects on free cholesterol and low-density lipoprotein (LDL) receptor activity. ACAT, acyl-CoA-cholesterol acyltransferase; LDL-C, LDL cholesterol; MUFA, monounsaturated fatty acid; PUFA, polyunsaturated fatty acids.

erroneous explanation of how dietary fatty acids either promote or prevent the development of cardiovascular atherosclerosis. The first is the fact that the propensity of a fatty acid in a food (e.g., oils, dairy) to oxidise in heated air, also called the "rancidity index" when applied to different oils, is directly proportional to the number of carbon double bonds in its chain, since these double initiate and fuel fat oxidation. Fatty acid-rich oils and foods therefore do show an increasing tendency to oxidise as their relative proportion of SFA to PUFA decreases. The second phenomenon is that fatty acids in the surface lipids of LDL must be oxidised to modify apoprotein B in LDL so it can be recognised by specific scavenger receptors on the surface of macrophages within the walls of arteries.' 'These cholesterol-loaded macrophages (foam cells) form atherosclerotic plaques that can rupture, causing an MI or heart attack. This oxidative modification of LDL occurs, in the main, once LDL has been sequestered in the artery wall, and is recognised as a pre-requisite step in the atherogenesis. However, despite erroneous claims that consuming large amounts of dietary SFA or PUFA will protect or promote against the development of CVD, respectively, via this oxidation processes, there is no convincing evidence to support the idea that PUFA increase and SFA decreases the oxidation of LDL or lipoprotein remnants (which do not need to be oxidised before entering macrophages). In reality, the oxidation of a fatty acid by air, in an oil or food, does not translate to the oxidative properties of fatty acids once they have been incorporated into a cell membrane or LDL in the body. If this were the case, SFA and highly polyunsaturated fatty acid-rich foods and oils would be associated with the prevention and promotion of CVD, when the opposite is true because the replacement of dietary SFA with PUFA is effective in reducing serum LDL cholesterol.

Dietary cholesterol in eggs

From a historical perspective, dietary sources of cholesterol, chiefly eggs, and to a lesser extent certain shell fish, have been restricted because of the over simplistic belief that the cholesterol content of these foods raises blood cholesterol and increases CVD risk. However, it has been established that dietary cholesterol exerts only a small, and clinically insignificant impact on serum LDL cholesterol over a normal range of dietary consumption (100–400 mg/day with one egg yolk containing between 150–250 mg cholesterol). As a result, most countries in the world have lifted restrictions on the intake of eggs. Persistent claims of associations between egg consumption and CVD in type 2 diabetes, and an increased incidence of diabetes, can be largely explained by eggs representing a marker of a dietary pattern that is inherently higher in energy and SFA, and by the clustering of other CVD risk factors in egg consumers. The consensus view is that up to seven eggs per week can be consumed safely, with the caveat that this advice must be accompanied by special emphasis on a healthy lifestyle in patients with established CVD or type-2 diabetes.

Portfolio Diet for reducing serum LDL cholesterol

The "Portfolio Diet" includes a collection of evidence-based dietary recommendations that target the lowering of serum LDL cholesterol. This was first proposed by Jenkins (1999), and later refined for the clinical management of hypercholesterolaemia by bodies such as HEART UK and others. The diet is based on the combined utility of weight loss, exchange of dietary fatty acids (SFA for PUFA/MUFA), inclusion of dietary soluble fibres (e.g., beta-glucan), plant stanols or sterols, and soy protein in reducing serum LDL-cholesterol by up to 30%. The rationale behind the effectiveness of this dietary approach is based on additive and/or synergistic mechanisms of action of its various components. These mechanisms include interruption of the enterohepatic circulation by active sequestration of bile acids and dietary and biliary cholesterol in the gut, and systemic upregulation of LDL receptors.

Plant sterols and soluble non-starch polysaccharides

These compounds may be grouped together, as at certain levels of intake they are both effective in reducing serum LDL cholesterol by limiting the resorption of dietary and biliary cholesterol, and bile acids, respectively, in the gut. This action interrupts the entero-hepatic circulation of these compounds, reducing the supply of cholesterol returning to the liver, and intracellular free cholesterol, which stimulates the production and activity of new LDL receptors. Plant sterols and their esters such as those incorporated into margarines (stanol esters), despite being nearly identical in structure to cholesterol, are poorly absorbed and interfere with the reabsorption of cholesterol originating from bile (~1g biliary cholesterol/day) and dietary sources (~300 mg/day) by either co-precipitation or competition. Margarines or spreads (30–40 g/day) containing plant sterols or their derivatives have been shown to reduce serum LDL cholesterol by up to 14% in controlled trials. Soluble fibres, as for example β-glucans found in oats and barley, act in a similar way, but by binding and preventing the absorption of bile acids (a modified form of cholesterol), and have been shown to be equally efficacious in reducing serum LDL cholesterol.

To place dietary influences on blood cholesterol in perspective of other cholesterol-lowering strategies, a meta-analysis of dietary intervention trials undertaken by the World Health Organization (WHO) revealed that dietary modification could achieve reductions in serum cholesterol of between only 4% and 5%. This finding contrasts with the greater efficacy of a targeted approach with the Portfolio diet (~30% reduction in LDL cholesterol), and especially the effects of cholesterol-lowering drugs (e.g., statins, PCSK9 inhibitors) that can reduce serum LDL cholesterol by in excess of 50–60%, and have proven efficacy in reducing the incidence of death from CVD. It also highlights the need to address other risk factors which are more responsive to dietary change.

The relative importance of blood cholesterol as distinct from cardio-metabolic risk factors for CVD

The majority of people with moderate hypercholesterolaemia (Total cholesterol 5.2–6.2 mmol/L, LDL-cholesterol 3.5–4 mmol/L), which represents up to 60% of some populations do not succumb to premature CHD. Conversely, most people who do suffer a premature cardiac event, do not have raised blood cholesterol. Total cholesterol 5.2–6.2 mmol/l)is associated with an absolute risk of CHD mortality of approximately 20%. The remaining 80% of overall risk can be attributed to other risk factors, a large part of which is often cardio-metabolic in origin. Cardio-metabolic risk can be described as collection of risk factors with a common metabolic origin(s) that increase risk of CVD. The sequelae can be explained in part, by the acquisition of excess body fat in the visceral cavity, and ectopic sites such as the liver. While this highlights the importance of energy restriction as being of paramount importance as a therapeutic modality, the quality of macronutrients may be critical in the development and management of cardio-metabolic risk associated with frank obesity and metabolic "obesity" (BMI>30 and <30, respectively).

Priorities in the dietary management of cardio-metabolic risk: quantity versus quality of dietary fat and carbohydrates

Excess body weight and obesity are major contributing factors to the development of cardio-metabolic risk. Contrary to popular belief, there is no evidence to support a single macronutrient theory for either the sustainable gain or loss of body weight, or the development and prevention of CVD in whole populations. There is evidence to suggest that extreme exclusions of either dietary carbohydrate or fat can assist weight loss, perhaps, in part, by increasing the degree of prescription and thus compliance to an energy restricted diet. There is also evidence to support physiological effects of mild ketosis induced by a high fat diet in the absence of carbohydrate, in suppressing appetite and sympathetic tone, which may facilitate a reduction in energy intake in the short term. Since a prolonged excess of both dietary fat and carbohydrate contributes to increased body weight and development of obesity in populations, the *sustained* reduction of energy intake and weight maintenance will require reduced intake of both of these nutrients. The underlying principle for a reduction in total fat intake is to reduce energy intake from the consumption of the most energy-dense macronutrient in order to prevent weight gain and ultimately obesity. The recommendation in the UK is to consume no more than 35% of total energy from fat. Since weight gain is associated with raised plasma TAGs and abnormalities in circulating lipoproteins, reducing total fat intake should, in theory, reduce blood lipids. However, in practice there is little evidence to support such an effect within populations. Meta-analyses have revealed that little benefit is to be gained, at least in terms of changes in serum lipids, by reducing total fat without altering the quality of dietary fat, possibly because different fatty acids exert different effects on CVD risk. The same applies to carbohydrates in respect of the opposing influences of excess free sugars and dietary fibre on increasing and decreasing cardio-metabolic risk, respectively.

The replacement of SFA with unsaturated fatty acids, (n-6 PUFA and MUFA) and the inclusion of adequate amounts of long chain n-3 PUFA, has been shown to produce favourable effects on cardio-metabolic risk factors, especially in individuals with a deficiency of these fatty acid in their tissues (low "n-3 index"). This includes effects on dyslipidaemia (e.g., reducing serum TAG in the post-absorotive and postprandial phases), vascular dysfunction, blood pressure and reducing depots of ectopic fat, most notably in the liver. Dietary free sugars (added sugars, mainly sucrose and fructose) may also contribute to cardio-metabolic risk through the direct metabolic effects of sugars at high level of intake (>20% total energy), and indirectly by contributing to body weight. Resistant starches and dietary fibre also have favourable effects in reducing cardio-metabolic risk.

Long chain n-3 PUFA

Long chain n-3 PUFA have been associated with a range of cardio-protective properties that come into effect at different levels of exposure (Mozaffarian D & Rimm EB *JAMA* 2006; 296: 1885-1899). Many of the beneficial effects of the these fatty acids impact on the more acute endpoints events of CHD, such as preventing thrombotic tendency, plaque rupture and arrhythmia, and are not ascribed to the longer term benefits on body fat depots and blood lipids. However, there is also convincing evidence to show that fish oil supplementation (1 g/day for three years) reduces the incidence of death from CHD in healthy, free-living subjects. This longer term benefit may be linked to the effects of eicosapentaenoic acid/docosahexaenoic acid on a host of other cardiometabolic risk factors, including plasma TAGs and lipoproteins.

Importantly, LC n-3s PUFA, either in supplements or oily fish, do not lower but increase serum LDL-cholesterol by between 5-10% in most intervention studies, especially in individuals with moderately raised serum TAG. This is not necessarily an adverse effect of these fatty acids, and can be explained, in part, by changes in the type and metabolic behavior of VLDL, a precursor of LDL, and increase in LDL particle size.

Long-chain n-3 PUFAs exert multiple effects on lipid metabolism, the most notable of which is the capacity to decrease post-absorptive plasma TAG levels by 20–30%. Fish oil-enriched diets have also been shown to attenuate the magnitude and duration of post-prandial lipemic response, following the ingestion of a fat-containing meal, by stimulating the activity of lipoprotein lipase

(LPL) in adipose tissue. These effects are accompanied by a beneficial reduction in the concentration of remnant lipoproteins that can deliver their cholesterol to the artery wall and lipids to ectopic sites like the liver, and increases in the particle size and composition of circulating LDL and HDL, all of which favour reduced CVD risk. Long chain n-3 PUFAs have potent metabolic effects in the liver, where they suppress the production of endogenous TAG by inhibiting the enzymes phosphatidic acid phosphatase and diacylglycerol acyltransferase. They may also selectively increase the degradation of apoB-100, further reducing the production of TAG-rich VLDLs. In intervention studies, LCn-3s have been associated with a relatively greater loss of liver fat than n-6 PUFA and SFA in non-alcoholic fatty liver disease (NAFLD). There is also evidence to suggest that people with NAFLD have a deficiency on LCn-3s in their liver and other tissues.

The current dietary recommendation for the intake of long-chain n-3 PUFAs (eicosapentaenoic acid/docosahexaenoic acid) in the UK is 450 mg/day (SACN, 2004). An aim of this recommendation was to increase intake by consuming two portions of fish per week, one of which should be oily (e.g., mackerel, sardines, salmon), though in reality, and depending on the source and composition of fish, two portions of oily fish (~120g) would be necessary to reach this target level of intake. This recommendation was based on evidence from a host of epidemiological and intervention studies, which showed that regular fish consumption could reduce the risk of sudden cardiac death.

Despite the established effects of long chain n-3 PUFA on cardio-metabolic risk factors, there is little evidence for the direct benefit of these fatty acids in reducing the morbidity and cardiovascular endpoints of CHD/CVD in populations. This has been confirmed in a meta-analyses of randomly controlled trials which concluded: "*We found high-quality evidence that long-chain omega-3 fats do not have important positive or negative effects on mortality or CVD events and moderate-quality evidence that they have little or no effect on other measures of cardiovascular health in primary or secondary prevention*".

Possible explanations for this apparent paradox are that the outcomes of this meta-analysis applied to capsule supplements and not to fish as food, which the study was unable to evaluate. Long chain n-3 PUFA produced clear benefits in CVD endpoints for some groups of individuals and no benefits in others, but these results effectively cancel each other out, so there is no overall effect. This is also seen in population studies in which a targeted response to long chain n-3 PUFA, is diluted-out by a lack of response in other members of the population without that particular condition requiring the treatment. This is analogous in some ways to treating a population of diseased and non-diseased people with a drug that exerts no effects on those without the disease. The benefits of long chain n-3 PUFA in reducing CVD are mediated through effects on cardiometabolic risk factors that may arise, in part, from a deficiency of these fatty acids, as measured by a low amounts of EPA and DHA in cell membranes ("n-3 index" %EPA+DHA in red blood cell membranes). It could be argued, that since meta-analyses are using clinical endpoints of CVD/CHD that do not discriminate between the metabolic origin of the disease, this helps to explain why the outcomes are equivocal and may potentially disadvantage those who could gain benefit from these fatty acids. Fortunately, the dietary recommendation to eat all fish, not just oily fish, is because of the epidemiological evidence, but also because of other, potentially beneficial components within fish other than LC n-3 PUFA (minerals, bioactive peptides).

Dietary carbohydrates: resistant starches, sugars and fibres

Carbohydrates produce significant effects on the metabolism of lipids in health and disease. A major report from SACN in the UK entitled: *Carbohydrates and Health* (2015) produced no evidence to link either the intake of total dietary carbohydrates or sugars with CVD or type 2 diabetes. Sugar sweetened beverages were shown to be significantly associated with the development of type 2 diabetes, and the intake of sugars was shown to make a significant contribution to energy intake and thus body weight. The intake of dietary fibre showed impressively strong and significant negative associations with the incidence of both CVD and type 2 diabetes. This evidence was used to inform two recommendations; to reduce intake of free (added) sugars to no more than 5% total energy intake (current intake in the UK ~12%), and to increase dietary fibre intake to 20g and 30g/day for women and men, respectively (current intake ~12g/day).

Free sugars, but more specifically fructose, has been vilified as being potentially "toxic" to health, "the new tobacco" and "alcohol without the buzz". These outlandish claims are based to a large extent on evidence from short term studies in which the participants were fed extremely high amounts of fructose (20–25% total energy), usually in liquid form. While the outcome of these studies was dramatic in demonstrating the acute, adverse effects of such high intakes of dietary fructose, in increasing post-prandial serum TAG, visceral adipose tissue, fat synthesis in the liver, and insulin resistance, it was also misleading in exaggerating the possible outcomes to the health of populations consuming much lower levels of fructose and sucrose. Dietary intake data in the UK and US indicates that the majority of people consume something closer to 12% as free sugars, only half of which is fructose. Although this may still be a detriment to cardio-metabolic health via its contribution to body weight over a much longer term than a matter of weeks, it is unlikely to exert the dramatic effects shown in these studies. The same dietary intake data reveals that smaller groups of individuals do consume free sugars at levels approaching 20% and beyond who may be susceptible to the direct adverse metabolic effects of free sugars. This applies especially to children and young adolescents who as such, represent the most important target group for the restriction of free sugars.

9.12 Perspectives on the future

With hindsight, it is possible to see how future perspectives from the earlier editions of this chapter panned out over the course of time, to either transform and advance nutritional practice or to be superseded by new evidence and new perspectives. What has become clearer in the intervening years is the recognition of critical stages of the human life cycle, at which dietary change is of increased importance in maintaining health by altering an often inevitable trajectory towards ill-health. The earliest origins of disease that may be influenced by diet begin before life, such as the imprinting of epigenetic signatures that can be inherited through generations, and influence of maternal diet on the developing fetus. Childhood and adolescence are periods when there is a propensity to develop obesity through inappropriate food choice and sedentary lifestyle, and have become a focus of concern for the prevention of disease co-morbidity in adult life. Middle-age can be a prolonged period when diet and lifestyle habits reach a steady state, but body burden of risk from a long term exposure to a diet insults manifests as the first and often fatal endpoints of chronic degenerative disease like CVD. Diet and lifestyle habits may then change radically as humans retire from working life and enter old age. At this stage, any metabolic dysfunction in lipid metabolism arising from excess body fat, especially visceral and ectopic fat, will be further compounded by the rapid, age-related loss of skeletal muscle and development of sarcopenic obesity.

What has also emerged in the intervening years is a greater need to understand the biological effects and impact on health of nutrients in whole foods within dietary patterns. Progress in this area should help to overcome the inherent difficulty in trying to translate nutrient-based dietary guidelines into whole food-based diets. It also draws attention to the effects of food processing in reducing nutrient content and removing the food matrix. The latter represents a vital component of whole foods that can alter the bioavailability and prevent the inappropriately rapid absorption and entry of nutrients, (chiefly sugar and fats), into the postprandial circulation.

Other perspectives on the future include the need to improve the ongoing inadequacy of our methods to measure dietary intake with greater accuracy and precision. In this respect, the exponential growth and application of digital technology has produced a quantum leap in our capacity to self-assess and manage our diet and lifestyle behaviours. There is also a need to move away from what has become a fashionable exclusion of single nutrients, typically fat, to promote weight loss. While there is evidence to support the physiological effects of excluding carbohydrates that could influence energy balance and facilitate weight loss, the exclusion of either fat or carbohydrate are equally efficacious in promoting weight loss and are less likely to be sustained in populations relative to diets with a balanced intake of macronutrients. Lastly, there is continued need to develop new phenomic-based technologies and biomarkers to tailor the dietary management of risk in individuals with increased susceptibility and resilience to disease.

Summary of priorities in nutrition and the metabolism of lipids

1 To increase knowledge, from primary randomly controlled trials, of the biological effects of dietary fatty acids, especially SFA and MUFA, in foods from animal (e.g., meat, dairy) and plant sources, and whole diets. Optimise macronutrient intake to reduce the impact of dietary fatty acids and carbohydrates on post-prandial lipid metabolism.
2 To gain a better understanding of the pathophysiological significance of body fat depots; the metabolic flexibility of subcutaneous adipose tissue, visceral AT as determinants of ectopic fat deposition in key metabolic organs (liver, pancreas) and skeletal muscle. How these fat depots are influenced by diet and determine different 'obese' phenotypes (e.g. metabolic or benign).
3 Develop biomarkers of variation in dietary responsiveness metabolic phenotypes or "metabotypes". Increase the application of metabolomics and phenomics to better understand qualitative and quantitative traits, including clinical, metabolic, biochemical, and imaging methodologies, for the refinement and characterisation of a phenotype.
4 Understanding difference in variation in the relationship between diet and lipid metabolism in males and females, and different ethnic groups.
5 Increased cross-disciplinary research between nutritional-lipid metabolism and: (i) behavioral psychology to understand psychobiological interactions between metabolic and behavioural origins of food choice and intake; ii) chrono-nutrition and meal timing and importance of mismatched biological and behavioural rhythms, and partial sleep deprivation to the control of energy intake and expenditure at critical stages of the human life cycle; iii) brain-gut-metabolic axis; bi-directional links between "i–ii" through interactions between diet, the microbiota (gut barrier function), brain and lipid metabolism.

This chapter has been revised and updated by Bruce Griffin based on the chapter in the second edition (2009) by Bruce Griffin and Stephen Cunnane.

References

Bloomfield(1960). The formation of Δ^9-unsaturated fatty acids. *J Biol Chem* **235**: 337–345.

Burr, M.M. and Burr, G.O. (1929). A new deficiency disease produced by the rigid exclusion of fat from the diet. *J Biol Chem* **82**: 345–367.

Goldstein, J.L. and Brown, M.S. (1977). Atherosclerosis: the LDL receptor hypothesis. *Metabolism* **26**: 1257–1275.

Hegsted, D.M., McGrandy, R.B., Myers, M.L. *et al.* (1965). Quantitative effects of dietary fat on serum cholesterol in man. *Am J Clin Nutr.* **17**: 281–295.

Keys, A., Anderson, J.T. and Grande, F. (1977). Prediction of serum cholesterol responses of man to changes in fats in the diet. *Lancet* **2**: 959–966.

Pett, K.D., Kahn, J., Willett, W.C. *et al.* (2017). Ancel Keys and the Seven Countries Study: *An Evidence-based Response to Revisionist Histories.* White Paper Commissioned by The True Health Initiative http://www.truehealthinitiative.org/

Ponticorvo, L., Rittenberg, D. and Bloch, K. (1949). The utilisation of acetate for the synthesis of fatty acids, cholesterol and protoporphyrin. *J Biol Chem* **179**: 839–842.

Scientific Advisory Committee on Nutrition (SACN) (2004). Report published for the Food Standards Agency and the Department of Health by TSO. ISBN 0-11-243083-X.

Willet, W.C., Stamfer, M.J., Manson, J.E. *et al.* (1993). Intake of trans fatty acids and risk of coronary heart disease among women, *Lancet* **341**: 581–585.

Zilversmit, D.B. (1979). Atherogenesis is a postprandial phenomenon. *Circulation.* **60**: 473–485.

Further reading

Cunnane, S.C. (1995). Alpha-linolenate acid in human nutrition. In: (Ed. S.C. Cunnane, L.U. Thompson) *Flaxseed in Human Nutrition.* Champaign, IL: AOCS Press, 99–127.

Dolecek, T.A. (1992). Epidemiological evidence of relationships between dietary polyunsaturated fatty acids and mortality in the Multiple Risk Factor Intervention Trial. *Proc Soc Exp Biol Med.* **200**: 177–182.

Durrington, P.N. (1995). *Hyperlipidaemia Diagnosis and Management*, 2e. Oxford: Elsevier Science.

Griffin, B.A. (2001). The effects of n-3 PUFA on LDL subfractions. *Lipids* **36**: S91–S97.

Griffin, B.A. (2008). How relevant is the ratio of dietary n-6 to n-3 polyunsaturated fatty acids to cardiovascular disease risk? Evidence from the OPTILIP Study. *Curr Opin Lipidol* **19**: 57–62.

Lands, W.E.M. (2001). Impact of daily food choices on health promotion and disease prevention. In: Hamazaki H, Okuyama H, eds. *Fatty Acids and Lipids: New Findings.* Basel, Karger. 1–5.

Lee, A. and Griffin, B.A. (2006). Dietary cholesterol, eggs and coronary heart disease in perspective. *Br Nutr Found Bull* **31**: 21–27.

Mangiapane, E.H. and Salter, A.M. (Eds). (1999). *Diet, Lipoproteins and Coronary Heart Disease. A Biochemical Perspective*. Nottingham: Nottingham University Press.

Simopoulos, A.P. (2001). Evolutionary aspects of diet and essential fatty acids. In: Hamazaki H, Okuyama H, eds. *Fatty Acids and Lipids: New Findings*. Basel: Karger. 18–27.

Willett, W.C. (2001). *Eat, Drink and Be Healthy: The Harvard Medical School Guide to Healthy Eating*. New York: Simon and Schuster.

10
The Vitamins

David A. Bender

Key messages

- The vitamins are a chemically disparate group of compounds with a variety of functions in the body.
- What they have in common is that they are organic compounds that are required for the maintenance of normal health and metabolic integrity.
- Vitamins are required in very small amounts, of the order of milligrams or micrograms per day, and thus can be distinguished from the essential fatty acids and the essential amino acids, which are required in larger amounts of grams per day.
- Where relevant, this chapter will deal with each of the vitamins under the following headings:
  - vitamers
  - absorption and metabolism
  - metabolic functions and other uses
  - deficiency
  - requirements
  - assessment of status
  - toxicity and drug interactions.

10.1 Introduction

In order to demonstrate that a compound is a vitamin, it is necessary to demonstrate both that deprivation of experimental subjects will lead to the development of a more or less specific clinical deficiency disease and abnormal metabolic signs, and that restoration of the missing compound will prevent or cure the deficiency disease and normalise metabolic abnormalities. It is not enough simply to demonstrate that a compound has a function in the body, since it may normally be synthesised in adequate amounts to meet requirements, or that a compound cures a disease, since this may simply reflect a pharmacological action and not indicate that the compound is a dietary essential.

The vitamins, and their principal functions and deficiency signs, are shown in Table 10.1; the curious nomenclature is a consequence of the way in which they were discovered at the beginning of the twentieth century. Early studies showed that there was something in milk that was essential, in very small amounts, for the growth of animals fed on a diet consisting of purified fat, carbohydrate, protein, and mineral salts. Two factors were found to be essential: one was found in the cream and the other in the watery part of milk. Logically, they were called factor A (fat-soluble, in the cream) and factor B (water-soluble, in the watery part of the milk). Factor B was identified chemically as an amine, and in 1913 the name "vitamin" was coined for these "vital amines."

Further studies showed that "vitamin B" was a mixture of a number of compounds, with different actions in the body, and so they were given numbers as well: vitamin B_1, vitamin B_2, and so on. There are gaps in the numerical order of the B vitamins. When what might have been called vitamin B_3 was discovered, it was found to be a chemical compound that was already known, nicotinic acid. It was therefore not given a number. Other gaps are because compounds that were assumed to be vitamins and were given numbers, such as B_4 and B_5, were later shown

Introduction to Human Nutrition, Third Edition. Edited on behalf of The Nutrition Society by Susan A. Lanham-New, Thomas R. Hill, Alison M. Gallagher and Hester H. Vorster.

Companion website: www.wiley.com/go/lanham-new/humannutrition

Table 10.1 The vitamins

Vitamin		Functions	Deficiency disease
A	Retinol β-carotene	Visual pigments in the retina; regulation of gene expression and cell differentiation; (β-carotene is an antioxidant)	Night blindness, xerophthalmia; keratinisation of skin.
D	Calciferol	Maintenance of calcium balance; enhances intestinal absorption of Ca^{2+} and mobilises bone mineral	Rickets = poor mineralisation of bone; osteomalacia = bone demineralisation
E	Tocopherols tocotrienols	Antioxidant, especially in cell membranes	Extremely rare - serious neurological dysfunction
K	Phylloquinone menaquinones	Coenzyme in formation of γ-carboxy-glutamate in proteins of blood clotting and bone matrix	Impaired blood clotting, haemorrhagic disease
B_1	Thiamin	Coenzyme in pyruvate and α-ketoglutarate dehydrogenases, and transketolase; role in nerve conduction	Peripheral nerve damage (beriberi) or central nervous system lesions (Wernicke-Korsakoff syndrome)
B_2	Riboflavin	Coenzyme in oxidation and reduction reactions; prosthetic group of flavoproteins	Lesions of corner of mouth, lips and tongue, sebhorroeic dermatitis
Niacin	Nicotinic acid nicotinamide	Coenzyme in oxidation and reduction reactions, functional part of NAD and NADP	Pellagra - photosensitive dermatitis, depressive psychosis,
B_6	Pyridoxine pyridoxal pyridoxamine	Coenzyme in transamination and decarboxylation of amino acids and glycogen phosphorylase; role in steroid hormone action	Disorders of amino acid metabolism, convulsions
B_{12}	Cobalamin	Coenzyme in transfer of one-carbon fragments and metabolism of folate	Pernicious anaemia = megaloblastic anaemia with degeneration of the spinal cord.
	Folic acid	Coenzyme in transfer of one-carbon fragments	Megaloblastic anaemia
H	Biotin	Coenzyme in carboxylation reactions in gluconeogenesis and fatty acid synthesis	Impaired fat and carbohydrate metabolism, dermatitis
	Pantothenic acid	Functional part of CoA and acyl carrier protein fatty acid synthesis and metabolism	Peripheral nerve damage (nutritional melalgia, "burning foot" syndrome)
C	Ascorbic acid	Coenzyme in hydroxylation of proline and lysine in collagen synthesis; anti-oxidant; enhances absorption of iron	Scurvy - impaired wound healing, loss of dental cement, subcutaneous hemorrhage

either not to be vitamins, or to be vitamins that had already been described by other workers and given other names.

Vitamins C, D, and E were named in the order of their discovery. The name "vitamin F" was used at one time for what we now call the essential fatty acids; "vitamin G" was later found to be what was already known as vitamin B_2. Biotin is still sometimes called vitamin H. Vitamin K was discovered by Henrik Dam, in Denmark, as a result of studies of disorders of blood coagulation, and he named it for its function: *koagulation* in Danish.

As the chemistry of the vitamins was elucidated, so they were given names as well, as shown in Table 10.1. When only one chemical compound has the biological activity of the vitamin, this is quite easy. Thus, vitamin B_1 is thiamin, vitamin B_2 is riboflavin, etc. With several of the vitamins, a number of chemically related compounds found in foods can be interconverted in the body, and all show the same biological activity. Such chemically related compounds are called vitamers, and a general name (a generic descriptor) is used to include all compounds that display the same biological activity.

It has long been known that intestinal bacteria synthesise relatively large amounts of some of the water-soluble vitamins; indeed they may synthesise amounts of folate and biotin almost equal to the normal dietary intake, and bacterial synthesis of thiamin, riboflavin, nicotinic acid, biotin, and folate can all be increased when the diet contains relatively large amounts of fermentable non-glycaemic carbohydrates (dietary fibre). This bacterial contribution to vitamin nutrition has largely been ignored, since conventional wisdom was that absorption occurs in the small, rather than large, intestine. However, specific high affinity carrier-mediated transport systems for thiamin, riboflavin, nicotinic acid, biotin and folate have been identified in the colon, suggesting that intestinal bacterial synthesis may indeed make a significant contribution to vitamin nutrition.

Some compounds have important metabolic functions, but are not considered to be vitamins, since, as far as is known, they can be synthesised in the body in adequate amounts to meet requirements. These include carnitine, choline, inositol, taurine, and ubiquinone.

Two compounds that are generally considered to be vitamins can be synthesised in the body, normally in adequate amounts to meet requirements: vitamin D, which is synthesised from 7-dehydrocholesterol in the skin on exposure to sunlight; and niacin, which is synthesised from the essential amino acid tryptophan. However, both were discovered as a result of studies of deficiency diseases that were, during the early twentieth century, significant public health problems: rickets (due to vitamin D deficiency and inadequate sunlight exposure) and pellagra (due to deficiency of both tryptophan and preformed niacin).

10.2 Vitamin A

Vitamin A was the first vitamin to be discovered, initially as an essential dietary factor for growth. It has a role in vision, as the prosthetic group of the light-sensitive proteins in the retina, and a major role in the regulation of gene expression and tissue differentiation. Deficiency is a major public health problem in large areas of the world, and prevention of vitamin A deficiency is one of the three micronutrient priorities of the World Health Organisation (WHO) (the other two are iron and iodine).

Vitamers and international units

Two groups of compounds, shown in Figure 10.1, have vitamin A activity: retinol, retinaldehyde, and retinoic acid (preformed vitamin A); and a variety of carotenes and related compounds (collectively known as carotenoids) that can be cleaved oxidatively to yield retinaldehyde, and hence retinol and retinoic acid. Those carotenoids that can be cleaved to yield retinaldehyde are known as provitamin A carotenoids.

Preformed vitamin A (mainly as retinyl esters) is found only in foods of animal origin. The richest source by far is liver, which may contain sufficient vitamin A to pose a potential problem for pregnant women, since retinol is teratogenic in excess. Carotenes are found in green, yellow, and red fruits and vegetables, as well as in liver, margarine, and milk and milk products. In addition to their role as precursors of vitamin A, carotenoids have potentially useful antioxidant action, and there is epidemiological evidence that diets that are rich in carotenoids (both those that are vitamin A active and those that are not) are associated with a lower incidence of cancer and cardiovascular disease. However, intervention studies with β-carotene have been disappointing, and it is not possible to determine desirable intakes of carotene other than as a precursor of vitamin A.

Retinoic acid is a metabolite of retinol; it has important biological activities in its own right and will support growth in vitamin A-deficient animals. The oxidation of retinaldehyde to retinoic acid is irreversible, so that retinoic acid cannot be converted *in vivo* to retinol, and does not support either vision or fertility in deficient animals.

Some 50 or more dietary carotenoids are potential sources of vitamin A: α-, β-, and γ-carotenes and cryptoxanthin are quantitatively the most important. Although it would appear from its structure that one molecule of β-carotene will yield two of retinol, this is not so in practice. Nutritionally, 6–12 μg of β-carotene is equivalent to 1 μg of preformed retinol. For other carotenes with vitamin A activity, 12–24 μg is equivalent to 1 μg of preformed retinol.

Conventionally, the total amount of vitamin A in foods is expressed as μg retinol equivalents, calculated from the sum of μg of preformed vitamin A + 1/6 × μg β-carotene + 1/12 × μg other provitamin A carotenoids. Recent studies on the absorption of carotenes and their bioefficacy as vitamin A precursors have led to the definition of retinol activity equivalents. 1 μg retinol activity equivalent = 1 μg preformed retinol, 12 μg β-carotene or 24 μg of other provitamin A carotenoids.

Before pure vitamin A was available for chemical analysis, the vitamin A content of foods was determined by biological assays and the results

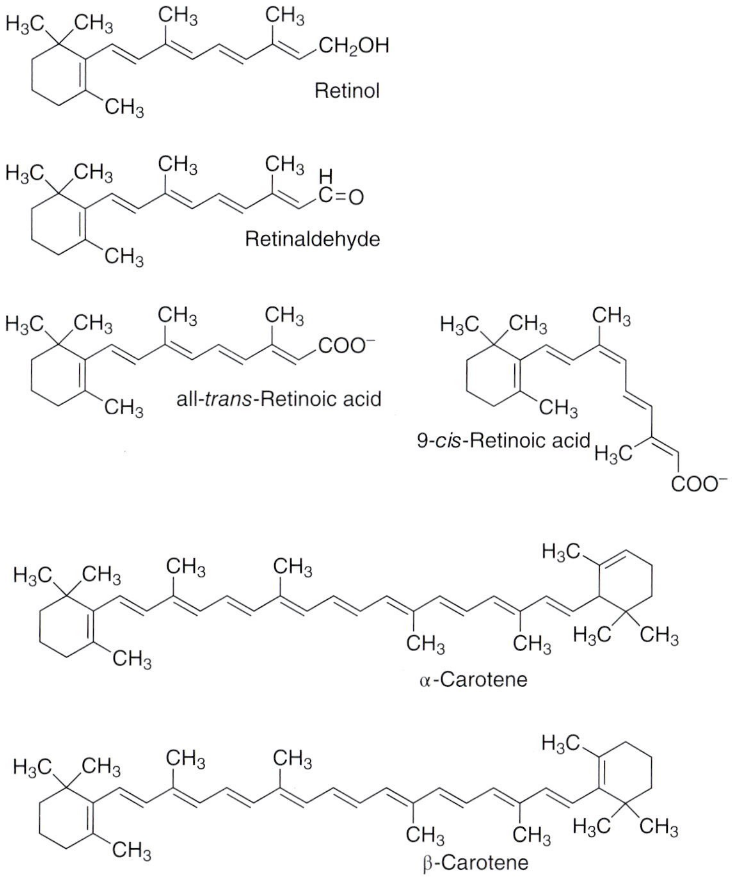

Figure 10.1 The major vitamin A vitamers and vitamin A active carotenoids.

were expressed in standardised international units (IU): 1 IU = 0.3 μg of retinol, or 1 μg of retinol = 3.33 IU. Although obsolete, IU are sometimes still used in food labelling.

Metabolism and storage of vitamin A and pro-vitamin A carotenoids

Retinol is absorbed from the small intestine dissolved in lipid. About 70–90% of dietary retinol is normally absorbed, and even at high levels of intake this falls only slightly. However, in people with a very low fat intake (less than about 10% of energy from fat), absorption of both retinol and carotene is impaired, and low-fat diets are associated with vitamin A deficiency.

Dietary retinyl esters are hydrolysed by lipases in the intestinal lumen and mucosal brush border membrane, absorbed in lipid micelles, then re-esterified to form retinyl palmitate before release into the circulation in chylomicrons. Assuming an adequate intake of fat, 70–90% of dietary retinol is absorbed.

Tissues can take up retinyl esters from chylomicrons, but most retinol is in the chylomicron remnants that are taken up by the liver. Here retinyl esters are hydrolysed, and the vitamin may either be secreted from the liver bound to retinol binding protein, or be transferred to stellate cells in the liver, where it is stored as retinyl esters in intracellular lipid droplets. Some 50–80% of the total body content of retinol is in the stellate cells of the liver, but a significant amount may also be stored in adipose tissue.

The main pathway for catabolism of retinol is oxidation to retinoic acid has important biological activities in its own right, distinct from the activities of retinol. The main excretory product of both retinol and retinoic acid is retinoyl glucuronide, which is secreted in the bile.

As the intake of retinol increases, and the liver concentration rises above 70 μmol/kg, a different pathway becomes increasingly important for the catabolism of retinol in the liver. This is a microsomal cytochrome P_{450}-dependent oxidation, leading to a number of polar metabolites that are excreted in the urine and bile. At high intakes this pathway becomes saturated, and excess retinol is toxic since there is no further capacity for its catabolism and excretion.

Carotene dioxygenase

Like retinol, carotenoids are absorbed dissolved in lipid micelles. The biological availability and absorption of dietary carotene varies between 5% and 60%, depending on the nature of the food, whether it is cooked or raw, and the amount of fat in the meal.

As shown in Figure 10.2, β-carotene and other provitamin A carotenoids are cleaved in the intestinal mucosa by carotene dioxygenase, yielding retinaldehyde, which is reduced to retinol, then esterified and secreted in chylomicrons together with retinyl esters formed from dietary retinol.

Only a proportion of carotene undergoes oxidation in the intestinal mucosa, and a significant amount enters the circulation in chylomicrons. Carotene in the chylomicron remnants is cleared by the liver; some is cleaved by hepatic carotene dioxygenase, again giving rise to retinaldehyde and retinyl esters; the remainder is secreted in very low-density lipoprotein (VLDL), and may be taken up and cleaved by carotene dioxygenase in other tissues.

Central oxidative cleavage of β-carotene, as shown in Figure 10.2, should yield two molecules of retinaldehyde, which can be reduced to retinol. However, as noted above, the biological

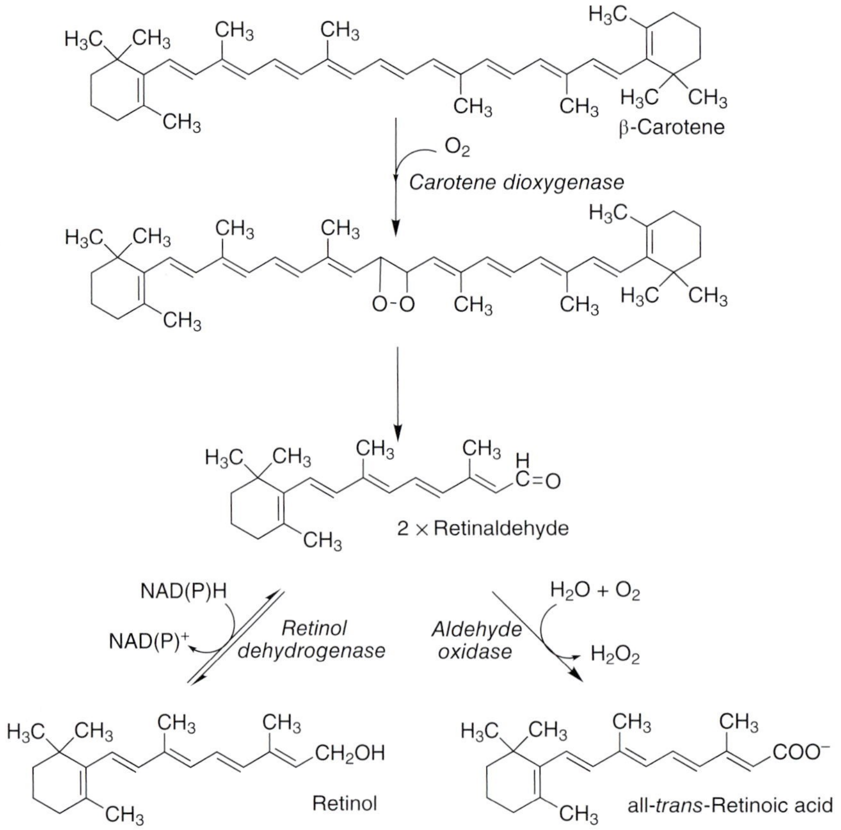

Figure 10.2 The oxidative cleavage of carotene to yield retinol and retinoic acid. Carotene dioxygenase (EC 1.13.11.21), retinol dehydrogenase (EC 1.1.1.105), retinaldehyde oxidase (EC 1.2.3.11).

activity of β-carotene, on a molar basis, is considerably lower than that of retinol, not twofold higher as might be expected. In addition to poor absorption of carotene, three factors may account for this.

- The intestinal activity of carotene dioxygenase is relatively low, so that a relatively large proportion of ingested β-carotene may be absorbed unchanged.
- Other carotenoids in the diet may inhibit carotene dioxygenase and reduce the formation of retinol.
- The principal site of carotene dioxygenase attack is the central bond of β-carotene, but asymmetric cleavage also occurs, leading to the formation of 8′-, 10′- and 12′-apo-carotenals, which are oxidised to yield retinoic acid, but are not precursors of retinol or retinaldehyde.

Plasma retinol binding protein

Retinol is released from the liver bound to an α-globulin, retinol binding protein (RBP); this serves to maintain the vitamin in aqueous solution, protects it against oxidation, and delivers the vitamin to target tissues. RBP is secreted from the liver as a 1:1 complex with the thyroxine-binding prealbumin, transthyretin. This is important to prevent urinary loss of retinol bound to the relatively small RBP, which would otherwise be filtered by the kidney, with a considerable loss of vitamin A from the body.

Cell surface receptors on target tissues take up retinol from the RBP–transthyretin complex, transferring it on to an intracellular RBP. The receptors also remove the carboxy-terminal arginine residue from RBP, so inactivating it by reducing its affinity for both transthyretin and retinol. As a result, apo-RBP is filtered at the glomerulus; most is reabsorbed in the proximal renal tubules and hydrolysed. The apoprotein is not recycled.

During the development of vitamin A deficiency in experimental animals, the plasma concentration of RBP falls, whereas the liver content of apo-RBP rises. The administration of retinol results in release of holo-RBP from the liver. This provides the basis of the relative dose–response (RDR) test for liver reserves of vitamin A.

Metabolic functions of vitamin A and carotenes

The first function of vitamin A to be defined was in vision, where it is retinaldehyde that is important; retinoic acid has a major function in regulation of gene expression and tissue differentiation. Vitamin A also acts as a carrier of mannosyl units in the synthesis of hydrophobic glycoproteins. Retinoic acid also has a role in modulating the actions of cell-surface acting hormones and neurotransmitters, acting to retinoylate cAMP-dependent protein kinases.

Vitamin A in vision

In the retina, retinaldehyde functions as the prosthetic group of the light-sensitive opsin proteins, forming rhodopsin (in rods) and iodopsin (in cones). Any one cone cell contains only one type of opsin, and hence is sensitive to only one colour of light. Colour blindness results from loss or mutation of one or other of the cone opsins.

In the pigment epithelium of the retina, all-*trans*-retinol is isomerised to 11-*cis*-retinol and then oxidised to 11-*cis*-retinaldehyde. This reacts with a lysine residue in opsin, forming the holoprotein rhodopsin. As shown in Figure 10.3, the absorption of light by rhodopsin causes isomerisation of the retinaldehyde bound to opsin from 11-*cis* to all-*trans*, and a conformational change in opsin. This results in the release of retinaldehyde from the protein and the initiation of a nerve impulse. The overall process is known as bleaching, since it results in the loss of the color of rhodopsin. The all-*trans*-retinaldehyde released from rhodopsin is reduced to all-*trans*-retinol, and joins the pool of retinol in the pigment epithelium for isomerisation to 11-*cis*-retinol and regeneration of rhodopsin. The key to initiation of the visual cycle is the availability of 11-*cis*-retinaldehyde, and hence vitamin A. In deficiency both the time taken to adapt to darkness and the ability to see in poor light are impaired.

The excited form of rhodopsin (metarhodopsin II) initiates a G-protein cascade leading to hyperpolarisation of the outer section membrane of the rod or cone, caused by the closure of sodium channels through the membrane, and the initiation of a nerve impulse.

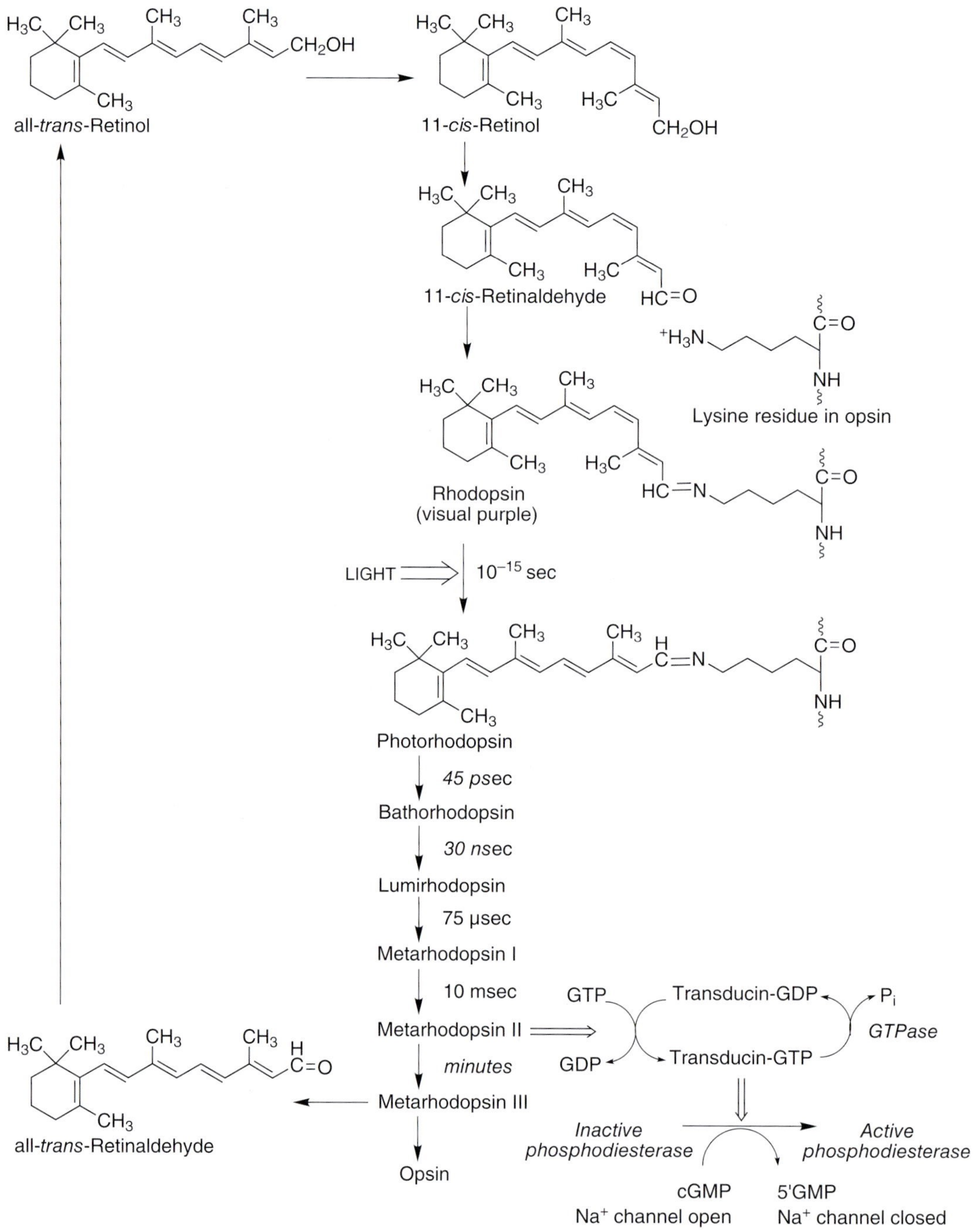

Figure 10.3 Role of vitamin A and the cyclic GMP cascade in the visual cycle. Retinol isomerase (EC 5.2.1.3), phosphodiesterase (EC 3.1.4.35).

Retinoic acid and the regulation of gene expression

Retinoic acid has a general role in growth and a specific morphogenic role in development and tissue differentiation. These functions are the result of nuclear actions, modulating gene expression by activation of nuclear receptor proteins that bind to response elements (control regions) of DNA, and regulate the transcription of specific genes. Both deficiency and excess of retinoic acid cause severe developmental abnormalities. Both all-*trans*-retinoic acid and 9-*cis*-retinoic acid are involved; they have different actions in different tissues.

There are two families of nuclear retinoid receptors: the retinoic acid receptors (RARs) bind all-*trans*-retinoic acid or 9-*cis*-retinoic acid; and the retinoid X receptors (RXRs) bind 9-*cis*-retinoic acid and some of the other physiologically active retinoids. RXR can form dimers with RARs, RXRs (homodimers), and the receptors for calcitriol (the active metabolite of vitamin D), thyroid hormone, long-chain polyunsaturated fatty acid (PUFA) derivatives [the peroxisome proliferators-activated receptor (PPAR)], and two orphan receptor for which the physiological ligands have not yet been identified (the COUP receptors).

The result of this is that a very large number of genes are sensitive to control by retinoic acid in different tissues, and at different stages in development, and retinoic acid is also essential for the normal responses to vitamin D, thyroid hormone and long-chain PUFA derivatives. Activation of PPAR receptors by binding to occupied RXR leads to increased expression of genes regulating lipid and carbohydrate metabolism, resulting in increased lipolysis and enhanced insulin responsiveness.

Unoccupied RXRs can form homodimers and heterodimers with calcitriol and other receptors; these bind to hormone response elements on DNA, but not only do not lead to activation of transcription, but downregulate it. This means that vitamin A deficiency has a more marked effect than that due simply to lack of occupied receptors, and will impair responses to vitamin D and thyroid hormone more markedly than might be expected simply from lack of 9-*cis*-retinoic acid to form active heterodimers.

Vitamin A in excess may also impair responsiveness to vitamin D and other hormones, since high concentrations of 9-*cis*-retinoic acid will lead to the formation of RXR–RXR homodimers, leaving too few RXRs to form heterodimers with vitamin D and other receptors. There is epidemiological evidence that habitually high intakes of vitamin A are associated with poor bone health in later life as a result of impaired responsiveness to vitamin D.

The antioxidant function of carotenes

At least *in vitro*, and under conditions of low oxygen availability, carotenes can act as radical-trapping antioxidants. There is epidemiological evidence that high intakes of carotene are associated with a low incidence of cardiovascular disease and some forms of cancer, although the results of intervention trials with β-carotene have been disappointing, with an increased incidence of lung cancer among those taking carotene supplements.

The problem is that although carotene is an antioxidant at a low partial pressure of oxygen, as occurs in most tissues, at a high partial pressure of oxygen, as occurs in the lungs, it is an autocatalytic pro-oxidant, acting as a source of oxygen radicals. It is also possible that the epidemiological association between high intakes of carotene and lower incidence of disease is epiphenomenonal, since plant foods that are the source of carotenes are also sources of a variety of potentially protective phytonutrients.

Vitamin A deficiency: night blindness and xerophthalmia

Worldwide, vitamin A deficiency is a major public health problem and the most important preventable cause of blindness; WHO estimated in 2005 that some 190 million children under 5 years old show subclinical deficiency (low serum retinol), 5.2 million suffer from night blindness, and 2.7 million have xerophthalmia. Globally, 19.1 million pregnant women have low serum retinol, and 9.8 million suffer from night blindness.

The earliest signs of clinical deficiency are associated with vision. Initially, there is a loss of sensitivity to green light; this is followed by impairment of the ability to adapt to dim light, then an inability to see at all in dim light: night blindness. More prolonged or severe deficiency leads to the condition called xerophthalmia: keratinisation of the cornea, followed by ulceration – irreversible damage to the eye that causes blindness. At the same time there are changes in the skin, with excessive formation of keratinised tissue.

Vitamin A also plays an important role in the differentiation of immune system cells, and mild deficiency, not severe enough to cause any disturbance of vision, leads to increased susceptibility to a variety of infectious diseases. A number of trials of vitamin A supplementation in areas of endemic deficiency have shown that it leads to a 20–35% reduction in childhood mortality.

The synthesis of RBP is reduced in response to infection (it is a negative acute-phase protein), so that there is a reduction in the circulating concentration of the vitamin, and hence further impairment of immune responses; a mild infection may trigger the development of xerophthalmia in children whose vitamin A status is marginal. There may also be urinary loss of vitamin A due to increased renal epithelial permeability and proteinuria, permitting loss of the vitamin bound to RBP-transthyretin.

Signs of vitamin A deficiency also occur in protein–energy malnutrition, regardless of whether or not the intake of vitamin A is adequate. This is due to impairment of the synthesis of plasma RBP; functional vitamin A deficiency can occur secondary to protein–energy malnutrition; even if liver reserves of the vitamin are adequate, it cannot be mobilised.

Various epithelia are affected by vitamin A deficiency, earlier than the more readily observed diagnostic changes in the eye. There is increased intestinal permeability to disaccharides, and later a reduction in the number of goblet cells and hence mucus secretion. There is also atrophy of respiratory epithelium, with loss of goblet cells, and keratinisation,

Vitamin A deficiency is also associated with reduced incorporation of iron into haemoglobin, and hence iron deficiency anaemia, with increased deposition of iron in liver and spleen. Conversely, iron deficiency leads to reduced plasma retinol concentrations and increased liver stores of vitamin A that are not adequately mobilised.

Vitamin A requirements and reference intakes

There have been relatively few studies of vitamin A requirements in which subjects have been depleted of the vitamin for long enough to permit the development of clear deficiency signs. Current estimates of requirements are based on the intakes required to maintain a concentration in the liver of 70 μmol retinol/kg, determined by measurement of the rate of metabolism of isotopically labeled vitamin A. This is adequate to maintain normal plasma concentrations of the vitamin, and people with this level of liver reserves can be maintained on a vitamin A-free diet for many months before they develop any detectable signs of deficiency.

The average requirement to maintain a concentration of 70 μmol/kg of liver is 6.7 μg retinol equivalents/kg body weight, and this is the basis for calculation of reference intakes.

Assessment of vitamin A status

The only direct assessment of vitamin A status is by liver biopsy and measurement of retinyl ester reserves. This is an invasive procedure that cannot be considered for routine investigations and population surveys. Status can also be assessed by clinical and functional tests, the plasma concentrations of retinol and RBP, and the response to a test dose of vitamin A, the relative dose response (RDR) test.

In field surveys, clinical signs of vitamin A deficiency, including Bitot's spots, corneal xerosis, corneal ulceration, and keratomalacia, can be used to identify those suffering from vitamin A deficiency. The earliest signs of corneal damage are detected by conjunctival impression cytology (CIC); however, abnormalities only develop when liver reserves are seriously depleted.

The ability to adapt to dim light is impaired early in deficiency, and dark adaptation time is sometimes used to assess vitamin A status. However, the test is not suitable for use on children (the group most at risk of deficiency) and the apparatus is not suited to use in the field.

The fasting plasma concentration of retinol remains constant over a wide range of intakes and only falls significantly when liver reserves are nearly depleted. Therefore, although less sensitive to subtle changes within the normal range than some methods of assessing nutritional status, measurement of plasma retinol provides a convenient and sensitive means of detecting people whose intake of vitamin A is inadequate to maintain normal liver reserves.

The RDR test is a test of the ability of a dose of retinol to raise the plasma concentration several hours after chylomicrons have been cleared from the circulation. It depends on the fact that apo-RBP accumulates in the liver in vitamin A deficiency. The RDR is the ratio of the plasma concentration of retinol 5 h after the dose to that immediately before it was given. An RDR greater than 20% indicates depletion of liver retinol to less than 70 μmol/kg.

Toxicity of vitamin A

There is only a limited capacity to metabolise vitamin A. Excessively high intakes lead to accumulation in the liver and other tissues, beyond the capacity of normal binding proteins, so that free, unbound, vitamin A is present. This leads to liver and bone damage, hair loss, vomiting, and headaches. Single doses of 60 mg of retinol are given to children in developing countries as a prophylactic against vitamin A deficiency: an amount adequate to meet the child's needs for four to six months. About 1% of children so treated show transient signs of toxicity, but this is considered an acceptable risk in view of the high prevalence and devastating effects of deficiency.

The chronic toxicity of vitamin A is a more general cause for concern; prolonged and regular intake of more than about 7.5–9 mg/day by adults (and significantly less for children) causes signs and symptoms of toxicity affecting:

- the central nervous system: headache, nausea, ataxia, and anorexia, all associated with increased cerebrospinal fluid pressure
- the liver: hepatomegaly with histological changes in the liver, increased collagen formation and hyperlipidemia
- bones: joint pains, thickening of the long bones, hypercalcaemia, and calcification of soft tissues
- skin: excessive dryness, scaling and chapping of the skin, desquamation and alopecia (hair loss).

The recommended upper limits of habitual intake of retinol, compared with reference intakes, are shown in Table 10.2. Habitual intakes of vitamin A around 1500 μg /day, albeit below these prudent upper levels of intake, may be associated with impaired responsiveness to vitamin D, poor mineralisation of bone, and the early development of osteoporosis and bone fracture, as a result of formation of RXR homodimers and consequent lack of RXR to dimerise with the vitamin D receptor.

Table 10.2 Tolerable upper levels of habitual intake of preformed retinol

	Tolerable upper limit	Reference intake	
	μg /day	μg /day	Ratio
Infants	900	350	2.6
1–3 years	1800	400	4.5
4–6 years	3000	500	6.0
6–12 years	4500	500	9.0
13–20 years	6000	600–700	8.6–10
Adult men	9000	700	12.9
Adult women	7500	600	12.5
Pregnant women	3000	700	4.3

Carotenoids do not cause hypervitaminosis A, because of the limited oxidation to retinol. Accumulation of even abnormally large amounts of carotene seems to have no short-term adverse effects, although plasma, body fat and skin can have a strong orange-yellow colour (hypercarotinaemia) following prolonged high intakes.

Teratogenicity of vitamin A

The synthetic retinoids (vitamin A analogues) used in dermatology are highly teratogenic. After women have been treated with them, it is recommended that contraceptive precautions be continued for 12 months, because of their retention in the body. By extrapolation, it has been assumed that retinol is also teratogenic. In case–control studies, intakes between 2400 and 3300 μg/day during pregnancy have been associated with birth defects. Other studies have not demonstrated any teratogenic effect at this level of intake, and it has been suggested that the threshold plasma concentration associated with teratogenic effects is unlikely to be reached with intakes below 7500 μg/day. Nevertheless, pregnant women are advised not to consume more than 3000 μg/day (American Pediatric Association recommendation) or 3300 μg (UK Department of Health recommendation).

Interactions of vitamin A with drugs and other nutrients

Historically, there was considerable confusion between vitamins A and D, and for many years it was not clear which acted in which system. By the 1950s it was believed that the problem had been solved, with clearly defined functions of vitamin A in vision, and vitamin D in calcium homeostasis and bone development. However, both have overlapping effects on a number of systems, including bone metabolism and immune system function. It is now known that this is the result of formation of RXR–vitamin D receptor heterodimers, so that in some systems both are required in appropriate amounts for normal regulation of gene expression.

Excessive alcohol consumption may precipitate vitamin A deficiency by reducing liver reserves of the vitamin as a result of both alcoholic liver damage and also induction of cytochrome P_{450}, which catalyses the catabolism of retinol. Habitual use of barbiturates may also lead to deficiency as a result of induction of cytochrome P_{450}.

Chlorinated hydrocarbons, as contained in agricultural pesticides, deplete liver retinol. Metabolites of polychlorinated biphenyls bind to the thyroxine binding site of transthyretin, and in doing so impair the binding of RBP. As a result there is free RBP-bound retinol in plasma, which is filtered at the glomerulus and hence lost in the urine.

10.3 Vitamin D

Vitamin D is not strictly a vitamin, since it can be synthesised in the skin, and indeed under most conditions (except in temperate regions) endogenous synthesis is the major source of the vitamin: it is only when sunlight exposure is inadequate that a dietary source is required. Its main function is in the regulation of calcium absorption and homeostasis; most of its actions are mediated by nuclear receptors that regulate gene expression. Deficiency, leading to rickets in children and osteomalacia in adults, continues to be a problem in northern latitudes, where sunlight exposure is poor.

There are relatively few dietary sources of vitamin D, mainly oily fish, with eggs, liver, and butter providing modest amounts; fortified milk, containing ergocalciferol, is available in some countries, and some other foods are fortified with the vitamin. No common plant foods contain vitamin D, apart from mushrooms that are grown in the light; most cultivated mushrooms are grown in the dark and so do not form vitamin D from ergosterol. As a result, strict vegetarians are especially at risk of deficiency, especially in northern latitudes with little sunlight exposure.

Although meat provides apparently negligible quantities of vitamin D, it may be an important source, since what is present is largely the final active metabolite, calcidiol, which is five times more potent on a molar basis than is cholecalciferol.

Vitamers and international units

The normal dietary form of vitamin D is cholecalciferol (also known as calciol). This is also the compound that is formed in the skin by ultraviolet (UV) irradiation of 7-dehydrocholesterol. Some foods are enriched or fortified with (synthetic) ergocalciferol, which undergoes the same metabolism as cholecalciferol and has the same biological activity. Early studies assigned the name vitamin D_1 to an impure mixture of products derived from the irradiation of ergosterol; when ergocalciferol was identified it was called vitamin D_2, and when the physiological compound was identified as cholecalciferol it was called vitamin D_3.

Like vitamin A, before the pure compound was isolated vitamin D was measured in international units of biological activity: 1 IU = 25 ng of cholecalciferol; 1 μg of cholecalciferol = 40 IU.

Absorption and metabolism

Vitamin D is absorbed in lipid micelles and incorporated into chylomicrons; therefore, people on a low-fat diet will absorb little of such dietary vitamin D as is available. Indeed, it is noteworthy that at the time that rickets was a major public health problem in Scotland, herrings (a rich source) were a significant part of the diet: it can only be assumed that the diet was so low in fat that the absorption of the vitamin was impaired.

Synthesis of vitamin D in the skin

As shown in Figure 10.4, the steroid 7-dehydrocholesterol (an intermediate in the

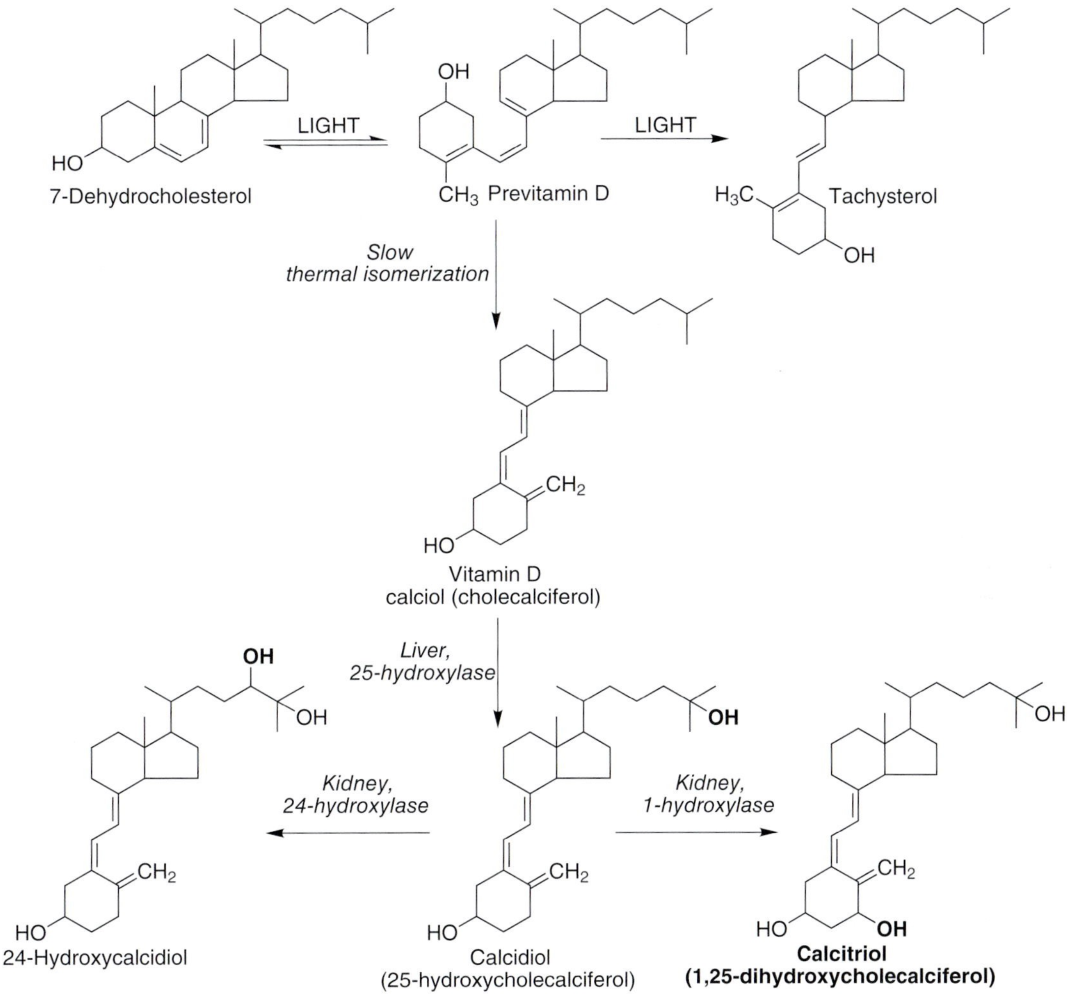

7-Dehydrocholesterol
LIGHT
Previtamin D
LIGHT
Tachysterol
Slow thermal isomerization
Vitamin D
calciol (cholecalciferol)
Liver, 25-hydroxylase
Kidney, 24-hydroxylase
Kidney, 1-hydroxylase
24-Hydroxycalcidiol
Calcidiol
(25-hydroxycholecalciferol)
Calcitriol
(1,25-dihydroxycholecalciferol)

Figure 10.4 Vitamin D synthesis and metabolism.

synthesis of cholesterol that accumulates in the skin but not other tissues) undergoes a non-enzymic reaction on exposure to UV light, yielding previtamin D, which undergoes a further reaction over a period of hours to form cholecalciferol, which is absorbed into the bloodstream.

In temperate climates there is a marked seasonal variation in the plasma concentration of vitamin D; it is highest at the end of summer and lowest at the end of winter. Although there may be bright sunlight in winter, beyond about 40° N or S there is very little UV radiation of the appropriate wavelength for cholecalciferol synthesis when the sun is low in the sky. By contrast, in summer, when the sun is more or less overhead, there is a considerable amount of UV light even on a moderately cloudy day, and can enough penetrate thin clothes to result in significant formation of vitamin D.

In northerly climates, and especially in polluted industrial cities with little sunlight, people may well not be exposed to enough UV light to meet their vitamin D needs, and they will be reliant on supplements and the few dietary sources of the vitamin.

Metabolism of cholecalciferol

Cholecalciferol, either synthesised in the skin or from foods, undergoes two hydroxylations to yield the active metabolite, 1,25-dihydroxyvitamin D or calcitriol, as shown in Figure 10.4. Ergocalciferol from fortified foods undergoes similar hydroxylation to yield ercalcitriol.

Table 10.3 Nomenclature of vitamin D metabolites

Trivial name	Recommended name	Abbreviation
vitamin D_3		
cholecalciferol	calciol	-
25-hydroxycholecalciferol	calcidiol	$25(OH)D_3$
1α-hydroxycholecalciferol	1(*S*)-hydroxycalciol	$1\alpha(OH)D_3$
24,25-dihydroxycholecalciferol	24(*R*)-hydroxycalcidiol	$24,25(OH)_2D_3$
1,25-dihydroxycholecalciferol	calcitriol	$1,25(OH)_2D_3$
1,24,25-trihydroxycholecalciferol	calcitetrol	$1,24,25(OH)_3D_3$
vitamin D_2		
ergocalciferol	ercalciol	-
25-hydroxyergocalciferol	ercalcidiol	$25(OH)D_2$
24,25-dihydroxyergocalciferol	24(*R*)-hydroxyercalcidiol	$24,25(OH)_2D_2$
1,25-dihydroxyergocalciferol	ercalcitriol	$1,25(OH)_2 D_2$
1,24,25-trihydroxyergocalciferol	ercalcitetrol	$1,24,25(OH)_3D_2$

The abbreviations shown in column 3 are not recommended, but are frequently used in the literature.

The nomenclature of the vitamin D metabolites is shown in Table 10.3.

The first stage in vitamin D metabolism occurs in the liver, where it is hydroxylated to form the 25-hydroxy derivative calcidiol. This is released into the circulation bound to a vitamin D binding globulin. There is little tissue storage of vitamin D; plasma calcidiol is the main storage form of the vitamin, and it is plasma calcidiol that shows the most significant seasonal variation in temperate regions. In human liver, concentrations of vitamin D do not exceed about 25 nmol/kg; although adipose tissue contains relatively large amounts of vitamin D, this is not readily available, and may represent sequestration of the vitamin rather than storage; there is an inverse relationship between the serum concentration of calcidiol and adiposity. There is some evidence of storage of calcidiol in muscle.

The second stage of vitamin D metabolism occurs in the kidney, where calcidiol undergoes either 1-hydroxylation to yield the active metabolite 1,25-dihydroxyvitamin D (calcitriol) or 24-hydroxylation to yield an apparently inactive metabolite, 24,25-dihydroxyvitamin D (24-hydroxycalcidiol). There is some evidence from animal studies that 24,25-dihydroxyvitamin D may have a metabolic function in bone healing.

Catabolism of vitamin D is by further oxidation to calcitroic acid, which is the main excretory product of the vitamin.

A number of tissues other than the kidney, including the bone, skin, placenta, breast, endothelial cells, pancreatic islets, and the parathyroid glands also express calcidiol 1-hydroxylase, and so can take up calcidiol from the circulation and produce the active hormone intracellularly, without relying on circulating calcitriol. Unlike the kidney, 1-hydroxylation in these tissues does not contribute to the plasma concentration of calcitriol. It serves to provide calcitriol for autocrine or paracrine actions of the hormone. This extrarenal formation of calcitriol may be important with respect to many of the metabolic effects of vitamin D insufficiency, since the circulating concentration of calcitriol is maintained in moderate deficiency, while the concentration of calcidiol falls.

Regulation of vitamin D metabolism

The main function of vitamin D is in the control of calcium homeostasis and, in turn, vitamin D metabolism in the kidney is regulated, at the level of 1- or 24-hydroxylation, by factors that respond to the plasma concentrations of calcium and phosphate. In tissues other than the kidney that hydroxylate calcidiol to calcitriol, the enzyme is not regulated in response to plasma calcium.

- Calcitriol acts to reduce its own synthesis and increase formation of 24-hydroxycalcidiol, by regulating the expression of the genes for the two hydroxylases.
- Parathyroid hormone is secreted in response to a fall in plasma calcium. In the kidney it acts to increase the activity of calcidiol 1-hydroxylase

and decrease that of 24-hydroxylase. In turn, both calcitriol and high concentrations of calcium repress the synthesis of parathyroid hormone; calcium also inhibits the secretion of the hormone from the parathyroid gland.

- Calcium exerts its main effect on the synthesis and secretion of parathyroid hormone. However, calcium ions also have a direct effect on the kidney, reducing the activity of calcidiol 1-hydroxylase.
- Phosphate also affects calcidiol metabolism; throughout the day there is an inverse fluctuation of plasma phosphate and calcitriol, and feeding people on a low-phosphate diet results in increased circulating concentrations of calcitriol.

Metabolic functions of vitamin D

Calcitriol acts to increase the plasma concentration of calcium by increasing intestinal absorption of calcium, reducing urinary excretion by increasing reabsorption in the distal renal tubule, and mobilising the mineral from bone.

Calcitriol binds to, and activates, nuclear receptors that modulate gene expression. For activity, the vitamin D receptor has to dimerise with the occupied vitamin A RXR receptor. Dimers formed with the unoccupied RXR receptor act to decrease gene expression; because of this, vitamin A deficiency leads to impaired vitamin D function. Excess vitamin A can also impair vitamin D function, since in the presence of large amounts of 9-*cis*-retinoic acid, RXR homodimers are formed, leaving insufficient RXR to form heterodimers with the vitamin D receptor.

There are several polymorphisms of the vitamin D receptor gene, which occur with different frequency in different population groups. Many of these polymorphisms affect functional vitamin D status; two variants have been associated with increased risk of stress fractures of bones.

More than 50 genes are known to be regulated by calcitriol, including: calcidiol 1- and 24-hydroxylases; calbindin, a calcium binding protein in the intestinal mucosa and other tissues; the vitamin K-dependent protein osteocalcin in bone; osteopontin, which permits the attachment of osteoclasts to bone surfaces; and the osteoclast cell membrane protein integrin. In addition, calcitriol affects the secretion of insulin and the synthesis and secretion of parathyroid and thyroid hormones – these actions may be secondary to changes in intracellular calcium concentrations resulting from induction of calbindin or changes in cytosolic calcium.

Calcitriol also has a role in the regulation of cell proliferation and differentiation, regulation of the cell cycle and apoptosis. Because of the role of vitamin D in cell differentiation, maternal vitamin D status in pregnancy is important in fetal development. The activity of calcidiol 1-hydroxylase in the kidney increases during the first trimester of pregnancy, and the placenta also expresses 1-hydroxylase, forming calcitriol from circulating calcidiol. There is also reduced expression of the 24-hydroxylase in the placenta, so ensuring an adequate supply of calcitriol to the developing fetus. Because of the role of vitamin D in insulin secretion (and possibly also insulin function and sensitivity), poor vitamin D status in pregnancy is associated with an increased risk of gestational diabetes.

Activated macrophages, T-lymphocytes and antigen-presenting cells express the vitamin D receptor and have calcidiol 1-hydroxylase, and therefore, can synthesise calcitriol from calcidiol, suggesting that in addition to its endocrine role, calcitriol may have a paracrine or autocrine role in the immune system. There is some evidence that vitamin D affects immune responsiveness, and poor vitamin D status is associated with increased risk of infection. However, there is no evidence from intervention trials that vitamin D supplementation reduces infection.

Calcitriol receptors have been identified in a variety of tumour cells. At low concentrations it is a growth promoter, while at higher concentrations it has both antiproliferative and pro-apoptotic actions in cancer cells in culture. There is an epidemiological association between low vitamin D status and prostate and colorectal cancer, but there is no evidence for a protective effect of vitamin D supplementation.

Epidemiological evidence suggests a link between obesity and vitamin D insufficiency. While it may be that obesity lowers vitamin D status because of sequestration of the vitamin in adipose tissue, adipocytes have vitamin D receptors. There is evidence that vitamin D suppresses adipocyte development from pre-adipocytes both through inhibition of gene expression and also competition with PPARγ, the master regulator of adipogenesis, for the available RXR for dimerisation. It is likely that vitamin D inadequacy is a factor in the development of the metabolic syndrome (the combination of insulin resistance, hyperlipidaemia and atherosclerosis associated with abdominal obesity). Epidemiological studies show an inverse relationship between vitamin D status and diabetes mellitus, and intervention trials have shown that calcitriol improves insulin sensitivity. Sunlight exposure, and hence vitamin D status, may be a factor in the difference in incidence of metabolic syndrome and atherosclerosis between northern and southern European countries.

In addition to its nuclear actions, calcitriol has two non-genomic actions:

- In intestinal mucosal cells it acts to recruit membrane calcium transport proteins from intracellular vesicles to the cell surface, resulting in a rapid increase in calcium absorption, before there has been induction of calbindin.
- In a variety of cells it acts via cell-surface receptors, leading to the opening of intracellular calcium channels and activation of protein kinase C and mitogen-activated protein kinases (MAP kinases). The effect of this is inhibition of cell proliferation, and induction of differentiation. Calcitriol affects the proliferation, differentiation and immune function of lymphocytes and monocytes.

Vitamin D deficiency: rickets and osteomalacia

Historically, rickets is a disease of toddlers, especially in northern industrial cities. Their bones are under-mineralised as a result of poor absorption of calcium in the absence of adequate amounts of calcitriol. When the child begins to walk, the long bones of the legs are deformed, leading to bow-legs or knock knees. More seriously, rickets can also lead to collapse of the ribcage and deformities of the bones of the pelvis. Similar problems may also occur in adolescents who are deficient in vitamin D during the adolescent growth spurt, when there is again a high demand for calcium for new bone formation.

Osteomalacia is the adult equivalent of rickets. It results from the demineralisation of bone, rather than the failure to mineralise it in the first place, as is the case with rickets. Women who have little exposure to sunlight are especially at risk from osteomalacia after several pregnancies, because of the strain that pregnancy places on their marginal reserve of calcium.

Osteomalacia also occurs in older people. Here again the problem may be inadequate exposure to sunlight, but there is also evidence that the capacity to form 7-dehydrocholesterol in the skin decreases with advancing age, so that older people are more reliant on the few dietary sources of vitamin D.

Although vitamin D is essential for prevention and treatment of osteomalacia in older people, there is less evidence that it is beneficial in treating the other common degenerative bone disease of advancing age, osteoporosis, which is due to a loss of bone matrix, rather than enhanced release of calcium from bone with no effect on the organic matrix, as is seen in osteomalacia. The result is negative calcium balance and loss of bone mineral, but secondary to the loss of organic matrix, owing to progressive loss of oestrogens and androgens, rather than failure of the vitamin D system.

Vitamin D requirements and reference intakes

Before anatomical deformities are apparent in vitamin D deficient children, bone density is lower than normal – radiological rickets. At an earlier stage of deficiency there is a marked elevation of plasma alkaline phosphatase released by osteoclast activity – biochemical rickets.

The plasma concentration of calcidiol is the most sensitive index of vitamin D status, and is correlated with elevated plasma parathyroid hormone and alkaline phosphatase activity. The reference range of plasma calcidiol is between 20–150 nmol/l, with a two-fold seasonal variation in temperate regions. Concentrations below

25 nmol/l are considered to indicate deficiency, and osteomalacia is seen in adults when plasma calcidiol falls below 10 nmol/l. A desirable plasma concentration of calcidiol is >25 nmol/l at any time of the year.

Early estimates of vitamin D requirements were based on the amount required by housebound elderly people to maintain the same plasma concentration of calcidiol as is seen in younger people at the end of winter. It was assumed that sunlight exposure met requirements for younger adults. The current view is that vitamin D synthesis in the skin through sunlight exposure in summer is insufficient to meet the requirements of the UK population for their needs during winter. Recent reviews show that vitamin D is important for aspects of musculoskeletal health other than reducing the risk of rickets and osteomalacia and recommendations for intake reflect this. In view of the importance of vitamin D for musculoskeletal health other than in preventing rickets and osteomalacia, reference intakes between 10 and 15 μg /day for all people aged over 4 years have been proposed by many countries. This will maintain a plasma concentration of calcidiol above 25 nmol/l throughout the year. There is insufficient evidence to make recommendations based on other health outcomes. These intakes are most unlikely to be achievable through diet without either widespread fortification of foods or the use of supplements; average intakes of vitamin D from unfortified foods are less than 4 μg/day.

The vitamin D content of human milk is probably inadequate to meet the requirements of breastfed infants without exposure to sunlight, especially during the winter, when the mother's reserves of the vitamin are low. Therefore, it is unlikely that an exclusively breast fed infant would maintain a serum calcidiol concentration above 25 nmol/l. The safe intake of 8.5 μg /day for non-breast fed infants is also recommended from birth for exclusively breast fed infants.

There is increasing evidence that high vitamin D status is associated with a lower incidence of various cancers, diabetes, and the metabolic syndrome, suggesting that desirable intakes are higher than current reference intakes. Widespread fortification of foods would improve vitamin D status, but might also put a significant proportion of the population at risk of hypervitaminosis and hypercalcaemia. Increased sunlight exposure will improve vitamin D status without the risks of toxicity, but excessive sunlight exposure is a cause of skin cancer.

Vitamin D toxicity

Toxicity is seen when plasma calcidiol exceeds 500 nmol/l. In children, clinical signs of rickets are seen when plasma calcidiol falls below 20 nmol/l. Intoxication with vitamin D causes weakness, nausea, loss of appetite, headache, abdominal pains, cramp and diarrhoea. More seriously, it also causes hypercalcaemia, with plasma concentrations of calcium between 2.75 and 4.5 mmol/l, compared with the normal range of 2.2–2.5 mmol/l. which results in calcinosis (deposition of calcium in soft tissues including kidney, heart, lungs and blood vessels), diffuse demineralisation of bones and irreversible renal and cardiovascular toxicity. Hypercalcaemia can also lead to hypercalcinuria, which may result in the precipitation of calcium phosphate in the renal tubules and the development of urinary calculi. Above a serum calcium concentration of 3.75 mmol/l, vascular smooth muscle may contract abnormally, leading to hypertension. Hypercalcaemia has been reported at plasma concentration above 375-500 nmol/l.

During the 1950s, rickets was more or less totally eradicated in Britain and other temperate countries. This was due to enrichment of a large number of infant foods with vitamin D. However, a small number of infants suffered from vitamin D poisoning, the most serious effect of which is an elevated plasma concentration of calcium. This can lead to contraction of blood vessels, and hence dangerously high blood pressure, and calcinosis – the calcification of soft tissues.

Some infants are sensitive to intakes of vitamin D as low as 45 μg/day. To avoid the serious problem of vitamin D poisoning in these susceptible infants, the extent to which infant foods are fortified with vitamin D has been reduced considerably. Unfortunately, this means that a proportion of infants (about 10%), who have relatively high requirements, are now at risk of developing rickets. The problem is to identify those who have higher requirements and provide them with supplements.

The tolerable upper level of intake is 100 μg/day for adults and 25 μg/day for infants. A small number of infants have been reported who developed hypercalcaemia at normal levels of vitamin D intake; they had defects in the 24-hydroxylase that inactivates calcitriol. Reports of hypercalcaemia in adults have involved intakes in excess of 1000 μg/day.

Although excess dietary vitamin D is toxic, excessive exposure to sunlight does not lead to vitamin D poisoning. There is a limited capacity to form 7-dehydrocholesterol in the skin, and a limited capacity to take up cholecalciferol from the skin. Furthermore, prolonged exposure of previtamin D to UV light results in further reactions to yield lumisterol and other biologically inactive compounds.

Interactions with drugs and other nutrients

As discussed above, vitamin D receptors form heterodimers with RXR, so that vitamin D-dependent functions require adequate, but not excessive, vitamin A status. A number of drugs, including barbiturates and other anticonvulsants, induce cytochrome P_{450}, resulting in increased catabolism of calcidiol (and retinol), and cause drug-induced osteomalacia. The antituberculosis drug isoniazid inhibits cholecalciferol 25-hydroxylase in the liver, and prolonged administration can lead to the development of osteomalacia.

Strontium is a potent inhibitor of the kidney 1-hydroxylase, and strontium intoxication can lead to the development of vitamin D-resistant rickets or osteomalacia. Although there is normally little exposure to potentially toxic intakes of strontium, its salts are sometimes used to treat chronic lead intoxication.

10.4 Vitamin E

Although vitamin E was identified as a dietary essential for animals in the 1920s, it was not until 1983 that it was clearly demonstrated to be a dietary essential for human beings. For a long time it was considered that, unlike the other vitamins, vitamin E had no specific functions; rather it was the major lipid-soluble radical trapping antioxidant in membranes. Many of its functions can be met by synthetic antioxidants; however, some of the effects of vitamin E deficiency in experimental animals do not respond to synthetic antioxidants. More recent studies have shown that vitamin E also has roles in cell signalling, by inhibition or inactivation of protein kinase C, and in modulation of gene expression, inhibition of cell proliferation and platelet aggregation. These effects are specific for α-tocopherol, and are independent of the antioxidant properties of the vitamin.

Vegetable oils are rich sources of vitamin E, but significant amounts are also found in nuts and seeds, most green leafy vegetables, and a variety of fish.

Vitamers and units of activity

Vitamin E is the generic descriptor for two families of compounds, the tocopherols and the tocotrienols (Figure 10.5). The different vitamers have different biological potency. The most active is α-tocopherol, and it is usual to express vitamin E intake in terms of mg α-tocopherol equivalents. This is the sum of mg α-tocopherol + 0.5 × mg β-tocopherol + 0.1 × mg γ-tocopherol + 0.3 × mg α-tocotrienol. The other vitamers have negligible vitamin activity.

The obsolete international unit of vitamin E activity is still sometimes used: 1 IU = 0.67 mg α-tocopherol equivalent; 1 mg α-tocopherol = 1.49 IU.

Synthetic α-tocopherol does not have the same biological potency as the naturally occurring compound. This is because the side-chain of tocopherol has three centres of asymmetry and when it is synthesised chemically the result is a mixture of the various isomers. In the naturally occurring compound all three centers of asymmetry have the *R*-configuration, and naturally occurring α-tocopherol is called all-*R*, or *RRR*-α-tocopherol.

Absorption and metabolism

Vitamin E is absorbed in micelles with other dietary lipids, but only 20–40% of a test dose is absorbed from the small intestine. Esters are hydrolysed in the intestinal lumen by pancreatic esterase, and also by intracellular esterases in the mucosal cells. In intestinal mucosal cells, all

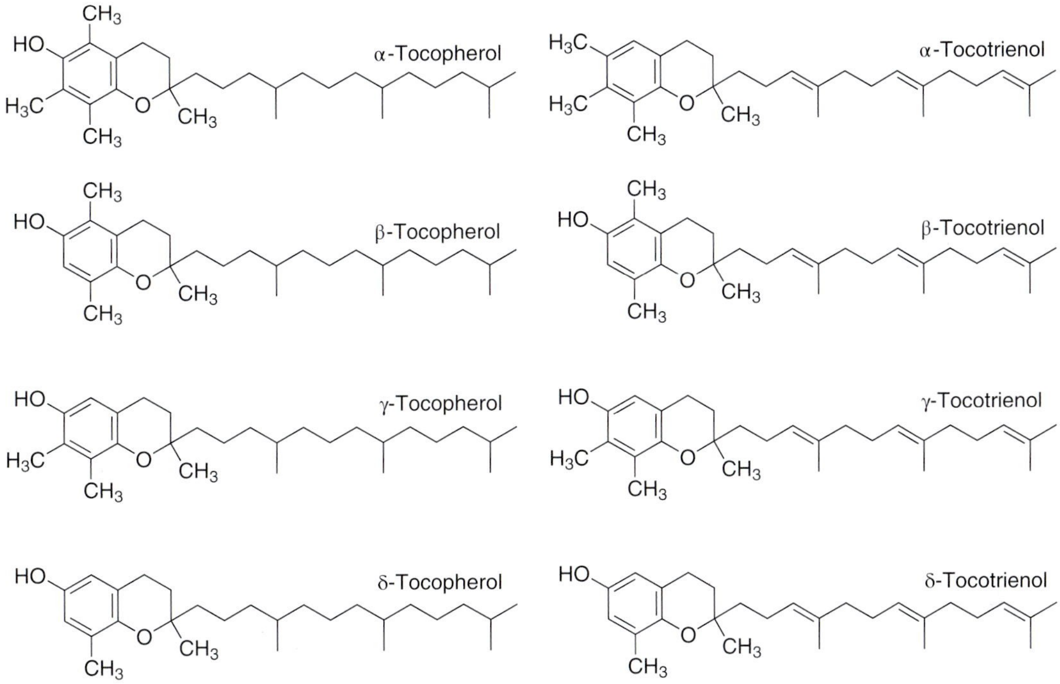

Figure 10.5 The vitamin E vitamers, tocopherols and tocotrienols.

vitamers of vitamin E are incorporated into chylomicrons, and tissues take up some vitamin E from chylomicrons. Most, however, goes to the liver in chylomicron remnants. α-Tocopherol, which binds to the liver α-tocopherol transfer protein, is then exported in very low density lipoprotein, and is available for tissue uptake. The other vitamers do not bind well to the α-tocopherol transfer protein, and much is not incorporated into VLDL, but is metabolised in the liver by cytochrome P_{450} linked ω-oxidation, followed by β-oxidation, then conjugated and excreted.

Tocopherol can undergo reversible oxidation to an epoxide, followed by ring cleavage to yield a quinone, which is reduced to the hydroquinone and conjugated with glucuronic acid, then excreted in the bile. There may also be significant excretion of the vitamin by the skin.

Metabolic functions of vitamin E

The main function of vitamin E is as a radical-trapping antioxidant in cell membranes and plasma lipoproteins. It is especially important in limiting radical damage resulting from oxidation of polyunsaturated fatty acids, by reacting with the lipid peroxide radicals before they can establish a chain reaction. The tocopheroxyl radical formed from vitamin E is relatively unreactive and persists long enough to undergo reaction to yield non-radical products. Commonly, the vitamin E radical in a membrane or lipoprotein is reduced back to tocopherol by reaction with vitamin C in plasma. The resultant monodehydroascorbate radical then undergoes enzymic or non-enzymic reaction to yield ascorbate and dehydroascorbate, neither of which is a radical.

The stability of the tocopheroxyl radical means that it can penetrate further into cells, or deeper into plasma lipoproteins, and potentially propagate a chain reaction. Therefore, although it is regarded as an antioxidant, vitamin E may, like other antioxidants, also have pro-oxidant actions at high concentrations. Also, much cell signalling for apoptosis is via radicals, and excessive quenching of these radicals may permit survival of seriously damaged cells. This may explain why, although epidemiological studies have shown a clear association between high blood concentrations of vitamin E and lower incidence of atherosclerosis, the results of intervention trials have generally been disappointing.

In many trials there has been increased all-cause mortality among those taking vitamin E and other antioxidant supplements.

The tocotrienols have lower vitamin activity than tocopherols, and indeed it is conventional to consider only γ-tocotrienol as a significant part of vitamin E intake. However, because of their unsaturated side-chain, the tocotrienols also have a hypocholesterolaemic action not shared by the tocopherols. They act to reduce the activity of 3-hydroxy-3-methylglutaryl-coenzyme A (HMG CoA) reductase, the rate-limiting enzyme in the pathway for synthesis of cholesterol, by repressing synthesis of the enzyme.

Non-antioxidant actions of vitamin E

α-Tocopherol (but not other vitamers) inhibits platelet aggregation and vascular smooth muscle proliferation. In monocytes it reduces formation of reactive oxygen species, cell adhesion to the endothelium and release of interleukins and tumour necrosis factor.

α-Tocopherol modulates transcription of a number of genes, including the scavenger receptor for oxidised LDL in macrophages and smooth muscle. As yet no response element for intracellular vitamin E binding protein has been identified on any of the proposed target genes. In experimental animals, vitamin E deficiency depresses immune system function, with reduced mitogenesis of B- and T-lymphocytes, reduced phagocytosis and chemotaxis and reduced production of antibodies and interleukin-2, suggesting a signalling role in the immune system.

Vitamin E modulates the activity of several signal transduction enzymes, leading to changes in gene expression. It may either bind directly to the enzymes, compete with substrates or may change their activity by a redox mechanism. Translocation of some of these enzymes to the plasma membrane is also regulated by vitamin E.

There is a structural similarity between α- and γ-tocopherols and the thiazolidinedione drugs that are used to treat insulin resistance, and act to increase insulin sensitivity via activation of PPARγ, leading to increased synthesis of adiponectin.

Vitamin E deficiency

In experimental animals vitamin E deficiency results in a number of different conditions.

- Deficient female animals suffer the death and resorption of the fetuses. This provided the basis of the original biological assay of vitamin E.
- In male animals, deficiency results in testicular atrophy and degeneration of the germinal epithelium of the seminiferous tubules.
- Both skeletal and cardiac muscle are affected in deficient animals. This necrotising myopathy is sometimes called nutritional muscular dystrophy – an unfortunate term, since there is no evidence that human muscular dystrophy is related to vitamin E.
- The integrity of blood vessel walls is affected, with leakage of blood plasma into subcutaneous tissues and accumulation under the skin of a green fluid: exudative diathesis.
- The nervous system is affected, with the development of central nervous system necrosis and axonal dystrophy. This is exacerbated by feeding diets rich in polyunsaturated fatty acids.

Dietary deficiency of vitamin E in human beings is unknown, although patients with severe fat malabsorption, cystic fibrosis, some forms of chronic liver disease or (very rare) congenital lack of plasma β-lipoprotein, suffer deficiency because they are unable to absorb the vitamin or transport it around the body. They suffer from severe damage to nerve and muscle membranes.

Premature infants are at risk of vitamin E deficiency, since they are often born with inadequate reserves of the vitamin. The red blood cell membranes of deficient infants are abnormally fragile, as a result of unchecked oxidative radical attack. This may lead to haemolytic anaemia if they are not given supplements of the vitamin.

Experimental animals that are depleted of vitamin E become sterile. However, there is no evidence that vitamin E nutritional status is in any way associated with human fertility, and there is certainly no evidence that vitamin E supplements increase sexual potency, prowess, or vigor.

Vitamin E requirements

It is difficult to establish vitamin E requirements, partly because deficiency is more or less unknown, but also because the requirement depends on the intake of polyunsaturated fatty acids (PUFA). It is generally accepted, albeit with little experimental evidence, that an acceptable intake of vitamin E is 0.4 mg α-tocopherol equivalent/g dietary PUFA.

Indices of vitamin E status

The plasma concentration of α-tocopherol is used to assess vitamin E status; since most vitamin E is transported in plasma lipoproteins, it is the concentration per gram total plasma lipid, or better, per mol cholesterol, that is useful, rather than the simple concentration.

Erythrocytes are incapable of *de novo* lipid synthesis, so peroxidative damage resulting from oxygen stress has a serious effect, shortening red cell life and possibly precipitating haemolytic anaemia in vitamin E deficiency. This has been exploited as a method of assessing status by measuring the haemolysis of red cells induced by dilute hydrogen peroxide relative to that observed on incubation in water. This gives a means of assessing the functional adequacy of vitamin E intake, albeit one that will be affected by other, unrelated, factors. Plasma concentrations of α-tocopherol below 2.2 mmol/mol cholesterol or 1.1 μmol/g total plasma lipid are associated with increased susceptibility of erythrocytes to induced haemolysis *in vitro*.

An alternative method of assessing functional antioxidant status, again one that is affected by both vitamin E and other antioxidants, is by measuring the exhalation of pentane arising from the catabolism of the products of peroxidation of n-6 PUFAs or ethane arising from n-3 PUFAs.

Higher levels of intake

There is good epidemiological evidence that higher intakes of vitamin E are associated with a lower risk of atherosclerosis and ischaemic heart disease. High concentrations of vitamin E will inhibit the oxidation of PUFAs in plasma lipoproteins, and it is this oxidation that is responsible for the development of atherosclerosis. The plasma concentrations of α-tocopherol that appear to be beneficial would require an intake of 17–40 mg/day, which is above what could be achieved by eating normal diets. Individual intervention trials of vitamin E supplements have generally been disappointing, and meta-analysis shows a significant increase in all-cause mortality among people taking vitamin E (and other antioxidant) supplements. This reflects the role of radicals in signalling for apoptosis, and the undesirability of excessive quenching of these radicals. However, it is also possible that the plasma concentration of α-tocopherol is a surrogate marker for some other protective factor in the diet.

Interactions with other nutrients

Vitamin C in plasma and extracellular fluid is important in reducing the tocopheroxyl radical in cell membranes and plasma lipoproteins back to tocopherol. There is also evidence that a variety of lipid-soluble antioxidants may be important in the antioxidant action of vitamin E in membranes and lipoproteins, including ubiquinone and synthetic antioxidants used in food processing, such as butylated hydroxytoluene and butylated hydroxyanisole. Synthetic antioxidants will prevent or cure a number of the signs of vitamin E deficiency in experimental animals.

There is a considerable overlap between the functions of vitamin E and selenium. Vitamin E reduces lipid peroxide radicals to unreactive hydroxy-fatty acids; the selenium-dependent enzyme glutathione peroxidase reduces hydrogen peroxide to water, thus lowering the intracellular concentration of potentially lipid-damaging peroxide. A membrane-specific isoenzyme of glutathione peroxidase will also reduce the tocopheroxyl radical back to tocopherol. Thus, vitamin E acts to remove the products of lipid peroxidation, whereas selenium acts both to remove the cause of lipid peroxidation and to recycle vitamin E.

10.5 Vitamin K

Vitamin K was discovered as a result of investigations into the cause of a bleeding disorder (haemorrhagic disease) of cattle fed on silage made from sweet clover and of chickens fed on a fat-free diet. The missing factor in the diet of the chickens was identified as vitamin K, whereas the problem in the cattle was that the feed contained dicumarol, an antagonist of the vitamin.

Since the effect of an excessive intake of dicumarol was severely impaired blood clotting, it was isolated and tested in low doses as an anticoagulant, for use in patients at risk of thrombosis. Although it was effective, it had unwanted side-effects, and synthetic vitamin K antagonists were developed for clinical use as anticoagulants. The most commonly used of these is warfarin, which is also used, in larger amounts, as a rodenticide.

Vitamers

Three compounds have the biological activity of vitamin K (Figure 10.6):

- phylloquinone, the normal dietary source, found in green leafy vegetables;
- menaquinones, a family of related compounds synthesised by intestinal bacteria, with differing lengths of the side-chain;
- menadiol and menadiol diacetate, synthetic compounds that can be metabolised to phylloquinone.

Dietary sources, bacterial synthesis and metabolism

Phylloquinone has a role in photosynthesis, and therefore it is found in all green leafy vegetables; the richest sources are spring (collard) greens, spinach, and Brussels sprouts. In addition, soybean, rapeseed, cottonseed, and olive oils are relatively rich in vitamin K, although other oils are not.

About 80% of dietary phylloquinone is normally absorbed into the lymphatic system in chylomicrons, and is then taken up by the liver from chylomicron remnants and released into the circulation in VLDL.

Menaquinones are synthesised by intestinal bacteria, but it is unclear how much they contribute to vitamin K nutrition, since they are extremely hydrophobic, and will only be absorbed from regions of the gastrointestinal tract where bile salts are present – mainly the terminal ileum. However, prolonged use of antibiotics can lead to vitamin K deficiency and the development of vitamin K responsive hypoprothrominaemia, as can dietary deprivation of phylloquinone. It is often suggested that about half of the requirement for vitamin K is met by intestinal bacterial synthesis, but there is little evidence for this, other than the fact that about

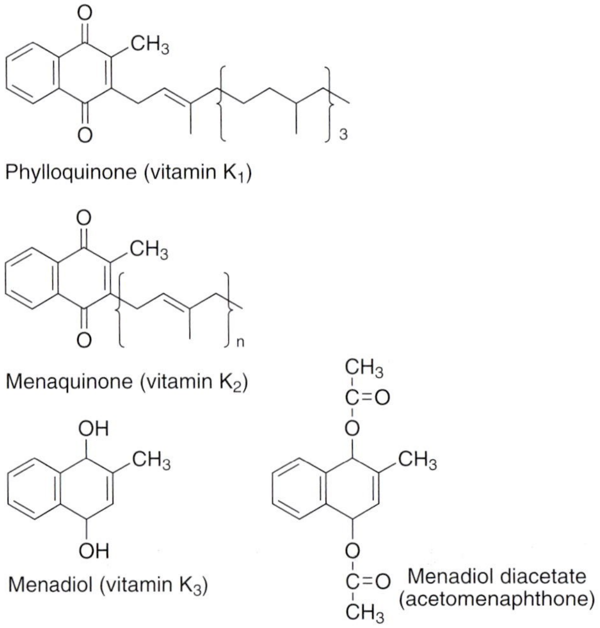

Phylloquinone (vitamin K_1)

Menaquinone (vitamin K_2)

Menadiol (vitamin K_3)

Menadiol diacetate (acetomenaphthone)

Figure 10.6 The vitamin K vitamers, phylloquinone (vitamin K1), menaquinone (vitamin K2), and menadiol (a synthetic compound, vitamin K3).

half of the vitamin K in liver is phylloquinone and the remainder a variety of menaquinones. It is not clear to what extent the menaquinones are biologically active.

The synthetic compound menadiol is absorbed largely into the hepatic portal system, and undergoes alkylation in the liver to yield menaquinone-4, which is released together with phylloquinone and other menaquinones in VLDLs.

Metabolic functions of vitamin K

Although it has been known since the 1920s that vitamin K was required for blood clotting, it was not until the 1970s that its precise function was established. It is the cofactor for the carboxylation of glutamate residues in the postsynthetic modification of proteins to form the unusual amino acid γ-carboxyglutamate, abbreviated to Gla (Figure 10.7).

In the presence of warfarin, vitamin K epoxide cannot be reduced back to the active hydroquinone, but accumulates and is excreted as a variety of conjugates. However, if enough vitamin K is provided in the diet, the quinone can be reduced to the active hydroquinone by the warfarin-insensitive enzyme, and carboxylation can continue, with stoichiometric utilisation of vitamin K and excretion of the epoxide. High doses of vitamin K are used to treat patients who have received an overdose of warfarin, and at least part of the resistance of some populations of rats to the action of warfarin is due to a high consumption of vitamin K from maram grass, although there are also genetically resistant populations of rodents.

Prothrombin and several other proteins of the blood clotting system (factors VII, IX and X, and proteins C and S) each contain between four and six γ-carboxyglutamate residues per mol. γ-Carboxyglutamate chelates calcium ions, and so permits the binding of the blood clotting proteins to lipid membranes. In vitamin K deficiency, or in the presence of an antagonist such as warfarin, an abnormal precursor of prothrombin (preprothrombin) containing little or no γ-carboxyglutamate is released into the circulation. Preprothrombin cannot chelate calcium or bind to phospholipid membranes, and so is unable to initiate blood clotting. Preprothrombin is sometimes known as PIVKA: the protein induced by vitamin K absence.

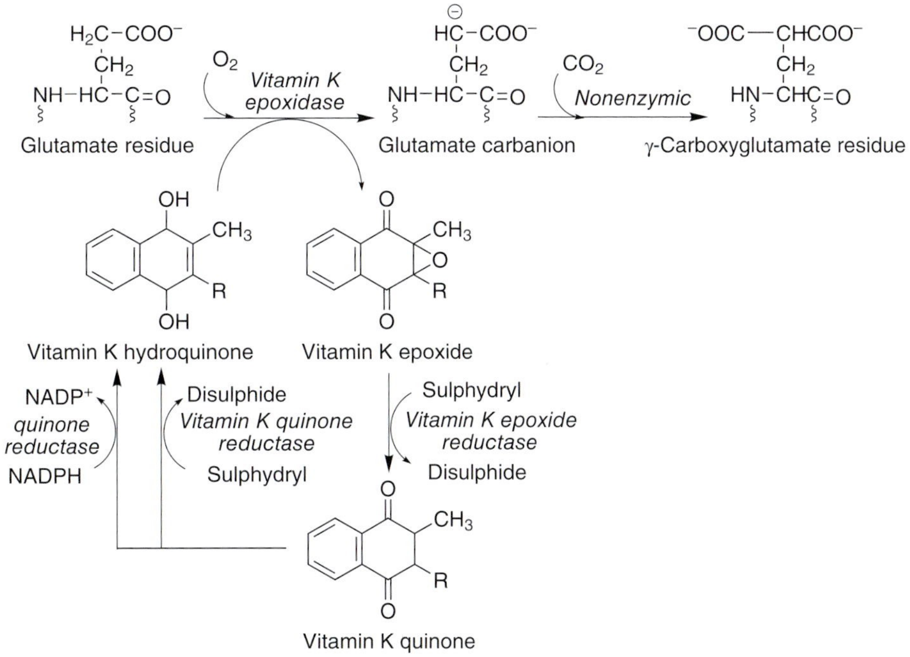

Figure 10.7 Role of vitamin K in the carboxylation of glutamate. Vitamin K epoxidase (EC 1.14.99.20), warfarin-sensitive epoxide/quinone reductase (EC 1.1.4.1), warfarin-insensitive quinone reductase (EC 1.1.4.2).

A specific vitamin K binding protein has been identified in the nucleus in osteoblasts, suggesting that the vitamin may also have direct nuclear actions. Phylloquinone, but not menaquinones, downregulates osteoclastic bone resorption by inducing apoptosis in osteoclasts.

It has long been known that treatment of pregnant women with warfarin can lead to bone abnormalities in the child: the fetal warfarin syndrome. Two proteins in bone matrix contain γ-carboxyglutamate: osteocalcin and a less well characterised protein simply known as bone matrix Gla protein. Osteocalcin is interesting in that as well as γ-carboxyglutamate, it also contains hydroxyproline, so its synthesis is dependent on both vitamins K and C; in addition, its synthesis is induced by vitamin D, and the release into the circulation of osteocalcin provides a sensitive index of vitamin D action. It constitutes some 1–2% of total bone protein, and modifies the crystallisation of bone mineral. The matrix Gla protein is found in a variety of tissues, and acts to prevent mineralisation of soft connective tissue.

The product of the growth arrest specific gene 6 (Gas6) is a γ-carboxyglutamate-containing protein that is important in the regulation of growth and development. The γ-carboxyglutamate region of Gas6 is required for binding to phosphatidylserine in cell membranes before interacting with a receptor tyrosine kinase, leading to the induction of mitogen-activated protein kinase (MAP kinase). Phosphatidylserine is normally deep in the membrane phospholipid bilayer, but it is exposed at the cell surface in senescent red blood cells and apoptotic cells, suggesting that Gas6 has a role in the recognition of cells that are to undergo phagocytosis, and hence regulation of apoptosis and cell survival.

The fetal warfarin syndrome involves neurological as well as bone abnormalities. The vitamin K-dependent carboxylase is expressed in different brain regions at different times during embryological development, and the product of the growth arrest-specific gene 6 (*Gas6*) is a Gla-containing growth factor that is important in the regulation of growth and development, and the regulation of apoptosis and cell survival.

Vitamin K deficiency and requirements

Vitamin K deficiency results in prolonged prothrombin time, and haemorrhagic disease, because of impaired synthesis of the vitamin K dependent blood clotting proteins. Osteocalcin synthesis is similarly impaired, and there is evidence that under-carboxylated osteocalcin is formed in people with marginal intakes of vitamin K who show no impairment of blood clotting. However, apart from deliberate experimental manipulation, vitamin K deficiency is unknown, and determination of requirements is complicated by the lack of information on the importance of menaquinones synthesised by intestinal bacteria.

The usual method of assessing vitamin K status, or monitoring the efficacy of anticoagulant therapy, is to measure the time taken for the formation of a fibrin clot in citrated plasma after the addition of calcium ions and thromboplastin to activate the extrinsic clotting system – the prothrombin time. The normal prothrombin time is 12–13 seconds; greater than 25 seconds is associated with severe bleeding. An alternative measure is the International Normalised Ratio (INR), which is the patient's prothrombin time / that of a control sample, raised to the power of the (standardised) sensitivity of the batch of thromboplastin used. In the absence of anticoagulant treatment, the INR is 0.8–1.2.

Measurement of plasma preprothrombin, most commonly by immunoassay using antisera against preprothrombin that do not react with prothrombin, provides an index of status, but measurement of under-carboxylated osteocalcin in plasma is more sensitive; it is detectable, and responds to supplements of vitamin K in people with normal clotting time and no detectable preprothrombin. The urinary excretion of γ-carboxyglutamate, as both the free amino acid and in small peptides, also reflects functional vitamin K status, since γ-carboxyglutamate released by the catabolism of proteins is neither reutilised nor metabolised.

The total body pool of vitamin K is 150–200 nmol (70–100 mg), with a half-life of 17 hours, suggesting a requirement for replacement of 50–70 mg/day. Preprothrombin is elevated at intakes between 40–60 mg/day, but not at intakes above 80 mg/day. An intake of 1 μg/kg body weight per day is considered adequate; this forms the basis of reference intakes of between 65 and 80 μg/day for adults.

Newborn infants have low plasma levels of prothrombin and the other vitamin K dependent clotting factors (about 30–60% of the adult concentrations, depending on gestational age). To a great extent this is the result of the relatively late development of liver glutamate carboxylase, but they are also short of vitamin K, as a result of the placental barrier that limits fetal uptake of the vitamin. This is probably a way of regulating the activity of Gas6 and other vitamin K dependent proteins in development and differentiation. Over the first six weeks of postnatal life the plasma concentrations of clotting factors gradually rise to the adult level; in the meantime infants are at risk of potentially fatal haemorrhage which was formerly called haemorrhagic disease of the newborn, and is now known as vitamin K deficiency bleeding in infancy. It is usual to give all newborn infants prophylactic vitamin K, either orally or by intramuscular injection. At one time menadione was used, but because of a possible association between menadione and childhood leukaemia, phylloquinone is preferred.

Toxicity and drug interactions

There is no evidence that phylloquinone has any significant toxicity. However, high intakes can overcome the effects of warfarin and other anticoagulants. This means that patients who are being treated with warfarin could overcome the beneficial effects of their medication if they took supplements of vitamin K. The danger is that if their dose of warfarin is increased to counteract the effects of the vitamin supplements and they then stop taking the supplements, they would be receiving considerably too much warfarin and would be at risk of haemorrhage.

It is unlikely that a normal diet could provide a sufficient excess of vitamin K to lead to problems, but habitual consumption of especially rich sources could result in intakes close to those that antagonise therapeutic warfarin. A diet containing relatively large amounts of foods prepared with vitamin K-rich oils may pose a risk.

10.6 Thiamin (vitamin B_1)

Historically, thiamin deficiency affecting the peripheral nervous system (beriberi) was a major public health problem in south-east Asia following the introduction of the steam-powered mill that made highly polished (and therefore thiamin-depleted) rice widely available. It is likely that this was due not only to loss of thiamin in the discarded rice bran, but also to loss of the fermentable carbohydrates in bran that promote the growth of intestinal bacteria. There are still sporadic outbreaks of deficiency among people whose diet is rich in carbohydrate and poor in thiamin. More commonly, thiamin deficiency affecting the heart and central nervous system is a problem in people with an excessive consumption of alcohol, to the extent that there was a serious suggestion in Australia at one time that thiamin should be added to beer. The structures of thiamin and the coenzyme thiamin diphosphate are shown in Figure 10.8.

Thiamin is widely distributed in foods, with pork being an especially rich source; potatoes, whole-grain cereals, meat, and fish are the major sources in most diets. Like other water-soluble vitamins, thiamin is readily lost by leaching into cooking water; furthermore, it is unstable to light, and although bread and flour contain significant amounts of thiamin, much of this can be lost when baked goods are exposed to sunlight in a shop window.

Thiamin is also destroyed by sulphites, and in potato products that have been blanched by immersion in sulphite solution there is little or no thiamin remaining. Polyphenols, including tannic acid in

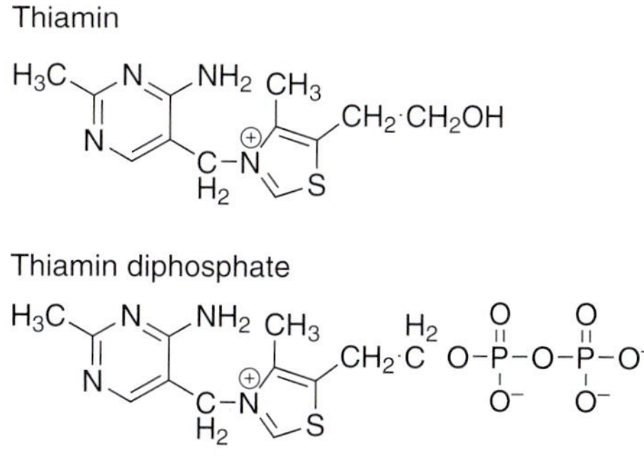

Thiamin

Thiamin diphosphate

Figure 10.8 Thiamin (vitamin B1) and the coenzyme thiamin diphosphate.

tea and betel nuts, also destroy thiamin, and have been associated with thiamin deficiency.

Thiaminases that catalyse base exchange or hydrolysis of thiamin are found in microorganisms (including some that colonise the gut), a variety of plants, and raw fish. The presence of thiaminase in fermented fish is believed to be a significant factor in the aetiology of thiamin deficiency in parts of southeast Asia.

Absorption and metabolism of thiamin

Dietary thiamin phosphates are hydrolysed by intestinal phosphatases, and thiamin is absorbed by active transport in the duodenum and proximal jejunum, and by carrier mediated transport in the colon. The active transport system is saturated at relatively low concentrations, so limiting the amount that can be absorbed. There is also active transport from the intestinal cells into the bloodstream; this is inhibited by alcohol, leading to thiamin deficiency in alcoholics. Much of the absorbed thiamin is phosphorylated in the liver, and both free thiamin and thiamin monophosphate circulate in plasma, bound to albumin. All tissues can take up both thiamin and thiamin monophosphate, and are able to phosphorylate them to the active di- and triphosphates.

Tissues take up both free thiamin and thiamin monophosphate, then phosphorylate them further to yield thiamin diphosphate (the active coenzyme) and, in the nervous system, thiamin triphosphate.

Some free thiamin is excreted in the urine, increasing with diuresis, and a significant amount may also be lost in sweat. Most urinary excretion is as thiochrome, the result of non-enzymic cyclisation, as well as a variety of products of side-chain oxidation and ring cleavage.

There is little storage of thiamin in the body, and biochemical signs of deficiency can be observed within a few days of initiating a thiamin-free diet.

Metabolic functions of thiamin

Thiamin has a central role in energy-yielding metabolism, and especially the metabolism of carbohydrates. Thiamin diphosphate (also known as thiamin pyrophosphate, see Figure 10.8) is the coenzyme for three oxidative decarboxylation reactions: pyruvate dehydrogenase in carbohydrate metabolism, α-ketoglutarate dehydrogenase in the citric acid cycle, and the branched-chain keto-acid dehydrogenase involved in the metabolism of leucine, isoleucine, and valine. These three enzymes are multienzyme complexes that catalyse oxidative decarboxylation of the substrate linked to reduction of enzyme-bound lipoamide, and eventually reduction of NAD^+ to NADH.

Thiamin diphosphate is also the coenzyme for transketolase, in the pentose phosphate pathway of carbohydrate metabolism. This is the major pathway of carbohydrate metabolism in some tissues, and an important alternative to glycolysis in all tissues, being the source of half of the NADPH required for fatty acid synthesis.

Thiamin triphosphate has a role in nerve conduction, as the phosphate donor for phosphorylation of a nerve membrane sodium transport protein.

Thiamin deficiency

The biological half-life of thiamin is 10–20 days, and deficiency can develop rapidly during depletion. Diuresis increases the excretion of the vitamin, and patients who are treated with diuretics are at risk of deficiency.

Thiamin deficiency can result in three distinct syndromes:

- a chronic peripheral neuritis, beriberi, which may or may not be associated with heart failure and oedema
- acute pernicious (fulminating) beriberi (shoshin beriberi), in which heart failure and metabolic abnormalities predominate, with little evidence of peripheral neuritis
- Wernicke's encephalopathy with Korsakoff's psychosis, a thiamin-responsive condition associated especially with alcohol and narcotic abuse.

In general, a relatively acute deficiency is involved in the central nervous system lesions of the Wernicke–Korsakoff syndrome, and a high energy intake, as in alcoholics, is also a predisposing factor. Dry beriberi is associated with a more prolonged, and presumably less severe, deficiency, and a generally low food intake, whereas higher carbohydrate intake and physical activity predispose to wet beriberi.

The role of thiamin diphosphate in pyruvate dehydrogenase means that in deficiency there is impaired conversion of pyruvate to acetyl-CoA, and hence impaired entry of pyruvate into the citric acid cycle. Especially in subjects on a relatively high carbohydrate diet, this results in increased plasma concentrations of lactate and pyruvate, which may lead to life-threatening lactic acidosis. The increase in plasma lactate and pyruvate after a test dose of glucose has been used as a means of assessing thiamin nutritional status.

Dry beriberi

Chronic deficiency of thiamin, especially associated with a high carbohydrate diet, results in beriberi, which is a symmetrical ascending peripheral neuritis. Initially, the patient complains of weakness, stiffness and cramps in the legs, and is unable to walk more than a short distance. There may be numbness of the dorsum of the feet and ankles, and vibration sense may be diminished. As the disease progresses, the ankle jerk reflex is lost, and the muscular weakness spreads upwards, involving first the extensor muscles of the foot, then the muscles of the calf, and finally the extensors and flexors of the thigh. At this stage there is pronounced toe and foot drop: the patient is unable to keep either the toe or the whole foot extended off the ground. When the arms are affected there is a similar inability to keep the hand extended: wrist drop.

The affected muscles become tender, numb, and hyperaesthetic. The hyperaesthesia extends in the form of a band around the limb, the so-called stocking and glove distribution, and is followed by anaesthesia. There is deep muscle pain, and in the terminal stages, when the patient is bed-ridden, even slight pressure, as from bedclothes, causes considerable pain.

Wet beriberi

The heart may also be affected in beriberi, with dilatation of arterioles, rapid blood flow, and increased pulse rate leading to right-sided heart failure and oedema, so-called wet beriberi. The signs of chronic heart failure may be seen without peripheral neuritis. The arteriolar dilatation probably results from high circulating concentrations of lactate and pyruvate as a result of impaired activity of pyruvate dehydrogenase.

Acute pernicious (fulminating) beriberi: shoshin beriberi

Heart failure without increased cardiac output, and no peripheral oedema, may also occur acutely, associated with severe lactic acidosis. This was a common presentation of deficiency in Japan, where it was called shoshin (meaning acute) beriberi; in the 1920s some 26 000 deaths a year were recorded.

With improved knowledge of the cause and improved nutritional status, the disease has become more or less unknown, although in the 1980s it reappeared among Japanese adolescents consuming a diet based largely on such high-carbohydrate, low-nutrient, foods as sweet carbonated drinks, "instant" noodles, and polished rice. It also occurs among alcoholics, when the lactic acidosis may be life-threatening, without clear signs of heart failure. Acute beriberi has also been reported when previously starved subjects are given intravenous glucose.

Wernicke–Korsakoff syndrome

Whereas peripheral neuritis, acute cardiac beriberi, and lactic acidosis occur in thiamin deficiency associated with alcohol abuse, the more usual presentation is as the Wernicke–Korsakoff syndrome, due to central nervous system lesions.

Initially, there is a confused state, Korsakoff's psychosis, which is characterised by confabulation and loss of recent memory, although memory for past events may be unimpaired. Later, clear neurological signs develop: Wernicke's encephalopathy. This is characterised by nystagmus and extraocular palsy. Post-mortem examination shows characteristic brain lesions.

Like shoshin beriberi, Wernicke's encephalopathy can develop acutely, without the more gradual development of Korsakoff's psychosis, among previously starved patients given intravenous glucose and seriously ill patients given parenteral hyperalimentation.

Thiamin requirements

Because thiamin has a central role in energy-yielding, and especially carbohydrate, metabolism, requirements depend mainly on carbohydrate intake, and have been related to "non-fat calories." In practice, requirements and reference intakes are calculated on the basis of total energy intake, assuming that the average diet provides 40% of energy from fat. For diets that are lower in fat, and hence higher in carbohydrate, thiamin requirements may be somewhat higher.

From depletion/repletion studies, an intake of at least 40 μg of thiamin /MJ (0.2 mg/1000 kcal) is required to prevent the development of deficiency signs and maintain normal urinary excretion, but an intake of 46 μg/MJ is required for a normal transketolase activation coefficient.

Reference intakes are calculated on the basis of 100 μg/MJ (0.5 mg/1000 kcal) for adults consuming more than 2000 kcal (8MJ) /day, with a minimum requirement for people with a low energy intake of 0.8–1.0 mg/day to allow for metabolism of endogenous substrates.

Assessment of thiamin status

The impairment of pyruvate dehydrogenase in thiamin deficiency results in a considerable increase in the plasma concentrations of lactate and pyruvate. This has been exploited as a means of assessing thiamin status, by measuring changes in the plasma concentrations of lactate and pyruvate after an oral dose of glucose and mild exercise. The test is not specific for thiamin deficiency since a variety of other conditions can also result in metabolic acidosis. Although it may be useful in depletion/repletion studies, it is little used nowadays in assessment of nutritional status.

Whole blood total thiamin below 150 nmol/l is considered to indicate deficiency. However, the changes observed in depletion studies are small. Even in patients with frank beriberi the total thiamin concentration in erythrocytes is only 20% lower than normal, so whole blood thiamin is not a sensitive index of status.

Although there are several urinary metabolites of thiamin, a significant proportion is excreted either unchanged or as thiochrome, and therefore the urinary excretion of the vitamin (measured as thiochrome) can provide information on nutritional status. Excretion decreases proportionally with intake in adequately nourished subjects, but at low intakes there is a threshold below which further reduction in intake has little effect on excretion.

The activation of apo-transketolase in erythrocyte lysate by thiamin diphosphate added *in vitro* has become the most widely used and accepted index of thiamin nutritional status. Apo-transketolase is unstable both *in vivo* and *in vitro*, so problems may arise in the interpretation of results, especially if samples have been stored for any appreciable time. An activation coefficient >1.25 is indicative of deficiency, and <1.15 is considered to reflect adequate thiamin status.

10.7 Riboflavin (vitamin B_2)

Riboflavin deficiency is a significant public health problem in many areas of the world. The vitamin has a central role as a coenzyme in energy-yielding metabolism, yet deficiency is rarely, if ever, fatal, since there is very efficient conservation and recycling of riboflavin in deficiency.

The structures of riboflavin and the riboflavin-derived coenzymes are shown in Figure 10.9.

Milk and dairy products are important sources, providing 25% or more of total riboflavin intake in most diets, and it is noteworthy that average riboflavin status in different countries reflects milk consumption to a considerable extent. Other rich sources are eggs, meat, and fish. In addition, because of its intense yellow color, riboflavin is widely used as a food colour (E101).

Photolysis of riboflavin leads to the formation of lumiflavin (in alkaline solution) and lumichrome (in acidic or neutral solution), both of which are biologically inactive. Exposure of milk in clear glass bottles to sunlight or fluorescent light can result in the loss of significant amounts of riboflavin. This is potentially nutritionally important. Lumiflavin and lumichrome catalyse oxidation of lipids (to lipid peroxides) and methionine (to methional), resulting in the development of an unpleasant flavor, known as the "sunlight" flavor.

Absorption and metabolism

Apart from milk and eggs, which contain relatively large amounts of free riboflavin bound to specific binding proteins, most of the vitamin in foods is as flavin coenzymes bound to enzymes, which are released when the protein is hydrolysed. Intestinal phosphatases then hydrolyse

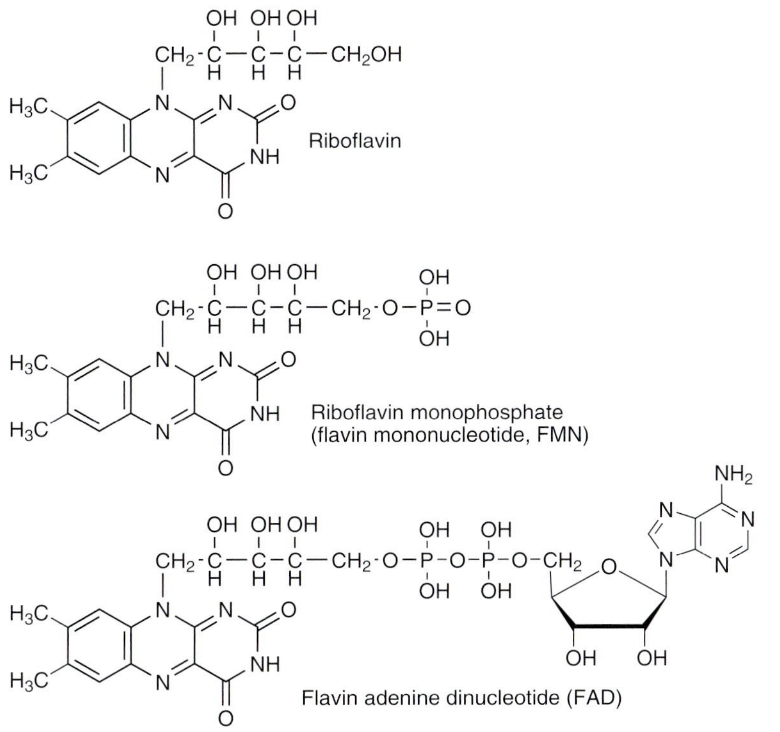

Figure 10.9 Riboflavin (vitamin B^{2}) and the flavin coenzymes, riboflavin monophosphate and flavin adenine dinucleotide.

the coenzymes to liberate riboflavin, which is absorbed in the upper small intestine. The absorption of riboflavin is limited and after moderately high doses only a small proportion is absorbed. Riboflavin synthesised by intestinal bacteria is absorbed in the colon by a carrier-mediated system

Much of the absorbed riboflavin is phosphorylated in the intestinal mucosa and enters the bloodstream as riboflavin phosphate, although this is not essential for absorption of the vitamin.

About 50% of plasma riboflavin is free riboflavin, which is the main transport form, with 44% as flavin adenine dinucleotide (FAD) and the remainder as riboflavin phosphate. The vitamin is largely protein-bound in plasma; free riboflavin binds to both albumin and α- and β-globulins; both riboflavin and the coenzymes also bind to immunoglobulins.

Uptake into tissues is by passive carrier-mediated transport of free riboflavin, followed by metabolic trapping by phosphorylation to riboflavin phosphate, and onward metabolism to FAD.

Riboflavin phosphate and FAD that are not bound to proteins are rapidly hydrolysed to riboflavin, which diffuses out of tissues into the bloodstream. Riboflavin and riboflavin phosphate that are not bound to plasma proteins are filtered at the glomerulus; renal tubular resorption is saturated at normal plasma concentrations. There is also active tubular secretion of the vitamin; urinary excretion of riboflavin after moderately high doses can be two- to threefold greater than the glomerular filtration rate.

Under normal conditions about 25% of the urinary excretion of riboflavin is as the unchanged vitamin, with a small amount as glycosides of riboflavin and its metabolites.

Riboflavin balance

There is no significant storage of riboflavin; apart from the limitation on absorption, any surplus intake is excreted rapidly, so that once metabolic requirements have been met urinary excretion of riboflavin and its metabolites reflects intake until intestinal absorption is saturated. In depleted animals, the maximum growth response is achieved with intakes that give about

75% saturation of tissues, and the intake to achieve tissue saturation is that at which there is quantitative excretion of the vitamin.

There is very efficient conservation of riboflavin in deficiency, and almost the only loss from tissues will be the small amount that is covalently bound to enzymes and cannot be salvaged for reuse. There is only a fourfold difference between the minimum concentration of flavins in the liver in deficiency and the level at which saturation occurs. In the central nervous system there is only a 35% difference between deficiency and saturation.

Metabolic functions of the flavin coenzymes

The metabolic function of the flavin coenzymes is as electron carriers in a wide variety of oxidation and reduction reactions central to all metabolic pathways, including the mitochondrial electron transport chain, and key enzymes in fatty acid and amino acid oxidation, and the citric acid cycle. The flavin coenzymes remain bound to the enzyme throughout the catalytic cycle. The majority of flavoproteins have FAD as the prosthetic group rather than riboflavin phosphate; some have both flavin coenzymes and some have other prosthetic groups as well.

Flavins can undergo a one-electron reduction to the semiquinone radical or a two-electron reduction to dihydroflavin. In some enzymes formation of dihydroflavin occurs by two single-electron steps, with intermediate formation of the semiquinone radical. Dihydroflavin can be oxidised by reaction with a substrate, $NAD(P)^+$, or cytochromes in a variety of dehydrogenases, or can react with molecular oxygen in oxygenases and mixed function oxidases (hydroxylases).

Flavins and oxidative stress

Reoxidation of the reduced flavin in oxygenases and mixed function oxidases proceeds by way of formation of the flavin radical and flavin hydroperoxide, with the intermediate generation of superoxide and perhydroxyl radicals and hydrogen peroxide. Because of this, flavin oxidases make a significant contribution to the total oxidant stress of the body. Overall, some 3–5% of the daily consumption of about 30 mol of oxygen by an adult is converted to singlet oxygen, hydrogen peroxide, and superoxide, perhydroxyl, and hydroxyl radicals, rather than undergoing complete reduction to water in the electron transport chain. There is thus a total production of some 1.5 mol of reactive oxygen species daily, potentially capable of causing damage to membrane lipids, proteins, and nucleic acids.

Riboflavin deficiency

Although riboflavin is involved in all areas of metabolism, and deficiency is widespread on a global scale, deficiency is not fatal. There seem to be two reasons for this. One is that, although deficiency is common, the vitamin is widespread in foods and most diets will provide minimally adequate amounts to permit maintenance of central metabolic pathways. The second, more important, reason is that in deficiency there is extremely efficient reutilisation of the riboflavin that is released by the turnover of flavoproteins, so that only a very small amount is metabolised or excreted.

Riboflavin deficiency is characterised by lesions of the margin of the lips (cheilosis) and corners of the mouth (angular stomatitis), a painful desquamation of the tongue, so that it is red, dry, and atrophic (magenta tongue), and a seborrhoeic dermatitis, with filiform excrescences, affecting especially the nasolabial folds, eyelids, and ears.

There may also be conjunctivitis with vascularisation of the cornea and opacity of the lens. This last is the only lesion of ariboflavinosis for which the biochemical basis is known: glutathione is important in maintaining the normal clarity of crystallin in the lens, and glutathione reductase is a flavoprotein that is particularly sensitive to riboflavin depletion.

The main metabolic effect of riboflavin deficiency is on lipid metabolism. Riboflavin-deficient animals have a lower metabolic rate than controls and require a 15–20% higher food intake to maintain body weight. Feeding a high-fat diet leads to more marked impairment of growth and a higher requirement for riboflavin to restore growth.

Neonatal hyperbilirubinaemia is usually treated by phototherapy. The peak wavelength for photolysis of bilirubin is the same as that for photolysis of riboflavin. Infants undergoing phototherapy show biochemical evidence of riboflavin depletion, but because photolysis products of riboflavin can cause damage to DNA, riboflavin supplements are not provided during phototherapy.

Resistance to malaria in riboflavin deficiency

Several studies have noted that in areas where malaria is endemic, riboflavin-deficient people are relatively resistant and have a lower parasite burden than adequately nourished people. The biochemical basis of this resistance to malaria in riboflavin deficiency is not known, but two possible mechanisms have been proposed.

- The malarial parasites may have a particularly high requirement for riboflavin. Some flavin analogues have antimalarial action.
- As a result of impaired antioxidant activity in erythrocytes, there may be increased fragility of erythrocyte membranes or reduced membrane fluidity. As in sickle cell trait, which also protects against malaria, this may result in exposure of the parasites to the host's immune system at a vulnerable stage in their development, resulting in the production of protective antibodies.

Riboflavin requirements

Estimates of riboflavin requirements are based on depletion/repletion studies to determine the minimum intake at which there is significant excretion of the vitamin. In deficiency there is virtually no excretion of the vitamin; as requirements are met, so any excess is excreted in the urine. On this basis the minimum adult requirement for riboflavin is 0.5–0.8 mg/day. At intakes of 1.1–1.6 mg/day urinary excretion rises sharply, suggesting that tissue reserves are saturated.

A more generous estimate of requirements, and the basis of reference intakes, is based on the activation coefficient of erythrocyte glutathione reductase. Normal values of the activation coefficient are seen in people whose habitual intake of riboflavin is between 1.2 and 1.5 mg/day.

Because of the central role of flavin coenzymes in energy-yielding metabolism, reference intakes are sometimes calculated on the basis of energy intake: 0.14–0.19 mg/MJ (0.6–0.8 mg/1000 kcal). However, in view of the wide range of riboflavin-dependent reactions, other than those of energy-yielding metabolism, it is difficult to justify this basis for the calculation of requirements.

Assessment of riboflavin nutritional status

The urinary excretion of riboflavin and its metabolites (either basal excretion or after a test dose) can be used as an index of status. However, riboflavin excretion is only correlated with intake in subjects who are in nitrogen balance. In subjects in negative nitrogen balance there may be more urinary excretion than would be expected, as a result of the catabolism of tissue flavoproteins, and loss of their prosthetic groups. Higher intakes of protein than are required to maintain nitrogen balance do not affect the requirement for riboflavin or indices of riboflavin nutritional status.

Glutathione reductase is especially sensitive to riboflavin depletion. The activity of the enzyme in erythrocytes can therefore be used as an index of riboflavin status. Interpretation of the results can be complicated by anaemia, and it is more usual to use the activation of erythrocyte glutathione reductase (EGR) by FAD added *in vitro*. An activation coefficient of 1.0–1.4 reflects adequate nutritional status, whereas >1.7 indicates deficiency.

Interactions with drugs and other nutrients

Phenothiazines such as chlorpromazine, used in the treatment of schizophrenia, and tricyclic antidepressant drugs such as imipramine, are structural analogues of riboflavin, and inhibit flavokinase. In experimental animals, administration of these drugs at doses equivalent to those used clinically results in an increase in the erythrocyte glutathione reductase activation coefficient and increased urinary excretion of riboflavin, with reduced tissue concentrations of riboflavin phosphate and FAD, despite feeding diets providing more riboflavin than is needed to meet requirements. Although there is no evidence that patients treated with these drugs for a prolonged period develop clinical signs of riboflavin deficiency, long-term use of chlorpromazine is associated with a reduction in metabolic rate.

Riboflavin deficiency is sometimes associated with hypochromic anaemia as a result of impaired iron absorption. A greater proportion of a test dose of iron is retained in the intestinal mucosal cells bound to ferritin, and hence lost in the faeces, rather than being absorbed, because the mobilisation of iron bound to ferritin in mucosal cells for transfer to transferrin requires oxidation by a flavin-dependent enzyme.

Riboflavin depletion decreases the oxidation of dietary vitamin B_6 to pyridoxal; pyridoxine oxidase is a flavoprotein and is very sensitive to riboflavin depletion. It is not clear to what extent there is functional vitamin B_6 deficiency in riboflavin deficiency. This is partly because vitamin B_6 nutritional status is generally assessed by the metabolism of a test dose of tryptophan, and kynurenine hydroxylase in the tryptophan oxidative pathway is a flavoprotein; riboflavin deficiency can therefore disturb tryptophan metabolism quite separately from its effects on vitamin B_6 nutritional status.

The disturbance of tryptophan metabolism in riboflavin deficiency, due to impairment of kynurenine hydroxylase, can also result in reduced synthesis of NAD from tryptophan, and may therefore be a factor in the aetiology of pellagra.

10.8 Niacin

Niacin is not strictly a vitamin, since it can be synthesised in the body from the essential amino acid tryptophan. Indeed, it is only when tryptophan intake is inadequate or its metabolism is impaired that dietary preformed niacin becomes important. Nevertheless, since niacin was discovered as a nutrient during studies of the deficiency disease pellagra, which was a major public health problem in the southern USA throughout the first half of the twentieth century, and continued to be a problem in parts of India and sub-Saharan Africa until the 1990s, it is regarded as a vitamin.

Vitamers and niacin equivalents

Two compounds, nicotinic acid and nicotinamide, have the biological activity of niacin. When nicotinic acid was discovered as the curative and preventive factor for pellagra, it was already known as a chemical compound, and was therefore never assigned a number among the B vitamins. The name niacin was coined in the USA when it was decided to enrich maize meal with the vitamin to prevent pellagra; it was considered that the name nicotinic acid was not desirable because of its similarity to nicotine. In the USA the term niacin is commonly used to mean specifically nicotinic acid, and nicotinamide is known as niacinamide; elsewhere "niacin" is used as a generic descriptor for both vitamers. Figure 10.10 shows the structures of

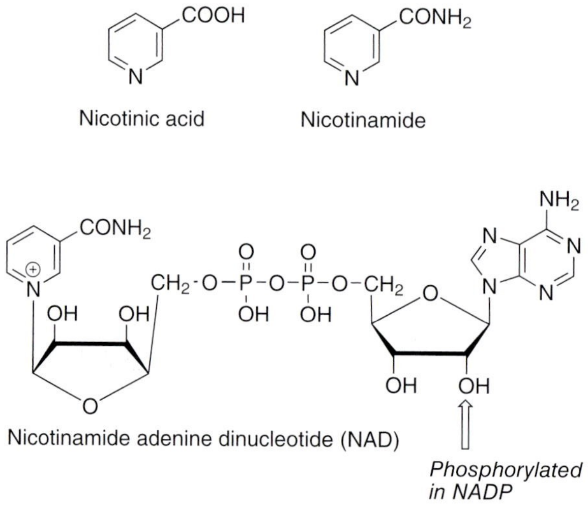

Nicotinic acid

Nicotinamide

Nicotinamide adenine dinucleotide (NAD)

Phosphorylated in NADP

Figure 10.10 The niacin vitamers, nicotinic acid and nicotinamide, and the coenzyme nicotinamide adenine dinucleotide.

nicotinic acid and nicotinamide, as well as coenzymes, NAD and NADP.

The nicotinamide ring of NAD can be synthesised in the body from the essential amino acid tryptophan. In adults almost all of the dietary intake of tryptophan, apart from the small amount that is used for net new protein synthesis, and synthesis of melatonin and the neurotransmitter serotonin, is metabolised by this pathway, and hence is potentially available for NAD synthesis.

Several studies have investigated the equivalence of dietary tryptophan and preformed niacin as precursors of the nicotinamide nucleotides, generally by determining the excretion of niacin metabolites in response to test doses of the precursors, in subjects maintained on deficient diets. The most extensive such study was that of Horwitt *et al.* in 1956. They found that there was a considerable variation between subjects in the response to tryptophan and niacin, and in order to allow for this individual variation they proposed the ratio of 60 mg of tryptophan equivalent to 1 mg of preformed niacin. Changes in hormonal status may result in considerable changes in this ratio, with between 7 and 30 mg of dietary tryptophan being equivalent to 1 mg of preformed niacin in late pregnancy.

The niacin content of foods is generally expressed as mg niacin equivalents; 1 mg niacin equivalent = mg preformed niacin + 1/60 × mg tryptophan. Because most of the niacin in cereals is biologically unavailable, it is conventional to ignore niacin in cereal products.

Because endogenous synthesis from tryptophan is more important than preformed dietary niacin, the main dietary sources of niacin are generally those that are also rich sources of protein. It is only when the dietary staple is a cereal such as maize, which is remarkably lacking in tryptophan, that problems of deficiency occur. Trigonelline (N^1-methylnicotinic acid) in coffee beans is demethylated to nicotinic acid during roasting, and moderate coffee consumption may meet a significant proportion of niacin requirements.

Unavailable niacin in cereals

Chemical analysis reveals niacin in cereals (largely in the bran), but this is biologically unavailable, since it is bound as niacytin – nicotinoyl esters to a variety of macromolecules. In wheat bran some 60% is esterified to polysaccharides, and the remainder to polypeptides and glycopeptides.

Treatment of cereals with alkali (e.g., by soaking overnight in calcium hydroxide solution, as is the traditional method for the preparation of tortillas in Mexico) and baking with alkaline baking powder releases much of the nicotinic acid. This may explain why pellagra has always been rare in Mexico, despite the fact that maize is the dietary staple. Up to 10% of the niacin in niacytin may be biologically available as a result of hydrolysis by gastric acid.

Absorption and metabolism

Niacin is present in tissues, and therefore in foods, largely as the nicotinamide nucleotides NAD and NADP. The postmortem hydrolysis of NAD(P) is extremely rapid in animal tissues, so it is likely that much of the niacin of meat (a major dietary source of the preformed vitamin) is free nicotinamide.

Nicotinamide nucleotides present in the intestinal lumen are not absorbed as such, but are hydrolysed to free nicotinamide. Many intestinal bacteria have nicotinamide deamidase activity, and a significant proportion of dietary nicotinamide may be deamidated in the intestinal lumen. Both nicotinic acid and nicotinamide are absorbed from the small intestine by a sodium-dependent saturable process, and by a sodium-independent process in the colon.

The nicotinamide nucleotide coenzymes can be synthesised from either of the niacin vitamers and from quinolinic acid, an intermediate in tryptophan metabolism. In the liver, synthesis of the coenzymes increases with increasing intake of tryptophan, but not preformed niacin. The liver exports nicotinamide, derived from turnover of coenzymes, for uptake by other tissues.

Catabolism of NAD(P)

The catabolism of NAD^+ is catalysed by four enzymes:

- NAD glycohydrolase, which releases nicotinamide and ADP-ribose;
- NAD pyrophosphatase, which releases nicotinamide mononucleotide; this can be either

hydrolysed by NAD glycohydrolase to release nicotinamide, or reutilised to form NAD;
- ADP-ribosyltransferases;
- poly(ADP-ribose) polymerase.

The activation of ADP-ribosyltransferase and poly(ADP-ribose) polymerase by toxins, oxidative stress or DNA damage may result in considerable depletion of intracellular NAD(P), and may indeed provide a protective mechanism to ensure that cells that have suffered very severe DNA damage die as a result of NAD(P) depletion. The administration of DNA-breaking carcinogens to experimental animals results in the excretion of large amounts of nicotinamide metabolites and depletion of tissue NAD(P); addition of the compounds to cells in culture has a similar effect. Chronic exposure to such carcinogens and mycotoxins may be a contributory factor in the aetiology of pellagra when dietary intakes of tryptophan and niacin are marginal.

Urinary excretion of niacin and metabolites

Under normal conditions there is little or no urinary excretion of either nicotinamide or nicotinic acid. This is because both vitamers are actively reabsorbed from the glomerular filtrate. It is only when the concentration is so high that the reabsorption mechanism is saturated that there is any significant excretion of niacin.

Nicotinamide in excess of requirements for NAD synthesis is methylated by nicotinamide *N*-methyltransferase. N^1-Methylnicotinamide is actively secreted into the urine by the proximal renal tubules. N^1-Methylnicotinamide can also be metabolised further, to yield methylpyridone-2- and 4-carboxamides.

Nicotinamide can also undergo oxidation to nicotinamide *N*-oxide when large amounts are ingested. Nicotinic acid can be conjugated with glycine to form nicotinuric acid (nicotinoylglycine) or may be methylated to trigonelline (N^1-methylnicotinic acid). It is not clear to what extent urinary excretion of trigonelline reflects endogenous methylation of nicotinic acid, since there is a significant amount of trigonelline in foods, which may be absorbed, but cannot be utilised as a source of niacin, and is excreted unchanged.

Metabolic functions of niacin

The best-defined role of niacin is in the metabolism of metabolic fuels, as the functional nicotinamide moiety of the coenzymes NAD and NADP, which play a major role in oxidation and reduction reactions. The oxidised coenzymes have a positive charge on the nicotinamide ring nitrogen and undergo a two-electron reduction. The oxidised forms are conventionally shown as $NAD(P)^+$ and the reduced forms either as $NAD(P)H_2$ or, more correctly, as NAD(P)H + H^+, since although it is a two-electron reduction, only one proton is incorporated into the ring, the other remaining associated with the coenzyme.

In general, NAD^+ acts as an electron acceptor in energy-yielding metabolism, being oxidised by the mitochondrial electron transport chain, while the major coenzyme for reductive synthetic reactions is NADPH. An exception to this general rule is the pentose phosphate pathway of glucose metabolism, which results in the reduction of $NADP^+$ to NADPH, and is the source of half the reductant for fatty acid synthesis.

In addition to its coenzyme role, NAD is the source of ADP-ribose for the ADP-ribosylation of a variety of proteins and poly(ADP-ribosylation) and hence activation of nucleoproteins involved in the DNA repair mechanism.

In the nucleus, poly(ADP-ribose)polymerase is activated by binding to breakage points in DNA. The enzyme is involved in activation of the DNA repair mechanism in response to strand breakage caused by radical attack or UV radiation. In cells that have suffered considerable DNA damage, the activation of poly (ADP-ribose) polymerase may deplete intracellular NAD to such an extent that ATP formation is impaired, leading to cell death.

ADP-ribose cyclase catalyses the formation of cyclic ADP-ribose from NAD, and of nicotinic acid adenine dinucleotide phosphate from NADP (by catalysing the exchange of nicotinamide for nicotinic acid). Both of these compounds act to raise cytosolic calcium concentrations by releasing calcium from intracellular stores, acting as second messengers in response to nitric oxide, acetylcholine, and other neurotransmitters.

The sirtuins are a family of enzymes that catalyse the deacetylation of lysine residues in histones and other proteins, and hence in epigenetic regulation of gene expression. The reaction involves the hydrolysis of NAD^+ and the formation of *O*-acetyl ADP-ribose and nicotinamide. Sirtuin activity is limited by the availability of NAD^+, and hence depends on niacin nutritional status and the ratio of NAD^+:NADH, and hence the energy state of the cell. There is evidence from animal studies that over-expression of some sirtuins is associated with increased life-span.

Pellagra: a disease of tryptophan and niacin deficiency

Pellagra became common in Europe when maize was introduced from the New World as a convenient high-yielding dietary staple, and by the late nineteenth century it was widespread throughout southern Europe, north and south Africa, and the southern USA. The proteins of maize are particularly lacking in tryptophan, and, as with other cereals, little or none of the preformed niacin is biologically available unless the cereal is treated with alkali before cooking, as in the traditional production of tortillas in Mexico.

Pellagra is characterised by a photosensitive dermatitis, resembling severe sunburn, typically with a butterfly-like pattern of distribution over the face, affecting all parts of the skin that are exposed to sunlight. Similar skin lesions may also occur in areas not exposed to sunlight, but subject to pressure, such as the knees, elbows, wrists, and ankles. Advanced pellagra is also accompanied by dementia (more correctly a depressive psychosis), and there may be diarrhoea. Untreated pellagra is fatal.

The depressive psychosis is superficially similar to schizophrenia and the organic psychoses, but clinically distinguishable by sudden lucid phases that alternate with the most florid psychiatric signs. It is probable that these mental symptoms can be explained by a relative deficit of the essential amino acid tryptophan, and hence reduced synthesis of the neurotransmitter 5-hydroxytryptamine (serotonin), and not to a deficiency of niacin *per se*.

Additional factors in the aetiology of pellagra

Pellagra also occurs in India among people whose dietary staple is jowar (*Sorghum vulgare*), even though the protein in this cereal contains enough tryptophan to permit adequate synthesis of NAD. Here the problem seems to be the relative excess of leucine in the protein, which can inhibit tissue uptake of tryptophan, and hence the synthesis of NAD from tryptophan. It is likely that leucine is a factor in the aetiology of pellagra only when the dietary intakes of both tryptophan and niacin are low, a condition that may occur when sorghum is the dietary staple, especially at times of food shortage.

Although the nutritional aetiology of pellagra is well established, and tryptophan or niacin will prevent or cure the disease, additional factors, including deficiency of riboflavin or vitamin B_6, both of which are required for synthesis of NAD from tryptophan, may be important when intakes of tryptophan and niacin are only marginally adequate.

During the first half of the twentieth century, of the 87 000 people who died from pellagra in the USA there were twice as many women as men. Reports of individual outbreaks of pellagra, both in the USA and more recently elsewhere, show a similar gender ratio. This may well be the result of inhibition of tryptophan metabolism by oestrogen metabolites, and hence reduced synthesis of NAD from tryptophan.

Several bacterial, fungal, and environmental toxins activate ADP-ribosyltransferase or poly(ADP-ribose) polymerase, and it is possible that chronic exposure to such toxins will deplete tissue NAD(P) and hence be a contributory factor in the development of pellagra when intakes of tryptophan and niacin are marginal.

Niacin requirements

On the basis of depletion/repletion studies in which the urinary excretion of niacin metabolites was measured after feeding tryptophan or preformed niacin, the average requirement for niacin is 1.3 mg of niacin equivalents/MJ energy expenditure, and reference intakes are based on 1.6 mg/MJ. Average intakes of tryptophan in Western diets will more than meet requirements without the need for a dietary source of preformed niacin.

Assessment of niacin status

Although the nicotinamide nucleotide coenzymes function in a large number of oxidation and reduction reactions, this cannot be exploited as a means of assessing the state of the body's niacin reserves, because the coenzymes are not firmly attached to their apoenzymes, as are thiamin pyrophosphate, riboflavin, and pyridoxal phosphate, but act as cosubstrates of the reactions, binding to and leaving the enzyme as the reaction proceeds. No specific metabolic lesions associated with NAD(P) depletion have been identified.

The two methods of assessing niacin nutritional status are measurement of the ratio of NAD/NADP in red blood cells and the urinary excretion of niacin metabolites, neither of which is wholly satisfactory.

Niacin toxicity

Nicotinic acid has been used to lower blood triacylglycerol and cholesterol in patients with hyperlipidaemia. However, relatively large amounts are required (of the order of 1–6 g/day, compared with reference intakes of 18–20 mg/day). At this level of intake, nicotinic acid causes dilatation of blood vessels and flushing, with skin irritation, itching, and a burning sensation. This effect wears off after a few days.

High intakes of both nicotinic acid and nicotinamide, in excess of 500 mg/day, cause liver damage, and prolonged use can result in liver failure. This is especially a problem with sustained-release preparations of niacin, which permit a high blood level to be maintained for a relatively long time.

10.9 Vitamin B_6

Apart from an outbreak in the 1950s, due to overheated infant milk formula, vitamin B_6 deficiency is unknown except under experimental conditions. Nevertheless, there is a considerable body of evidence that marginal status and biochemical deficiency may be relatively widespread in developed countries.

Vitamin B_6 is widely distributed in a variety of foods. However, a considerable proportion of the vitamin in plant foods may be present as glucosides, which are probably not biologically available, although a proportion may be hydrolysed by intestinal bacteria.

When foods are heated, pyridoxal and pyridoxal phosphate can react with the ε-amino groups of lysine to form a Schiff base (aldimine). This renders both the vitamin B_6 and the lysine biologically unavailable; more importantly, the pyridoxyl-lysine released during digestion is absorbed and has antivitamin B_6 antimetabolic activity. Overall, it is estimated that some 70–80% of dietary vitamin B_6 is available.

Vitamers

The generic descriptor vitamin B_6 includes six vitamers: the alcohol pyridoxine, the aldehyde pyridoxal, the amine pyridoxamine, and their 5′-phosphates. There is some confusion in the older literature, because at one time "pyridoxine," which is now used specifically for the alcohol, was used as a generic descriptor, with "pyridoxol" as the specific name for the alcohol. The vitamers are metabolically interconvertible and, as far as is known, they have equal biological activity; they are all converted in the body to the metabolically active form, pyridoxal phosphate. 4-Pyridoxic acid is a biologically inactive end-product of vitamin B_6 metabolism.

Absorption and metabolism

The phosphorylated vitamers are dephosphorylated by membrane-bound alkaline phosphatase in the intestinal mucosa; pyridoxal, pyridoxamine, and pyridoxine are all absorbed rapidly by passive diffusion. Intestinal mucosal cells have pyridoxine kinase and pyridoxine phosphate oxidase (Figure 10.11), so that there is net accumulation of pyridoxal phosphate by metabolic trapping. Much of the ingested pyridoxine is released into the portal circulation as pyridoxal, after dephosphorylation at the serosal surface. Unlike other B vitamins, there seems to be no limit on the amount of vitamin B_6 that is absorbed.

Most of the absorbed vitamin is taken up by the liver by passive diffusion, followed by metabolic trapping as phosphate esters, which do not cross cell membranes, then oxidation to

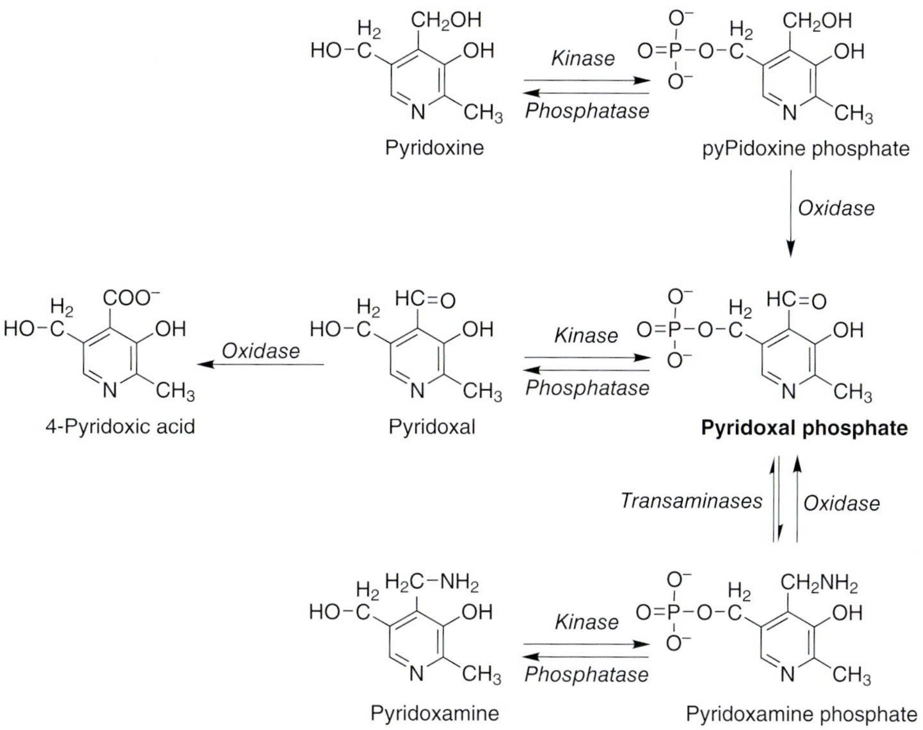

Figure 10.11 Interconversion of the vitamin B_6 vitamers. Pyridoxal kinase (EC 2.7.1.38), pyridoxine phosphate oxidase (EC 1.1.1.65), pyridoxamine phosphate oxidase (EC 1.4.3.5).

pyridoxal phosphate. The liver exports both pyridoxal phosphate (bound to albumin) and pyridoxal (which binds to both albumin and haemoglobin). Free pyridoxal remaining in the liver is rapidly oxidised to 4-pyridoxic acid, which is the main excretory product.

Extrahepatic tissues take up pyridoxal and pyridoxal phosphate from the plasma. The phosphate is hydrolysed to pyridoxal, which can cross cell membranes, by extracellular alkaline phosphatase, then trapped intracellularly by phosphorylation. Tissue concentrations of pyridoxal phosphate are controlled by the balance between phosphorylation and dephosphorylation.

Some 80% of the body's total vitamin B_6 is pyridoxal phosphate in muscle, mostly associated with glycogen phosphorylase. This does not function as a reserve of the vitamin and is not released from muscle in times of deficiency; it is released into the circulation (as pyridoxal) in starvation, when glycogen reserves are exhausted and there is less requirement for phosphorylase activity. Under these conditions it is available for redistribution to other tissues, and especially the liver and kidneys, to meet the increased need for transamination of amino acids to provide substrates for gluconeogenesis.

Metabolic functions of vitamin B_6

Pyridoxal phosphate is a coenzyme in three main areas of metabolism:

- in a wide variety of reactions of amino acids, especially transamination, in which it functions as the intermediate carrier of the amino group, and decarboxylation to form amines
- as the cofactor of glycogen phosphorylase in muscle and liver, where it is the phosphate group that is catalytically important
- in the regulation of the action of steroid hormones. Pyridoxal phosphate acts to remove the hormone–receptor complex from DNA binding, and so terminate the action of the hormones. In vitamin B_6 deficiency there is increased sensitivity and responsiveness of target tissues to low concentrations of steroid hormones, including oestrogens, androgens, and cortisol.

Vitamin B_6 deficiency

Deficiency of vitamin B_6 severe enough to lead to clinical signs is extremely rare, and unequivocal deficiency has only been reported in one outbreak, during the 1950s, when babies were fed on a milk preparation that had been severely overheated during manufacture. Many of the affected infants suffered convulsions, which ceased rapidly following the administration of vitamin B_6.

The cause of the convulsions was severe impairment of the activity of the pyridoxal phosphate-dependent enzyme glutamate decarboxylase, which catalyses the synthesis of the inhibitory neurotransmitter γ-aminobutyric acid (GABA), together with accumulation of hydroxykynurenine as a result of impaired activity of kynureninase, which is also pyridoxal phosphate dependent.

Moderate vitamin B_6 deficiency results in a number of abnormalities of amino acid metabolism, especially of tryptophan and methionine. In experimental animals, a moderate degree of deficiency leads to increased sensitivity of target tissues to steroid hormone action. This may be important in the development of hormone-dependent cancer of the breast, uterus, and prostate, and may therefore affect the prognosis. Vitamin B_6 supplementation may be a useful adjunct to other therapy in these common cancers; certainly, there is evidence that poor vitamin B_6 nutritional status is associated with a poor prognosis in women with breast cancer.

Vitamin B_6 depletion may result from the prolonged administration of drugs that can form biologically inactive adducts with pyridoxal, such as penicillamine and the anti-tuberculosis drug isoniazid. Drug-induced vitamin B_6 deficiency frequently manifests as the tryptophan-niacin deficiency disease pellagra because synthesis of the nicotinamide nucleotide coenzymes from tryptophan is pyridoxal phosphate dependent.

Vitamin B_6 requirements

Most studies of vitamin B_6 requirements have followed the development of abnormalities of tryptophan and methionine metabolism during depletion, and normalisation during repletion with graded intakes of the vitamin. Although the tryptophan load test is unreliable as an index of vitamin B_6 nutritional status in field studies, under the controlled conditions of depletion/repletion studies it gives a useful indication of the state of vitamin B_6 nutrition.

Since the major role of vitamin B_6 is in amino acid metabolism it is likely that protein intake will affect vitamin B_6 requirements. Adults maintained on vitamin B_6-deficient diets develop abnormalities of tryptophan and methionine metabolism more quickly, and their blood vitamin B_6 falls more rapidly, when their protein intake is relatively high (80 – 160 g/day in various studies) than on low protein intakes (30 – 50 g/day). Similarly, during repletion of deficient subjects, tryptophan and methionine metabolism and blood vitamin B_6 are normalised more rapidly at low than at high levels of protein intake.

From such studies the average requirement for vitamin B_6 is estimated to be 13 μg/g dietary protein, and reference intakes are based on 15–16 μg/g dietary protein.

Requirements of infants

Estimation of the vitamin B_6 requirements of infants presents a problem, and there is a clear need for further research. Human milk, which must be assumed to be adequate for infant nutrition, provides only some 2.5–3 μg of vitamin B_6/g protein. This is very much lower than the requirement of adults, although there is no reason why infants should have a lower requirement.

Based on the body content of 3.7 μg (15 nmol) of vitamin B_6/g body weight, and the rate of weight gain, a minimum requirement for infants over the first six months of life is 100 μg/day to establish tissue reserves, and an additional 20% to allow for metabolic turnover. Even if the mother receives daily supplements of 2.5 mg of vitamin B_6 throughout lactation, thus more than doubling her normal intake, the infant's intake ranges from 100 to 300 μg/day over the first six months of life. At one month this is only 8.5 μg/g protein, rising to 15 μg/g by two months.

Assessment of vitamin B_6 status

There are a number of indices of vitamin B_6 status available: plasma concentrations of the vitamin, plasma concentration and urinary excretion of 4-pyridoxic acid, activation of erythrocyte aminotransferases by pyridoxal phosphate added *in vitro*, and the ability to metabolise test doses of tryptophan and methionine. Where more than one index has been used in population studies there is poor agreement between different methods.

Fasting plasma total vitamin B_6 (measured microbiologically), or more specifically pyridoxal phosphate, is widely used as an index of vitamin B_6 nutritional status. Despite the fall in plasma pyridoxal phosphate in pregnancy, which has been widely interpreted as indicating vitamin B_6 depletion or an increased requirement, the plasma concentration of pyridoxal phosphate plus pyridoxal is unchanged. This suggests that determination of plasma pyridoxal phosphate alone may not be a reliable index of vitamin B_6 nutritional status.

Low serum albumin will lead to a low plasma concentration of pyridoxal phosphate, because it is transported bound to albumin, and a high circulating activity of alkaline phosphatase will also lead to low concentrations of pyridoxal phosphate, because it is hydrolysed to pyridoxal. In chronic diseases there is also a low plasma concentration of pyridoxal phosphate because of reduced serum albumin; there is no evidence of increased catabolism of the vitamin in inflammatory disease. There is also redistribution of vitamin B_6 to sites of inflammation, to permit increased activity of tryptophan catabolism (initiated by indoleamine dioxygenase), and metabolism of immunomodulatory sphingolipids, as well as increased activity of serine hydroxymethyltransferase for immune cell proliferation. By contrast, elevated plasma inorganic phosphate leads to an increased concentration of pyridoxal phosphate because of inhibition of alkaline phosphatase by phosphate.

About half of the normal dietary intake of vitamin B_6 is excreted as 4-pyridoxic acid. Urinary excretion of 4-pyridoxic acid will largely reflect the recent intake of the vitamin rather than the underlying nutritional status.

Coenzyme saturation of transaminases

The most widely used method of assessing vitamin B_6 status is by the activation of erythrocyte transaminases by pyridoxal phosphate added *in vitro*. An activation coefficient for alanine transaminase >1.25, or for aspartate transaminase >1.8, is considered to indicate deficiency.

The tryptophan load test

The tryptophan load test for vitamin B_6 nutritional status (the ability to metabolise a test dose of tryptophan) is one of the oldest metabolic tests for functional vitamin nutritional status. It was developed as a result of observation of the excretion of an abnormal coloured compound, later identified as the tryptophan metabolite xanthurenic acid, in the urine of deficient animals.

Kynureninase (see Figure 10.12) is a pyridoxal phosphate-dependent enzyme, and its activity falls markedly in vitamin B_6 deficiency, at least partly because it undergoes a slow mechanism-dependent inactivation that leaves catalytically inactive pyridoxamine phosphate at the active site of the enzyme. The enzyme can only be reactivated if there is an adequate supply of pyridoxal phosphate. This means that in vitamin B_6 deficiency there is a considerable accumulation of both hydroxykynurenine and kynurenine, sufficient to permit greater metabolic flux than usual through kynurenine transaminase, resulting in increased formation of kynurenic and xanthurenic acids.

Xanthurenic and kynurenic acids, and kynurenine and hydroxykynurenine, are easy to measure in urine, so the tryptophan load test [the ability to metabolise a test dose of 2–5 g (150–380 μmol/kg body weight) of tryptophan] has been widely adopted as a convenient and sensitive index of vitamin B_6 nutritional status. However, because glucocorticoid hormones induce tryptophan dioxygenase, especialy under conditions of stress, abnormal results of the tryptophan load test must be regarded with caution, and cannot necessarily be interpreted as indicating vitamin B_6 deficiency. Increased entry of tryptophan into the pathway will overwhelm the capacity of kynureninase, leading to increased formation of xanthurenic and kynurenic acids. Similarly, oestrogen metabolites inhibit kynureninase, leading to results that have been misinterpreted as vitamin B_6 deficiency.

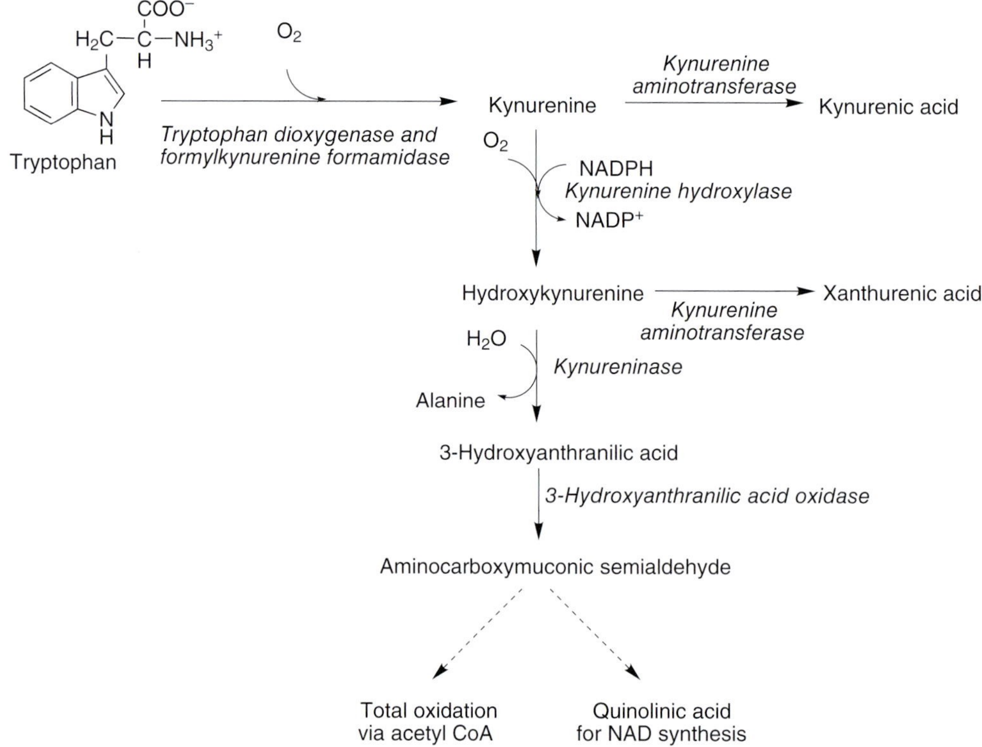

Figure 10.12 Oxidative pathway of tryptophan: the basis of the tryptophan load test. Tryptophan dioxygenase (EC 1.13.11.11), formylkynurenine formamidase (EC 3.5.1.9), kynurenine hydroxylase (EC 1.14.13.9), kynureninase (EC 3.7.1.3).

The methionine load test

The metabolism of methionine includes two pyridoxal phosphate-dependent steps: cystathionine synthetase and cystathionase (see Figure 10.16). Cystathionase activity falls markedly in vitamin B_6 deficiency, and as a result there is an increase in the urinary excretion of homocysteine and cystathionine, both after a loading dose of methionine and under basal conditions. However, homocysteine metabolism is more affected by folate status than by vitamin B_6 status and, like the tryptophan load test, the methionine load test is probably not reliable as an index of vitamin B_6 status in field studies.

Non-nutritional uses of vitamin B_6

Several studies have suggested that oral contraceptives cause vitamin B_6 deficiency. As a result of this, supplements of vitamin B_6 of 50–100 mg/day, and sometimes higher, have been used to overcome the side-effects of oral contraceptives. Similar supplements have also been recommended for the treatment of the premenstrual syndrome, although there is little evidence of efficacy from placebo-controlled trials.

All of the studies that suggested that oral contraceptives cause vitamin B_6 deficiency used the metabolism of tryptophan as a means of assessing vitamin B_6 nutritional status. When other biochemical markers of status were also assessed, they were not affected by oral contraceptive use. Furthermore, most of these studies were performed using the now obsolete high-dose contraceptive pills. Oral contraceptives do not cause vitamin B_6 deficiency. The problem is that oestrogen metabolites inhibit kynureninase and reduce the activity of kynurenine hydroxylase. This results in the excretion of abnormal amounts of tryptophan metabolites, similar to what is seen in vitamin B_6 deficiency, but for a different reason.

Doses of 50–200 mg of vitamin B_6/day have an antiemetic effect, and the vitamin is widely used, alone or in conjunction with other antiemetics, to minimise the nausea associated with radiotherapy and to treat pregnancy sickness. There is no evidence that vitamin B_6 has any beneficial effect in pregnancy sickness, or that women who suffer from morning sickness have lower vitamin B_6 nutritional status than other pregnant women.

Doses of vitamin B_6 of 100 mg/day have been reported to be beneficial in the treatment of the carpal tunnel syndrome or tenosynovitis. However, most of the reports originate from one centre and there appears to be little independent confirmation of the usefulness of the vitamin in this condition.

Vitamin B_6 toxicity

In experimental animals, doses of vitamin B_6 of 50 mg/kg body weight cause histological damage to dorsal nerve roots, and doses of 200 mg/kg body weight lead to the development of signs of peripheral neuropathy, with ataxia, muscle weakness, and loss of balance. The clinical signs of vitamin B_6 toxicity in animals regress within three months after withdrawal of these massive doses, but sensory nerve conduction velocity, which decreases during the development of the neuropathy, does not recover fully.

Sensory neuropathy has been reported in patients taking 2–7 g of pyridoxine/day. Although there was some residual damage, withdrawal of these extremely high doses resulted in a considerable recovery of sensory nerve function. Other reports have suggested that intakes as low as 50 mg/day are associated with neurological damage, although these studies were based on patients reporting symptoms rather than objective neurological examination. There have been no reports of nerve damage in children with vitamin B_6-dependent homocystinuria, or other inborn errors of metabolism, who take 200–300 mg/day.

10.10 Vitamin B_{12}

Dietary deficiency of vitamin B_{12} occurs only in strict vegans, since the vitamin is found almost exclusively in animal foods. However, functional deficiency (pernicious anaemia, with spinal cord degeneration) as a result of impaired absorption is relatively common, especially in older people with atrophic gastritis.

Structure and vitamers

The structure of vitamin B_{12} is shown in Figure 10.13. The term corrinoid is used as a generic descriptor for cobalt-containing compounds of this general structure that, depending on the substituents in the pyrrole rings, may or may not have vitamin activity. The term "vitamin B_{12}" is used as a generic descriptor for the cobalamins, that is, those corrinoids having the biological activity of the vitamin. Some of the corrinoids that are growth factors for microorganisms not only have no vitamin B_{12} activity, but may be antimetabolites of the vitamin.

Although cyanocobalamin was the first form in which vitamin B_{12} was isolated, it is not an important naturally occurring vitamer, but rather an artifact due to the presence of cyanide in the charcoal used in the extraction procedure. It is more stable to light than the other vitamers, and hence is used in pharmaceutical preparations. Photolysis of cyanocobalamin in solution leads to the formation of aquocobalamin or hydroxocobalamin, depending on pH. Hydroxocobalamin is also used in pharmaceutical preparations, and is better retained after parenteral administration than is cyanocobalamin.

Vitamin B_{12} is found only in foods of animal origin, although it is also formed by bacteria. There are no plant sources of this vitamin. This means that strict vegetarians (vegans), who eat no foods of animal origin, are at risk of developing dietary vitamin B_{12} deficiency, although the small amounts of vitamin B_{12} formed by bacteria on the surface of fruits may be adequate to meet requirements. Preparations of vitamin B_{12} made by bacterial fermentation that are ethically acceptable to vegans are readily available.

There are claims that yeast and some plants (especially some algae) contain vitamin B_{12}. This seems to be incorrect. The problem is that the officially recognised, and legally required, method of determining the vitamin in food analysis is a microbiological assay using organisms for which vitamin B_{12} is an essential growth factor. However, these organisms can also use some corrinoids that have no vitamin activity. Therefore, analysis reveals the presence of something that appears to be vitamin B_{12}, but in fact is not the active vitamin and is useless in human

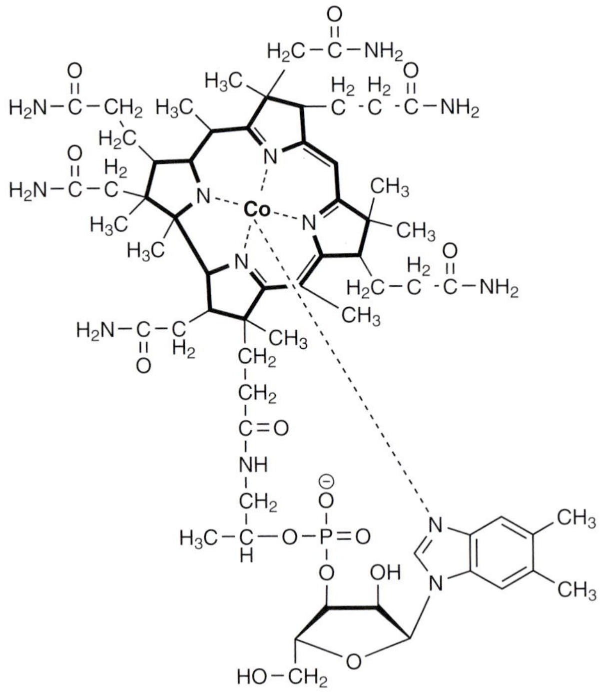

Figure 10.13 Vitamin B_{12}. Four coordination sites on the central cobalt atom are occupied by nitrogen atoms of the ring, and one by the nitrogen of the dimethylbenzimidazole side-chain. The sixth coordination site may be occupied by cyanide (cyanocobalamin), a hydroxyl ion (hydroxocobalamin), water (aquocobalamin), or a methyl group (methylcobalamin).

nutrition. Biologically active vitamin B_{12} has been identified in some preparations of algae, but this seems to be the result of faecal bacterial contamination of the lakes where the algae were harvested.

Absorption and metabolism of vitamin B_{12}

Very small amounts of vitamin B_{12} can be absorbed by passive diffusion across the intestinal mucosa, but under normal conditions this is insignificant; the major route of vitamin B_{12} absorption is by attachment to a specific binding protein in the intestinal lumen.

This binding protein is intrinsic factor, so called because in the early studies of pernicious anaemia it was found that two curative factors were involved: an extrinsic or dietary factor, which is now known to be vitamin B_{12}, and an intrinsic or endogenously produced factor. Intrinsic factor is a small glycoprotein secreted by the parietal cells of the gastric mucosa, which also secrete hydrochloric acid.

Gastric acid and pepsin play a role in vitamin B_{12} nutrition, serving to release the vitamin from protein binding, so making it available. Atrophic gastritis is a relatively common problem of advancing age; in the early stages there is failure of acid secretion but more or less normal secretion of intrinsic factor. This can result in vitamin B_{12} deficiency due to failure to release the vitamin from dietary proteins, although the absorption of free vitamin B_{12} (as in supplements or fortified foods) is unaffected. In the stomach, vitamin B_{12} binds to cobalophilin, a binding protein secreted in the saliva.

In the duodenum cobalophilin is hydrolysed, releasing vitamin B_{12} to bind to intrinsic factor. Pancreatic insufficiency can therefore be a factor in the development of vitamin B_{12} deficiency, since failure to hydrolyse cobalophilin will result in the excretion of cobalophilin-bound vitamin B_{12} rather than transfer to intrinsic factor. Intrinsic factor binds the various vitamin B_{12} vitamers, but not other corrinoids.

Vitamin B_{12} is absorbed from the distal third of the ileum. There are intrinsic factor–vitamin

B_{12} binding sites on the brush border of the mucosal cells in this region; neither free intrinsic factor nor free vitamin B_{12} interacts with these receptors.

In plasma, vitamin B_{12} circulates bound to transcobalamin II, which is required for tissue uptake of the vitamin. Although transcobalamin II is the metabolically important pool of plasma vitamin B_{12}, it accounts for only 10–15% of the total circulating vitamin. The majority is bound to haptocorrin (transcobalamin I). The function of haptocorrin is not well understood; it does not seem to be involved in tissue uptake or inter-organ transport of the vitamin. A third plasma vitamin B_{12}-binding protein, transcobalamin III, provides a mechanism for returning vitamin B_{12} and its metabolites from peripheral tissues to the liver.

Enterohepatic circulation of vitamin B_{12}

There is a considerable enterohepatic circulation of vitamin B_{12}. Transcobalamin III is rapidly cleared by the liver, with a plasma half-life of the order of 5 min. This provides a mechanism for returning vitamin B_{12} and its metabolites from peripheral tissues to the liver, as well as for clearance of other corrinoids without vitamin activity, which may arise from either foods or the products of intestinal bacterial action, and be absorbed passively across the lower gut.

These corrinoids are then secreted into the bile, bound to cobalophilins; 3–8 μg (2.25–6 nmol) of vitamin B_{12} may be secreted in the bile each day, about the same as the dietary intake. Like dietary vitamin B_{12} bound to salivary cobalophilin, the biliary cobalophilins are hydrolysed in the duodenum, and the vitamin binds to intrinsic factor, so permitting reabsorption in the ileum. Although cobalophilins and transcobalamin III have low specificity, and will bind a variety of corrinoids, intrinsic factor binds only cobalamins, and so only the biologically active vitamin is reabsorbed.

Metabolic functions of vitamin B_{12}

There are two vitamin B_{12}-dependent enzymes in human tissues: methionine synthase, which catalyses the transfer of the methyl group from methyltetrahydrofolate to homocysteine and methylmalonyl CoA mutase, which catalyses the rearrangement of methylmalonyl CoA, an intermediate in the metabolism of valine, cholesterol and odd-carbon fatty acids, to succinyl CoA.

Vitamin B_{12} deficiency: pernicious anaemia

Vitamin B_{12} deficiency causes pernicious anaemia; the release into the bloodstream of immature precursors of red blood cells (megaloblastic anaemia). Vitamin B_{12} deficiency causes functional folate deficiency; this is what disturbs the rapid multiplication of red blood cells, causing immature precursors to be released into the circulation.

The other clinical feature of vitamin B_{12} deficiency, which is rarely seen in folic acid deficiency, is degeneration of the spinal cord; hence the name "pernicious" for the anaemia of vitamin B_{12} deficiency. The spinal cord degeneration is due to a failure of the methylation of one arginine residue in myelin basic protein. About one-third of patients who present with megaloblastic anaemia due to vitamin B_{12} deficiency also have spinal cord degeneration, and about one-third of deficient people present with neurological signs but no anaemia.

Although moderate vitamin B_{12} deficiency is relatively common in older people, intervention trials of vitamin B_{12} supplementation in people without clinical signs of anaemia or neurological damage do not show any improvement in either neurological or cognitive function

The most common cause of pernicious anaemia is failure of the absorption of vitamin B_{12}, rather than dietary deficiency. Classical pernicious anaemia is due to failure of intrinsic factor secretion, commonly the result of autoimmune disease, with production of antibodies against either the gastric parietal cells or intrinsic factor. Atrophic gastritis with increasing age also leads to progressive failure of vitamin B_{12} absorption.

Dietary deficiency of vitamin B_{12} does occur, rarely, in strict vegetarians (vegans). The rarity of vitamin B_{12} deficiency among people who have no apparent dietary source of the vitamin suggests that bacterial contamination of water and foods with vitamin B_{12}-producing organisms may provide minimally adequate amounts of the vitamin. The fruit bat develops vitamin B_{12} deficiency when fed on washed fruit under laboratory conditions, but in the wild microbial contamination of the outside of the fruit provides an adequate intake of the vitamin.

Drug-induced vitamin B_{12} deficiency

Nitrous oxide inhibits methionine synthetase, by oxidising the cobalt of methylcobalamin. Patients with hitherto undiagnosed vitamin B_{12} deficiency can develop neurological signs after surgery when nitrous oxide is used as the anaesthetic agent, and there are a number of reports of neurological damage due to vitamin B_{12} depletion among dental surgeons and others occupationally exposed to nitrous oxide.

The histamine H_2 receptor antagonists and proton pump inhibitors used to treat gastric ulcers and gastro-oesophageal reflux act by reducing the secretion of gastric acid, and may result in impairment of the absorption of protein-bound vitamin B_{12}. However, a number of studies have shown that even prolonged use of these drugs does not lead to significant depletion of vitamin B_{12} reserves.

Vitamin B_{12} requirements

Most estimates of vitamin B_{12} requirements are based on the amounts given parenterally to maintain normal health in patients with pernicious anaemia due to a failure of vitamin B_{12} absorption. This over-estimates normal requirements, because of the enterohepatic circulation of vitamin B_{12} in people lacking intrinsic factor, or secreting anti-intrinsic factor antibodies, the vitamin that is excreted in the bile will be lost in the faeces, whereas normally it is almost completely reabsorbed.

The total body pool of vitamin B_{12} is of the order of 2.5 mg (1.8 μmol), with a minimum desirable body pool of about 1 mg (0.3 μmol). The daily loss is about 0.1% of the body pool in subjects with normal enterohepatic circulation of the vitamin; on this basis requirements are about 1–2.5 μg/day and reference intakes for adults range between 1.4 μg and 2.0 μg.

Assessment of vitamin B_{12} status

Total serum vitamin B_{12}, measured by radioligand binding assay, has been used to assess status. A serum concentration below 110 pmol/l is associated with megaloblastic bone marrow, incipient anaemia and myelin damage. Below 150 pmol/l there are early bone marrow changes, abnormalities of the dUMP suppression test and methylmalonic aciduria after a valine load. This is considered to be the lower limit of adequacy. However, most serum vitamin B_{12} is present bound to haptocorrin, which has no known function. Holotranscobalamin II is the form of the vitamin that is available for tissue uptake, and contains about 6 – 20% of plasma vitamin B_{12}. Transcobalamin II is depleted of vitamin B_{12} before deficiency develops, and measurement of holotranscobalamin II provides an index of depletion or negative balance.

The Schilling test for vitamin B_{12} absorption

The absorption of vitamin B_{12} can be determined by the Schilling test. An oral dose of [^{57}Co] or [^{58}Co]-vitamin B_{12} is given with a parenteral flushing dose of 1 mg of non-radioactive vitamin to saturate body reserves, and the urinary excretion of radioactivity is followed as an index of absorption of the oral dose. Normal people excrete 16–45% of the radioactivity over 24 h, whereas patients lacking the intrinsic factor excrete less than 5%.

The test can be repeated, giving the intrinsic factor orally together with the radioactive vitamin B_{12}; if the impaired absorption was due to a simple lack of intrinsic factor, and not to anti-intrinsic factor antibodies in the saliva or gastric juice, then a normal amount of the radioactive material should be absorbed and excreted.

Methylmalonic aciduria

Methylmalonyl-CoA is formed as an intermediate in the catabolism of valine and by the carboxylation of propionyl-CoA arising in the catabolism of isoleucine, cholesterol, and (rare) fatty acids with an odd number of carbon atoms. Normally, it undergoes vitamin B_{12}-dependent rearrangement to succinyl-CoA, catalysed by methylmalonyl-CoA mutase. Vitamin B_{12} deficiency leads to an accumulation of methylmalonyl-CoA, which is hydrolysed to methylmalonic acid, which is excreted in the urine. Urinary excretion of methylmalonic acid, especially after a loading dose of valine, provides a means of assessing vitamin B_{12} nutritional status. However, up to 25% of patients with confirmed pernicious anaemia excrete normal amounts of methylmalonic acid even after a dose of valine.

10.11 Folic acid and the folates

Folic acid derivatives function in the transfer of one-carbon fragments in a wide variety of biosynthetic and catabolic reactions; it is therefore metabolically closely related to vitamin B_{12}. Deficiency of either causes megaloblastic anaemia, and the haematological effects of vitamin B_{12} deficiency are due to disturbance of folate metabolism.

Apart from liver, the main dietary sources of folate are fruits and vegetables. Although folate is widely distributed in foods, dietary deficiency is not uncommon, and a number of commonly used drugs can cause folate depletion. More importantly, there is good evidence that intakes of folate considerably higher than normal dietary levels reduce the risk of neural tube defects, and, where cereal products are not fortified with folic acid by law, pregnant women are recommended to take supplements. There is also evidence that high intakes of folate may be effective in reducing plasma homocysteine in subjects genetically at risk of hyperhomocystinaemia (some 10–20% of the population), which may reduce the risk of ischaemic heart disease and stroke.

Vitamers and dietary equivalence

As shown in Figure 10.14, folic acid consists of a reduced pterin linked to *p*-aminobenzoic acid, forming pteroic acid. The carboxyl group of the *p*-aminobenzoic acid moiety is linked by a peptide bond to the α-amino group of glutamate,

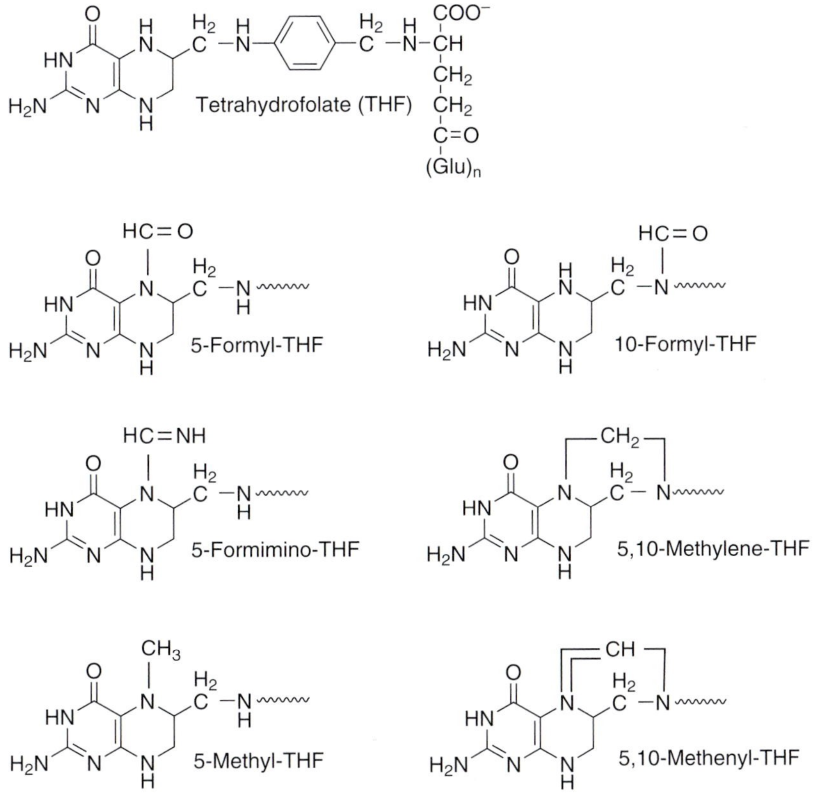

Tetrahydrofolate (THF)

5-Formyl-THF

10-Formyl-THF

5-Formimino-THF

5,10-Methylene-THF

5-Methyl-THF

5,10-Methenyl-THF

Figure 10.14 Tetrahydrofolate (folic acid) and the one-carbon substituted folate derivatives.

forming pteroyl-glutamate (PteGlu). The coenzymes may have up to seven additional glutamate residues linked by γ-peptide bonds, forming pteroyldiglutamate ($PteGlu_2$), pteroyltriglutamate ($PteGlu_3$), etc., collectively known as folate or pteroyl polyglutamate conjugates ($PteGlu_n$).

"Folate" is the preferred trivial name for pteroyl-glutamate, although both "folate" and "folic acid" may be used as a generic descriptor to include various polyglutamates. $PteGlu_2$ is sometimes referred to as folic acid diglutamate, $PteGlu_3$ as folic acid triglutamate, and so on.

Tetrahydrofolate can carry one-carbon fragments attached to N-5 (formyl, formimino, or methyl groups), *N*-10 (formyl),or bridging *N*-5–*N*-10 (methylene or methenyl groups). 5-Formyl-tetrahydrofolate is more stable to atmospheric oxidation than is folate, and is therefore commonly used in pharmaceutical preparations; it is also known as folinic acid, and the synthetic (racemic) compound as leucovorin.

The extent to which the different forms of folate can be absorbed varies; on average only about half of the folate in the diet is available, compared with more or less complete availability of the monoglutamate. To permit calculation of folate intakes, the dietary folate equivalent has been defined as 1 μg mixed food folates or 0.6 μg free folic acid. On this basis, total dietary folate equivalents = μg food folate + 1.7 × synthetic (free) folic acid.

Absorption and metabolism of folate

About 80% of dietary folate is as polyglutamates; a variable amount may be substituted with various one-carbon fragments or be present as dihydrofolate derivatives. Folate conjugates are hydrolysed in the small intestine by conjugase (pteroylpolyglutamate hydrolase), a zinc-dependent enzyme of the pancreatic juice, bile, and mucosal brush border; zinc deficiency can impair folate absorption.

Free folate, released by conjugase action, is absorbed by active transport in the jejunum. The folate in milk is mainly bound to a specific binding protein; the protein–tetrahydrofolate complex is absorbed intact, mainly in the ileum, by a mechanism that is distinct from the active transport system for the absorption of free folate. The biological availability of folate from milk is considerably greater than that of unbound folate. Folate synthesised by intestinal bacteria is absorbed by carrier-mediated diffusion in the colon.

Much of the dietary folate undergoes methylation and reduction within the intestinal mucosa, so that what enters the portal bloodstream is largely 5-methyl-tetrahydrofolate. Other substituted and unsubstituted folate monoglutamates, and dihydrofolate, are also absorbed; they are reduced and methylated in the liver, then secreted in the bile. The liver also takes up various folates released by tissues; again, these are reduced, methylated and secreted in the bile.

Folic acid, as used in food fortification and supplements, is a poor substrate for reduction in the intestinal mucosa, and undergoes reduction and methylation mainly in the liver.

The total daily enterohepatic circulation of folate is equivalent to about one-third of the dietary intake. Despite this, there is very little faecal loss of folate; jejunal absorption of methyl-tetrahydrofolate is a very efficient process, and the faecal excretion of some 450 nmol (200 μg) of folates per day represents synthesis by intestinal flora and does not reflect intake to any significant extent.

Tissue uptake of folate

Methyl-tetrahydrofolate circulates bound to albumin, and is available for uptake by extrahepatic tissues, where it is trapped by formation of polyglutamates, which do not cross cell membranes.

The main circulating folate is methyl-tetrahydrofolate, which is a poor substrate for polyglutamylation; demethylation by the action of methionine synthetase is required for effective metabolic trapping of folate. In vitamin B_{12} deficiency, when methionine synthetase activity is impaired, there will therefore be impairment of the uptake of folate into tissues.

Folate excretion

There is very little urinary loss of folate, only some 5–10 nmol/day. Not only is most folate in plasma bound to proteins (either folate binding protein for unsubstituted folates or albumin for methyl-tetrahydrofolate), and thus protected from glomerular filtration, but the renal brush border has a high concentration of folate binding protein, which acts to reabsorb any filtered in the urine.

The catabolism of folate is largely by cleavage of the C-9–N-10 bond, catalysed by carboxypeptidase G. The *p*-aminobenzoic acid moiety is amidated and excreted in the urine as *p*-acetamidobenzoate and *p*-acetamidobenzoyl-glutamate; pterin is excreted either unchanged or as a variety of biologically inactive compounds.

Metabolic functions of folate

The metabolic role of folate is as a carrier of one-carbon fragments, both in catabolism and in biosynthetic reactions. These may be carried as formyl, formimino, methyl or methylene residues. The major sources of these one-carbon fragments and their major uses, as well as the interconversions of the substituted folates, are shown in Figure 10.15.

The major point of entry for one-carbon fragments into substituted folates is methylene-tetrahydrofolate, which is formed by the catabolism of glycine, serine, and choline. Serine is the most important source of substituted folates for biosynthetic reactions, and the activity of serine hydroxymethyltransferase is regulated by the state of folate substitution and the availability of folate. The reaction is freely reversible, and under appropriate conditions in liver it functions to form serine from glycine as a substrate for gluconeogenesis.

Methylene-, methenyl-, and 10-formyl-tetrahydrofolates are freely interconvertible. This means that when one-carbon folates are not required for synthetic reactions, the oxidation of formyl-tetrahydrofolate to carbon dioxide and folate provides a means of maintaining an adequate tissue pool of free folate.

By contrast, the reduction of methylenetetrahydrofolate to methyl-tetrahydrofolate is irreversible, and the only way in which free folate can be formed from methyl-tetrahydrofolate is by the reaction of methionine synthetase.

Thymidylate synthetase and dihydrofolate reductase

The methylation of dUMP to thymidine monophosphate (TMP), catalysed by thymidylate synthetase, is essential for the synthesis of DNA, although preformed TMP arising from the catabolism of DNA can be reutilised.

The methyl donor for thymidylate synthetase is methylene-tetrahydrofolate; the reaction

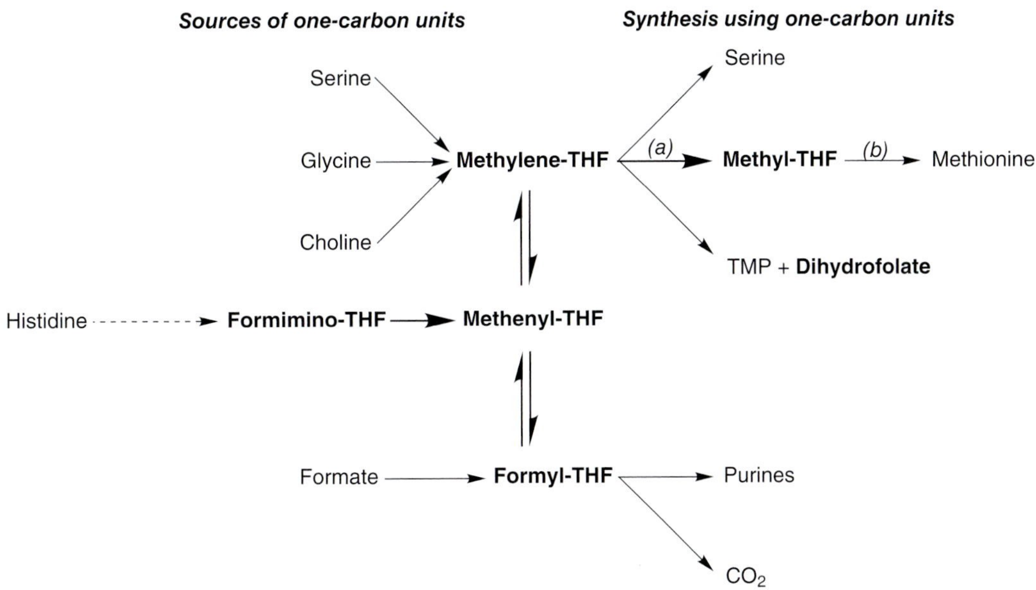

Figure 10.15 Interconversion of the principal one-carbon substituted folates; sources of one-carbon fragments are shown on the left, and pathways in which one-carbon units are used and free tetrahydrofolate is regenerated on the right. (a) Methylene-tetrahydrofolate reductase (EC 1.5.1.20); (b) methionine synthetase (EC 2.1.1.13).

involves reduction of the one-carbon fragment to a methyl group at the expense of the folate, which is oxidised to dihydrofolate. Dihydrofolate is then reduced to tetrahydrofolate by dihydrofolate reductase.

Thymidylate synthase and dihydrofolate reductase are especially active in tissues with a high rate of cell division, and hence a high rate of DNA replication and a high requirement for thymidylate. Because of this, inhibitors of dihydrofolate reductase have been exploited as anti-cancer drugs (e.g., methotrexate). Chemotherapy consists of alternating periods of administration of methotrexate to inhibit tumor growth, and folate (normally as 5-formyl-tetrahydrofolate, leucovorin) to replete tissues and avoid folate deficiency; this is known as leucovorin rescue.

Methionine synthetase and the methyl-folate trap

In addition to its role in the synthesis of proteins, methionine, as the *S*-adenosyl derivative, acts as a methyl donor in a wide variety of biosynthetic reactions. As shown in Figure 10.16, the resultant homocysteine may be either metabolised to yield cysteine or remethylated to yield methionine.

Two enzymes catalyse the methylation of homocysteine to methionine:

- Methionine synthetase is a vitamin B_{12}-dependent enzyme, for which the methyl donor is methyl-tetrahydrofolate.
- Homocysteine methyltransferase utilises betaine (an intermediate in the catabolism of choline) as the methyl donor, and is not vitamin B_{12} dependent.

Both enzymes are found in most tissues, but only the vitamin B_{12}-dependent methionine synthetase is found in the central nervous system.

The reduction of methylene-tetrahydrofolate to methyl-tetrahydrofolate is irreversible, and the major source of folate for tissues is methyl-tetrahydrofolate. The only metabolic role of methyl-tetrahydrofolate is the methylation of homocysteine to methionine, and this is the only way in which methyl-tetrahydrofolate can

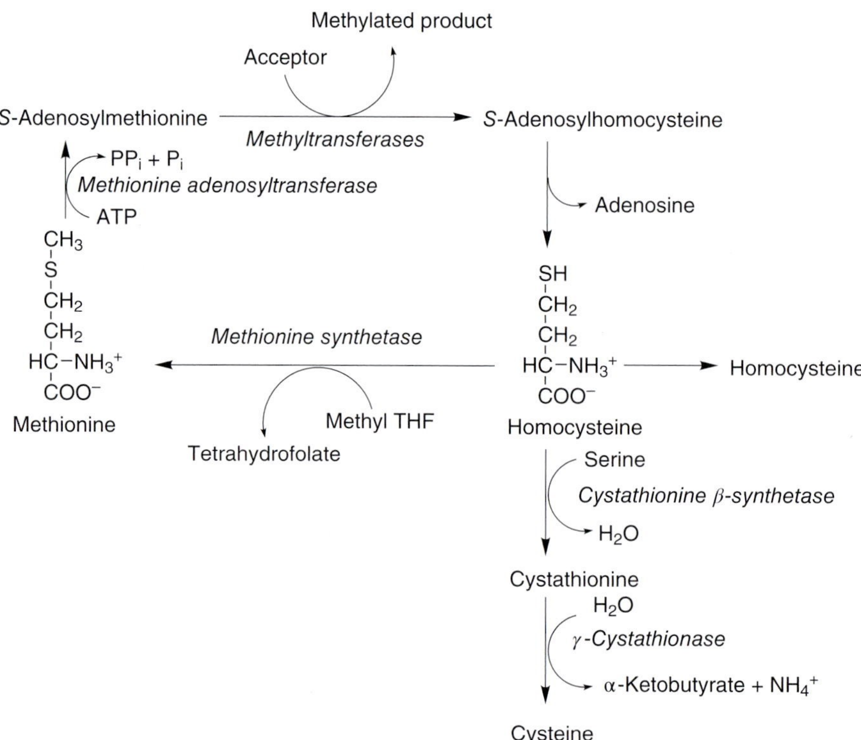

Figure 10.16 Methionine metabolism. Methionine synthetase (EC 2.1.1.13), methionine adenosyltransferase (EC 2.5.1.6), cystathionine synthetase (EC 4.2.1.22), cystathionase (EC 4.4.1.1).

be demethylated to yield free folate in tissues. Methionine synthetase thus provides the link between the physiological functions of folate and vitamin B_{12}. Impairment of methionine synthetase activity in vitamin B_{12} deficiency will result in the accumulation of methyl-tetrahydrofolate, which can neither be utilised for any other one-carbon transfer reactions nor be demethylated to provide free folate.

This functional deficiency of folate is exacerbated by low tissue concentrations of methionine and an accumulation of homocysteine, since the transulphuration pathway to form cysteine from homocysteine is regulated by the availability of cysteine: it is a biosynthetic pathway rather than a pathway for disposal of methionine and homocysteine.

Methylene-tetrahydrofolate reductase and hyperhomocysteinaemia

Elevated blood homocysteine is a significant risk factor for atherosclerosis, thrombosis, and hypertension, independent of factors such as dietary lipids and plasma lipoproteins. About 10–15% of the population, and almost 30% of people with ischaemic heart disease, have an abnormal variant of methylene-tetrahydrofolate reductase, which is unstable, and loses activity more quickly than normal. As a result, people with the abnormal form of the enzyme have an impaired ability to form methyl-tetrahydrofolate (the main form in which folate is taken up by tissues) and suffer from functional folate deficiency. Therefore, they are unable to remethylate homocysteine to methionine adequately and develop hyperhomocysteinaemia.

People with the abnormal variant of methylene-tetrahydrofolate reductase do not develop hyperhomocysteinaemia if they have a relatively high intake of folate. This seems to be due to the methylation of folate in the intestinal mucosa during absorption; intestinal mucosal cells have a rapid turnover (some 48 h between proliferation in the crypts and shedding at the tip of the villus), and therefore it is not important that methylene-tetrahydrofolate reductase is less stable than normal, as there is still an adequate activity of the enzyme in the intestinal mucosa to maintain a normal circulating level of methyl-tetrahydrofolate. Also, like many enzymes, methylene tetrahydrofolate reductase may be more stable in the presence of its substrate. Hence, it is possible that high tissue levels of methylene tetrahydrofolate (resulting from a high folate status) may protect the enzyme and enhance its stability

This has led to the suggestion that supplements of folate will reduce the incidence of cardiovascular disease. However, a number of intervention trials with folate supplements have shown no reduction in death from myocardial infarction, nor any decrease in all-cause mortality, despite a significant decrease in plasma homocysteine. Similarly, in countries where there has been mandatory enrichment of flour with folate for some years, there is no evidence of reduced mortality from cardiovascular disease. It is possible that elevated plasma homocysteine is not so much a cause of atherosclerosis (although there are good mechanisms to explain why it might be atherogenic) as the result of impaired kidney function due to early atherosclerosis. If this is so, the lowering of plasma homocysteine by increasing folate intake would not be expected to affect the development of atherosclerosis.

Folate in pregnancy

The development of the brain and spinal cord begins around day 18 of gestation; closure begins about day 21 and is complete by day 24. This is before the woman knows she is pregnant. The closed neural tube stimulates the development of the bony structures that will become the spinal cord and skull. Bone does not form over unclosed regions, leading to the congenital defects collectively known as neural tube defects, anencephaly and spina bifida, which affect between 0.5 and 8 per 1000 live births, depending on genetic and environmental factors.

During the 1980s a considerable body of evidence accumulated that spina bifida and other neural tube defects (which occur in about 0.75–1% of pregnancies) were associated with low intakes of folate, and that increased intake during pregnancy might be protective. It is now established that supplements of folate begun periconceptually result in a significant reduction in the incidence of neural tube defects, and it is recommended that intakes be increased by 400 μg/day before conception. The studies were conducted using folate monoglutamate and it is unlikely that an equivalent increase in intake could be achieved from unfortified foods. In many countries there is mandatory enrichment of flour with folic acid, and there has been a 25–50% decrease in the number of infants born with neural tube defects since the introduction of fortification. The true benefit is greater than this, since some affected fetuses abort spontaneously and there are few data on the number of therapeutic terminations of pregnancy for neural tube defects detected by antenatal screening. Where folate enrichment is not mandatory, the advice is that all women who are planning pregnancy should take supplements of 400 μg/day.

Folate and cancer

Much of the regulation and silencing of gene expression that underlies tissue differentiation involves methylation of CpG islands in DNA, and there is evidence that some cancers (and especially colorectal cancer) are associated with under-methylation of CpG islands as a result of low folate status. A number of small studies have suggested that folate supplements may be protective against colorectal cancer, but no results from large-scale randomised controlled trials have yet been reported, and to date there is no evidence of a decrease in colorectal cancer in countries where folate enrichment of flour is mandatory. Indeed, there is some evidence of a transient increase in colorectal cancer as a result of folate-induced transformation of precancerous polyps.

Folate deficiency: megaloblastic anaemia

Dietary deficiency of folic acid is not uncommon (some 8–10% of the population of developed countries have low folate stores) and, as noted above, deficiency of vitamin B_{12} also leads to functional folic acid deficiency. In either case, it is cells that are dividing rapidly, and therefore have a large requirement for thymidine for DNA synthesis, that are most severely affected. These are the cells of the bone marrow that form red blood cells, the cells of the intestinal mucosa and the hair follicles. Clinically, folate deficiency leads to megaloblastic anaemia, the release into the circulation of immature precursors of red blood cells.

There may also be a low white cell and platelet count, as well as hyper-segmented neutrophils. Deficiency is frequently accompanied by depression, insomnia, forgetfulness and irritability, and sometimes cognitive impairment and dementia. Suboptimal folate status is also associated with increased incidence of neural tube defects, hyperhomocysteinaemia leading to increased risk of cardiovascular disease and altered methylation of DNA, which may increase cancer risk.

Megaloblastic anaemia is also seen in vitamin B_{12} deficiency, where it is due to functional folate deficiency as a result of trapping folate as methyl-tetrahydrofolate. However, the neurological degeneration of pernicious anaemia is rarely seen in folate deficiency, and indeed a high intake of folate can mask the development of megaloblastic anemia in vitamin B_{12} deficiency, so that the presenting sign is irreversible nerve damage.

Folate requirements

Depletion/repletion studies to determine folate requirements using folate monoglutamate suggest a requirement of the order of 80–100 μg (170– 220 nmol) /day. The total body pool of folate in adults is some 17 μmol (7.5 mg), with a biological half-life of 101 days. This suggests a minimum requirement for replacement of 37 μg (85 nmol)/day. Studies of the urinary excretion of folate metabolites in subjects maintained on folate-free diets suggest that there is catabolism of some 80 μg (170 nmol) of folate/day.

Because of the problems in determining the biological availability of the various folate polyglutamate conjugates found in foods, reference intakes allow a wide margin of safety, and are based on an allowance of 3 μg (6.8 nmol)/kg body weight.

Assessment of folate status

Measurement of the serum or red blood cell concentration of folate is the method of choice, and radioligand binding assays have been developed. There are problems involved in radioligand binding assays for folate, and in some centres microbiological determination of plasma or whole blood folates is preferred. Serum folate below 7 nmol/l or erythrocyte folate below 320 nmol/l indicates negative folate balance and early depletion of body reserves. At this stage the first bone marrow changes are detectable.

Histidine metabolism: the formiminoglutamate (FIGLU) test

The ability to metabolise a test dose of histidine provides a sensitive functional test of folate nutritional status; formiminoglutamate (FIGLU) is an intermediate in histidine catabolism, and is metabolised by the folate-dependent enzyme formiminoglutamate formiminotransferase. In folate deficiency the activity of this enzyme is impaired, and FIGLU accumulates and is excreted in the urine, especially after a test dose of histidine: the so-called FIGLU test.

Although the FIGLU test depends on folate nutritional status, the metabolism of histidine will also be impaired, and hence a positive result obtained, in vitamin B_{12} deficiency, because of the secondary deficiency of free folate. About 60% of vitamin B_{12}-deficient subjects show increased FIGLU excretion after a histidine load.

The dUMP suppression test

Rapidly dividing cells can either use preformed thymidine triphosphate (TMP) for DNA synthesis, or synthesise it *de novo* from deoxyuridine monophosphate (dUMP). Stimulated lymphocytes incubated *in vitro* with [^{3}H]-TMP will incorporate the label into DNA. In the presence of adequate amounts of methylene-tetrahydrofolate, the addition of dUMP as a substrate for thymidylate synthetase reduces the incorporation of [^{3}H]-TMP as a result of dilution of the pool of labelled material by newly synthesised TMP and inhibition of thymidylate kinase by TMP.

In normal cells the incorporation of [^{3}H]-thymidine into DNA after preincubation with dUMP is 1.4–1.8% of that without preincubation. By contrast, cells that are deficient in folate form little or no thymidine from dUMP, and hence incorporate nearly as much of the [^{3}H]-thymidine after incubation with dUMP as they do without preincubation.

Either a primary deficiency of folic acid or functional deficiency secondary to vitamin B_{12} deficiency will have the same effect. In folate deficiency, addition of any biologically active form of folate, but not vitamin B_{12}, will normalise the dUMP suppression of [^{3}H]-thymidine incorporation. In vitamin B_{12} deficiency, addition of vitamin B_{12} or methylene-tetrahydrofolate, but not methyl-tetrahydrofolate, will normalise dUMP suppression.

Drug–nutrient interactions of folate

Several folate antimetabolites are used clinically, as cancer chemotherapy (e.g., methotrexate), and as antibacterial (trimethoprim) and antimalarial (pyrimethamine) agents. Drugs such as trimethoprim and pyrimethamine act by inhibiting dihydrofolate reductase, and they owe their clinical usefulness to a considerably higher affinity for the dihydrofolate reductase of the target organism than for the human enzyme; nevertheless, prolonged use can result in folate deficiency.

A number of anticonvulsants used in the treatment of epilepsy, including diphenylhydantoin (phenytoin), and sometimes phenobarbital and primidone, can also cause folate deficiency. Although overt megaloblastic anaemia affects only some 0.75% of treated patients, there is some degree of macrocytosis in 40%. The megaloblastosis responds to folic acid supplements, but in about 50% of such patients treated with relatively high supplements for 1–3 years there is an increase in the frequency of epileptic attacks.

Folate toxicity

There is some evidence that folate supplements in excess of 400 μg/day may impair zinc absorption. In addition, there are two potential problems that have to be considered when advocating either widespread use of folate supplements or enrichment of foods with folate for protection against neural tube defect and possibly cardiovascular disease and cancer.

Folate supplements will mask the megaloblastic anaemia of vitamin B_{12} deficiency, so that the presenting sign is irreversible nerve damage. This is especially a problem for older people, who may suffer impaired absorption of vitamin B_{12} as a result of atrophic gastritis. This problem might be overcome by adding vitamin B_{12} to foods as well as folate. Whereas gastric acid is essential for the release of vitamin B_{12} bound to dietary proteins, crystalline vitamin B_{12} used in food enrichment is free to bind to cobalophilin without the need for gastric acid. An intake of

1000 μg/day is considered unlikely to mask the development of megaloblastic anaemia in elderly people, and this can be considered to be an upper level of habitual intake.

Antagonism between folic acid and the anticonvulsants used in the treatment of epilepsy is part of their mechanism of action; about 2% of the population have (drug-controlled) epilepsy. Large supplements of folic acid (in excess of 5000 μg/day) may antagonise the beneficial effects of some anticonvulsants and may lead to an increase in the frequency of epileptic attacks. There is, however, no evidence of a significant problem in countries where enrichment of flour has been mandatory for some years.

10.12 Biotin

Biotin was originally discovered as part of the complex called *bios*, which promoted the growth of yeast and, separately, as vitamin H, the protective or curative factor in "egg white injury," the disease caused in human beings and experimental animals being fed diets containing large amounts of uncooked egg white. The structures of biotin, biocytin, and carboxy-biocytin (the active metabolic intermediate) are shown in Figure 10.17.

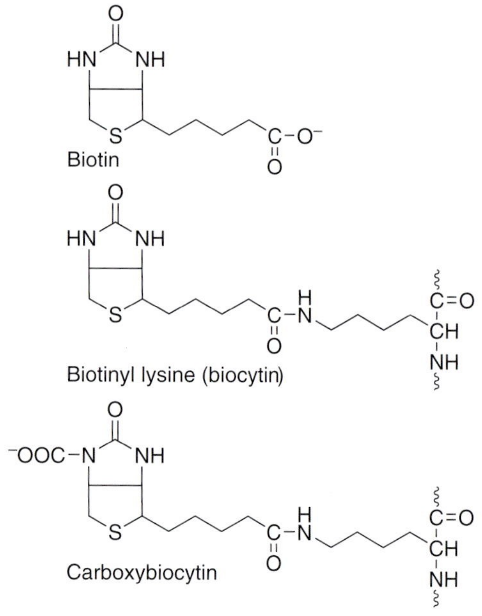

Figure 10.17 Biotin, biotinyl-lysine (biocytin) and the role of biocytin as a carbon dioxide carrier.

Biotin is widely distributed in many foods. It is synthesised by intestinal flora, and in balance studies the total output of biotin in urine plus faeces is three to six times greater than the intake, reflecting bacterial synthesis; it can be absorbed in the colon. However, there is some evidence that suboptimal biotin status may be relatively common.

Absorption and metabolism of biotin

Most biotin in foods is present as biocytin (ε-amino-biotinyllysine), which is released on proteolysis, then hydrolysed by biotinidase in the pancreatic juice and intestinal mucosal secretions, to yield free biotin. The extent to which bound biotin in foods is biologically available is not known.

Free biotin is absorbed from the small intestine by active transport. Biotin circulates in the bloodstream both free and bound to a serum glycoprotein that has biotinidase activity, catalysing the hydrolysis of biocytin.

Biotin enters tissues by a saturable transport system and is then incorporated into biotin-dependent enzymes as the ε-amino-lysine peptide, biocytin. Unlike other B vitamins, where concentrative uptake into tissues can be achieved by facilitated diffusion followed by metabolic trapping, the incorporation of biotin into enzymes is relatively slow, and cannot be considered part of the uptake process. On catabolism of the enzymes, biocytin is hydrolysed by biotinidase, permitting reutilisation.

Metabolic functions of biotin

Biotin functions to transfer carbon dioxide in a small number of carboxylation reactions. The reactive intermediate is 1-*N*-carboxy-biocytin (Figure 10.17), formed from bicarbonate in an ATP-dependent reaction. A single enzyme acts on the apoenzymes of acetyl-CoA carboxylase, pyruvate carboxylase, propionyl-CoA carboxylase, and methylcrotonyl-CoA carboxylase to form the active holoenzymes from (inactive) apoenzymes and free biotin.

Biotin also has a role in the control of the cell cycle, and acts via cell surface receptors to regulate the expression of key enzymes involved in glucose metabolism. In response to mitogenic stimuli there is a considerable increase in the tissue uptake of biotin, much of which is used to biotinylate histones and other nuclear proteins.

Biotin deficiency and requirements

Biotin is widely distributed in foods and deficiency is unknown, except among people maintained for many months on total parenteral nutrition, and a very small number of people who eat abnormally large amounts of uncooked egg. Avidin, a protein in egg white, binds biotin extremely tightly and renders it unavailable for absorption. Avidin is denatured by cooking and then loses its ability to bind biotin. The amount of avidin in uncooked egg white is relatively small, and problems of biotin deficiency have only occurred in people eating a dozen or more raw eggs a day, for some years.

The few early reports of human biotin deficiency are all of people who consumed large amounts of uncooked eggs. They developed a fine scaly dermatitis and hair loss (alopecia). Histology of the skin showed an absence of sebaceous glands and atrophy of the hair follicles. Provision of biotin supplements of 200–1000 μg/day resulted in cure of the skin lesions and regrowth of hair, despite continuing the abnormal diet providing large amounts of avidin. There have been no studies of providing modest doses of biotin to such patients, and none in which their high intake of uncooked eggs was not either replaced by an equivalent intake of cooked eggs (in which avidin has been denatured by heat, and the yolks of which are a good source of biotin) or continued unchanged, so there is no information from these case reports of the amounts of biotin required for normal health. More recently, similar signs of biotin deficiency have been observed in patients receiving total parenteral nutrition for prolonged periods after major resection of the gut. The signs resolve following the provision of biotin, but again there have been no studies of the amounts of biotin required; intakes have ranged between 60 μg/day and 200 μg/day.

Glucose metabolism in biotin deficiency

Biotin is the coenzyme for pyruvate carboxylase, one of the key enzymes of gluconeogenesis, and deficiency can lead to fasting hypoglycaemia. In addition, biotin acts via cell surface receptors to induce the synthesis of phosphofructokinase and pyruvate kinase (key enzymes of glycolysis), phospho-enolpyruvate carboxykinase (a key enzyme of gluconeogenesis) and glucokinase.

Rather than the expected hypoglycaemia, biotin deficiency may sometimes be associated with hyperglycaemia as a result of the reduced synthesis of glucokinase. Glucokinase is the high K_m isoenzyme of hexokinase that is responsible for uptake of glucose into the liver for glycogen synthesis when blood concentrations are high. It also acts as the sensor for hyperglycaemia in the β-islet cells of the pancreas; metabolism of the increased glucose 6-phosphate formed by glucokinase leads to the secretion of insulin. There is some evidence that biotin supplements can improve glucose tolerance in diabetes.

Lipid metabolism in biotin deficiency

The skin lesions of biotin deficiency are similar to those seen in deficiency of essential fatty acids, and serum linoleic acid is lower than normal in biotin-deficient patients owing to impairment of the elongation of PUFAs as a result of reduced activity of acetyl-CoA carboxylase.

The impairment of lipogenesis also affects the tissue fatty acid composition, with an increase in the proportion of palmitoleic acid, mainly at the expense of stearic acid, apparently as a result of increased fatty acid desaturase activity in biotin deficiency. Although dietary protein and fat intake also affect tissue fatty acid composition, the ratio of palmitoleic to stearic acid may provide a useful index of biotin nutritional status in some circumstances.

Biotin deficiency also results in an increase in the normally small amounts of odd-chain fatty acids (mainly C15:0 and C17:0) in triacylglycerols, phospholipids, and cholesterol esters. This is a result of impaired activity of propionyl-CoA carboxylase, leading to an accumulation of propionyl-CoA, which can be incorporated into lipids in competition with acetyl-CoA.

Safe and adequate levels of intake

There is no evidence on which to estimate requirements for biotin. Average intakes are between 10 and 200 μg/day. Since dietary deficiency does not occur, such intakes are obviously more than adequate to meet requirements.

10.13 Pantothenic acid

Pantothenic acid (sometimes known as vitamin B_5, and at one time called vitamin B_3) has a central role in energy-yielding metabolism as the functional moiety of coenzyme A (CoA) and in the biosynthesis of fatty acids as the prosthetic group of acyl carrier protein. The structures of pantothenic acid and CoA are shown in Figure 10.18.

Pantothenic acid is widely distributed in all foodstuffs; the name derives from the Greek for "from everywhere", as opposed to other vitamins that were originally isolated from individual especially rich sources. As a result, deficiency has not been unequivocally reported in human beings except in specific depletion studies, most of which have used the antagonist ω-methyl-pantothenic acid.

Absorption, metabolism, and metabolic functions of pantothenic acid

About 85% of dietary pantothenic acid is as CoA and phosphopantetheine. In the intestinal lumen these are hydrolysed to pantetheine; intestinal mucosal cells have a high pantetheinase activity and rapidly hydrolyse pantetheine to pantothenic acid. The intestinal absorption of pantothenic acid seems to be by simple diffusion and occurs at a constant rate throughout the length of the small intestine; bacterial synthesis may contribute to pantothenic acid nutrition.

The first step in pantothenic acid utilisation is phosphorylation. Pantothenate kinase is rate limiting, so that, unlike vitamins that are accumulated by metabolic trapping, there can be significant accumulation of free pantothenic acid in tissues. It is then used for synthesis of CoA and the prosthetic group of acyl carrier protein. Pantothenic acid arising from the turnover of CoA and acyl carrier protein may be either reused or excreted unchanged in the urine.

Coenzyme A and acyl carrier protein

All tissues are capable of forming CoA from pantothenic acid. CoA functions as the carrier of fatty acids, as thioesters, in mitochondrial β-oxidation and esterification reactions. In fatty acid oxidation, the resultant two-carbon fragments, as acetyl-CoA, then undergo oxidation in the citric acid cycle. CoA also functions as a carrier in the transfer of acetyl (and other fatty acyl) moieties in a variety of biosynthetic and catabolic reactions, including:

- cholesterol and steroid hormone synthesis
- long-chain fatty acid synthesis from palmitate and mitochondrial elongation of PUFAs
- acylation of serine, threonine, and cysteine residues on proteolipids, and acetylation of neuraminic acid.

Fatty acid synthesis is catalysed by a cytosolic multienzyme complex in which the growing

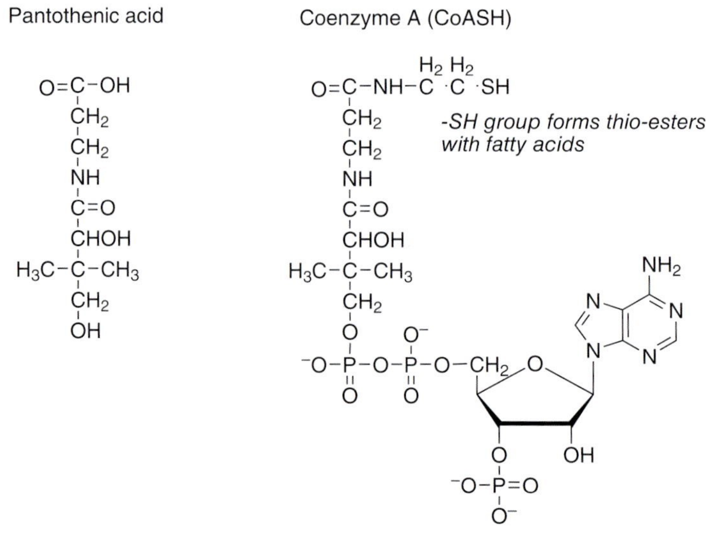

Pantothenic acid

Coenzyme A (CoASH)

-SH group forms thio-esters with fatty acids

Figure 10.18 Pantothenic acid and coenzyme A.

fatty acyl chain is bound by thioester linkage to an enzyme-bound 4′-phosphopantetheine residue, rather than to free CoA, as in β-oxidation. This component of the fatty acid synthetase complex is the acyl carrier protein.

Pantothenic acid deficiency and safe and adequate levels of intake

Prisoners of war in the Far East in the 1940s, who were severely malnourished, showed, among other signs and symptoms of vitamin deficiency diseases, a new condition of paraesthesia and severe pain in the feet and toes, which was called the "burning foot syndrome" or nutritional melalgia. Although it was tentatively attributed to pantothenic acid deficiency, no specific trials of pantothenic acid were conducted, rather the subjects were given yeast extract and other rich sources of all B vitamins as part of an urgent program of nutritional rehabilitation.

Experimental pantothenic acid depletion, together with the administration of ω-methylpantothenic acid, results in the following signs and symptoms after two to three weeks:

- neuromotor disorders, including paraesthesia of the hands and feet, hyperactive deep tendon reflexes, and muscle weakness. These can be explained by the role of acetyl-CoA in the synthesis of the neurotransmitter acetylcholine, and impaired formation of threonine acyl esters in myelin. Dysmyelination may explain the persistence and recurrence of neurological problems many years after nutritional rehabilitation in people who had suffered from burning foot syndrome
- mental depression, which again may be related to either acetylcholine deficit or impaired myelin synthesis
- gastrointestinal complaints, including severe vomiting and pain, with depressed gastric acid secretion in response to gastrin
- increased insulin sensitivity and a flattened glucose tolerance curve, which may reflect decreased antagonism by glucocorticoids
- decreased serum cholesterol and decreased urinary excretion of 17-ketosteroids, reflecting the impairment of steroidogenesis
- decreased acetylation of *p*-aminobenzoic acid, sulfonamides and other drugs, reflecting reduced availability of acetyl-CoA for these reactions
- increased susceptibility to upper respiratory tract infections.

There is no evidence on which to estimate pantothenic acid requirements. Average intakes are between 3 mg/day and 7 mg/day, and since deficiency does not occur, such intakes are obviously more than adequate to meet requirements.

Non-nutritional uses of pantothenic acid

The blood concentration of pantothenic acid has been reported to be low in patients with rheumatoid arthritis; some workers have reported apparently beneficial effects of supplementation, but these reports remain unconfirmed and there are no established pharmacological uses of the vitamin.

Pantothenic acid deficiency in rats leads to a loss of fur colour and at one time pantothenic acid was known as the "anti-grey hair factor." There is no evidence that the normal graying of hair with age is related to pantothenic acid nutrition, nor that pantothenic acid supplements have any effect on hair colour. Its use in shampoo is not based on any evidence of efficacy.

Pantothenic acid has very low toxicity; intakes of up to 10 g/day of calcium pantothenate (compared with a normal dietary intake of 2–7 mg/day) have been given for up to six weeks with no apparent ill-effects.

10.14 Vitamin C (ascorbic acid)

Ascorbic acid is a vitamin for only a limited number of vertebrate species: human beings and the other primates, the guinea pig, bats, the passeriform birds, and most fishes. Ascorbate is synthesised as an intermediate in the gulonolactone pathway of glucose metabolism; in those vertebrate species for which it is a vitamin, one enzyme of the pathway, gulonolactone oxidase, is absent.

The vitamin C deficiency disease, scurvy, has been known for many centuries and was described in the Ebers papyrus of 1500 BCE and by Hippocrates. The Crusaders are said to have lost more men through scurvy than were killed in battle, while in some of the long voyages of exploration of the fourteenth and fifteenth centuries up to 90% of the crew died from scurvy. Cartier's expedition to Quebec in 1535 was struck by scurvy; the local native Americans taught him to use an infusion of swamp spruce leaves to prevent or cure the condition.

Recognition that scurvy was due to a dietary deficiency came relatively early. James Lind demonstrated in 1757 that orange juice and lemon juice were protective, and Cook kept his crew in good health during his circumnavigation of the globe (1772–1775) by stopping frequently to take on fresh fruit and vegetables. In 1804 the British Navy decreed a daily ration of lemon or lime juice for all ratings, a requirement that was extended to the merchant navy in 1865.

The structure of vitamin C is shown in Figure 10.19; both ascorbic acid and dehydroascorbic acid have vitamin activity. Monodehydroascorbate is a stable radical formed by reaction of ascorbate with reactive oxygen species, and can be reduced back to ascorbate by monodehydroascorbate reductase. Alternatively, 2 mol of monodehydroascorbate can react together to yield 1 mol each of ascorbate and dehydroascorbate. Dehydroascorbate may either be reduced to ascorbate or undergo hydration to diketogulonate and onward metabolism.

Vitamin C is found in fruits and vegetables. Very significant losses occur as vegetables wilt, or when they are cut, as a result of the release of ascorbate oxidase from the plant tissue. Significant losses of the vitamin also occur in cooking, both through leaching into the cooking water and also atmospheric oxidation, which continues when foods are left to stand before serving.

Absorption and metabolism of vitamin C

There is active transport of the vitamin at the intestinal mucosal brush border membrane. Both ascorbate and dehydroascorbate are absorbed across the buccal mucosa by carrier-mediated passive processes. Intestinal absorption of dehydroascorbate is carrier mediated, followed by reduction to ascorbate before transport across the basolateral membrane.

Some 80–95% of dietary ascorbate is absorbed at usual intakes (up to about 100 mg/day). The fractional absorption of larger amounts of the vitamin is lower, and unabsorbed ascorbate from very high doses is a substrate for intestinal bacterial metabolism, causing gastrointestinal discomfort and diarrhoea.

About 70% of blood ascorbate is in plasma and erythrocytes, which do not concentrate the vitamin from plasma. The remainder is in white cells, which have a marked ability to concentrate it. Both ascorbate and dehydroascorbate circulate in free solution, and also bound to albumin. About 5% of plasma vitamin C is normally dehydroascorbate. Both vitamers are transported into cells by glucose transporters, and concentrations of glucose of the order of those seen in diabetic hyperglycaemia inhibit tissue uptake of ascorbate.

There is no specific storage organ for ascorbate; apart from leukocytes (which account for only 10% of total blood ascorbate), the only tissues showing a significant concentration of the vitamin are the adrenal and pituitary glands. Although the concentration of ascorbate in muscle is relatively low, skeletal muscle contains much of the body's pool of 900– 1500 mg (5–8.5 mmol).

Diketogulonate arising from dehydroascorbate can undergo metabolism to xylose, thus providing a route for entry into central

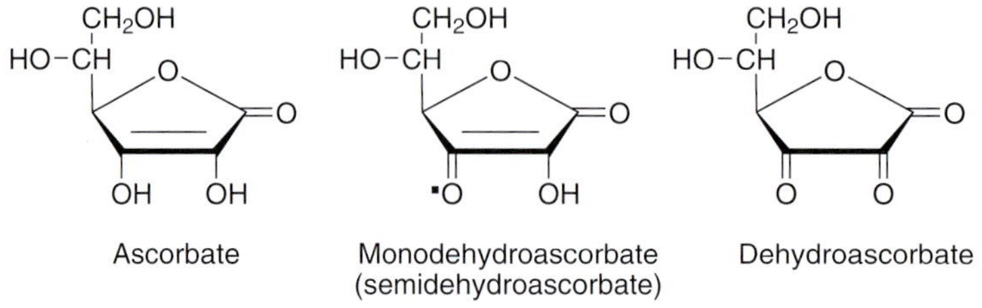

CH_2OH
HO–CH
OH OH
Ascorbate

CH_2OH
HO–CH
•O OH
Monodehydroascorbate (semidehydroascorbate)

CH_2OH
HO–CH
O O
Dehydroascorbate

Figure 10.19 Vitamin C (ascorbic acid, monodehydroascorbate and dehydroascorbate).

carbohydrate metabolic pathways via the pentose phosphate pathway. However, oxidation to carbon dioxide is only a minor fate of ascorbate in human beings. At usual intakes of the vitamin, less than 1% of the radioactivity from [^{14}C]-ascorbate is recovered as carbon dioxide. Although more $^{14}CO_2$ is recovered from subjects receiving high intakes of the vitamin, this is the result of bacterial metabolism of unabsorbed vitamin in the intestinal lumen.

The fate of the greater part of ascorbic acid is excretion in the urine, either unchanged or as dehydroascorbate and diketogulonate. Both ascorbate and dehydroascorbate are filtered at the glomerulus then reabsorbed. When glomerular filtration of ascorbate and dehydroascorbate exceeds the capacity of the transport systems, at a plasma concentration of ascorbate between 70 and 85 μmol/l, the vitamin is excreted in the urine in amounts proportional to intake.

Metabolic functions of vitamin C

Ascorbic acid has specific roles in two groups of enzymes: the copper-containing hydroxylases and the 2-oxoglutarate-linked iron-containing hydroxylases. It also increases the activity of a number of other enzymes *in vitro*, although this is a non-specific reducing action rather than reflecting any metabolic function of the vitamin. In addition, it has a number of non-enzymic effects due to its action as a reducing agent and oxygen radical quencher.

Copper-containing hydroxylases

Dopamine β-hydroxylase is a copper-containing enzyme involved in the synthesis of the catecholamines norepinephrine (noradrenaline) and epinephrine (adrenaline) from tyrosine in the adrenal medulla and central nervous system. The enzyme contains Cu^{+}, which is oxidised to Cu^{2+} during the hydroxylation of the substrate; reduction back to Cu^{+} specifically requires ascorbate, which is oxidised to monodehydroascorbate.

Some peptide hormones have a carboxy-terminal amide that is hydroxylated on the α-carbon by a copper-containing enzyme, peptidylglycine hydroxylase. The α-hydroxyglycine residue then decomposes non-enzymically to yield the amidated peptide and glyoxylate. The copper prosthetic group is oxidised in the reaction, and, as in dopamine β-hydroxylase, ascorbate is specifically required for reduction back to Cu^{+}.

Oxoglutarate-linked iron-containing hydroxylases

Several iron-containing hydroxylases share a common reaction mechanism, in which hydroxylation of the substrate is linked to decarboxylation of 2-oxoglutarate. Many of these enzymes are involved in the modification of precursor proteins to yield the final, mature, protein. This is a process of postsynthetic modification of an amino acid residue after it has been incorporated into the protein during synthesis on the ribosome.

- Proline and lysine hydroxylases are required for the postsynthetic modification of procollagen in the formation of mature, insoluble, collagen, and proline hydroxylase is also required for the postsynthetic modification of the precursor proteins of osteocalcin and the C1q component of complement.
- Aspartate β-hydroxylase is required for the postsynthetic modification of the precursor of protein C, the vitamin K-dependent protease that hydrolyses activated factor V in the blood-clotting cascade.
- Trimethyl-lysine and γ-butyrobetaine hydroxylases are required for the synthesis of carnitine.

Ascorbate is oxidised during the reaction of these enzymes, but not stoichiometrically with the decarboxylation of 2-oxoglutarate and hydroxylation of the substrate. The purified enzyme is active in the absence of ascorbate, but after some 5–10 s (about 15–30 cycles of enzyme action) the rate of reaction begins to fall. At this stage the iron in the catalytic site has been oxidised to Fe^{3+}, which is catalytically inactive; activity is restored only by ascorbate, which reduces it back to Fe^{2+}. The oxidation of Fe^{2+} is the consequence of a side-reaction rather than the main reaction of the enzyme, which explains how 15–30 cycles of enzyme activity can occur before there is significant loss of activity in the absence of ascorbate, and why the consumption of ascorbate is not stoichiometric.

Pro-oxidant and antioxidant roles of ascorbate

Ascorbate can act as a radical-trapping antioxidant, reacting with superoxide and a proton to yield hydrogen peroxide, or with the hydroxyl radical to yield water. In each instance the product is the monodehydroascorbate radical. Thus, as well as reducing the tocopheroxyl (vitamin E) radical formed by interaction of α-tocopherol in membranes with lipid peroxides, ascorbate acts to trap the oxygen radicals that would otherwise react to form lipid peroxides.

At high concentrations, ascorbate can reduce molecular oxygen to superoxide, being oxidised to monodehydroascorbate. At physiological concentrations of ascorbate, both Fe^{3+} and Cu^{2+} ions are reduced by ascorbate, yielding monodehydroascorbate. Fe^{2+} and Cu^{+} are readily reoxidised by reaction with hydrogen peroxide to yield hydroxide ions and hydroxyl radicals. Cu^{+} also reacts with molecular oxygen to yield superoxide. Thus, as well as its antioxidant role, ascorbate has potential pro-oxidant activity. However, because at high levels of intake the vitamin is excreted quantitatively, is it unlikely that tissue concentrations will rise high enough for there to be significant formation of oxygen radicals.

Vitamin C deficiency: scurvy

Historically, the vitamin C deficiency disease scurvy was a common problem at the end of winter, when there had been no fresh fruit and vegetables for many months.

Although there is no specific organ for storage of vitamin C in the body, signs of deficiency do not develop in previously adequately nourished subjects until they have been deprived of the vitamin for four to six months, by which time plasma and tissue concentrations have fallen considerably. The earliest signs of scurvy in volunteers maintained on a vitamin C-free diet are skin changes, beginning with plugging of hair follicles by horny material, followed by enlargement of the hyperkeratotic follicles, and petechial haemorrhage with significant extravasation of red cells, presumably as a result of the increased fragility of blood capillaries.

At a later stage there is also haemorrhage of the gums, beginning in the interdental papillae and progressing to generalised sponginess and bleeding. This is frequently accompanied by secondary bacterial infection and considerable withdrawal of the gum from the necks of the teeth. As the condition progresses, there is loss of dental cement, and the teeth become loose in the alveolar bone and may be lost.

Wounds show only superficial healing in scurvy, with little or no formation of (collagen-rich) scar tissue, so that healing is delayed and wounds can readily be reopened. The scorbutic scar tissue has only about half the tensile strength of that normally formed.

Advanced scurvy is accompanied by intense pain in the bones, which can be attributed to changes in bone mineralisation as a result of abnormal collagen synthesis. Bone formation ceases and the existing bone becomes rarefied, so that the bones fracture with minimal trauma.

The name scurvy is derived from the Italian *scorbutico*, meaning an irritable, neurotic, discontented, whining, and cranky person. The disease is associated with listlessness and general malaise, and sometimes changes in personality and psychomotor performance, and a lowering of the general level of arousal. These behavioral effects can be attributed to impaired synthesis of catecholamine neurotransmitters, as a result of low activity of dopamine β-hydroxylase.

Most of the other clinical signs of scurvy can be accounted for by the effects of ascorbate deficiency on collagen synthesis, as a result of impaired proline and lysine hydroxylase activity. Depletion of muscle carnitine, due to impaired activity of trimethyllysine and γ-butyrobetaine hydroxylases, may account for the lassitude and fatigue that precede clinical signs of scurvy.

Anaemia in scurvy

Anaemia is frequently associated with scurvy, and may be either macrocytic, indicative of folate deficiency, or hypochromic, indicative of iron deficiency.

Folate deficiency may be epiphenomenal, since the major dietary sources of folate are the same as those of ascorbate. However, some patients with clear megaloblastic anaemia respond to the administration of vitamin C alone, suggesting that there may be a role of ascorbate in the maintenance of normal pools of reduced folates, although there is no evidence that any of the reactions of folate is ascorbate dependent.

Iron deficiency in scurvy may well be secondary to reduced absorption of inorganic iron and impaired mobilisation of tissue iron reserves. At the same time, the haemorrhages of advanced scurvy will cause a significant loss of blood.

There is also evidence that erythrocytes have a shorter half-life than normal in scurvy, possibly as a result of peroxidative damage to membrane lipids owing to impairment of the reduction of tocopheroxyl radical by ascorbate.

Vitamin C requirements

Vitamin C illustrates extremely well how different criteria of adequacy, and different interpretations of experimental data, can lead to different estimates of requirements, and to reference intakes ranging between 30 and 90 mg/day for adults.

The requirement for vitamin C to prevent clinical scurvy is less than 10 mg/day. However, at this level of intake wounds do not heal properly because of the requirement for vitamin C for the synthesis of collagen. An intake of 20 mg/day is required for optimum wound healing. Allowing for individual variation in requirements, this gives a reference intake for adults of 30 mg/day, which was the British recommended daily allowance (RDA) until 1991.

The 1991 British reference nutrient intake (RNI) for vitamin C is based on the level of intake at which the plasma concentration rises sharply, showing that requirements have now been met, tissues are saturated and there is spare vitamin C being transported between tissues, available for excretion. This criterion of adequacy gives an RNI of 40 mg/day for adults.

The alternative approach to determining requirements is to estimate the total body content of vitamin C, then measure the rate at which it is metabolised, by giving a test dose of radioactive vitamin. This is the basis of both the former US RDA of 60 mg/day for adults and the Netherlands RDA of 80 mg/day. Indeed, it also provides an alternative basis for the RNI of 40 mg/day.

The problem lies in deciding what is an appropriate body content of vitamin C. The studies were performed on subjects whose total body vitamin C was estimated to be 1500 mg at the beginning of a depletion study. However, there is no evidence that this is a necessary, or even a desirable, body content of the vitamin. It is simply the body content of the vitamin of a small group of people eating a self-selected diet relatively rich in fruit and vegetables. There is good evidence that a total body content of 900 mg is more than adequate. It is three times larger than the body content at which the first signs of deficiency are observed, and will protect against the development of any signs of deficiency for several months on a completely vitamin C-free diet.

There is a further problem in interpreting the results. The rate at which vitamin C is metabolised varies with the amount consumed. This means that as the experimental subjects become depleted, so the rate at which they metabolise the vitamin decreases. Thus, calculation of the amount that is required to maintain the body content depends on both the way in which the results obtained during depletion studies are extrapolated to the rate in subjects consuming a normal diet and the amount of vitamin C in that diet.

An intake of 40 mg/day is more than adequate to maintain a total body content of 900 mg of vitamin C (the British RNI). At a higher level of habitual intake, 60 mg/day is adequate to maintain a total body content of 1500 mg (the former US RDA). Making allowances for changes in the rate of metabolism with different levels of intake, and allowing for incomplete absorption of the vitamin gives the Netherlands RDA of 80 mg/day.

The current US reference intake (75 mg for women and 90 mg for men) is based on intakes required to saturate leukocytes with vitamin C.

Assessment of vitamin C status

Urinary excretion of ascorbate falls to undetectably low levels in deficiency, and therefore very low excretion will indicate deficiency. However, no guidelines for the interpretation of urinary ascorbate have been established.

It is relatively easy to assess the state of body reserves of vitamin C by measuring the excretion after a test dose. A subject who is saturated will excrete more or less the whole of a test dose of 500 mg of ascorbate over 6 h. A more precise method involves repeating the loading test daily until more or less complete recovery is achieved, thus giving an indication of how depleted the body stores were.

The plasma concentration of vitamin C falls relatively rapidly during experimental depletion studies to undetectably low levels within four weeks of initiating a vitamin C-free diet, although clinical signs of scurvy may not develop for a further three to four months, and tissue concentrations of the vitamin may be as high as 50% of saturation. In field studies and surveys, subjects with plasma ascorbate below 11 μmol/l are considered to be at risk of developing scurvy, and anyone with a plasma concentration below 6 μmol/l would be expected to show clinical signs.

The concentration of ascorbate in leukocytes is correlated with the concentrations in other tissues, and falls more slowly than the plasma concentration in depletion studies. The reference range of leukocyte ascorbate is 1.1–2.8 pmol/10^6 cells; a significant loss of leukocyte ascorbate coincides with the development of clear clinical signs of scurvy.

Without a differential white cell count, leukocyte ascorbate concentration cannot be considered to give a meaningful reflection of vitamin C status. The different types of leukocyte have different capacities to accumulate ascorbate. This means that a change in the proportion of granulocytes, platelets, and mononuclear leukocytes will result in a change in the total concentration of ascorbate/10^6 cells, although there may well be no change in vitamin nutritional status. Stress, myocardial infarction, infection, burns, and surgical trauma all result in changes in leukocyte distribution, with an increase in the proportion of granulocytes, and hence an apparent change in leukocyte ascorbate. This has been widely misinterpreted to indicate an increased requirement for vitamin C in these conditions.

Urinary excretion of hydroxyproline-containing peptides is reduced in people with inadequate vitamin C status, but a number of other factors that affect bone and connective tissue turnover confound interpretation of the results. Excretion of compounds derived from collagen cross-links provides a more useful index, but is affected by copper status. There is increased formation of 8-hydroxyguanine (a marker of oxidative radical damage) in DNA during vitamin C depletion, suggesting that measurement of 8-hydroxyguanine excretion may provide a way of estimating requirements to meet a biomarker of optimum status.

Possible benefits of high intakes of vitamin C

There is evidence from a variety of studies that high vitamin C status and a high plasma concentration of the vitamin is associated with reduced all-cause mortality.

At intakes above about 100–120 mg/day the body's capacity to metabolise vitamin C is saturated, and any further intake is excreted in the urine unchanged. Therefore, it would not seem justifiable to recommend higher levels of intake. However, in addition to its antioxidant role and its role in reducing the tocopheroxyl radical, and thus sparing vitamin E, vitamin C is important in the absorption of iron, and in preventing the formation of nitrosamines. Both of these actions depend on the presence of the vitamin in the gut together with food, and intakes totaling more than 100 mg/day may be beneficial.

Iron absorption

Inorganic dietary iron is absorbed as Fe^{2+} and not as Fe^{3+}; ascorbic acid in the intestinal lumen will both maintain iron in the reduced state and chelate it, thus increasing the amount absorbed. A dose of 25 mg of vitamin C taken together with a meal increases the absorption of iron by around 65%, while a 1 g dose gives a ninefold increase. This occurs only when ascorbic acid is present together with the test meal; neither intravenous administration of vitamin C nor intake several hours before the test meal has any effect on iron absorption. Optimum iron absorption may therefore require significantly more than 100 mg of vitamin C/day.

Inhibition of nitrosamine formation

The safety of nitrates and nitrites used in curing meat, a traditional method of preservation, has been questioned because of the formation of nitrosamines by reaction between nitrite and amines naturally present in foods under the acid conditions in the stomach. In experimental animals nitrosamines are potent carcinogens, and some authorities have limited the amounts of these salts that are permitted, although there is no evidence of any hazard to human beings from endogenous nitrosamine formation. Ascorbate can prevent the formation of nitrosamines by reacting non-enzymically with nitrite and other nitrosating reagents, forming NO, NO_2, and N_2. Again, this is an effect of ascorbate present in the stomach at the same time as the dietary nitrites and amines, rather than an effect of vitamin C nutritional status.

Pharmacological uses of vitamin C

Several studies have reported low ascorbate status in patients with advanced cancer, which is perhaps an unsurprising finding in seriously ill patients. With very little experimental evidence, it has been suggested that very high intakes of vitamin C (of the order of 10 g/day or more) may be beneficial in enhancing host resistance to cancer and preventing the development of the acquired immunodeficiency syndrome (AIDS) in people who are human immunodeficiency virus (HIV) positive. In controlled studies with patients matched for age, gender, site and stage of primary tumors and metastases, and previous chemotherapy, there was no beneficial effect of high-dose ascorbic acid in the treatment of advanced cancer.

High doses of vitamin C have been recommended for the prevention and treatment of the common cold, with some evidence that the vitamin reduces the duration of symptoms. However, the evidence from controlled trials is unconvincing.

Toxicity of vitamin C

Regardless of whether or not high intakes of ascorbate have any beneficial effects, large numbers of people habitually take between 1 and 5 g/day of vitamin C supplements (compared with reference intakes of 40–90 mg/day) and some take considerably more. There is little evidence of significant toxicity from these high intakes. Once the plasma concentration of ascorbate reaches the renal threshold, it is excreted more or less quantitatively with increasing intake, and there is no evidence that higher intakes increase the body pool above about 110 μmol/kg body weight. Unabsorbed ascorbate in the intestinal lumen is a substrate for bacterial fermentation, and may cause diarrhoea and intestinal discomfort.

Ascorbate can react non-enzymically with amino groups in proteins to glycate them, in the same way as occurs in poorly controlled diabetes mellitus, and there is some evidence of increased cardiovascular mortality associated with vitamin C supplements in diabetics.

Up to 5% of the population are at risk from the development of renal oxalate stones. The risk is from both ingested oxalate and that formed endogenously, mainly from the metabolism of glycine. High intakes of ascorbate lead to acidification of the urine, which will increase the risk of forming oxalate and urate renal stones, but reduce the risk of forming phosphate stones.

10.15 Perspectives on the future

Current estimates of requirements and reference intakes of vitamins are based on the amounts required to prevent or reverse subtle indices of deficiency, and can thus be considered to be amounts required to prevent deficiency, but possibly not to promote optimum nutritional status and health. There is currently very little evidence on which to base reference intakes above those required to prevent (subtle biochemical) deficiency, but indices of enhanced immune system function and whole-body oxidative stress and other biomarkers may do so in due course.

There are several compounds that have clearly defined functions in the body but can be synthesised in apparently adequate amounts, so that they are not considered to be dietary essentials. These substances have been receiving increasing attention, and these, in addition to other compounds, are likely to continue to stimulate interest and discussion in the future.

Bioflavonoids

The most studied flavonoids are hesperitin and quercitin. Because they are biologically active, they are commonly called bioflavonoids. Most fruits and green leafy vegetables contain relatively large amounts of flavonoids; altogether some 2000 have been identified, and average intakes of flavonoids from a mixed diet are of the order of 1 g/day.

There is no evidence that bioflavonoids are dietary essentials, but they have potentially useful antioxidant actions. Oxidation of flavonoids may serve to protect susceptible nutrients from damage in foods and the intestinal lumen, and they may also act as antioxidants in plasma and tissues. Epidemiological evidence suggests that the intake of flavonoids is inversely correlated with mortality from coronary heart disease.

Carnitine

Carnitine has a central role in the transport of fatty acids across the mitochondrial membrane. It is synthesised in both liver and skeletal muscle by methylation of lysine, followed by two vitamin C-dependent hydroxylations. In experimental animals, deficiency of lysine has little effect on plasma and tissue concentrations, but methionine deficiency can lead to carnitine depletion, and carnitine has a methionine-sparing effect in methionine-deficient animals. Deficiency of vitamin C may result in impaired synthesis of carnitine in species for which ascorbate is a vitamin.

The administration of the anticonvulsant valproic acid can lead to carnitine depletion. This results in impaired β-oxidation of fatty acids and ketogenesis, and hence a nonketotic hypoglycaemia, with elevated plasma, non-esterified fatty acids, and triacylglycerols. There may also be signs of liver dysfunction, with hyperammonaemia and encephalopathy. The administration of carnitine supplements in these conditions has a beneficial effect.

Although carnitine is not generally nutritionally important, it may be required for premature infants, since they have a limited capacity to synthesise it. There is some evidence that full-term infants may also have a greater requirement for carnitine than can be met by endogenous synthesis; infants fed on carnitine-free soya-milk formula have higher plasma concentrations of non-esterified fatty acids and triacylglycerols than those receiving carnitine supplements. Carnitine depletion, with disturbed lipid metabolism, has also been reported in adults maintained for prolonged periods on total parenteral nutrition. There is some evidence that supplements of carnitine may increase the ability of muscle to oxidise fatty acids, and so increase physical work capacity, although other studies have shown no effect.

Choline

Choline is important as a base in phospholipids: both phosphatidylcholine (lecithin) in all cell membranes and sphingomyelin in the nervous system. In addition, acetylcholine is a transmitter in the central and parasympathetic nervous systems and at neuromuscular junctions. There is some evidence that the availability of choline may be limiting for the synthesis of acetylcholine in the central nervous system under some conditions. In animals, deficiency of choline results in fatty infiltration of the liver, apparently as a result of impairment of the export of lipoproteins from hepatocytes; prolonged deficiency may result in cirrhosis. The kidney can also be affected, with tubular necrosis and interstitial hemorrhage, probably as a result of lysosomal membrane disruption.

There is no evidence that choline is a dietary essential for human beings, and no condition similar to the effects of choline deficiency in experimental animals has been reported. Since phosphatidylcholine is found in all biological membranes, dietary deficiency is unlikely to occur except when people are maintained on defined diets free from phospholipids. Plasma concentrations fall during long-term total parenteral nutrition, and it is possible that the impaired liver function seen in such patients is partly the result of choline depletion.

Inositol

The main function of inositol is in phospholipids; phosphatidylinositol constitutes some 5–10% of the total membrane phospholipids. In addition to its structural role in membranes, phosphatidylinositol has a major function in the intracellular responses to hormones and neurotransmitters, yielding two intracellular second messengers, inositol trisphosphate, and diacylglycerol.

There is no evidence that inositol is a dietary essential. Infants may have a higher requirement than can be met by endogenous synthesis. Untreated diabetics have high plasma concentrations of free inositol and high urinary excretion of inositol, associated with relatively low intracellular concentrations, suggesting that elevated plasma glucose may inhibit tissue uptake of inositol. There is some evidence that impaired nerve conduction velocity in diabetic neuropathy in both patients and experimental animals is associated with low intracellular concentrations of inositol, and inositol supplements may improve nerve conduction velocity. However, high intracellular concentrations of inositol also impair nerve conduction velocity, and supplements may have a deleterious effect.

Taurine

Until about 1976 it was assumed that taurine was an end-product of cysteine metabolism, the only function of which was the conjugation of bile acids. The occurrence of changes in the electrical activity of the retina in children maintained on long-term total parenteral nutrition without added taurine has shown that it has physiological functions, and has raised the question of whether or not it should be regarded as a dietary essential, especially under conditions of low availability of the sulphur amino acids.

Ubiquinone (coenzyme Q, "vitamin Q")

Ubiquinone is one of the electron carriers in mitochondria. Therefore, it has an essential function in all energy-yielding metabolism and may also have a general antioxidant role in membranes. Like vitamin E, it can be anchored in membranes by the hydrophobic tail, with the reactive quinone group at the membrane surface. Ubiquinone is readily synthesised in the body, and there is no evidence that it is a dietary essential, or that supplements serve any useful purpose, although they may have non-specific antioxidant actions and so spare vitamin E.

"Phytoceuticals"

In addition to the compounds with clearly defined metabolic functions discussed above, various compounds naturally present in foods, and especially in foods of plant origin, have potentially beneficial effects, although they are not nutrients. Collectively, they are known as phytoceuticals (substances of plant origin with potential pharmaceutical action) or nutraceuticals. The following are examples of phytoceuticals:

- Many glucosinolates and glycosides either inhibit the enzymes of phase I metabolism of foreign compounds (the reactions that activate many potential carcinogens) or induce the reactions leading to conjugation and excretion of foreign compounds.
- Terpenes that are found in the volatile (essential) oils of herbs and spices are potentially active as lipid-soluble antioxidants, as are many of the carotenoids that are not active as precursors of vitamin A.
- Squalene, which is a precursor of cholesterol synthesis, may have a hypocholesterolaemic action, by reducing the activity of the rate-limiting enzyme of cholesterol synthesis, hydroxymethylglutaryl-CoA reductase. However, squalene can also be metabolised to yield additional cholesterol.
- Various water-soluble compounds, including polyphenols, anthocyanins, and flavonoids, have antioxidant actions.
- Several plants (especially soyabeans) contain compounds with oestrogenic action (phytoestrogens) that also have anti-oestrogenic action and appear to be protective against the development of hormone-dependent cancer of the breast and uterus.

Further reading

Bender, D.A. (2003). *Nutritional Biochemistry of the Vitamins*, 2e. Cambridge University Press.

Food Safety Authority of Ireland. (2018). The Safety of Vitamins and Minerals in Food Supplements – Establishing Tolerable Upper Intake Levels and a Risk Assessment Approach for Products Marketed in Ireland.

Institute of Medicine (IOM). (1998). Dietary Reference Intakes for Thiamin, Riboflavin, Niacin, Vitamin B6, Folate, Vitamin B12, Pantothenic Acid, Biotin, and Choline.

Institute of Medicine (IOM). (2001). Dietary Reference Intakes for Vitamin C, Vitamin E, Selenium, and Carotenoids.

Institute of Medicine (IOM). (2001). Dietary Reference Intakes for Vitamin A, Vitamin K, Arsenic, Boron, Chromium, Copper, Iodine, Iron, Manganese, Molybdenum, Nickel, Silicon, Vanadium, and Zinc.

Institute of Medicine (IOM). (2011). Dietary Reference Intakes for Calcium and Vitamin D. Washington, DC: The National Academies Press.

11
Minerals and Trace Elements

JJ. Strain, Alison J. Yeates, and Kevin D. Cashman

Key messages

- This chapter defines the essential minerals and trace elements.
- It describes the functions and routes of metabolism within the body of each of the minerals and trace elements in turn.
- Dietary requirements and dietary sources are discussed for each mineral.
- Health effects and symptoms of both inadequate and toxic intakes are described.
- Methods of assessing the body status of each mineral and trace element are reviewed.

11.1 Introduction

Essential minerals, including the trace elements, are inorganic elements (see Figure 11.1) that have a physiological function within the body. These must be supplied in the diet (food and fluids) and vary from grams per day for the major (macro) minerals through milligrams to micrograms per day for the trace elements.

It has been proposed that the environment (most probably in the primordial sea around hydrothermal vents) in which living organisms evolved was a primary determinant of which elements became essential for life by providing structural integrity and catalytic ability to the first complex organic molecules. As life evolved from the oceans on to land, a natural selection process may have resulted in some elements becoming relatively more important because of superior catalytic abilities over other elements. In any event, the uneven distribution of elements in a land-based environment meant that efficient homeostatic mechanisms had to be in place to conserve essential elements and to eliminate excesses of essential and nonessential elements. The processes of absorption from the gastrointestinal tract and excretion with body fluids, therefore, are major ways in which the concentration and amount of an element can be controlled in the body. In addition, storage in inactive sites or in an unreactive form can prevent an element from causing adverse effects in the body, and release from storage can be important in times of dietary insufficiency.

All elements have the potential to cause toxic symptoms, whereas some, the known essential elements in Figure 11.1, have the potential to cause deficiency symptoms in animals. Even so, deficiencies of only four of these inorganic elements are known to be prevalent in human populations. Two of these deficiencies, iodine and iron, are widespread in human populations whereas the other two, zinc and selenium, only occur in some population groups under specially defined conditions. Overt clinical signs of deficiency of any of the other inorganic elements are exceptional in humans and mainly occur secondary to other clinical conditions. Such observations do not preclude the possibility that suboptimum status of the great majority of the elements indicated in Figure 11.1 is important in human nutrition. Indeed, there is an increasing

Introduction to Human Nutrition, Third Edition. Edited on behalf of The Nutrition Society by Susan A. Lanham-New, Thomas R. Hill, Alison M. Gallagher and Hester H. Vorster.

Companion website: www.wiley.com/go/lanham-new/humannutrition

1a	2a	3a	4a	5a	6a	7a	8			1b	2b	3b	4b	5b	6b	7b	8b
1 H																	
3 Li	4 Be											5 B	6 C	7 N	8 O	9 F	10 Ne
11 Na	12 Mg											13 Al	14 Si	15 P	16 S	17 Cl	18 Ar
19 K	20 Ca	21 Sc	22 Ti	23 V	24 Cr	25 Mn	26 Fe	27 Co	28 Ni	29 Cu	30 Zn	31 Ga	32 Ge	33 As	34 Se	35 Br	36 Kr
37 Rb	38 Sr	39 Y	40 Zr	41 Nb	42 Mo	43 Tc	44 Ru	45 Rh	46 Pd	47 Ag	48 Cd	49 In	50 Sn	51 Sb	52 Te	53 I	54 Xe
55 Cs	56 Ba	57 La	72 Hf	73 Ta	74 W	75 Re	76 Os	77 Ir	78 Pt	79 Au	80 Hg	81 Tl	82 Pb	83 Bi	84 Po	85 At	86 Rn
87 Fr	88 Ra	89 Ac	104	105	106												
Lanthanides		58 Ce	59 Pr	60 Nd	61 Pm	62 Sm	63 Eu	64 Gd	65 Tb	66 Dy	67 Ho	68 Er	69 Tm	70 Yb	71 Lu		
Actinides		90 Th	91 Pa	92 U	93 Np	94 Pu	95 Am	96 Cm	97 Bk	98 Cf	99 Es	100 Fm	101 Md	102 No	103 Lr		

Figure 11.1 The periodic table of the elements. The widely accepted or putative essential elements are encircled.

awareness of the potential role of suboptimal as well as supra-optimal nutritional status of minerals and trace elements in the development of degenerative age-related diseases, such as coronary heart disease, cancer, and osteoporosis. Moreover, other elements, which currently have no published dietary recommendations but are highlighted in Figure 11.1, might prove to be essential for the optimum health and well-being of humans. These elements are discussed briefly in section 11.16 below.

Major constraints to the elucidation of the potential roles of minerals and trace elements in the onset of degenerative diseases include difficulties in assessing status, and thereby defining requirements, and myriad interactions among minerals and other nutrient and non-nutrients in the diet. Sometimes, natural experiments of genetic disorders can throw light on the potential roles of minerals in disease processes and genetic issues will also be discussed as appropriate in the following sections.

11.2 Calcium

Calcium is a metallic element, fifth in abundance in the Earth's crust, of which it forms more than 3%. Calcium is never found in nature uncombined; it occurs abundantly as chalk, granite, eggshell, seashells, "hard" water, bone, and limestone. Calcium was among the first materials known to be essential in the diet. All foods of vegetable origin contain small but useful amounts of calcium. Animals concentrate calcium in milk, and milk and dairy products are the most important food sources of calcium for many human populations.

Absorption, transport, and tissue distribution

The adult human body contains about 1000–1200 g of calcium, which amounts to about 1–2% of body weight and thus making it the most abundant mineral in the body. Of this, 99% is found in mineralised tissues, such as bones and teeth, where it is present mainly as calcium hydroxyapatite [$Ca_{10}(PO_4)_6(OH)_2$], providing rigidity and structure. The remaining 1% is found in blood, extracellular fluid (ECF), muscle, and other tissues, but while quantitatively small, this calcium plays critical roles in these soft tissues (see below). In fact, due to calcium's involvement in these critical metabolic functions, soft tissue calcium concentrations are maintained at the expense of bone (see below). Calcium is present in blood as free Ca^{2+} ions (ionised calcium) and bound to proteins, in about equal proportions, and about 10% complexed to citrate, phosphate, sulfate and carbonate.

Calcium is under close homeostatic control, with processes such as absorption, excretion and secretion, and storage in bone being involved in maintaining the concentration of ionised calcium in the plasma within a tightly regulated range (between 1.1 and 1.4 mmol/l). This tight regulation of plasma calcium concentration is achieved through a complex physiological system comprising the interaction of the calcitropic hormones, such as parathyroid hormone (PTH), 1,25-dihydroxycholecalciferol [$1,25(OH)_2D_3$] and calcitonin, with specific target tissues (kidney, bone, and intestine) that serve to increase or to decrease the entry of calcium into plasma (Figure 11.2). Only in extreme circumstances, such as severe malnutrition or hyperparathyroidism, is the serum ionised calcium concentration below or above the normal range. The secretion of these hormones is governed wholly, or in part, by the plasma concentration of ionised calcium, thus forming a negative feedback system. PTH and $1,25(OH)_2D_3$ are secreted when plasma calcium is low, whereas calcitonin is secreted when plasma calcium is high.

Calcium in food occurs as salts or associated with other dietary constituents in the form of complexes of calcium ions. Calcium must be released in a soluble, and probably ionised, form before it can be absorbed. Calcium is absorbed in the intestine by two routes, transcellular (meaning across or through the cell) and paracellular (meaning between cells) (Figure 11.3). The transcellular route involves active transport of calcium by the mucosal calcium transport protein, calbindin, and is saturable and subject to physiological and nutritional regulation via $1,25(OH)_2D_3$. The paracellular route involves passive calcium transport through the tight junctions between

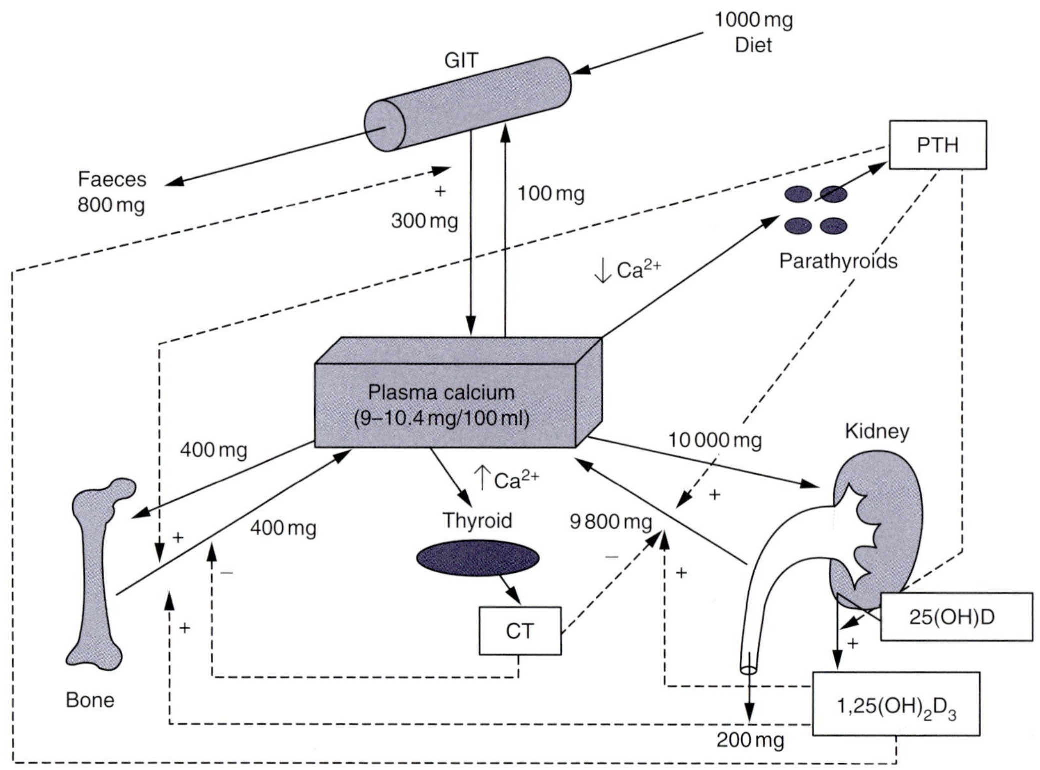

Figure 11.2 Homeostatic regulation of serum calcium, showing the integration of calcitropic hormone action at the tissue level. CT, calcitonin; PTH, parathyroid hormone; $1,25(OH)_2D_3$, 1,25-dihydroxycholecalciferol (to convert calcium from mg/day to mmol/day, multiply by 40).

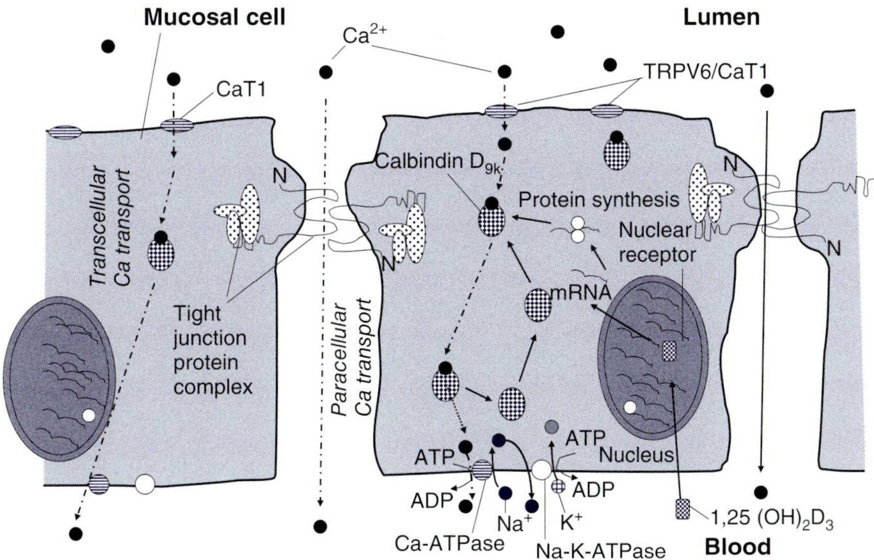

Figure 11.3 Calcium transport across the intestinal mucosal lining: paracellular calcium transport (between mucosal cells) and transcellular calcium transport (across the mucosal cell).

mucosal cells; it is non-saturable, essentially independent of nutritional and physiological regulation, and concentration dependent. Most calcium absorption in humans occurs in the small intestine, but there is some evidence for a small colonic component. Transcellular calcium absorption responds to calcium needs, as reflected by changes in plasma calcium concentration, by hormone-mediated up- or down-regulation of calbindin in mucosal cells; for example, reduced plasma calcium evokes a PTH-mediated increase in plasma $1{,}25(OH)_2D_3$, which stimulates increased calbindin synthesis but also likely the brush border-based epithelial entry channel (TRPV6) and basolateral-based pump (PMCA1b) in intestinal mucosal cells and thus facilitating the uptake, transport and extrusion of calcium from the mucosal cell.

On average, around 25% of the calcium is absorbed from a mixed diet by healthy adults. However, fractional calcium absorption varies with the intake of the mineral. It also varies considerably throughout the lifespan, being higher during periods of rapid growth and lower in old age. The efficiency of calcium absorption is also influenced by a number of other physiological and dietary factors (Table 11.1).

Unabsorbed dietary calcium is lost in faeces, whereas the main routes of endogenous calcium excretion are urine, faeces, and skin and sweat (sometimes referred to as the dermal losses) (Figure 11.2). These endogenous losses amass to about 240 mg calcium each day and these basal losses need to be replenished to maintain homeostasis (or constant body calcium levels).

Metabolic function and essentiality

Calcium is required for normal growth and development of the skeleton. During skeletal growth over the first two decades, calcium accumulates in the skeleton at an average rate of 150 mg/day. It is estimated that 40% of the total bone mass is accrued during the pubertal period alone and thereafter, in the twenties, the maximum genetically programmed amount of bone mass is achieved (this is called the peak bone mass [PBM]). During maturity, the body, and therefore the skeleton, is more or less in calcium equilibrium. From the age of about 50 years in men and from the menopause in women, bone balance becomes negative and bone is lost from all skeletal sites. This bone loss is associated with a marked rise in fracture rates in both sexes, but particularly in women. Adequate calcium intake is critical to achieving optimal PBM and modifies the rate of bone loss associated with aging. Extra-skeletal calcium (while only

Table 11.1 Factors affecting calcium absorption

Increased absorption	Decreased absorption
Physiological factors	
Vitamin D adequacy	Vitamin D deficiency
Increased mucosal mass	Decreased mucosal mass
Calcium deficiency	Menopause
Phosphorus deficiency	Old age
Pregnancy	Decreased gastric acid (without a meal)
Lactation	Rapid intestinal transit time
Disease states (e.g., hyperparathyroidism, sarcoidosis, idiopathic hypercalciuria)	Disease states (e.g., malabsorption syndrome, celiac disease, Crohn's disease, chronic renal failure, diabetes, hypoparathyroidism, primary biliary cirrhosis)
Dietary factors	
Lactose (in infants)	Phytate
Casein phosphopeptides (?)[a]	Oxalate
Nondigestible oligosaccharides	Large calcium load
Small calcium load	High habitual calcium intake
Low habitual calcium intake	Ingestion without a meal
Ingestion with a meal	

[a] Conflicting data in the literature.

representing around 1% of total body calcium) acts as an essential intracellular messenger in cells and tissues and it plays a key role in mediating vascular contraction and vasodilatation, muscle contraction, enzyme activation, membrane transport nerve transmission, glandular secretion, amongst others. Ionised calcium is the most common signal transduction element in the human body.

Deficiency symptoms

Because of the small metabolic pool of calcium (less than 0.1% in the ECF compartment) relative to the large skeletal reserve, for all practical purposes metabolic calcium deficiency probably never exists, at least not as a nutritional disorder. An inadequate intake or poor intestinal absorption of calcium causes the circulating ionised calcium concentration to decline acutely, which triggers an increase in PTH synthesis and release. PTH acts on three target organs (either directly or indirectly) to restore the circulating calcium concentration to normal (Figure 11.2). At the kidney, PTH promotes the reabsorption of calcium in the distal tubule. PTH affects the intestine indirectly by stimulating the production of 1,25(OH)$_2$D$_3$ (in the kidney), which, in turn, leads to increased calcium absorption. PTH also induces bone resorption (by signaling osteoclasts, or bone resorbing cells), thereby releasing calcium into blood. Owing to the action of PTH and 1,25(OH)$_2$D$_3$ on the target tissues, plasma calcium concentrations are restored within minutes to hours.

If, however, there is a continual inadequate intake or poor intestinal absorption of calcium (e.g., because of vitamin D deficiency), circulating calcium concentration is maintained largely at the expense of skeletal mass, that is, from an increased rate of bone resorption. This PTH-mediated increase in bone resorption is one of several important causes of reduced bone mass and osteoporosis. The cumulative effect of calcium depletion (by whatever mechanism) on the skeleton over many years contributes to the increasing frequency of osteoporotic fractures with age. Prolonged inadequate calcium intake in younger people reduces the rate of accretion of the skeleton and may prevent the attainment of the genetically determined maximal PBM. This may increase the risk of osteoporosis as the PBM in adulthood is predictive of bone mass in later life. Chronic inadequate intake or poor intestinal absorption of calcium may also play some role in the etiologies of other potential adverse health outcomes, such as increased risk of colorectal cancer, cardiovascular disease (even though calcium supplementation has been associated with increased risk), hypertension, preeclampsia as well as obesity. The evidence-base for these non-skeletal health effects is less developed than that for bone health and in some cases there is a need to show cause and effect relationship.

Toxicity

The available data on the adverse effects of high calcium intakes in humans are primarily from the intake of calcium from nutrient supplements. The three most widely studied and biologically important are:

- kidney stone formation (nephrolithiasis);
- the syndrome of hypercalcemia and renal insufficiency, with or without alkalosis (referred to historically as milk alkali syndrome associated with peptic ulcer treatments);
- the effect on absorption of other essential minerals, e.g., iron and zinc.

Some evidence links higher calcium intake (particularly from supplementation) with increased risk of prostate cancer as well as vascular and soft tissue calcification, but these are not conclusive. High calcium intake can also cause constipation.

Assessing status

There is, as yet, no biochemical indicator that reflects calcium nutritional status. Blood calcium concentration, for example, is not a good indicator because it is tightly regulated. Estimates of calcium deficiency are based largely on adequacy of dietary intake relative to requirements. In particular, the proportion of the population, or population subgroup, with calcium intakes below the Estimated Average Requirement (EAR; the nutrient intake value that is estimated to meet the requirement of 50% of the individuals in a life-stage and sex group; estimates vary between 750 and 1000 mg/day depending on age and sex-group) has been used as a benchmark of inadequacy of intake. On that basis, it has been estimated that 3.5 billion people are at risk of calcium deficiency globally due to inadequate dietary supply, with about 90% of those at risk of calcium deficiency in Africa and Asia where inadequate calcium intakes are widespread. In industrialised countries significant proportions of some population groups fail to achieve the recommended calcium intakes. For example, in the USA 38% of the population aged ≥2 years has inadequate calcium intake with lowest intakes relative to needs in adolescent females and older adults. In fact, calcium is one of the four shortfall nutrients of public health concern as designated in the *2015–2020 Dietary Guidelines for Americans.*

Bone mineral content (BMC, which is the amount of mineral at a particular skeletal site such as the femoral neck, lumbar spine, or total body) and bone mineral density (BMD, which is BMC divided by the area of the scanned region) can be used to assess the response to changes in intake over a relatively long period of time (>1 year), but not to measure calcium status *per se.*

Dietary sources and requirements

Milk and milk products are the most important dietary sources of calcium for most people in Western countries, with cereal products and fruits and vegetables each making a much smaller contribution (Table 11.2). For example, the contribution of dairy products to total calcium intake has been estimated as 73% in the Netherlands, 72% in the USA, 51–52% in Germany, 44% in the UK and 38% in Ireland. Tinned fish, such as sardines, are rich sources of calcium but do not make a significant contribution to intake for most people. In general, foods of plant origin are not very rich sources of calcium. However, owing to the level of consumption, foods of plant origin make a significant contribution to total calcium intake. For example, in the USA, cereals contribute about 25–27% of total calcium intake, whereas in the UK cereals and cereal products contribute about 29-31% of total calcium intake in adults with about 16-17% from bread because of calcium fortification of white flour. Increased availability of calcium-fortified foods and dietary supplements containing calcium salts is leading to a wider range of rich dietary sources of calcium. Contributions from nutritional supplements or medicines may be significant for some people.

Table 11.2 Calcium and phosphorus contents of some common foods

		Range (mg/100g)	
Food source	Description	Ca	P
Cheese	Hard, from milk (e.g., Cheedar/Gouda)	739/773	505/498
Cheese	Soft, from milk (e.g., Cottage/Feta)	127/360	171/280
Milk	Cow's (3.5, 1.0 and 0.1% fat)	120–125	94–96
Yoghurt	Whole milk, fruit	122	96
Ice cream	Dairy, vanilla	104	85
Eggs	Chicken, raw, whole	46	179
Chicken, duck, turkey	Raw	5–12	160–220
Beef, lamb, pork	Raw	5–12	79–200
Cod, plaice	Raw	1217	157–169–180
Sardines	Tinned, in oil	500	520
Wheat flour	Wholemeal	32	281
Wheat flour	White flour	96–280	114–463
Bread	White	121–177	89–101
Bread	Brown/wholemeal	186/106	157/202
Spinach	Raw	170	45
Watercress	Raw	170	52
Broccoli	Green, raw	48	81
Carrots	old, raw	26	16
Rice	Raw, white	1–16	101–117
Potatoes	Raw, old	7	34
Tofu	Soyabean, steamed, or fried	Variable; depends use of coagulant	95–270

Data from Finglas *et al.* (2015). Reproduced with permission from the Royal Society of Chemistry.

Given the high proportion of body calcium which is present in bone, and the importance of bone as the major reservoir for calcium, development and maintenance of bone is the major determinant of calcium needs. Thus, unlike other nutrients, the requirement for calcium is considered to relate not to the maintenance of the metabolic function of the nutrient but to the maintenance of an optimal reserve and the support of the reserve's function (i.e., bone integrity). Calcium requirements, therefore, vary throughout an individual's life, with greater needs during the periods of rapid growth in childhood and adolescence, during pregnancy and lactation, and in later life. There are important genetic and environmental influences of calcium requirements. Genetic influences include such factors as bone architecture and geometry, and responsiveness of bone to hormones that mediate the function of bone as the body's calcium reserve. Environmental influences include factors such as dietary constituents and the degree of mechanical loading imposed on the skeleton in everyday life. Because of their effects on urinary calcium losses, high intakes of both sodium and protein increase dietary calcium requirements.

There is considerable disagreement over human calcium requirements, and this is reflected in the wide variation in estimates of daily calcium requirements made by different expert authorities. For example, expert committees in the USA, UK and the EU have established very different recommendations for calcium intake (Table 11.3). Much of this divergence arises because of different interpretations of available human calcium balance data for ages 1–50 years as well as the US recommendations also using bone loss data from observational and clinical trial evidence for the 50+ age groups.

Based largely on the data concerning the association of high calcium intakes with hypercalcemia and renal insufficiency in adults, the US Institute of Medicine in 2011 established

Table 11.3 Recommended calcium intakes in the UK, USA and Europe

UK RNI (1998)[a]		US RDA (2011)[b]		EC PRI (2015)[c]	
Age group (years)	mg/day	Age group (years)	mg/day	Age group (years)	mg/day
0–1	525	0–0.5	200*	7–11 months	280**
1–3	350	0.5–1	260*	1–3	450
4–6	450	1–3	700	4–10	800
7–10	550	4–8	1000		
11–14 M	1000	9–13	1300	11–17	1150
15–18 M	1000	14–18	1300	11–17	1150
11–14 F	800	19–30	1000		
15–18 F	800	31–50	1000		
19–50	700	51–70 (M)	1000	≥25	950
>50	700	51–70 (F)	1200		
		>70	1200		
		Pregnancy		Pregnancy	
Pregnancy	NI	14–18	1300	18–24	1000
		19–50	1000	≥25	950
Lactation	+550	Lactation		Lactation	
		14–18	1300	18–24	1000
		19–50	1000	≥25	950

[a] Reference nutrient intake (RNI); UK Department of Health (1991).
[b] Recommended Daily Allowance (RDA); US Institute of Medicine (2011). *Reflect Adequate Intakes and not RDA values.
[c] Population Reference Intake (PRI); European Food Safety Authority (2015). **Reflects an Adequate Intake and not PRI value.
Estimates of Ca requirements refer to both males and females unless stated otherwise.
M, requirements for males; F, requirements for females; NI, no increment.

tolerable upper intake levels (ULs) of calcium of 2000, 2500 and 3000 mg/day for older adults (51+ years), children (1–8 years) and adults (19–50 years, including pregnancy and lactation), and adolescents (9–18 years), respectively. The European Food Safety Authority (EFSA) in 2012 established a UL for calcium of 2,500 mg for adults, and for pregnant and lactating women, and considered that the available data are insufficient to set a UL for infants, children or adolescents.

Micronutrient interactions

There is considerable evidence from studies on experimental animals that excessive calcium intake can impair the nutritional status of other nutrients, particularly iron, zinc, and magnesium, but data on humans are not clear. While calcium interacts with magnesium and phosphorus, and reduces their absorption, there is no evidence that high calcium intakes are associated with depletion of the affected nutrient. Calcium inhibits the absorption of iron in a dose-dependent and dose-saturable fashion. However, the available human data fail to show cases of iron deficiency or even decreased iron stores as a result of high calcium intake. There is some evidence that high dietary calcium intakes reduce zinc absorption and balance in humans and may increase the zinc requirement. Overall, the available data on the interaction of calcium with these nutrients do not show any clinically or functionally significant depletion of the affected nutrient in humans and, in the context of risk assessment, these interactions should probably not be considered adverse effects of calcium. However, such interactions deserve further investigation. It is well established that a deficiency of vitamin D (arising from a lack of exposure to sunlight, inadequate dietary intake, or both) can result in a reduced efficiency of intestinal calcium absorption that, in turn, can lead to a decrease in serum ionised calcium.

11.3 Magnesium

Like calcium, magnesium is an alkaline earth metal. Magnesium is the eighth most abundant element in the Earth's crust. Like calcium, its oxidation state is +2 and, owing to its strong reactivity, it does not occur in the native metallic state, but rather as the free cation (Mg^{2+}) in aqueous solution or as the mineral part of a large variety of compounds, including chlorides carbonates and hydroxides.

Magnesium was first shown to be an essential dietary component for rats in 1932 and later for humans. This essentiality is a reflection of the role that magnesium plays in the stabilisation of adenosine triphosphate (ATP) and other molecules. Since then, nutritionists have come to realise that frank magnesium deficiency is rare and that it only occurs in clinical settings as a secondary consequence of another disease. More recently, moderate or marginal deficiency has been proposed as a risk factor for chronic diseases such as osteoporosis, cardiovascular disease, diabetes, and cancer. These associations are controversial.

Absorption, transport and tissue distribution

Magnesium is the second most common cation found in the body (about 25 g). It is evenly distributed between the skeleton (50–60% of total) and the soft tissues (40–50% of total). In the skeleton, about one-third of the magnesium is on the surface of bone. This magnesium pool is thought to be exchangeable and thus may serve to maintain serum or soft-tissue magnesium concentrations in times of need. Body magnesium is most closely associated with cells; only 1% of total body magnesium is extracellular. Within the cell, magnesium is found in all of the compartments.

Magnesium homeostasis is maintained by controlling the efficiency of intestinal absorption and magnesium losses through the urine. The latter process is a stronger regulatory control mechanism for magnesium. Magnesium absorption is presumed to occur throughout the small intestine of humans. In normal, healthy individuals, magnesium absorption is typically between 40% and 50%, but figures from 10 to 70% have also been reported. Magnesium crosses the intestinal epithelium by three different mechanisms: passive diffusion, solvent drag (i.e., following water movement) and active transport. Regulation of intestinal nutrient absorption is generally thought to occur only for the active component of absorption. The mechanisms controlling intestinal magnesium absorption are unclear at this time. Because of the chemical similarity of magnesium to calcium, scientists have examined whether vitamin D status regulates magnesium absorption. It appears that only large changes in vitamin D status lead to alterations in magnesium absorption. Only limited information is available on the influence of dietary components on magnesium in humans. Phosphate may be an inhibitor of magnesium absorption. Free phosphate may form insoluble salt complexes with magnesium; phosphate groups in phytate may also inhibit magnesium absorption. Fibre-rich foods have been shown to lower magnesium bioavailability. However, it is not clear whether this was an independent effect of fibre or a reflection of the phytate content of these foods. Protein and fructose may enhance magnesium absorption.

As mentioned above, the kidney is the principal organ involved in magnesium homeostasis. The renal handling of magnesium in humans is a filtration– reabsorption process. Approximately 70% of serum magnesium is ultrafiltrable, and the normal healthy kidney reabsorbs about 95% of filtered magnesium. When an individual is fed a low-magnesium diet, renal output of magnesium is reduced. Excessive magnesium loss via urine is a clinical condition contributing to magnesium depletion in patients with renal dysfunction.

Metabolic function and essentiality

Magnesium is essential for a wide range of fundamental cellular reactions, and is a cofactor for more than 300 enzymatic reactions, acting either on the substrate or on the enzyme itself as a structural or catalytic component. As ATP utilisation is involved in many metabolic pathways, magnesium is essential in the intermediary metabolism for the synthesis of carbohydrates, lipids, nucleic acids, and proteins. Magnesium plays a role in modulating membrane permeability and electrical characteristics. Magnesium also plays an important role in the development and maintenance of bone; about 60% of total body magnesium is present in bone. Magnesium has also been demonstrated to enhance the condensation of chromatin, and given the role of chromosomal condensation in the regulation of gene activity, magnesium depletion could indirectly affect gene transcription.

Deficiency symptoms

Magnesium homeostasis can be maintained over a wide range of intakes in normal, healthy individuals. Thus, magnesium deficiency does not appear to be a problem in healthy people. Frank magnesium deficiency is only seen in humans under two conditions: as a secondary complication of a primary disease state (diseases of cardiovascular and neuromuscular function, endocrine disorders, malabsorption syndromes, muscle wasting) and resulting from rare genetic abnormalities of magnesium homeostasis. Symptoms of frank magnesium deficiency include:

- progressive reduction in plasma magnesium (10–30% below controls) and red blood cell magnesium (slower and less extreme than the fall in plasma magnesium)
- hypocalcemia and hypocalciuria
- hypokalemia resulting from excess potassium excretion and leading to negative potassium balance
- all of which can lead to neurological or cardiac symptoms.

All of these symptoms are reversible with dietary magnesium repletion. Disrupted calcium metabolism is also evident from the effect of magnesium depletion on serum PTH and $1,25(OH)_2D_3$ concentrations.

Scientists have attempted to demonstrate that suboptimal intake of magnesium [e.g., below the Recommended Dietary Allowance (RDA; the nutrient intake value that is sufficient to meet the requirement of nearly all (97–98%) individuals in a life-stage and sex group) but not frank deficiency] is a contributor to the development of chronic disease such as cardiovascular disease, type 2 diabetes mellitus, hypertension, metabolic syndrome, eclampsia and pre-eclampsia, cancer, and osteoporosis. However, the results of studies in this area are ambiguous. The lack of consistent positive findings may reflect the lack of sensitive and reliable tools for assessing magnesium status, the failure to account for magnesium intake from water (in earlier dietary studies), or the difficulty in attributing causality to a single nutrient owing to the apparent heterogeneity of causes arising from epidemiological data relating to most chronic diseases.

Toxicity

Very large doses of magnesium-containing laxatives and antacids (typically providing more than 5000 mg magnesium/day) have been associated with magnesium toxicity. Symptoms of magnesium toxicity can include hypotension, nausea, vomiting, facial flushing, retention of urine, ileus, depression, and lethargy before progressing to muscle weakness, difficulty breathing, extreme hypotension, irregular heartbeat, and cardiac arrest. The risk of magnesium toxicity increases with impaired renal function or kidney failure because the ability to remove excess magnesium is reduced or lost.

Assessing status

Estimating magnesium requirements and establishing magnesium–disease relationships depend on accurate and specific indicators of magnesium status. Several such indicators have been described. All of these are based on measurement of the magnesium content in various body pools. Analysis of total magnesium in serum is often used as an indicator of magnesium status, although only about 1% of total body magnesium is present in ECF. It has been suggested that the concentration of ionised magnesium in serum may be a more reliable and relevant determinant of magnesium deficiency. In addition, intracellular magnesium concentration (usually measured in accessible tissues such as erythrocytes and lymphocytes) provides a more accurate assessment of body magnesium status than does the concentration of magnesium in serum. The dietary balance approach is considered to be the best available method for estimating magnesium requirements. Although this method is a powerful research tool for the study of magnesium homeostasis, it is time, resource, and labor intensive, and these limit its application to large populations. None of the currently available procedures is perfect for all circumstances and no single method is considered satisfactory. The percentage of the population or population subgroups with intakes of magnesium below the EAR (265 and 350 mg/day for adult women and men, respectively) can be used as an index of inadequacy of intake. For example, in the USA 44.8% of the population aged ≥2 years has a magnesium intake below the EAR. This also appears to be the case for several European populations. However, while the public health relevance of these observations is currently being debated, the fact that there is not a universally accepted reliable magnesium status assessment tool makes it difficult to determine the actual consequence of this apparent low intake.

Requirements and dietary sources

The current US RDA, established in 1997, for adult women is 320 mg/day and for adult men is 420 mg/day. More recently, EFSA in 2015 established Adequate Intakes (AIs; typically established when an EAR and Population Reference Intake [PRI, which is an RDA-equivalent] cannot be derived) of 300 mg/day for adult females and 350 mg/day for adult males.

For those who want to increase their magnesium intake, a number of high magnesium foods and dietary practices will lead to adequate intake. Foods with a high magnesium content include whole grains, legumes, green leafy vegetables; meat, fruits, and dairy products have an intermediate magnesium content (Table 11.4).

Table 11.4 Magnesium content of some common foods

Food source	Description	Mg content (mg/100 g)
Beef	Average, raw, Fat/Lean	9/22
Lamb	Average, raw, Fat/Lean	9/22
Pork	Average, raw, Fat/Lean	9/24
Chicken	Meat, average, raw	26
White fish	Raw, Cod/plaice	25/21
Eggs	Chicken, whole, raw	13
Cheese	Soft and hard varieties	7–41
Wheat flour	Brown/wholemeal flour	72/83
Wheat flour	White flour	23–26
Milk	Cow's (3.5, 1.0 and 0.1% fat)	11–12
Yoghurt	Whole milk, fruit	13
Carrots	Raw	9
Broccoli	Raw	22
Cabbage	Raw	14
Rice	Raw, white	21–25
Potatoes	Raw, old, no skin	21

Source: Data from Finglas *et al.* (2015). Reproduced with permission from the Royal Society of Chemistry.

Cereals and cereal products are the most important dietary sources of magnesium (contributing 28–29%) for adults and older adults in the UK. The poorest sources of magnesium are refined foods. Although high levels of calcium, phosphate, or fibre may lead to reduced bioavailability of magnesium, differences in bioavailability of magnesium from various food sources do not appear to be a significant barrier to achieving adequate magnesium status. Drinking water can also be a source of magnesium, but the amount of magnesium in water varies by source (can range from 1 to 120 mg/l).

Magnesium, when ingested as a naturally occurring substance in foods, has not been demonstrated to exert any adverse effects in people with normal renal function. However, adverse effects of excess magnesium intake (e.g., diarrhea, nausea, abdominal cramping) have been observed with intakes from non-food sources such as various magnesium salts used for pharmacological purposes. For this reason, the US Food and Nutrition Board established the tolerable UL for adolescents and adults as 350 mg of non-food magnesium. EFSA in 2006 established a UL for magnesium of 250 mg/day for adults, including pregnant and lactating women, and children from four years on, but considered that the available data are insufficient to set a UL for infants or children aged one to three years; thus, no UL could be established for these age groups. This UL does not include Mg normally present in foods and beverages.

Micronutrient interactions

As mentioned above, phosphorus as phosphate, especially in phytate, may decrease intestinal magnesium absorption. In general, calcium intake in the usual dietary range does not affect magnesium absorption, but calcium intakes in excess of 2.6 g have been reported to reduce magnesium balance. Magnesium intake in the usual dietary range does not appear to alter calcium balance.

11.4 Phosphorus

Phosphorus is the 11th most abundant element in the Earth's crust. Phosphorus is never found free in nature because of its high reactivity, but is widely distributed in combination with minerals. Phosphate rock, which contains the mineral apatite, an impure tricalcium phosphate, is an important source of the element. Phosphorus is most commonly found in nature in its pentavalent form in combination with oxygen as phosphate (PO_4^{3-}). Phosphorus (as phosphate) is an essential constituent of all known protoplasm and is uniform across most plant and animal tissues. A practical consequence is that, as organisms consume other organisms lower in the food chain (whether animal or plant), they automatically obtain their phosphorus.

Absorption, transport, and tissue distribution

Phosphorus makes up about 0.65–1.1% of the adult body (~600 g). In the adult body 85% of phosphorus is in bone and teeth (in the form of hydroxyapatite) and the remaining 15% is distributed in soft tissues where it is integral to diverse functions ranging from transfer of genetic information to energy utilisation. Total phosphorus concentration in whole blood is 13 mmol/l, most of which is in the phospholipids of erythrocytes and plasma lipoproteins, with approximately 1 mmol/l present as inorganic phosphate. This inorganic component, while constituting only a minute percentage of body phosphorus (<0.1%), is of critical importance. In adults, this component makes up about 15 mmol in total and is located mainly in the blood and ECF. It is into the inorganic compartment that phosphate is inserted on absorption from the diet and resorption from bone, and from this compartment that most urinary phosphorus and hydroxyapatite mineral phosphorus are derived (Figure 11.4). This compartment is also the primary source from which the cells of all tissues derive both structural and high-energy phosphate.

Food phosphorus is a mixture of inorganic and organic forms. Intestinal phosphatases hydrolyze the organic forms contained in ingested protoplasm and, thus, most phosphorus absorption occurs as inorganic phosphate. On a mixed diet, absorption of total phosphorus ranges from 55% to 80% in adults. There is no evidence that this absorption varies with dietary intake. Furthermore, there appears to be no apparent adaptive mechanism that improves phosphorus absorption at low intakes. This

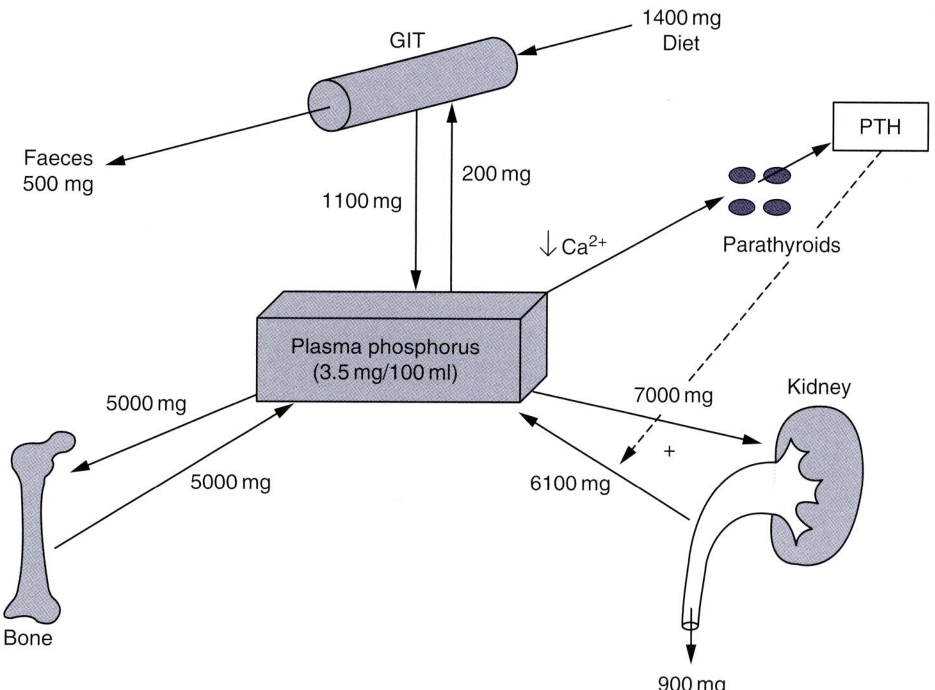

Figure 11.4 Homeostatic regulation of serum phosphorus. PTH, parathyroid hormone.

situation is in sharp contrast to calcium, for which absorption efficiency increases as dietary intake decreases and for which adaptive mechanisms exist that improve absorption still further at habitual low intakes. While a portion of phosphorus absorption is by way of a saturable, active transport facilitated by 1,25$(OH)_2D_3$ the fact that fractional phosphorus absorption is virtually constant across a broad range of intakes suggests that the bulk of phosphorus absorption occurs by passive, concentration-dependent processes. Phosphorus absorption is reduced by ingestion of aluminum-containing antacids and by pharmacological doses of calcium carbonate. There is, however, no significant interference with phosphorus absorption by calcium at intakes within the typical adult range. Excretion of endogenous phosphorus is mainly through the kidneys. Inorganic serum phosphate is filtered at the glomerulus and reabsorbed in the proximal tubule. In the healthy adult, urine phosphorus is essentially equal to absorbed dietary phosphorus, minus small amounts of phosphorus lost in shed cells of skin and intestinal mucosa.

Metabolic function and essentiality

Structurally, phosphorus occurs as hydroxyapatite in calcified tissues and as phospholipids, which are a major component of most biological membranes, and as nucleotides and nucleic acid. Other functional roles of phosphorus include:

- buffering of acid or alkali excesses, hence helping to maintain normal pH
- as an integral component of ATP, the temporary storage and transfer of the energy derived from metabolic fuels
- by phosphorylation of sugars, proteins and enzymes, and hence activation of many catalytic proteins and other molecules
- intracellular signaling processes by way of phosphorus-containing compounds

As phosphorus is not irreversibly consumed in these processes and can be recycled indefinitely, the actual functions of dietary phosphorus are first to support tissue growth (either during individual development or through pregnancy and lactation), and second to replace excretory and dermal levels. In both processes, it is necessary to maintain a normal level of inorganic phosphate in the ECF, which would otherwise be depleted of phosphorus by growth and excretion.

Deficiency symptoms

Inadequate phosphorus intake is expressed as hypophosphatemia (i.e., serum phosphorus concentrations below 0.8 mmol/l in adults). Only limited quantities of phosphate are stored within cells, and most tissues depend on ECF inorganic phosphate for their metabolic phosphate. When ECF inorganic phosphate levels are low, cellular dysfunction follows. At a whole organism level, the effects of hypophosphataemia include anorexia, anaemia, muscle weakness, bone pain, rickets and osteomalacia, general debility, increased susceptibility to infection, paresthesia, ataxia, confusion, and even death. The skeleton will exhibit either rickets in children or osteomalacia in adults. In both groups, the disorder consists of a failure to mineralise forming growth plate cartilage or bone matrix, together with impairment of chrondroblast and osteoblast function. These severe manifestations of hypophosphataemia are usually confined to situations in which serum phosphate concentrations falls below approximately 0.3 mmol/l. Phosphorus is so ubiquitous in various foods that near total starvation is required to produce dietary phosphorus deficiency. Thus, hypophosphataemia occurs only rarely because of inadequate dietary phosphorus intake, and is almost always due to metabolic disorders. In the USA, only 5.3% of the population aged ≥2 years has a phosphorus intake below the EAR.

Toxicity

Serum inorganic phosphate rises as total phosphorus intake increases. Excess phosphorus intake from any source is expressed as hyperphosphataemia and, essentially, all the adverse effects of phosphorus excess are owing to the elevated inorganic phosphate in the ECF. The principal effects that have been attributed to hyperphosphataemia are:

- adjustments in the hormonal control system regulating the calcium economy
- ectopic (metastatic) calcification, particularly of the kidney

- in some animal models, increased porosity of the skeleton
- a suggestion that high phosphorus intakes could decrease calcium absorption by complexing calcium in the chyme.

Assessing status, requirements, and dietary sources

Historically, dietary phosphorus recommendations have been tied to those for calcium, usually on an equimass or equimolar basis, and this approach was used in the USA, EU, and UK in establishing RDAs, PRIs, and Reference Nutrient Intakes (RNIs), respectively, for phosphorus. However, in 1997 the US Food and Nutrition Board suggested that a calcium–phosphorus concept of defining phosphorus requirements is of severely limited value, in that there is little merit in having the ratio "correct" if the absolute quantities of both nutrients are insufficient to support optimal growth. Therefore, because the phosphorus intake directly affects serum inorganic phosphate, and because both hypophosphataemia and hyperphosphataemia directly result in dysfunction or disease, the US Food and Nutrition Board considered that the most logical indicator of nutritional adequacy of phosphorus intake in adults is inorganic phosphate. If serum inorganic phosphate is above the lower limits of normal for age, the phosphorus intake may be considered adequate to meet cellular and bone formation needs of healthy individuals. The US RDAs for phosphorus, established in 1997, are infants 100 mg (first 6 months), 275 mg (7–12 months), children 460 mg (1–3 years), 500 mg (4–8 years), 1250 mg (9–18 years), adults 700 mg, pregnant women 1250 mg (<18 years), 700 mg (19–50 years), and lactating women 1250 mg (<18 years), 700 mg (19–50 years). More recently, EFSA, in 2015, considered that as there was no reliable biomarker of phosphorus intake and status, they used the approximate molar ratio of calcium to phosphorus in the whole body (1.4:1) to derive an AI for phosphorus (as data was insufficient to derive an EAR or PRI). The molar ratio used in combination with the PRIs for calcium yielded AIs of 640 and 550 mg/day for adolescents and adults, respectively.

Phosphates are found in foods as naturally occurring components of biological molecules and as food additives in the form of various phosphate salts. The phosphorus content of cow's milk and other dairy produce is higher than that of most other foods in a typical diet (Table 11.2). The same is true for diets high in colas and a few other soft drinks that use phosphoric acid as an acidulant. While concern about high phosphorus intake has been raised in recent years because of a probable population level increase in phosphorus intake through such sources as cola beverages and food phosphate additives, EFSA in 2006 concluded that the available data are not sufficient to establish an UL for phosphorus.

Micronutrient interactions

It has been reported that intakes of polyphosphates, such as are found in food additives, can interfere with the absorption of iron, copper, and zinc.

11.5 Sodium and chloride

Sodium is the sixth most abundant element in the Earth's crust and salt (sodium chloride) makes up about 80% of the dissolved matter in seawater. Although there is a wide variety of sodium salts, many of which are used as additives in food processing (e.g., sodium nitrate and monosodium glutamate), sodium chloride is the major source of sodium in foods. As sodium and chloride intakes in humans are so closely matched, both will be considered together. One g (17nmol) of salt provides 0.4g sodium and 0.6g chloride.

Salt was of major importance in early civilisations and in prehistory. Humans have special taste and salt appetite systems, which led to special culinary uses for salt and made it a much sought-after commodity. Nowadays, salt is still used widely to modify flavor, to alter the texture and consistency of food, and to control microbial growth (Table 11.5).

Absorption, transport and tissue distribution

Sodium is the major extracellular electrolyte and exists as the fully water-soluble cation. Chloride is also mainly found in ECF and is fully water

Table 11.5 Sodium-containing additives used in food processing

Additive	Use
Sodium citrate	Flavoring, preservative
Sodium chloride	Flavoring, texture, preservative
Sodium nitrate	Preservative, color fixative
Sodium nitrite	Preservative, color fixative
Sodium tripoliphosphate	Binder
Sodium benzoate	Preservative
Sodium eritrobate	Antioxidant
Sodium propionate	Preservative
Monosodium glutamate	Flavor enhancer
Sodium aluminosilicate	Anticaking agent
Sodium aluminum phosphate acidic	Acidity regulatory, emulsifier
Sodium cyclamate	Artificial sweetener
Sodium alginate	Thickener and vegetable gum
Sodium caseinate	Emulsifier
Sodium bicarbonate	Yeast substitute

soluble as the chloride anion. Both ions are readily absorbed from the digestive tract. Glucose and anions such as citrate, propionates, and bicarbonate enhance the uptake of sodium. The "average" 70 kg male has about 90 g of sodium with up to 75% contained in the mineral apatite of bone. Plasma sodium is tightly regulated through a hormone system, which also regulates water balance, pH, and osmotic pressure. Angiotensin and aldosterone both act to conserve sodium by increasing sodium reabsorption by the kidney. Sodium depletion stimulates the renal production of renin, which generates active angiotensin in the circulation. The latter stimulates vasoconstriction, which increases blood pressure, decreases water loss, and stimulates aldosterone release from the adrenal cortex. Atrial natriuretic hormone counteracts the sodium retention mechanisms by suppressing renin and aldosterone release and by inducing water and sodium excretion. It also decreases blood pressure and antagonises angiotensin. A raised plasma sodium concentration stimulates the renal reabsorption of water and decreases urinary output via antidiuretic hormone from the posterior pituitary. In contrast to sodium, chloride is passively distributed throughout the body and moves to replace anions lost to cells via other processes.

The main excretory route for both sodium and chloride is the urine. Sweat loss of these ions tends to be very low except with severe exertion in hot climates. Faecal losses are also low in healthy individuals.

Metabolic function and essentiality

The sodium cation is an active participant in the regulation of osmotic and electrolyte balances, whereas the chloride anion is a passive participant in this regulatory system. Each ion, however, has other functions within the body.

Sodium is involved in nerve conduction, active cellular transport and the formation of mineral apatite of bone. Central to its role in water balance, nerve conduction, and active transport is the plasma membrane enzyme sodium–potassium-ATPase (Na^+/K^+-ATPase). This enzyme pumps sodium out of the cell and at the same time returns potassium to the intracellular environment while ATP is hydrolyzed. Signal transmission along nerve cells, active transport of nutrients into the enterocyte and muscle contraction/ relaxation all depend on the Na^+/K^+-ATPase pump. In the muscle there is an additional pump, the sodium–calcium system. The ATP utilised by the sodium pump makes up a substantial part of the total metabolic activity and thermogenesis.

Among the main functions of the chloride anion are as dissociated hydrochloric acid in the stomach and in the chloride shift in the erythrocyte plasma membrane, where it exchanges with the bicarbonate ion.

Deficiency symptoms

Obligatory losses of sodium are very low, and plasma sodium or chloride depletion is difficult to induce. Low plasma sodium or chloride is normally not diet related but rather caused by a variety of clinical conditions, including major trauma and cachexia and overuse of diuretics. Loss of sodium can also ensue because of excessive water intake, anorexia nervosa, ulcerative colitis, liver disease, congestive heart failure with oedema, and severe infection and diarrhoea. Acute diarrhoea is the most common cause of sodium deficiency, and oral rehydration depends on the efficient enteric uptake of sodium from isotonic glucose/saline solutions and saves many lives worldwide. Vomiting, chronic renal disease, renal failure, and chronic respiratory acidosis can result in chloride depletion. Sodium deficiency or hyponatremia, defined as a serum concentration <135nmol/l, produces severe neurological symptoms progressing from malaise, nausea, vomiting, and headache to lethargy, impaired consciousness, seisures, and coma.

Toxicity

Excessive salt intakes are usually excreted efficiently in healthy individuals, whereas high plasma sodium and chloride are commonly caused by diabetes insipidus, brainstem injury, and dehydration through either excessive sweating or low water intake. There are accumulating data from epidemiological studies and controlled clinical trials to indicate an adverse effect of sodium intake on blood pressure, and up to 50% of patients with essential hypertension are sodium or salt sensitive. Lowering blood pressure reduces morbidity and mortality of cardiovascular disease. The mechanism linking salt intake with blood pressure is unclear but probably relates to sodium homeostasis. Extracellular sodium concentrations may adversely affect vascular reactivity and growth and stimulate myocardial fibrosis. Low-sodium diets differ in nutrient composition from the prevailing diet, and animal experimentation indicates that low potassium or calcium intake encourages a salt-induced increase in blood pressure, as does feeding simple carbohydrates (sucrose, glucose, or fructose). Copper deficiency in rats has been demonstrated to increase blood pressure independently of sodium intake. Epidemiological and other studies indicate that heavy metals, such as lead and mercury, may also contribute to increased blood pressure.

Efficient sodium conservation mechanisms mean that current sodium intakes in many populations are unnecessarily high and are probably much higher than the generally lower sodium diets eaten during the long period of human evolution. Clinical studies indicate that a high-sodium diet increases calcium excretion and measures of bone resorption; thereby suggesting a possible role for high salt intakes in osteoporosis.

Cross-cultural epidemiology suggests that high salt intakes are associated with gastric cancer, whereas a low-salt diet is regarded as having a potentially favourable effect in asthma patients.

Genetics

Blood pressure responses to dietary sodium vary among individuals and hypertension results from complex interactions between environmental and genetic factors. Common genetic variants can affect blood pressure responses to dietary sodium interventions and include polymorphisms in the renin-angiotensin converting enzyme (ACE) gene, angiotensin receptor genes, epithelial sodium channel genes, beta-receptor gene, endothelial nitric oxide synthase gene and the adiponectin gene. The genetic basis leading to sodium or salt sensitivity, therefore, appears to be complex.

Assessing status

The tight regulation of plasma sodium and, in turn, chloride ensures that fluctuations in the plasma concentration of these ions are minimised and changes only occur in certain pathological circumstances. Measurements of plasma sodium, therefore, are of little consequence as far as nutritional status is concerned. Total body (excluding bone) sodium, however, is increased in malnutrition and trauma and this total exchangeable sodium can be measured, with some technical difficulty, using radioisotopes.

Salt intakes are notoriously difficult to measure, and urinary sodium excretion is considered to be a valid measure of sodium intake under circumstances where little sodium is lost in sweat. Sodium in urine is easily measured, but the collection of complete 24 h urinary samples is difficult because of subject compliance, and the completeness of these collections should be validated using a marker such as para-amino benzoic acid. Lithium (as carbonate) fused with sodium chloride can act as a reliable tracer to estimate discretionary salt (cooking and table) intakes. Spot urine samples are generally unreliable.

Requirements and dietary sources

Normal sodium (mostly from salt) intake varies from about 2 g/day to 14 g/day, with chloride (mostly from salt) intakes generally slightly in excess of sodium (Table 11.6). Snack and processed foods have more added salt than unprocessed foods. The amount of discretionary salt

Table 11.6 Salt intake as NaCl (g/day)

Before 1982	Year	Intake	From 1988	Year	Intake
Communities not using added salt					
Brazil (Yanomamo Indian)	1975	0.06			
New Guinea (Chimbus)	1967	0.40			
Solomon Islands (Kwaio)		1.20			
Botswana (Kung bushmen)		1.80			
Polynesia (Pukapuka)		3.60			
Alaska (Eskimos)	1961	4.00			
Marshall Islands in the Pacific		7.00			
Salt-using communities					
Kenya (Sambura nomads)		5–8	Mexico (Tarahumsa Indian)		3–10
Mexico (Tarahumsa Indian)	1978	5–8	Mexico, rural (Nalinalco)	1992	5.7
			Mexico, urban (Tlaplan)	1991	7.18
Denmark		9.8	Denmark	1988	8.00
Canada (Newfoundland)		9.9	Canada		8–10
New Zealand		10.1			
Sweden (Göteborg)		10.2			
USA (Evans Country, Georgia)		10.6	USA (Chicago)		7.7
Iran		10.9			
Belgium	1966	11.4	Belgium	1988	8.4
UK (Scotland)		11.5			
Australia		12.0			
India (north)		12–15	India		9–11.4
Federal Republic of Germany		13.1			
Finland (east)		14.3	Finland		10.6
Bahamas		15–30			
Kenya (Samburus, army)	1969	18.6			
Korea		19.9			
Japan					
Japan (farmers)	1955	60.3	Japan	1988	8–15
Japan (Akita)		27–30			
Japan	1964	20.9			

added in cooking or at the table is very variable. Discretionary salt intakes can vary from less than 10% to 20–30% of total salt intake and these figures emphasise the major effect of processed foods on total salt intakes in most populations (Table 11.7). The UL set by IOM is 2.3 g/d.

Micronutrient interactions

The major interactions between sodium (and chloride) and other micronutrients are with respect to potassium and calcium. Data from animals (and some clinical studies) indicate that dietary potassium and calcium potentiate increases in blood pressure in salt-sensitive experimental models. There is evidence to suggest that the sodium to potassium ratio correlates more strongly with blood pressure than does either nutrient alone. As indicated previously, the metabolism of sodium, chloride, and potassium is closely related, and sodium and calcium ions have a close metabolic relationship within cells.

11.6 Potassium

Potassium, sodium, and chloride make up the principal electrolytes within the body. In contrast to sodium and chloride, nutritional issues with potassium are mainly concerned with the possibility of under consumption.

Absorption, transport, and tissue distribution

Potassium is the major intracellular electrolyte and exists as the fully water-soluble cation. More than 90% of dietary potassium is absorbed from the digestive tract.

Few dietary components affect absorption of potassium, although olive oil can increase and

Table 11.7 Salting (mg/100 g fresh weight) of foods in Western societies

	Na	K	Ca	Mg
Maize-based products				
Corn	4	284	55	41
Tortilla, rural	11	192	177	65
Breakfast cereals	866	101	3	11
Processed snacks	838	197	102	56
Wheat-based products				
Natural cereals	39	1166	94	343
Tortillas, wheat	622	73	11	17
Breakfast cereals	855	869	81	236
Processed bread (urban)	573	126	47	31
Salted bread, made locally (rural)	410	92	10	74
Sweet bread, made locally (rural)	97	93	87	18
Processed bread (rural)	344	79	213	18
Processed biscuits	582	80	16	17
Pulses				
Unprocessed, cooked	53	373	50	41
Processed, canned	354	371	27	79

Reproduced from Sánchez-Castillo and James in Sadler *et al. Encyclopedia of Human Nutrition*, copyright 1999 with permission of Elsevier.

dietary fiber decrease absorption to some extent. The "average" 70 kg man contains about 120 g of potassium, depending on muscle mass, with men having proportionally greater muscle mass, and hence potassium, than women. Almost all of the body potassium is exchangeable, intracellular concentration being more than 30 times the concentration of the ECF. Potassium is distributed within the body in response to energy-dependent sodium redistribution. Various hormonal and other factors regulate potassium homeostasis, both within cells and with the external environment. Hyperkalaemia (too much potassium in the ECF) stimulates insulin, aldosterone, and epinephrine (adrenaline) secretions, which promote the uptake of potassium by body cells. The aldosterone hormone also stimulates potassium excretion by the kidney and, at the same time, conserves sodium. Hypokalaemia has opposite effects, such that more potassium is released from cells. As with sodium, the kidney regulates potassium balance. Urine is the major excretory route in healthy people, with only small amounts lost in the faeces and minimal amounts in sweat.

Metabolic function and essentiality

Potassium, sodium, and chloride are the major determinants of osmotic pressure and electrolyte balance. The concentration difference of potassium and sodium across cell membranes is maintained by the Na^+/K^+-ATPase pump and is critical for nerve transmission and muscle function. The physiological importance of potassium in the body covers many systems including cardiovascular, respiratory, digestive, renal, and endocrine. In addition, potassium is a cofactor for enzymes involved in *inter alia* energy metabolism, glycogenesis, and cellular growth and division.

Deficiency symptoms

The low concentration of potassium in plasma is tightly regulated. Hypokalaemia, however, can result from either excessive uptake of potassium by cells or potassium depletion from the body. Insulin excess, catecholamine increases, Cushing's disease (excess steroids), diuretics that enhance potassium loss, chronic renal disease, diarrhoea, vomiting, and laxative abuse can result in hypokalaemia. Low potassium intakes are unlikely to lead to clinical potassium depletion and hypokalaemia except during starvation and anorexia nervosa.

The activity of nerves and muscles is affected in potassium depletion, and other clinical sequelae involve cardiac (including cardiac arrest), renal, and metabolic alterations. Potassium supplementation may have a role to play in treating chronic heart failure, and increased potassium intakes can decrease blood pressure via antagonistic metabolic interactions with sodium, resulting in increased sodium excretion, and also via a direct vasodilatory effect. Increased potassium intake is potentially beneficial to most people for the prevention and control of hypertension and stroke and does not impair renal control of potassium balance. Oral administration of potassium salts has been shown to improve calcium and phosphorus balance, reduce bone resorption and increase the rate of bone formation.

Toxicity

Hyperkalaemia, as a result of either a shift of potassium from cells to the ECF or excessive potassium retention, can be caused by major trauma and infection, metabolic acidosis, Addison's disease (aldosterone insufficiency) and chronic renal failure. Overuse of potassium supplements can also result in potassium excess. As with potassium depletion, the most important clinical consequence of potassium excess is cardiac arrest.

Genetics

Genetic factors may contribute to the blood pressure response to dietary potassium intake. Gene variants for kinases controlling electrolyte homeostasis may modulate the effect of dietary intake of potassium on blood pressure. It is likely that genes that modulate the response of blood pressure to dietary sodium intake will also play a role with respect to potassium intake.

Assessing status

The plasma concentration of potassium is not a reliable index of whole-body potassium status. Total body potassium can be measured by ^{42}K dilution or by whole body counting of the naturally abundant ^{40}K to determine the amount of lean body tissue. More direct measures of tissue potassium can be obtained by muscle biopsies.

Requirement and dietary sources

Because of potential beneficial antagonistic effects against high salt intakes, intakes of potassium of around 3.5g/day are considered to be optimal, although chronic intakes above 5.9 g/day may be dangerous for individuals with impaired renal function. Potassium, like sodium and chloride, is naturally widely distributed in foods (Table 11.8). Food processing (through leaching) may decrease potassium content as well as increasing salt content. Legumes, nuts, dried fruit, and fresh fruit, especially bananas, melons, avocados, and kiwi fruit, are rich sources of potassium. Major vegetable sources of potassium are potatoes and spinach, although cereal and dairy products, which have a lower potassium content but are consumed in large quantities, are also important dietary sources. In addition, meat and fish contain appreciable quantities of potassium. People who eat large quantities of fruit and vegetables may have dietary intakes of potassium exceeding 6 g/day.

Table 11.8 Sodium and potassium content of various foods (mg/100 g edible portion)

Food	Na	K
Legumes		
Red kidney beans	18	1370
Soyabeans	5	1730
Lentils	12	940
Dried fruit		
Raisins	60	1020
Figs	62	970
Nuts		
Walnuts	7	450
Almonds	14	780
Fruit and vegetables		
Banana	1	400
Melon	5–32	100–210
Potato	11	320
Spinach	140	500
Meat and fish		
Beef, veal, lamb	52–110	230–260
Chicken	81	320
Herring	120	320
Halibut	60	410
Tuna	47	400
Mussels	290	320
Miscellaneous		
Cow's milk	55	140
Chocolate	11	300

Reproduced from Sánchez-Castillo and James in Sadler *et al. Encyclopedia of Human Nutrition,* copyright 1999 with permission of Elsevier.

Micronutrient interactions

As might be expected from the close metabolic interactions among the major electrolytes, potassium and sodium dietary interactions are important in determining the risk of coronary heart disease and stroke. Another potentially important interaction concerns calcium. Potassium appears to have positive effects on calcium balance by regulating the acid–base balance and ameliorating any effects of sodium on calcium depletion.

11.7 Iron

The core of the Earth is thought to be largely composed of iron and iron makes up 4.7% of the Earth's crust placing it in 4th place in term of most abundant elements. Because iron is easy to obtain, its discovery is lost in the history of man, many thousands of years ago. The early Greeks were aware of the health-giving properties of iron. Iron has been used for centuries as a health tonic. It is therefore paradoxical that although the need for iron was discovered long ago and although it is the most common and cheapest of all metals, iron deficiency is the most frequent deficiency disorder in the world and the main remaining nutritional deficiency in Europe. Iron can exist in oxidation states ranging from −2 to +6. In biological systems, these oxidation states occur primarily as the ferrous (Fe^{2+}) and ferric (Fe^{3+}) forms and these are interchangeable.

Absorption, transport, and tissue distribution

The iron content of a typical 75 kg adult man and 55 kg adult women is approximately 4.5 and 3 g, respectively. Of this content, approximately two-thirds is utilised as functional iron such as haemoglobin (60%), myoglobin (5%), and various haem (cytochromes and catalase) and non-haem (NADH hydrogenase, succinic dehydrogenase, aconitase) enzymes (5%). The remaining iron is found in body storage as ferritin and to a lesser extent hemosiderin, the two major iron storage proteins. Only very minor quantities of iron (<0.1%) are found associated with transferrin, the main iron transport protein in the body.

The metabolism of iron differs from that of other minerals in one important respect: there is no physiological mechanism for iron excretion. The body has three unique mechanisms for maintaining iron balance and preventing iron deficiency and iron overload:

- storage of iron (with ferritin being an important reversible storage protein for iron)
- reutilisation of iron (especially of iron in erythrocytes); about 25 mg of systemic iron recycled daily.
- regulation of iron absorption.

In theory, therefore, when the body needs more iron, absorption is increased, and when the body is iron sufficient, absorption is restricted. This control is not perfect but is still of great importance for the prevention of iron deficiency and excess. Iron from food is absorbed mainly in the duodenum by an active process that transports iron from the gut lumen into the mucosal cell. When required by the body for metabolic processes, iron passes directly through the mucosal cell into the bloodstream, where Fe^{3+} is transported by transferrin, together with the iron released from old blood cells (i.e., the efficient iron recycling system, Figure 11.5), to the bone marrow (80%) and other tissues (20%). If iron is not required by the body, iron in the mucosal cell is stored as ferritin and is excreted in faeces when the mucosal cell is exfoliated (sloughed off). Any absorbed iron in excess of needs is stored as ferritin or hemosiderin in the liver, spleen, or bone marrow. Iron can be released from these iron stores for utilisation in times of high need, such as during pregnancy.

Dietary iron consists of haem iron (formed when iron combines with protoporphyrin IX; Figure 11.6) and non-haem iron. Haem iron is absorbed by a different mechanism from non-haem iron. The haem molecule is absorbed intact into the mucosal cell, where iron is released by the enzyme haem oxygenase. Its absorption is little influenced by the composition of the meal, and varies from 15% to 35% depending on the iron status of the consumer (Table 11.9). Although haem iron represents only 10–15% of dietary iron intake in populations with a high meat intake, it could contribute 40% or more of the total absorbed iron

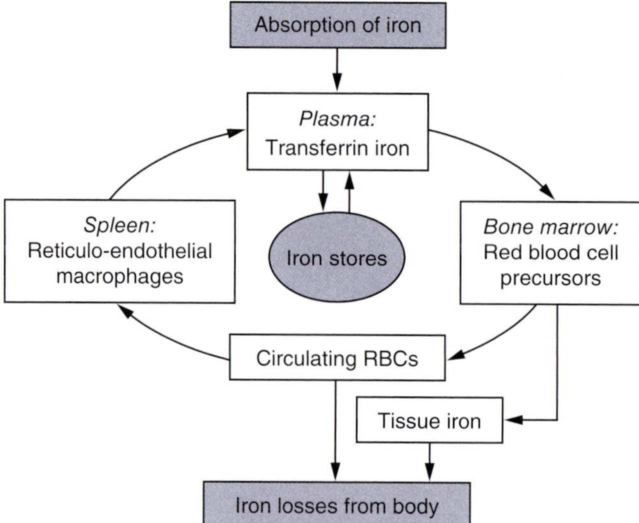

Figure 11.5 Metabolism of iron. There is a main internal loop with a continuous reutilisation of iron and an external loop represented by iron losses from the body and absorption from the diet. Source: Adapted from Hallberg *et al.* (1993) with permission of Elsevier.

Figure 11.6 Structure of haem iron.

(Figure 11.7). Many poorer regions of the world consume little animal tissue and rely entirely on non-haem iron. The absorption of non-haem iron is strongly influenced by dietary components, which bind iron in the intestinal lumen. The complexes formed can be either insoluble or so tightly bound that the iron is prevented from being absorbed. Alternatively, the complexes can be soluble and iron absorption is facilitated. Under experimental conditions, non-haem iron absorption can vary widely from less than 1% to more than 90%, but under more typical dietary conditions it is usually in the region of 1–20%. The main inhibitory substances and enhancers of iron absorption are shown in Table 11.9.

Table 11.9 Factors affecting (a) haem and (b) non-haem iron absorption

Increased absorption	Decreased absorption
(a) Haem	
Physiological factors	
Low iron status	High iron status
Dietary factors	
Low haem iron intake	High haem iron intake
Meat	Calcium
(b) Non-haem	
Physiological factors	
Depleted iron status	Replete iron status
Pregnancy	Achlorhydria (low gastric acid)
Disease states (aplastic anaemia, haemolytic anaemia, haemochromatosis)	
Dietary factors	
Ascorbic acid	Phytate
Meat, fish, seafood	Iron-binding phenolic compounds
	Calcium

Metabolic function and essentiality

Iron acts as a catalytic center for a broad spectrum of metabolic functions. As present in haemoglobin, iron is required for the transport of oxygen, critical for cell respiration. As myoglobin, iron is required for short-term oxygen storage in muscle. Iron is also a component of various tissue enzymes, such as the cytochromes,

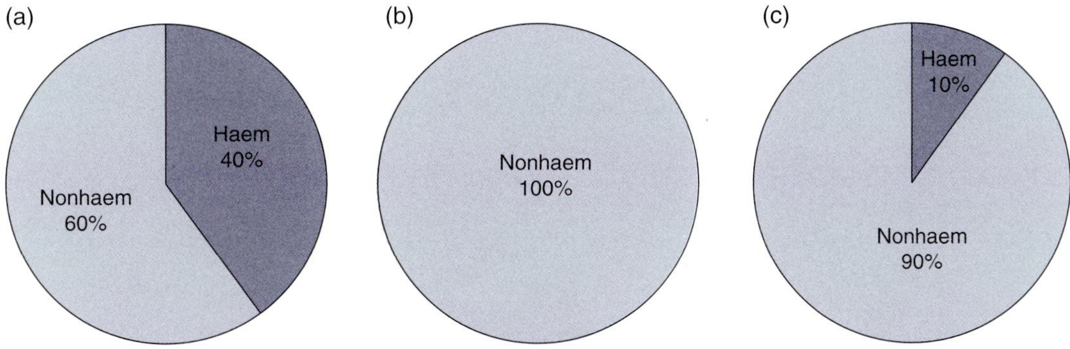

Figure 11.7 Haem and nonhaem iron in foods: (a) foods of animal origin; (b) foods of plant origin; (c) dietary iron intake from all foods, daily average.

that are critical for energy production, and enzymes necessary for immune system functioning. Therefore, these iron-containing molecules ensure that body fuels, such as carbohydrate, fat, and protein are oxidised to provide the energy necessary for all physiological processes and movement. The importance of iron as an element necessary for life derives from its redox reactivity as it exists in two stable, interchangeable forms of iron, Fe^{2+} and Fe^{3+}. This reaction is an essential part of the electron transport chain, responsible for the generation of ATP during the oxidation of substances in intermediary metabolism and for the reductions necessary in the synthesis of larger molecules from their components.

Deficiency symptoms

The progression from adequate iron status to iron-deficiency anaemia develops in three overlapping stages. The first stage consists of depletion of storage iron, which is characterised by a decrease in serum ferritin, which, in turn, reflects the size of the iron stores in the liver, bone marrow, and spleen. The second stage is a decrease in transported iron and is characterised by a decline in serum iron and an increase in the total iron-binding capacity, as transferrin has more free binding sites than in normal iron status. The third stage develops when the supply of iron is insufficient to provide for enough haemoglobin for new erythrocytes and insufficient to fulfill other physiological functions. During the last stage, free protoporphyrin, destined for haemoglobin, increases in plasma two- to five-fold, indicating a lack of tissue iron. The harmful consequences of iron deficiency occur mainly in conjunction with anaemia. Iron deficiency anaemia is most common in infants, preschool children, adolescents, and women of child-bearing age, particularly in developing countries. Globally, the World Health Organisation (WHO) estimated that anaemia due to iron deficiency affects 1.62 billion people, which corresponds to 24.8% of the population. The highest prevalence is in preschool-age children (47.4%), and the lowest prevalence is in men (12.7%). However, the population group with the greatest number of individuals affected is non-pregnant women (468.4 million) (Figure 11.8). Not unsurprisingly, the WHO global nutrition targets for 2025 is to reduce anaemia in women of reproductive age by 50%.

The functional effects of iron deficiency anaemia result from both a reduction in circulating haemoglobin and a reduction in iron-containing enzymes and myoglobin. Both factors presumably play a role in the fatigue, restlessness, and impaired work performance associated with iron deficiency anaemia. Other functional defects include disturbances in normal thermoregulation and impairment of certain key steps in the immune response. For example, there is evidence that iron deficiency anaemia is associated with lower T- and B-lymphocyte, macrophage, and neutrophil function. Although the phagocytic uptake of neutrophils is usually normal, the intracellular killing mechanism is usually defective. This abnormality is thought to be owing to a defect in the generation of reactive

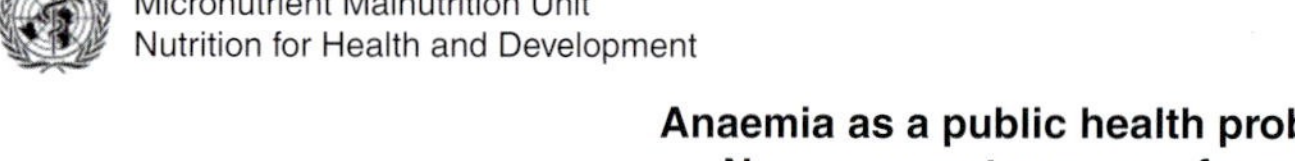

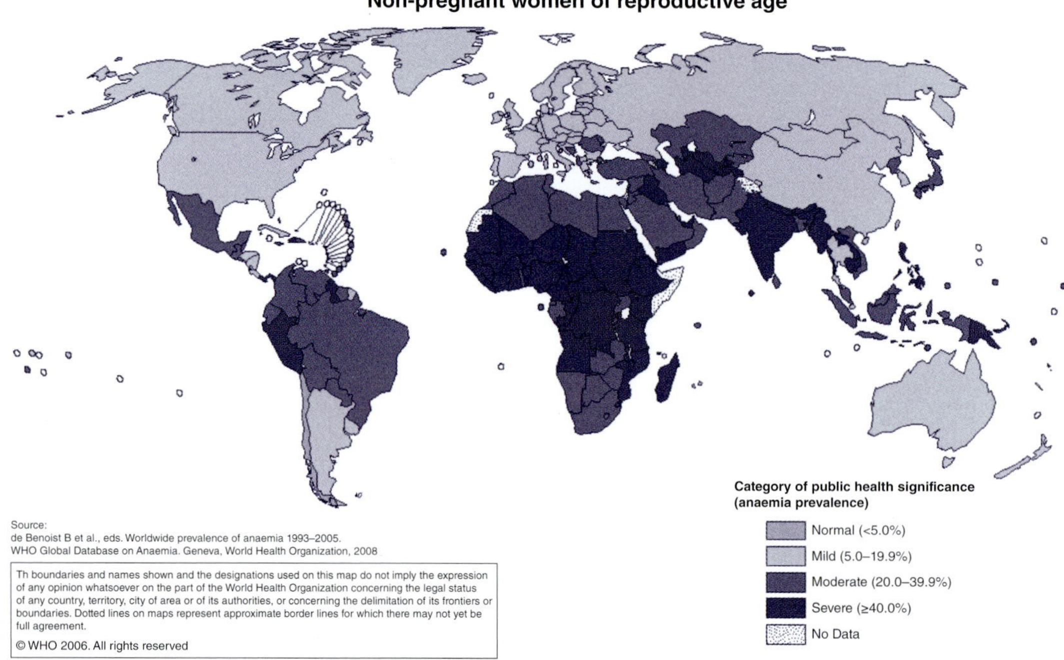

Figure 11.8 The World Health Organization's worldwide prevalence of anaemia in pregnant women. With permission the WHO. Source: de Benoist B. *et al.*, eds. Worldwide prevalence of anaemia 1993-2005. WHO Global Database on Anaemia Geneva, World Health Organization, 2008.

oxygen intermediates resulting from a decrease in the iron-containing enzyme myeloperoxidase. Iron deficiency anaemia can also have an adverse effect on psychomotor and mental development in children, and the mortality and morbidity of mother and infant during pregnancy.

Toxicity

The very effective regulation of iron absorption prevents overload of the tissues by iron from a normal diet, except in individuals with genetic defects, as in primary idiopathic hemochromatosis. This hereditary disorder of iron metabolism is characterised by an abnormally high iron absorption owing to a failure of the iron absorption control mechanism at the intestinal level. High deposits of iron in the liver and the heart can lead to cirrhosis, hepatocellular cancer, congestive heart failure, and eventual death. Sufferers of this disorder can develop iron overload through consumption of a normal diet, but would be at much higher risk if consuming iron-fortified foods. Thus, early detection of the disease via genetic screening followed by regular blood removal has proven to be a successful treatment.

Excess iron via overuse of iron supplements could pose a possible health risk. The mechanism of cellular and tissue injury resulting from excess iron is not fully understood. Liabilities may include increased risks for bacterial infection, neoplasia, arthropathy, cardiomyopathy, and endocrine dysfunctions. However, there is still much debate as to the strength of evidence to support a relationship between dietary iron intake and cancer or cardiovascular disease.

Gastrointestinal distress does not occur from consuming a diet containing naturally occurring or fortified iron. Individuals taking iron at high levels (>45 mg/day) may encounter gastrointestinal side-effects (constipation, nausea, vomiting, and diarrhea), especially when taken on an empty stomach.

Assessing status

Several different laboratory methods must be used in combination to diagnose iron deficiency anaemia correctly. The most commonly used methods to assess iron status include:

- serum ferritin
- transferrin saturation
- erythrocyte protoporphyrin
- mean corpuscular volume
- serum transferrin receptor
- haemoglobin or packed cell volume.

Iron deficiency anaemia is usually defined as a haemoglobin level below the cut-off value for age and sex (typically 12 g/100 ml for women and 13 g/100 for men) plus at least two other abnormal iron status measurements. The most commonly used are probably low serum ferritin (15 μg/l as a threshold), high protoporphyrin, and high serum transferrin receptor.

Requirements and dietary sources

Daily (absorbed or physiological) iron requirements are calculated from the amount of dietary iron necessary to cover basal iron losses (cells from the skin and the interior surfaces of the body), menstrual losses, and growth needs. They vary according to age and sex, and, in relation to body weight, they are highest for the young infant. An adult man has obligatory iron losses of around 1 mg of iron/day, largely from the gastrointestinal tract (exfoliation of epithelial cells and secretions), skin, and urinary tract. Thus, to remain replete with regard to iron, an average adult man needs to absorb (i.e., internalise) only 1 mg of iron from the diet on a daily basis. Similar obligatory iron losses for women amount to around 0.8 mg/day. However, adult women of reproductive age experience additional iron loss owing to menstruation, which raises the median daily iron requirement for absorption to 1.4 mg, while at the 90th percentile the requirement is at least 2.4 mg iron (to compensate for their high menstrual losses). Pregnancy creates an additional demand for iron, especially during the second and third trimesters, leading to daily requirements of 4–6 mg. Growing children and adolescents require 0.5 mg iron/day in excess of body losses to support growth. Physiological iron needs can be translated into dietary requirements by taking into account the efficiency at which iron is absorbed from the diet (typically around 10–18%). These dietary requirements, stratified by sex and age grouping, from the US, UK and European authorities, are shown in Table 11.10.

Based largely on the data on gastrointestinal effects following supplemental elemental iron intake in apparently healthy adults, the US Food and Nutrition Board established a tolerable UL of iron of 45 mg/day. EFSA in 2006 concluded that the available data are not sufficient to establish an UL for iron.

Iron is widely distributed in meat (especially offal), eggs, vegetables, and cereals, but the concentrations in milk, fruit, and vegetables are low (Table 11.11). However, in addition to the iron content *per se* of the individual food, the bioavailability of iron from those foods also needs to be taken account of.

Micronutrient interactions

The fact that serum copper has been found to be low in some cases of iron deficiency anaemia suggests that iron status has an effect on copper metabolism. Copper deficiency impinges on iron metabolism, causing an anaemia that does not respond to iron supplementation. Interactions between iron and copper seem to be owing to impaired utilisation of one in the absence of the other. As mentioned above, calcium can inhibit iron absorption under certain circumstances. In aqueous solutions iron impairs zinc absorption, but this interaction does not take place when iron is added to an animal protein meal, indicating different uptake mechanisms for solutions and solid foods.

11.8 Zinc

The natural abundance of zinc in the Earth's crust is 0.02%. The principal ores of zinc are sphalerite or blende (sulfide), smithsonite (carbonate), calamine (silicate), and franklinite (zinc iron oxide). Zinc is used to form numerous alloys with other metals.

Brass, nickel, silver, typewriter metal, commercial bronze, spring brass, German silver, soft

Table 11.10 Recommended iron intakes in the UK, USA, and Europe

UK RNI (1991)[a]		US RDA (2001)[b]		EC PRI (2015)[c]	
Age group (years)	mg/day	Age group (years)	mg/day	Age group (years)	mg/day
0–3 (months)	1.7	0–0.5	0.27*	7–11 months	11
4–6 (months)	4.3	0.5–1	11	1–6	7
7–12 months	7.8	1–3	7	7–11	11
1–3	6.9	4–8	10	12–17 (M)	11
4–6	6.1	9–13 (M)	8	12–17 (F)	13
7–10	8.7	9–13 (F)	8	≥18 (M)	11
11–14 (M)	11.3	14–18 (M)	11	≥18 (F)	
11–14 (F)	14.8	14–18 (F)	15	Premenopausal	16
15–18 (M)	11.3	14–18 (F)	15	Postmenopausal	11
15–18 (F)	14.8	19+ (M)	8		
19–50 (M)	8.7	19–50 (F)	18		
19–50 (F)	14.8	>50 (F)	8		
50+	8.7				
		Pregnancy			
Pregnancy	NI	<18	27	Pregnancy	NI
		19–50	1000		
Lactation	+550	Lactation		Lactation	NI
		<18	10		
		19–50	9	≥	

[a] Reference nutrient intake (RNI); UK Department of Health (1991).
[b] Recommended Daily Allowance (RDA); US Institute of Medicine (2011). *Reflects an Adequate Intake and not an RDA value.
[c] Population Reference Intake (PRI); European Food Safety Authority (2015). Estimates of Ca requirements refer to both males and females unless stated otherwise.
M, requirements for males; F, requirements for females; NI, no increment.

Table 11.11 Iron content of some common foods

Food source	Description	Fe content (mg/100 g)
Liver	Fried, calf/lamb	12.2/7.7
Beef	Lean, average, raw	2.7
Black (blood) sausage	Dry-fried	12.3
Chicken	Meat, average, raw	0.7
White fish	Raw, Cod/plaice,	0.1/0.1
Eggs	Chicken, whole, raw	1.7
Baked beans	Canned in tomato sauce	1.4
Red kidney beans	Dried, raw	6.4
Wheat flour	Brown/wholemeal	2.4/2.5
Wheat flour	White flour	1.7–1.9
Milk	Cow's (3.5, 1 and 0.1% fat)	0.02–0.03
Broccoli	Raw	1.1
Carrots	Raw, old	0.2
Cauliflower	Raw	0.4
Rice	Raw, white	0.3–1.7
Potatoes	Raw, no skins	0.3

Data from Finglas *et al.* (2015). Reproduced with permission from Royal Society of Chemistry.

solder, and aluminum solder are some of the more important alloys. Large quantities of zinc are used to produce die castings, used extensively by the automotive, electrical, and hardware industries. Zinc is also extensively used to galvanise other metals, such as iron to prevent corrosion. Zinc oxide is widely used in the manufacture of paints, rubber products, cosmetics, pharmaceuticals, floor coverings, plastics, printing inks, soap, storage batteries, textiles, electrical equipment, and other products. Zinc sulfide is used in making luminous dials, X-ray and television screens, and fluorescent lights. The chloride and chromate are also important compounds. In biological systems zinc is virtually always in the divalent (+2) state. Unlike iron, zinc does not exhibit any direct redox chemistry.

Absorption, transport, and tissue distribution

Zinc is ubiquitous in the body. It is the most abundant intracellular trace element, with >3000 known zinc or zinc-dependent proteins in the

Table 11.12 Approximate zinc content of major organs and tissues in the adult man

Tissue	Total Zn content (g)	Percentage of body Zn (%)
Skeletal muscle	1.53	~57
Bone	0.77	29
Skin	0.16	6
Liver	0.13	5
Brain	0.04	1.5
Kidneys	0.02	0.7
Heart	0.01	0.4
Hair	<0.01	~0.1
Blood (plasma)	<0.01	~0.1

Modified from Mills CF, ed, *Zinc in Human Biology*, copyright 1998 with kind permission of Springer Science + Business Media.

body. An adult human contains about 2 g of zinc, of which about 60% and 30% are in skeletal muscle and bone, respectively, and 4–6% is present in skin (Table 11.12). Zinc turnover in these tissues is slow and, therefore, the zinc in these tissues is not accessible at times of deprivation. Because zinc is essential for the synthesis of lean tissue, it is while this is occurring that it may become a limiting nutrient. Although some zinc may be available in short-term zinc deprivation from a mobile hepatic pool, it is generally assumed that the body has no specific zinc reserve and is dependent on a regular supply of the element.

With essential roles in many fundamental cellular processes (see below), it is not surprising that whole-body zinc content is tightly controlled. The gastrointestinal system plays a central role in zinc homeostasis. Zinc in foods is absorbed via a carrier-mediated transport process, which under normal physiological conditions appears not to be saturated. Exogenous zinc is absorbed throughout the small intestine. Proximal intestinal absorption is efficient, but it has a large enteropancreatic circulation; the net intestinal absorption of zinc is achieved by the distal small intestine. Zinc is transported in the plasma by albumin and α_2-macroglobulin, but only 0.1% of body zinc is found in plasma. Body zinc content is regulated by homeostatic mechanisms over a wide range of intakes by changes in fractional absorption (normally 20–40%) and urinary (0.5 mg/day) and intestinal (1–3 mg/day) excretion. For example, during periods of

Table 11.13 Factors affecting zinc absorption

Increased absorption	Decreased absorption
Physiological factors	
Depleted zinc status	Replete zinc status
	Disease state (acrodermatitis enteropathica)
Dietary factors	
Low zinc intake	High zinc intake
Certain organic acids	Phytate
Certain amino acids	Certain metals
Human milk	

low zinc intake, absorption is enhanced and secretion of endogenous zinc into the gastrointestinal lumen is suppressed. In contrast, high zinc intake is associated with decreased absorption and enhanced secretion of endogenous zinc. Within cells, fluctuations in zinc content are modulated by changes in the amount of metallothioneins, a class of proteins with high affinity for metals, and also by a variety of zinc transporter proteins (ZnT) found throughout cells. Although ZnT are very important for generating and maintaining zinc gradients across membranes and within cellular compartments, little is known about many aspects of their functions and regulatory modes of action.

The bioavailability of dietary zinc depends on dietary enhancers and inhibitors and host-related factors (Table 11.13). Diets can be roughly classified as having a low, medium, or high bioavailability, according to the content of zinc, phytate, and animal protein. From a mixed animal and plant product diet, 20–30% zinc absorption can be expected. The lowest absorption, 10–15%, is seen from diets prevalent in developing countries that are based on cereals and legumes with a high phytate content and with negligible amounts of animal protein.

Metabolic function and essentiality

Zinc has three major groups of functions in the human body: catalytic, structural, and regulatory. Most biochemical roles of zinc reflect its involvement in the folding and activity of a large number (up to 10%) of proteins and over 100 different zinc metalloenzymes have been identified, including RNA nucleotide polymerase I and II, alkaline phosphatase and carbonic anhydrases. Important structural roles for zinc are in the zinc finger motif in proteins, but also in metalloenzymes, including the antioxidant enzyme, copper/zinc superoxide dismutase (Cu/Zn-SOD). Zinc is also required by protein kinases that participate in signal transduction processes and as a stimulator of transacting factors responsible for regulating gene expression. Adequate zinc is required to maintain optimal functionality of the innate and adaptive immune responses.

Deficiency symptoms

The clinical manifestations of severe zinc deficiency in humans are growth retardation, sexual and skeletal immaturity, neuropsychiatric disturbances, dermatitis, alopecia, impaired immune response and loss of appetite. Many of these features, by and large, represent the dependence on zinc of tissues with a high rate of turnover. However, severe zinc deficiency in humans is rare, and more interest has been focused on marginal zinc deficiency. Marginal zinc deficiency is more difficult to diagnose, has non-specific features and often occurs with other micronutrient deficiencies including iron. The current understanding of zinc deficiency is largely based on responses to zinc supplementation. Zinc supplementation has been reported to stimulate growth and development in infants and young children, and reduce morbidity (diarrhoea and respiratory infections) in children, particularly in developing countries and can increase both innate and adaptive immunity. In women, low serum zinc concentration during pregnancy was found to be a significant predictor of low birth weight, and low maternal zinc intake has been associated with an approximately twofold increased risk of low birth weight and increased risk of preterm delivery in poor urban women. Furthermore, there is also evidence that low maternal zinc status is associated with reduced cognitive ability of children. Deficiency of zinc, through reduced antioxidant activity and impaired immune response (including a decreased production of certain cytokines), results in an increased susceptibility to infectious disease; most evident as diarrhoea, pneumonia and malaria amongst children suffering from zinc deficiency and the cycle of malnutrition–infection in developing countries. Emerging evidence suggests that patients with autoimmune disease are more likely to have low zinc status than healthy control subjects, indicating a further link between zinc deficiency and altered immunity. Those at risk of deficiency include infants, pregnant and lactating women, those on low zinc and low protein (e.g., vegetarian) diets including patients receiving parenteral nutrition and individuals with conditions which may impair absorption of zinc from the intestine (e.g., coeliac disease and Crohn's disease).

Toxicity

Gross acute zinc toxicity has been described following the drinking of water that has been stored in galvanised containers or the use of such water for renal dialysis. Symptoms include nausea, vomiting, and fever, and are apparent after acute ingestion of 2 g or more. The more subtle effects of moderately elevated intakes, not uncommon in some populations, are of greater concern, because they are not easily detected. Prolonged intakes of supra-physiological intakes of zinc (75–300 mg/day) have been associated with impaired copper utilisation (producing features such as microcytic anaemia and neutropenia), impaired immune responses and a decline of high-density lipoproteins, but some have argued that even short-term intakes of about 25–50 mg zinc/day may interfere with the metabolism of both iron and copper.

Genetics

Polymorphisms in genes encoding various zinc-transporters have been associated with a reduced zinc status in various tissues. However, there is insufficient evidence to suggest a clear relationship between genetic variation in these genes with clinical outcomes.

Acrodermatitis enteropathica, a rare, inborn, autosomal recessive disease, is a disorder of primary zinc malabsorption. It is characterised by alopecia; vesicular, pustular and/or eczematoid skin lesions, specifically of the mouth, face, hands, feet and groin; growth retardation; mental apathy; diarrhoea and secondary malabsorption, defects in cellular and phagocytic immune function; and intercurrent infections. It is believed that a SNP in the Zn transporter SLC39A4 plays a role in the pathogenesis of this condition. The disorder responds very well to zinc therapy.

Assessing status

Measurement of zinc in plasma is the most commonly used biomarker to measure zinc status. However high heterogeneity in plasma zinc concentrations between studies call for a degree of caution in interpreting values, as other factors including pregnancy, inflammation and time of day are all known to influence plasma zinc concentrations. In healthy individuals 24 hour urinary zinc excretion and hair zinc concentrations are correlated with dietary zinc, but may not be useful among those with inadequate zinc status. The development of zinc deficiency is different from that of many other nutrients because a functional reserve or store of zinc does not seem to be available when zinc intake is inadequate. Homeostatic mechanisms respond to dietary intakes and help preserve endogenous losses via the kidneys and the gastrointestinal tract. When homeostatic mechanisms fail owing to sustained inadequate zinc tissue concentrations, the clinical symptoms of zinc deficiency develop. Stable isotope technology may be useful for evaluating potential biomarkers in future large scale studies. Current evidence also indicates that metallothionein expression in peripheral blood mononuclear cells (PBMCs) may be a sensitive indicator of dietary zinc intake.

Requirements and dietary sources

In view of the absence of specific and sensitive biomarkers of zinc status, the US RDA for zinc was originally based on data derived from metabolic balance studies. Such studies are technically difficult to perform and it is uncertain whether information from these studies reflects true requirements. A different approach, using the factorial method, was proposed for estimates of zinc requirements and future RDAs by the World Health Organization. Factorial calculations to estimate zinc requirements require knowledge of obligatory losses, tissue composition, and needs for growth and tissue repair. Current RDAs for zinc (recommended by the US Institute of Medicine in 2001 are infants 3 mg (7 months–3 years of age), young children 5 mg (4–8 years), older boys and girls 8mg (9–13 years), teenage boys 11mg (14–18 years), adult men 11 mg (19 years and more), teenage girls 9 mg (14–18 years), adult women 8 mg (19 years and older), pregnant women 13 and 11 mg (younger than 18 years and 19–50 years, respectively) and lactating women 14 and 12 mg (younger than 18 years and 19–50 years, respectively). More recently, EFSA in 2015 established recommendations for dietary zinc necessary to meet physiological requirements which took into account the inhibitory effect of dietary phytate on zinc absorption. Recommendations were established for phytate intake levels of 300, 600, 900 and 1200 mg/day, which cover the range of mean/median intakes observed in European populations. For adult males, the PRIs were 9.4, 11.7, 14.0, and 16.3 mg/day, at phytate intake levels of 300, 600, 900 and 1200 mg/day, respectively, whereas the equivalent PRIs for adult females at the same phytate intake levels were 7.5, 9.3, 11.0, and 12.7 mg/day, respectively.

The US Food and Nutrition Board reported that there was no evidence of adverse effects from intake of naturally occurring zinc in food; however, they derived a tolerable UL of 40 mg/day for adults older than 19 years, which applies to total zinc intake from food, water, and supplements (including fortified foods). Data on reduced copper status in humans were used to derive this UL for zinc. Using similar data but different uncertainty factors, the UL for total zinc intake was set at 25 mg/day in the EU.

The zinc content of some common foods is given in Table 11.14, whereas Table 11.15 classifies foods based on zinc energy density. The bioavailability of zinc in different foods varies widely, from 5% to 50%. Meat, seafood (in particular oysters) and liver are good sources of bioavailable zinc. It has been estimated that approximately 70% of dietary zinc in the US diet is provided by animal products. In meat products, the zinc content to some extent follows the colour of the meat, so that the highest content, approximately 50 mg/kg, is found in lean red meat, at least twice that in chicken. However, in many parts of the world, most zinc is provided by cereals. In cereals, most of the zinc is found in the outer fibre-rich part of the kernel. The degree of refinement, therefore, determines the total zinc content. Wholegrain products provide 30–50 mg/ kg, but a low extraction rate wheat flour contains 8–10 mg/kg. The bioavailability

Table 11.14 Zinc content of some common foods

Food source	Description	Zn content (mg/100 g)
Liver	Raw, calf	7.8
Beef	Lean (from six different cuts)	4.3
Lamb	Lean (from six different cuts)	4.0
Pork	Lean (from three different cuts)	2.4
Chicken	Raw, meat only	1.1
Cod, plaice, whiting	Raw	0.3–0.5
Muscles	Boiled	2.1
Oysters	Raw	90–200
Crab	Boiled	5.5
Eggs	Chicken, whole, raw	1.3
Cheese	Soft and hard varieties	0.5–5.3
Pulses	Raw	0.2–5.0
Wheat flour	Whole flour	2.9
Wheat flour	White flour	0.6–0.9
Milk	Cow's (3.9, 1.6 and 0.1% fat)	0.4
Yoghurt	Whole milk	0.5–0.7
Green leafy vegetables	Raw	0.2–0.6
Rice	Raw, white, polished	1.8
Potatoes	Raw	0.2–0.3

Data from Holland *et al.* (1995). Reproduced with permission from HMSO.

Table 11.15 Classification of foods based on zinc energy density

Zinc energy	mg Zn/ 1000 kcal	Foods
Very poor	0–2	Fats, oils, butter, cream cheese, confectionery, soft/alcoholic drinks, sugar, preserves
Poor	1–5	Fish, fruit, refined cereal products, biscuits, cakes, tubers, sausage
Rich	4–12	Whole grains, pork, poultry, milk, low-fat cheese, yoghurt, eggs, nuts
Very rich	12–882	Lamb, leafy and root vegetables, crustaceans, beef kidney, liver, heart, molluscs

Adapted from Solomons, N.W. (2001) Dietary sources of zinc and factors affecting its bioavailability. *Food and Nutrition Bulletin, 22*, 138–54

of zinc can be low from plant-based diets, in particular from wholegrain cereals and legumes, owing to the high content of phytic acid, a potent inhibitor of zinc absorption.

Micronutrient interactions

A decrease in copper absorption has been reported in the presence of excessive zinc. Data indicate that the level necessary to impair bioavailability is >40–50 mg/ day; therapeutic supplemental intakes (150 mg/day) over extended periods produce symptoms of copper deficiency. As mentioned above, iron under certain circumstances impairs zinc absorption. For example, iron supplementation in pregnancy can negatively impact plasma zinc concentrations. Animal studies have suggested an interaction between calcium and zinc in phytate-rich diets, but this has not been confirmed in human studies.

11.9 Copper

Copper occurs in the environment in three oxidation states. Copper (0) metal is used widely in the building industry (e.g., water pipes, electrical wires) because of its properties of malleability, ductibility, and high thermal and electrical conductivity. Brass, an alloy of copper and zinc, is used for cooking utensils and musical instruments, and bronze, an alloy of copper and tin, has been used in castings since early times. Copper-based alloys and amalgams are used in dental bridges and crowns, and copper is a constituent of intrauterine contraceptive devices. Copper compounds are widely used in the environment as fertilisers and nutritional supplements and, because of their microbicidal properties, as fungicides, algicides, insecticides, and wood preservatives. Other industrial uses include dye manufacturing, petroleum refining, water treatment, and metal finishing. Copper compounds in the cuprous (1) state are easily oxidised to the more stable cupric (2) state, which is found most often in biological systems.

The most important copper ores are chalcocite (Cu_2S), chalcopyrite ($CuFeS_2$), and malachite [$CuCO_3 \cdot Cu(OH)_2$]. Copper concentrations in soil vary from 5 to 50 mg Cu/kg and in natural water from 4 to 10 μg Cu/l. Concentrations of copper in water, however, depend on acidity, softness, and the extent of copper pipes, and municipal water supplies can contain appreciably higher concentrations. The taste threshold of copper ranges from 1 to 5 mg Cu/l, producing a slight blue–green color at concentrations >5 mg/l copper. Acute copper toxicity symptoms, mainly nausea and gastrointestinal irritation, can occur at concentrations of >4 mg/l copper.

Absorption, transport, and tissue distribution

About 50–75% of dietary copper is absorbed, mostly via the intestinal mucosa, from a typical diet. The amount of dietary copper appears to be the primary factor influencing absorption, with decreases in the percentage absorption as the amount of copper ingested increases. High intakes of several nutrients can also influence copper bioavailability. These include antagonistic effects of zinc, iron, molybdenum, ascorbic acid, sucrose, and fructose, although evidence for some of these is mainly from animal studies. Drugs and medication, such as penicillamine and thiomolybdates, restrict copper accumulation in the body and excessive use of antacids can inhibit copper absorption. Although high intakes of sulfur amino acids can limit copper absorption, absorption of copper is promoted from high-protein diets.

Ionic copper can be released from partially digested food particles in the stomach, but immediately forms complexes with amino acids, organic acids, or other chelators. Soluble complexes of these and other highly soluble species of the metal, such as the sulfate or nitrate, are readily absorbed. Regulation of absorption at low levels of copper intake is probably by a saturable active transport mechanism, while passive diffusion plays a role at high levels of copper intake. The major regulator of copper elimination from the body is biliary excretion. Most biliary copper is not reabsorbed and is eliminated in the faeces. The overall effect of these regulatory mechanisms is a tight homeostasis of body copper status. Little copper is lost from the urine, skin, nails, and hair.

After absorption from the intestinal tract, ionic copper (2) is transported tightly bound to albumin and transcuprein to the liver via the portal blood-stream, with some going directly to other tissues, especially the kidney. Hepatic copper is mostly incorporated into ceruloplasmin, which is then released into the blood and delivered to other tissues. Uptake of copper by tissues can occur from various sources, including ceruloplasmin, albumin, transcuprein, and low molecular weight copper compounds. Chaperone proteins bind the copper and transfer bound copper across the cell membrane to the intracellular target proteins, for example cytochrome c oxidase. The ATPase proteins may form part of the transfer process.

The body of a healthy 70 kg adult contains a little over 0.1 g of copper, with the highest concentrations found in the liver, brain, heart, bone, hair, and nails. Over 25% of body copper resides in the muscle, which forms a large part of the total body tissue. Figure 11.9 provides an overview of whole body copper pools and fluxes. Storage of copper is very important to the neonate. At birth, infant liver concentrations are

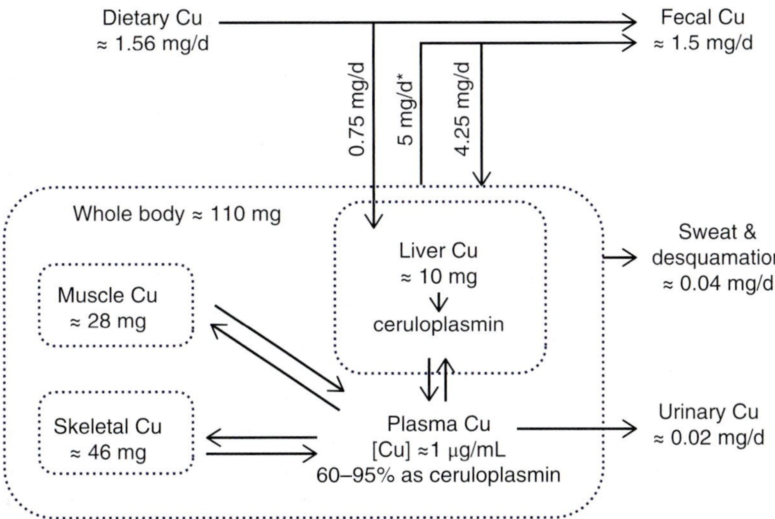

Figure 11.9 Whole body Cu pools and fluxes. Source: Bost *et al.*, 2016.

some five to 10 times the adult concentration and these stores are used during early life when copper intakes from milk are low.

Metabolic functions and essentiality

Copper is a component of several enzymes, cofactors, and proteins in the body. These enzymes and proteins have important functions in processes fundamental to human health (Table 11.16). These include a requirement for copper in the proper functioning of the immune, nervous and cardiovascular systems, for bone health, for iron metabolism and formation of red blood cells, and in the regulation of mitochondrial and other gene expression. In particular, copper functions as an electron transfer intermediate in redox reactions and as a cofactor in several copper-containing metalloenzymes. As well as a direct role in maintaining cuproenzyme activity, changes in copper status may have indirect effects on other enzyme systems that do not contain copper.

Deficiency symptoms

Owing to remarkable homeostatic mechanisms, clinical symptoms of copper deficiency occur in humans only under exceptional circumstances. Infants are more susceptible to overt symptoms of copper deficiency than are any other population group. Among the predisposing factors of

Table 11.16 Copper-binding proteins. Source: Danzeisen R *et al.* How reliable and robust are current biomarkers for copper status? Br J Nutr 2007; 98: 676-683. https://www.cambridge.org/core/journals/british-journal-of-nutrition/article/how-reliable-and-robust-are-current-biomarkers-for-copper-status/7F0E9CDB9D598E4E686D533F84F21FCC

Protein	Function
Cu-requiring enzymes	
Extracellular	
Cp	Plasma multi-copper oxidase necessary for Fe mobilisation; Cu binding and transport in plasma
Extracellular Cu, Zn SOD3	Involved in defence against reactive oxygen species
PAM	Peptide post-translational activation, modification of many important neuropeptides
Amine oxidases	A group of enzymes oxidising primary monoamines, diamines and histamine
Lysyl oxidase	Deaminates lysine and hydroxylysine residues in collagen or elastin; involved in formation of cross-links
Intracellular	
CCO	Mitochondrial protein and component of the electron transfer chain
Tyrosinase	Catalyst of melanin and other pigment production
Dopamine β mono-oxygenase	Involved in catecholamine metabolism, catalyses oxidation of 3,4-dihydroxyphenylethylamine to yield noradrenaline
Intracellular Cu, Zn SOD1	Involved in defence against reactive oxygen species
Phenylalanine hydroxylase	Catalyse of the oxidation of phenylalanine to tyrosine
Hephaestin	Intracellular multi-copper ferroxidase
Cu-binding or –transporting proteins	
Extracellular	
Albumin	Cu binding in plasma
Transcuprein	Cu binding and transport in plasma
Blood clotting factors V and VIII	Blood clotting
Intracellular	
Metallothionein	Cu storage and superoxide scavenging
Glutathione	Metal detoxification
Cartilage matrix glycoprotein	Contributes to the structural integrity of connective tissues
ATP7A	Cu transporter
ATP7B	Cu transporter
Ctr1	Plasma membrane Cu transporter
Intracellular Cu chaperones	
ATOX1	Delivery of Cu to the Cu ATPase ATP7A (Menkes protein) and ATP7A (Wilson protein)
CCS	Delivery of Cu to SOD1
Cox17	Delivery of C to mitochrondria (chaperone for CCO)

Cp, ceruloplasmin; SOD, superoxide dismutase; PAM, peptidylglycine α-amidating mono-oxygenase; CCO, cytochrome C oxidase; Ctr, Cu transporter; CCS, Cu chaperone for superoxide dismutase.

copper deficiency are prematurity, low birth weight, and malnutrition, especially when combined with feeding practices such as cow's milk or total parenteral nutrition. Feeding high sucrose or fructose diets in animal models increase the severity of copper deficiency symptoms. The most frequent symptoms of copper deficiency in humans are anaemia, neutropenia, and bone fractures, while less frequent symptoms are hypopigmentation, impaired growth, increased incidence of infections, and abnormalities of glucose and cholesterol metabolism and of electrocardiograms. Various attempts have been made to relate these symptoms to alterations in copper metalloenzymes (see Table 11.16) and non-copper enzymes that may be copper responsive, and to identify the role of copper as an antioxidant, in carbohydrate metabolism, immune function, bone health, and cardiovascular mechanisms. Notwithstanding the rarity of frank copper deficiency in human populations, some have speculated that suboptimal copper intakes over long periods may be involved in the precipitation of chronic diseases, such as cardiovascular disease and osteoporosis. The pathological significance of subtle changes, in the longer term, in those systems that respond to copper deficiency have yet to be defined for humans.

Toxicity

Acute copper toxicity in humans is rare and usually occurs from contamination of drinking water, beverages, and foodstuffs from copper pipes or containers, or from accidental or deliberate ingestion of large amounts of copper salts. Symptoms include vomiting, diarrhoea, haemolytic anaemia, renal and liver damage, sometimes (at about 100 g or more) followed by coma and death. Clinical symptoms of chronic copper toxicity appear when the capacity for protective copper binding in the liver is exceeded. These symptoms include hepatitis, liver cirrhosis, and jaundice.

Consumption of formula milks, heavily contaminated with copper after boiling or storage in brass vessels, is usually a feature of Indian childhood cirrhosis, which occurs in early-weaned infants between the ages of six months and five years. Symptoms include abdominal distension, irregular fever, excessive crying, and altered appetite, followed by jaundice and often death. Some believe that a genetic disorder enhances susceptibility to this toxicity syndrome, associated with excessive dietary exposure to copper and massive accumulation of liver copper.

Genetics

Several disorders result in deficiency or toxicity from exposure to copper intakes that are adequate or tolerated by the general population. The most important of these are Menkes' syndrome, an X-linked copper deficiency that is usually fatal in early childhood; Wilson's disease, an autosomal recessive disorder resulting in copper overload; and aceruloplasminaemia, an autosomal recessive disorder of iron metabolism. All three disorders are characterised by low serum copper and ceruloplasmin.

Menkes' syndrome, which affects 1 in 300 000 in most populations, is caused by mutations in the gene that encodes a novel member of the family of cation-transporting p-type ATPases. The gene is expressed in extrahepatic tissues, and symptoms result from an inability to export copper from cells, particularly from intestinal cells and across the placenta. The syndrome has three forms, classic, mild, and occipital horn. Among the symptoms of the classic (most severe) Menkes' syndrome are abnormal myelination with cerebellar neurodegeneration (giving progressive mental retardation), abnormal (steely, kinky) hair, hypothermia, hypopigmentation, seizures, convulsions, failure to thrive, and connective tissue abnormalities resulting in deformities in the skull, long bones and ribs, and twisted, tortuous arteries. Death usually occurs in the severe forms before three years of age.

Wilson's disease, which affects 1 in 30 000 in most populations, is caused by numerous (over 100 recognised) mutations in the gene for a copper-transporting ATPase. The defect results in impaired biliary excretion of copper and accumulation of copper in the liver and brain of homozygous individuals or compound heterozygotes. Abnormalities in copper homeostasis, however, may also occur in heterozygous carriers, who may make up 1–2% of the population. The age of onset is from childhood onwards and patients may present in three different ways: with hepatic symptoms (liver cirrhosis and fatty infiltration in the latter stages), with neurological symptoms (degeneration of the basal ganglia resulting in defective movement, slurred speech, difficulty swallowing, face and muscle spasms, dystonia, and poor motor control), or with psychiatric and behavioral problems (including depression and schizophrenia, loss of emotional control, temper tantrums, and insomnia). Kayser–Fleischer rings (corneal copper deposits) in the eyes are generally present in neurological or psychiatric presentations. The phenotypic differences between Wilson's disease and Menkes' syndrome are probably owing to the tissue-specific expression of the ATPase genes.

If Wilson's disease is diagnosed early, copper chelation therapy, usually with D-penicillamine, can be beneficial, although neurological symptoms are often irreversible and liver disease may be advanced at the time of diagnosis. Zinc supplements limit copper absorption and subsequent accumulation, and this is the treatment of choice for maintenance therapy.

Aceruloplasminaemia, which affects about 1 in 2 million individuals, is caused by mutations in the ceruloplasmin gene. Ceruloplasmin is involved in iron metabolism and, in this disease, there is an accumulation of ferrous iron within the recticuloendothelial system with pathogenesis mainly linked to the slow accumulation of iron in the brain, rather than other tissues. Symptoms include dementia, speech problems, retinal degeneration, poor muscle tone, and diabetes. Early therapy with the high-affinity iron chelator desferoxamine can relieve some of the symptoms.

Disruption of copper metabolism may be involved in other neurodegenerative diseases such as the accumulation of amyloid β-protein in Alzheimer's disease and the accumulation of modified prion protein in human prion disease.

About 10% of motor neuron disease cases are familial and 20% of these are owing to autosomal dominant inheritance of mutations in the Cu/Zn-SOD (*SODI*) gene. It is unclear how changes in activity of this copper enzyme might be involved in the progressive muscle weakness and atrophy of motor neuron disease or in Down's syndrome, where additional Cu/Zn-SOD activity results from the *SODI* gene being present in the extra chromosome 21.

Assessing status

It is possible to diagnose severe copper deficiency in infants from plasma or serum copper, ceruloplasmin protein, and neutrophils. These measures, however, cannot be used to detect suboptimal copper status in individuals, as such measures are insensitive to small changes in copper status and there are intractable problems in interpretation. Ceruloplasmin, the major copper protein in plasma or serum, is an acute-phase reactant and is raised by cigarette smoking, oral contraceptives, oestrogens, pregnancy, infections, inflammation, haematological diseases, hypertension, diabetes, cardiovascular diseases, cancer, and cirrhosis, and after surgery and exercise. Even though the effects of inflammation in increasing plasma or serum copper is well known, there are continued reports in the literature indicating a putative causal association between high body copper and cancer and other chronic diseases whereas the possibility of reverse causation would be a more logical conclusion from such observations.

Currently, there is no adequate measure of suboptimal (or supra-optimal) copper status and this is a major barrier to determining precise dietary requirements for copper and the possible role of suboptimal or supra-optimal copper status in the etiology of chronic disease. Table 11.17 gives some of the functional indices (classified as molecular, biochemical, and physiological) that might be used to define suboptimal or supra-optimal status in humans. A valid functional index of copper status in humans must respond sensitively, specifically, and predictably to changes in the concentration and supply of dietary copper or copper stores, be accessible for measurement and measurable, and impact directly on health. As such, indices in Table 11.17 have not been validated and many lack sensitivity and specificity. Perhaps, the best way forward is to use a combination of measures.

Requirements and dietary sources

Although copper is the third most abundant trace element, after iron and zinc, in the body, precise dietary requirements for copper are still subject to conjecture because of the difficulty in assessing copper status. Current estimates suggest that the requirements for copper

Table 11.17 Putative functional indices of copper status

Molecular indices
Changes in activity/concentration of Cu-metalloproteins
Ceruloplasmin oxidase
Ceruloplasmin protein
Superoxide dismutase
Cytochrome c oxidase
Lysyl oxidase
Diamine oxidase
Dopamine β-monooxgenase
Peptidylgycine α-amidating monooxgenase
Tyrosinase
Factor V
Factor VIII
Transcuprein
Biochemical indices
Pyridinium cross-links of collagen
Various measures of oxidative stress (TBARS)
Catecholamines
Encephalins
Polyamines
Physiological indices
Immune function
Haemostasis
Cholesterol metabolism
Glucose tolerance
Blood pressure
Arterial compliance
Arterial plaque
DNA damage and repair
Bone density

for the great majority of adults are below about 1.5 mg copper/day, while most people can tolerate 3 mg copper/day or more over the long term and 8–10 mg copper/day or more in the shorter term (over several months). Using similar data from copper supplementation trials where there was an absence of any adverse effects on liver function, UL for copper was derived to be 10 mg/day in the US and 5 mg/day in the EU; the difference owing to the use of different uncertainty factors in the derivation.

Estimates of average intakes of copper are about 1.5 and 1.2 mg copper/day for men and women, respectively, on mixed diets, with higher intakes for those on vegetarian diets or those consuming water with appreciable concentrations of copper. Particularly rich food sources of copper include offal, seafood, nuts, seeds, legumes, wholegrain cereals, and chocolate. Milk and dairy products are very low in copper and infants are at risk of copper deficiency if they are fed exclusively on cow's milk.

Micronutrient interactions

The major micronutrient interactions with copper are those involving zinc and iron, high intakes of which can restrict copper utilisation in infants and adults. The mechanism by which zinc appears to exert on antagonistic effect on copper status is through the induction of metallothionein synthesis by zinc in mucosal cells in the intestine. Metallothionein has a particularly strong affinity for copper. Metallothionein-bound copper is not available for transport into the circulation and is eventually lost in the faeces when the mucosal cells are sloughed off. Molybdenum also has a strong interaction with copper and thiomolybdates are potent systemic copper antagonists. Although both cadmium and lead can inhibit copper utilisation, this inhibition only occurs at dietary intakes of these heavy metals above those normally consumed by humans. Vitamin E, selenium, and manganese have metabolic interactions with copper as antioxidants, but data on beneficial interactions of these on symptoms of copper deficiency are largely confined to animal studies. Copper deficiency exerts an effect on iodine metabolism resulting in hypothyroidism, at least in animal models.

11.10 Selenium

Selenium is a nonmetallic element that has similar chemical properties to sulfur and has four natural oxidation states (0, −2, +4, +6). It combines with other elements to form inorganic selenides [sodium selenide (−2) Na_2Se], selenites [sodium selenite (+4) Na_2SeO_3] and selenates [sodium selenate (+6) Na_2SeO_4], and with oxygen to form oxides [selenium (+4) dioxide SeO_2] and oxyacids [selenic (+6) acid H_2SeO_4]. Selenium replaces sulphur to form a large number of organic selenium compounds, particularly as selenocysteine, the twenty-first amino acid. Selenium is a component of selenoproteins, where it also occurs as selenides on the side-chains of selenocysteine at physiological pH. Selenium also displaces sulfur to form the amino acid selenomethionine. Elemental selenium is stable and has three allotropic forms, deep red crystals, red amorphous powder, and the black vitreous form.

Selenium has many industrial uses, e.g., in electronics, glass, ceramics, pigments, as alloys in steel, as catalysts in pharmaceutical production, in rubber vulcanisation and in agriculture, as feed supplements and fertilisers. Because of its increasing use, selenium has become a potential health and environmental hazard. The primary pathway of exposure to selenium for the general population is food, followed by water (predominantly inorganic selenate and selenite), and air (mainly as elemental particulate selenium from combustion of fossil fuels and from volcanic gas).

Absorption, transport, and tissue distribution

Absorption of dietary selenium takes place mainly in the small intestine, where some 50–80% is absorbed. Organic forms of selenium (with selenomethionine and selenocysteine making up the major forms in food) are more readily absorbed than inorganic forms and selenium compounds from plants are generally more bioavailable than those from animals, and particularly from fish. Selenium-containing supplements generally provide a mixture of various organic selenium species. Some naturally occurring inorganic and organic compounds of selenium are given in Table 11.18.

The bioavailability of selenium from water (mainly inorganic selenates) and supplements is lower than from food. The overall bioavailability of selenium from the diet depends on a number of factors, including selenium status, lipid composition, and metals.

Inorganic forms of selenium are passively transported across the intestinal brush border, whereas organic forms (selenomethionine and probably selenocysteine) are actively transported. On reaching the bloodstream, selenium is transported largely bound to protein (mainly very low-density β-lipoprotein with a small amount bound to albumin) for deposition in various organs. Liver and kidney are the major target organs when selenium intake is high but, at lower intakes, the selenium content of the liver is decreased. Heart and muscle tissue are other target organs, with the latter, because of its total bulk, accounting for the greatest proportion of body selenium. The total body content of selenium can vary from about 3 mg to 15 mg depending on dietary intakes. Mounting evidence points to the need to determine selenium species in foodstuffs in order to characterise dietary intakes and status, although this presents an analytical challenge.

Table 11.18 Some naturally occurring inorganic and organic compounds of selenium

Selenite {SeO_3^{2-}]
Selenate {SeO_4^{2-}]
Methylselenol (CH_3SH)
Dimethylselenide (CH_3-Se-CH_3)
Trimethyselenonium ion [$(CH_3)_3$-Se^+]
Selenocysteine
Selenomethionine
Se-Methyl-selenocysteine

In the body, dietary selenium can be bound to selenium binding proteins but can also be directly incorporated into selenoproteins during translation at the ribosome complex using a transfer RNA specific for the amino acid selenocysteine; thus, selenocysteine can be considered as the twenty-first amino acid in terms of ribosome-mediated protein synthesis.

The major excretion routes of selenium are in urine (mainly as trimethylselenonium ion (TMSe)), in faeces (via biliary pancreatic and intestinal secretions, together with unabsorbed dietary selenium), and in breath (as volatile dimethylselenide). Unlike copper, and particularly iron, which have inefficient excretion mechanisms, selenium is rapidly excreted in the urine. Figure 11.10 gives an overall view of selenium metabolism and excretion.

Metabolic function and essentiality

Selenocysteine is a component of at least 30 selenoproteins, some of which have structural roles and others have important enzymatic functions (Table 11.19). Selenocysteine is generally at the active site of those selenoproteins with catalytic activity, and functions as a redox center for the selenium-dependent glutathione peroxidases (GPx1, GPx2, GPx3, GPx4 and GPx6), iodothyronine deiodinases (DIO types I, II, and III), and thioredoxin reductases (TXNRD1, TXNRD2 and TXNRD3). The glutathione peroxidase isozymes, which account for about 36% of total body selenium, differ in their tissue expression (cystolic,

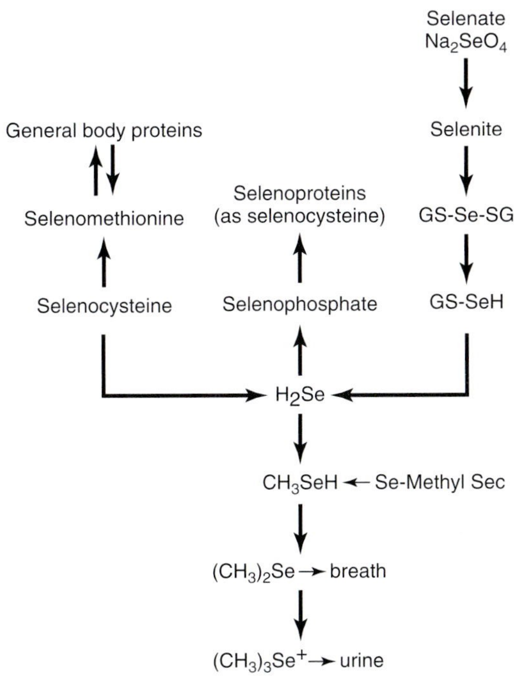

Figure 11.10 Selenium metabolism and excretion.

extracellular, and gastrointestinal) and map to different chromosomes. Selenoprotein P (SELENOP) and methionine sulfoxide reductase B (MSRB1) also act as antioxidant enzymes, with SELENOP serving to supply extrahepatic tissues with selenium. Additional functions of selenoproteins include thyroid hormone metabolism, calcium homeostasis, skeletal muscle regeneration, cell maintenance and immunity. The biosynthesis, and therefore function of, selenoproteins depends upon dietary availability of selenium.

Deficiency symptoms

Keshan's disease is a cardiomyopathy that affects children and women of child-bearing age and occurs in areas of China where the soil is deficient in selenium. Despite the strong evidence for an etiological role for selenium in Keshan's disease (i.e., the occurrence of the disease only in those regions of China with low selenium soils and, hence, low amounts of selenium in the food chain, and only in those individuals with

Table 11.19 Selenoproteins

Selenoprotein	Function
Glutathione peroxidases (GPx1, GPx2, GPx3, GPx4 and GPx6; cystolic, gastrointestinal, extracellular and phospholipid hydroperoxide, respectively)	Antioxidant enzymes: remove hydrogen peroxide, and lipid and phospholipid hydroperoxides (thereby maintaining membrane integrity, modulating eiconsanoid synthesis, modifying inflammation, and likelihood of propagation of further oxidative damage to biomolecules, such as lipids, lipoproteins and DNA)
(Sperm) mitochondrial capsule selenoprotein	Form of glutathione peroxidase (GPx4): shields developing sperm cells from oxidative damage and later polymerises into structural protein required for stability/motility of mature sperm
Iodothyronine deiodinases (three isoforms: DIO1, DIO2 and DIO3)	Production and regulation of level of active thyroid hormone, T_3, from thyroxine T_4
Thioredoxin reductases (three isoforms: TXNRD1, TXNRD2 and TXNRD3)	Reduction of nucleotides in DNA synthesis; regeneration of antioxidant systems; maintenance of intracellular redox state, critical for cell viability and proliferation; regulation of thioredoxin
Selenophosphate synthetase, SPS2	Required for biosynthesis of selenophosphate, the precursor of selenocysteine, and therefore for selenoprotein synthesis
Selenoprotein P (SELENOP)	Found in plasma and associated with endothelial cells; appears to protect endothelial cells against damage from lipid hydroperoxides; selenium transport
Selenoprotein W	Needed for skeletal and cardiac muscle function
Selenoprotein N	Found in most tissues, but main function largely unknown; possible role in muscle development
Selenoprotein S	Membrane protein widely expressed; involved in inflammatory response and regulation of cytokines
Selenoprotein K	Membrane protein localised to endoplasmic reticulum; possible antioxidant role
Selenoprotein R	Widely expressed; antioxidant role; involved in protein repair
Selenoprotein H	Widely expressed; DNA binding protein with roles in regulation of glutathione synthesis genes
Selenoprotein I	Largely unknown

Reprinted with permission from Elsevier (Rayman, MP Lancet, 2000, *356*, pp. 233–241 with adaptations from Fairweather-Tait SJ, Collings R and Hurst R, 2010, AJCN 91(suppl):1484S- 91S.).

poor selenium status together with the prevention of the disease in an at-risk population by supplementation with selenium), there are certain epidemiological features of the disease that are not readily explained solely on the basis of selenium deficiency. A similar situation occurs with Kashin–Beck disease, a chronic osteoarthropathy that most commonly affects growing children and occurs in parts of Siberian Russia and in China, where it overlaps with Keshan's disease. Although oral supplementation with selenium is effective in preventing the disease, it is likely that other factors, apart from selenium deficiency, are involved in the etiology of Kashin–Beck disease. There are also some selenium-responsive conditions with symptoms similar to Keshan's disease that occur in patients receiving total parenteral nutrition.

One explanation for the complex etiology of selenium-responsive diseases in humans is that low selenium status may predispose to other deleterious conditions, most notably the increased incidence, virulence, or disease progression of a number of viral infections. For example, in a selenium-deficient animal model, harmless coxsackie virus can become virulent and cause myocarditis, not only in the selenium-deficient host, but also when isolated and injected into selenium-replete animals. A coxsackie virus has been isolated from the blood and tissues of patients with Keshan's disease and the infection may be responsible for the cardiomyopathy of that disease. It has been speculated that similar events linked with other RNA viruses may explain the emergence of new strains of influenza virus in China and the postulated crossing-over of the human immunodeficiency virus (HIV) to humans in the selenium-deficient population of Zaire. Many human viral pathogens (e.g., HIV, coxsackie, hepatitis, and measles viruses) can synthesise viral selenoproteins and, thereby, lower the selenium available to the host. In any event, selenium deficiency is accompanied by loss of immunocompetence, with the impairment of both cell-mediated immunity and B-cell function.

Covert suboptimal selenium status may be widespread in human populations, as selenium supplementation in subjects considered to be selenium replete had marked immunostimulant effects, including increased proliferation of activated T-cells. The best evidence of the effect of selenium on immune responsiveness comes from human supplementation studies of immune-compromised elderly adults and cancer patients which studied doses of selenium between 100 and 400 μg per day. A range of immunostimulant effects were found, most notably an increase in CD4+ T cell subsets and increased cytotoxicity of natural killer cells. In general, a high selenium diet is believed to favour the differentiation of CD4+ cells into T-helper-1 (Th1) rather than T-helper-2 (Th2) cells which may benefit an individual fighting an active infection.

The most recent review and meta-analysis of prospective observational studies has reported lower cancer incidence and mortality associated with higher selenium intakes, particularly from studies of stomach, bladder and prostate cancers. However, reviews of RCT evidence are less clear. The results of two large trials – the Nutritional Prevention of Cancer Trial (NPCT) and the Selenium and Vitamin E Cancer Trial (SELECT) suggest potentially harmful effects of high selenium exposure. In the latter trial of 35 533 American men, supplementation with 200 μg per day selenium failed to show any significant risk reduction for prostate cancer as a result of selenium with vitamin E supplementation. Despite much criticism over their methodological design, it is clear that further research is required to understand more on the potential explanation for the null findings of these large trials which contrast with observational evidence. The proposed mechanisms for a cancer chemoprotective effect of selenium include antioxidant protection and reduction of inflammation; inactivation of protein kinase C; altered carcinogen metabolism; reduction in DNA damage, stimulation of DNA repair (p53), and alteration in DNA methylation; cell cycle effects; enhanced apoptosis and inhibition of angiogenesis.

The evidence for suboptimal selenium status increasing the risk of cardiovascular disease is more fragmentary, but it has been proposed that optimising the activity of the seleno-dependent glutathione peroxidases and, thereby, increasing antioxidant activity may be a factor. As selenium has well-recognised antioxidant and anti-inflammatory roles, other oxidative stress or inflammatory conditions (e.g., rheumatoid arthritis, ulcerative colitis, pancreatitis, and asthma) may benefit from selenium supplementation. In addition, some, but certainly not all, studies have suggested beneficial (possibly antioxidant) effects of selenium on mood and reproduction in humans. There is some evidence that a low maternal selenium status in pregnancy may affect infant cognitive development.

The evidence, however, supporting a role for optimum selenium status preventing or ameliorating most inflammatory conditions is not strong and may be confounded by other dietary antioxidants, particularly vitamin E, compensating for low selenium status.

Toxicity

It has been suggested that there is a U-shaped relationship between selenium intake and toxicity in humans, possibly owing to the narrow range of selenium intakes required to saturate selenoenzyme activity. Indeed there is a narrow margin, perhaps not much more than three- or fourfold, between beneficial and harmful intakes of selenium. The dose necessary to cause chronic selenosis in humans is not well defined, but the World Health Organization recommends that daily intakes should not exceed 70 μg/d and suggests intakes above 400-700 μg/d may be toxic. Excessive consumption can stimulate free radical and DNA damage, as well as interfere with thyroid function. Symptoms of chronic selenium toxicity include brittle hair and nails, skin lesions with secondary infections, and garlic odour on the breath, resulting from the expiration of dimethyl selenide. Toxicity depends on the chemical form of selenium, with most forms having low toxicity, but also on genotype and the presence of other compounds, which may have synergistic or antagonistic effects. Data from animal studies indicate that selenite and selenocysteine are a little more toxic than selenomethionine and much more toxic than other organic selenium compounds (dimethyl selenide, trimethyselenonium ion, selenoethers, selenobetaine). Methylation in the body is important for detoxification of the element.

Genetics

Although no important genetic diseases affecting selenium status are apparent, polymorphisms in gene sequences of some selenoenzymes may determine selenium utilisation and metabolic needs, dietary requirements and hence, risk of disease. These polymorphisms may explain the significant variation among individuals in the extent of the response to supplementation of selenoenzyme activities. For example, genetic variation in SELENOP and the glutathione peroxidases may influence selenium status or response to supplementation, while individuals with a genetic polymorphism in the indolethylamine N-methyltransferase encoding gene (*INMT*) are known to excrete higher amounts of selenium via the kidneys as TMSe. There is some evidence that individuals with some of these genetic variants may require additional selenium for their needs.

Assessing status

Plasma or whole blood, hair, and toenail selenium concentrations can indicate changes in selenium status in humans. Plasma and serum selenium concentrations respond rapidly to changes in selenium intakes (Figure 11.11), whereas erythrocyte selenium and indeed toenail concentrations are indices of longer term or chronic intake. The most sensitive method for measuring selenium content in tissues is by inductively coupled plasma mass spectrometry (ICP-MS). Dietary intake data, however, are insufficient to determine selenium status in individuals because of uncertainties about bioavailability and variations in the content and form of selenium in foodstuffs.

Although plasma (or preferably platelet) glutathione peroxidase activities have been used as functional indices to estimate selenium sufficiency, it has not been established how these measurements relate to other biochemical functions of selenium, such as thyroid metabolism, or immune function and their health sequelae. For example, at higher levels of selenium intake (90–100 μg/L), glutathione peroxidase activities plateau but immunoenhancement may be evident at supplementation levels higher than those needed to optimise the selenoenzyme activity. Plasma SELENOP concentration has

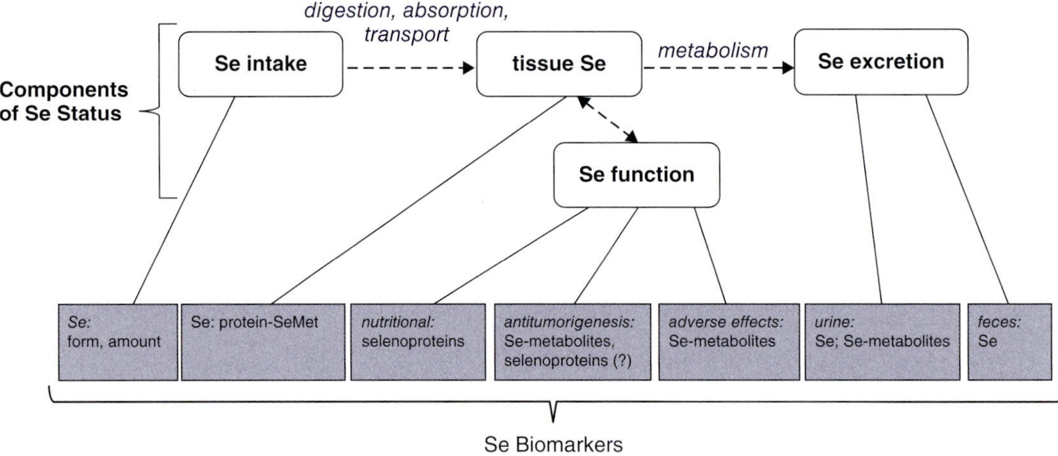

Figure 11.11 Selenium biomarkers and relationships with status. Source: Combs *et al.*, 2015.

been suggested a more suitable marker than plasma GPx activity.

Although diet is the most important source of selenium, other factors such as sex, age, BMI, education, smoking, and socioeconomic status may also be important in determining status.

Requirements and dietary sources

Dietary intakes of selenium vary widely with geographical spread, with China known to have the highest intake in some regions. Requirements for selenium have been estimated at intakes required to saturate plasma glutathione peroxidase activity (which corresponds to lower status and intake than that needed to saturate platelet glutathione peroxidase activity) in the vast majority (97.5%) of all individuals in a population. The RDAs for both men and women is 55 μg/day in the USA. In the UK, the RNI has thus been set at 75 and 60 μg/day selenium for men and women, respectively. Blood selenium concentrations in the UK population have declined by approximately 50% over the past 30 years and current UK intakes are only about 50% of the RNI. More recently, EFSA (in 2014) re-evaluated their recommendations for selenium and concluded that there was insufficient evidence to derive average requirements and PRIs, so instead used the selenium intake – plasma glutathione peroxidase activity relationship data to derive AIs. EFSA also considered it unnecessary to give sex-specific values. For adults, the AI for selenium was set at 70 μg/day, which was unchanged for pregnancy but increased to 85 μg/day for lactation. As explained previously, however, there is uncertainty as to what constitutes optimum selenium status and the intakes of selenium in various dietary regimens needed to achieve optimum status. Optimum status may not necessarily be reflected in saturated glutathione peroxidase activity. The UL for adults is set at 400 μg/day in the USA and at 300 μg/day in the EU. Table 11.20 shows the estimated intake of selenium from different foods in the UK diet (2006).

Selenium enters the food chain through plants that, in general, largely reflect concentrations of the element in the soil on which the plants were grown. The absorption of selenium by plants, however, is dependent not only on soil selenium content but also on pH, microbial activity, rainfall, and the chemical form of selenium. Selenomethionine is the predominant form in cereals, with wheat making the major contribution to overall intakes because of high quantities of wheat consumed as bread and other baked products. Wheat is the most efficient accumulator of selenium within the common cereal crops (wheat > rice > maize > barley > oats). Brazil nuts contain high concentrations of selenium, as selenomethionine, because of the seleniferous soils in the Andes Mountains but also the efficiency of accumulation of selenium by the plant. The major species in non-selenium-accumulating plant foods are selenite

Table 11.20 Estimated selenium intake from different foods in the UK

Food	Estimated contribution to total selenium intake µg/day (%)	Selenium content (µg/100g fresh weight)
Miscellaneous cereals	9 (16)	7
Meat products	8.5 (15)	14
Bread	6.4 (11)	6
Beverages	6.3 (11)	<0.5
Fish	5.9 (10)	42
Milk	3.4 (6)	1.4
Poultry	3.2 (6)	17
Carcass meat	2.8 (50	14
Eggs	2.5 (4)	19
Dairy products	2.5 (4)	3
Sugars & preserves	1.7 (3)	<3
Other vegetables	1.36 (3)	1.8
Potatoes	1.1 (2)	<1
Nuts	0.9 (2)	30
Offal	0.8 (1)	77
Oils & fats	0.7 (1)	<3
Canned vegetables	0.5 (1)	1.4
Fresh fruit	0.4 (1)	<0.5
Fruit products	0.3 (<1)	<0.5
Green vegetables	0.2 (<1)	0.7
Total	39 (100	-

Table adapted from *Food Standards Agency Survey* information sheet of the 2006 Total Diet Study (2009).

and to a lesser extent, selenocysteine. There are major varietal differences in selenium uptake and for wheat, tomatoes, soybean, and onions, there are up to fourfold differences in uptake of selenium from soils amongst cultivars. The ability of plants to accumulate selenium has been useful for agronomic biofortification, which differs from food fortification where the nutrient is added during food processing. The Finnish Policy (1984) has led to a 10-fold increase in cereal grain selenium concentration as well as marked increases in fruit and vegetables and meat concentrations as a result of adding selenium to fertilisers used for grain production and horticulture and fodder crop and hay production. The resulting increase in the selenium status of the population is largely owing to wheat (bread) consumption but the biofortification of vegetables may also have an impact on public health as, in contrast to wheat, where the major selenocompound is selenomethionine, seleno-methylselenocysteine is the predominant form in vegetables. Seleno-methylselenocysteine may have important cancer chemoprotective effects (see also Figure 11.12)

Fish, shellfish, and offal (liver, kidney) are rich sources of selenium, followed by meat and eggs. Animal sources, however, have lower bioavailability of selenium than do plant sources. The major forms of selenium in animal foodstuffs are selenomethionine and selenocysteine. However there are wide variations as a result of farming practice, where supplemented animal feeds and fertilisers are the main source in the animal diet. In general, supplementation of the animal diet with organic selenium species results in meat of a higher selenium concentration.

Micronutrient interactions

Selenium is an antioxidant nutrient and has important interactions with other antioxidant micronutrients, especially vitamin E (Figure 11.12). Vitamin E, as an antioxidant, can ameloriate some of the symptoms of selenium deficiencies in animals. Copper deficiency also increases oxidative stress, and the expression of glutathione peroxidase genes is decreased in the copper-deficient animal.

The metabolic interactions between selenium and other micronutrients, however, extend beyond those between selenium, vitamin E, and other antioxidants. Peripheral deiodination of thyroxine (T_4), the predominant hormone secreted by the thyroid, to the more biologically active triiodothyronine (T_3) in extrathyroidal tissues is accomplished through the selenium-dependent deiodinase enzymes. Selenium deficiency, therefore, can contribute to iodine deficiency disorders, and goitre complications have been noted in up to 80% of Keshan's disease casualties after autopsy. Moreover, higher serum T_4 concentrations were found in patients with subacute Keshan's disease and in children with latent Keshan's disease compared with the respective controls. All thyroid hormone concentrations in these studies were within normal ranges, suggesting that selenium deficiency, or even suboptimal selenium status, was blocking optimum thyroid and iodine metabolism.

Excess selenium intake interferes with zinc bioavailability, decreases tissue iron stores, and increases copper concentrations in the heart, liver, and kidney. Vitamins C and E, sulphur

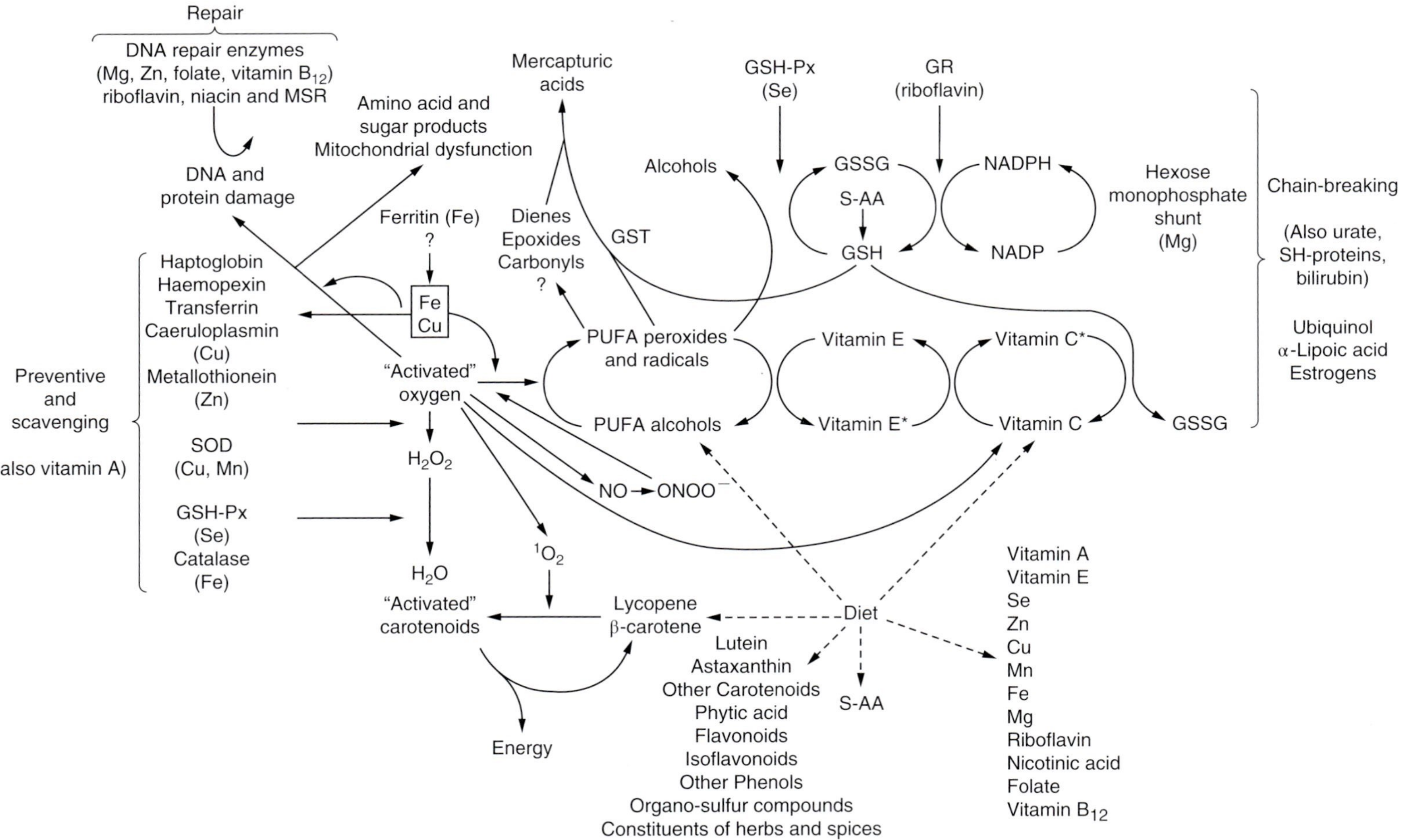

GR, glutathione reductase (EC1.6.4.2); GSH, reduced glutathione; GSH-Px glutathione peroxidase (EC1.11.1.9); GSSG, oxidized glutathione; GST, glutathione-S-transferase (EC 2.5.1.18); MSR, methionine sulfoxide reductase (EC1.8.4.5); PUFA, polyunsaturated fatty acids; S-AA, sulfur amino acids; SH-proteins, sulfydryl proteins; SOD, superoxide dismutase (EC1.15.1.1); [Fe Cu], transition metal-catalyzed oxidant damage to biomolecules. ? Biological relevance.

Figure 11.12 Antioxidant defense system. Source: From Strain and Benzie, 1999.

amino acids and sulphate can decrease the toxicity of selenium. Conversely, selenium modifies the toxicity of many heavy metals. The interaction between selenium and arsenic is particularly well-known, with evidence that selenium may decrease arsenic toxicity. In seafoods, selenium is combined with inorganic mercury or organic methyl mercury (MeHg) and this interaction may be one of the factors that decreases the bioavailability of selenium in these foods. It is known that both species of mercury can readily bind to selenium and subsequently reduce the amount available for synthesis and activity of selenoproteins. The most obvious impact of this binding is impaired redox homeostasis and increased oxidative stress. However, increased dietary intakes of selenium can overcome this decreased bioavailability. Well-known antagonistic interactions of selenium with both mercury and arsenic suggest that selenium can promote detoxification effects with respect to these toxins. Selenite is given as an antidote in cases of excessive inorganic mercury exposure through industrial sources in order to prevent the neurotoxic effects of this metal.

11.11 Iodine

Iodine is a nonmetallic element of the halogen group with common oxidation states of −1 (iodides), +5 (iodates), and +7 (periodates), and less common states of +1 (iodine monochloride) and +3 (iodine trichloride). Elemental iodine (0) is a soft blue–black solid, which sublimes readily to form a violet gas.

The principal industrial uses of iodine are in the pharmaceutical industry, medical and sanitary uses (e.g., iodised salt, water treatment, protection from radioactive iodine, and disinfectants), as catalysts (synthetic rubber, acetic acid synthesis), and in animal feeds, herbicides, dyes, inks, colorants, photographic equipment, lasers, metallurgy, conductive polymers, and stabilisers (nylon). Naturally occurring iodine minerals are rare and occur usually in the form of calcium iodates. Commercial production of iodine is largely restricted to extraction from Chilean deposits of nitrates (saltpeter) and iodine in caliche (soluble salts precipitated by evaporation), and from concentrated salt brine in Japan. Iodine is the least abundant halogen in the Earth's crust, at concentrations of 0.005%.

The concentration of iodine (as iodide and iodate) in the oceans is high, at about 0.06 mg/l. Iodine volatilises from the surface of the oceans and sea spray as salt particles, iodine vapor or methyl iodide vapor and is deposited back to the land in rainfall (0.0018–0.0085 mg iodine/l). The content of iodine in soils varies widely by geographical location and is a determinant of the prevalence of iodine deficiency in many populations. Iodine deficient soils are common in inland and mountainous areas and in regions with frequent flooding. The pH and organic composition of the soil may also affect the mobilisation of iodine into the food chain. There is a large variation of iodine content in drinking water (0.0001– 0.1 mg iodine/l).

Absorption, transport, and tissue distribution

Iodine, usually as an iodide or iodate compound in food and water, is rapidly absorbed in the intestine and circulates in the blood to all tissues in the body. The sodium +/iodide-symporter (NIS) is a plasma membrane glycoprotein expressed in intestinal epithelial cells which mediate iodine absorption. It also regulates the active uptake of iodine from the circulation by the thyroid gland, which traps most (about 80%) of the ingested iodine, but salivary glands, the gastric mucosa, choroid plexus, and the lactating mammary gland also concentrate the element by a similar active transport mechanism. Several sulphur-containing compounds, thiocyanate, isothiocyanate, and goitrin inhibit this active transport by competing for uptake with iodide at the NIS. These active goitrogens are released by plant enzymes from thioglucosides or cyanogenic glucosides found in cassava, kale, cabbage, sprouts, broccoli, kohlrabi, turnips, swedes, rapeseed, and mustard. The most important of these goitrogen-containing foods is cassava, which can be detoxified by soaking in water. Tobacco smoke also contributes thiocyanate and other antithyroid compounds to the circulation. These goitrogens are more of a concern among populations with suboptimal iodine intake; however, their goitrogenic activity can be overcome by iodine supplementation.

Metabolic functions and essentiality

Iodine is an essential micronutrient which cannot be replaced by any other nutrient in the body and must be obtained through the diet. Iodine is a constituent of the thyroid hormones, thyroxine (T_4) and triiodothyronine (T_3), which have key modifying or permissive roles in development and growth. Although T_4 is quantitatively predominant, T_3 is the more active. Adequate amounts of thyroid hormones are necessary for reproductive function, metabolic regulation, fetal growth and brain development. The mechanism of action of thyroid hormones appears to involve binding to nuclear receptors throughout the body that, in turn, alter gene expression in the pituitary, liver, heart, kidney, and, most crucially, brain cells. Overall, thyroid hormones stimulate enzyme synthesis, oxygen consumption, and basal metabolic rate and, thereby, affect the heart rate, respiratory rate, mobilisation, and metabolism of carbohydrates, lipogenesis and a wide variety of other physiological activities. It is probable that iodine has additional roles to those of thyroid hormone activity, for example in antibiotic and anticancer activity, but these roles are poorly understood.

Once iodide (−1) is trapped from the circulation and actively transported into the thyroid gland cells by the NIS, wherein it is oxidised by the enzymes thyroperoxidase (TPO) and hydrogen peroxidase (H202) to I_2 (0) and reacts with tyrosine in thyroglobulin protein to form the hormone precursors monoiodotyrosine (MIT) and diiodotyrosine (DIT). The iodinated compounds, in turn, couple to form T_3 and T_4, which are secreted from the thyroid into the circulation (Figure 11.13).

Flavonoids, found in many plants, including pearl millet, and phenol derivatives, released into water from soil humus, inhibit thyroid peroxidase and the organification of iodide. The concentration of iodine in the thyroid gland also affects the uptake of iodide into the follicle, the ratio of T_3 to T_4, and the rate of release of these hormones into the circulation. This process is also under hormonal control by the hypothalamus of the brain, which produces thyroid-releasing hormone, which then stimulates the pituitary gland to secrete thyroid-stimulating hormone (TSH), which, in turn, acts on the thyroid gland to produce more thyroid hormones.

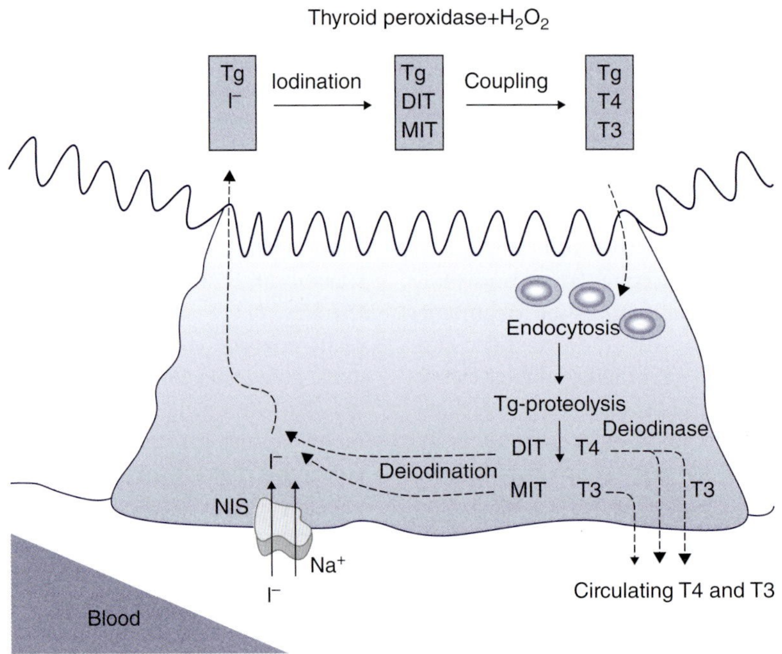

Figure 11.13 Iodine metabolism in the thyroid cell. Source: Zimmermann, 2008.

Almost all of the thyroid hormones released from the thyroid are bound to transport proteins, mainly thyroxine-binding globulin. The longer half-life of T_4 ensures that there is a reservoir for conversion to the more active T_3 with a much shorter half-life of 1 day. The deiodination of T_4 to T_3 takes place in extrathyroidal tissues (mainly the liver) by the deiodinase enzymes. Excretion of iodine is predominantly in the urine.

Deficiency symptoms

A deficiency of iodine causes a wide spectrum of disorders from mild goitre (a larger thyroid gland than normal) to the most severe forms of endemic congenital hypothyroidism (cretinism) (severe, irreversible mental, and growth retardation). Collectively, these manifestations of iodine deficiency are termed iodine deficiency disorders (IDDs) and symptoms differ depending on the life stage at which iodine deficiency occurs. Children are most vulnerable to the effects of iodine deficiency but the most severe disorders (congenital hypothyroidism) arise if the developing fetus suffers from iodine deficiency. This increased severity is because adequate thyroid hormones are required for the processes of neuronal migration and myelination of the fetal brain in early gestation. The fetus is entirely dependent on the mother for thyroid hormones which cross the placenta. An inadequate supply, as a result of insufficient maternal iodine intake, can cause irreversible structural changes in the developing brain's cerebral cortex. Maternal hypothyroidism is the most common cause of congenital hypothyroidism.

The clinical features of endemic congenital hypothyroidism are either a predominant neurological syndrome with severe to profound mental retardation, including defects of hearing and speech (often deaf–mutism), squint, and disorders of stance and gait of varying degrees (neurological congenital hypothyroidism), or predominant features of hypothyroidism and stunted growth with less severe mental retardation (myxedematous congenital hypothyroidism). Profound hypothyroidism is biochemically defined as high serum TSH and very low T_4 and T_3, and is accompanied by a low basal metabolic rate, apathy, slow reflex relaxation time with slow movements, cold intolerance, and myxoedema (skin and subcutaneous tissue are thickened because of an accumulation of mucin, and become dry and swollen). Although congenital hypothyroidism is the severest form of IDD, varying degrees of intellectual or growth retardation are apparent when iodine deficiency occurs in the fetus, infancy or childhood and adolescence. In adulthood, the consequences of iodine deficiency are more serious in women, especially during pregnancy, than in men.

The mildest form of IDD, goitres, range from those only detectable by touch (palpation) to very large goitres that can cause breathing problems. The enlargement of the thyroid gland to produce goitre arises from stimulation of the thyroid cells by TSH and, without the ability to increase hormone production owing to iodine deficiency, and the gland becomes hyperplastic.

Apart from congenital hypothyroidism, hypothyroidism, and goitre, other features linked to IDDs are decreased fertility rates, increased stillbirth and spontaneous abortion rates, and increased perinatal and infant mortality. The public health significance of iodine deficiency cannot be underestimated, with over 1 billion people (worldwide, but mostly in Asia and Africa) estimated to be living in iodine-deficient areas and, therefore, at risk of IDDs. In recent years, iodine deficiency has re-emerged in industrialised countries including many European countries. Figure 11.14 shows the global incidence and severity of inadequate iodine nutrition in countries where national monitoring of urinary iodine concentration data exist for school-age children and adults.

Estimates of those with IDDs demonstrate the scale of the problem, with 200–300 million goitrous people, over 40 million affected by some degree of mental impairment and some 7 million people with congenital hypothyroidism. The eradication of iodine deficiency remains a significant public health challenge and requires a multidisciplinary approach. Fortunately, the implementation of public health programs introducing synthetic forms of iodine into the diet, predominantly through the addition of potassium iodide to salt, have proven largely successful in reducing the global incidence of iodine deficiency in recent decades. Treatment with iodine supplementation in older children and adults can reverse many of the clinical

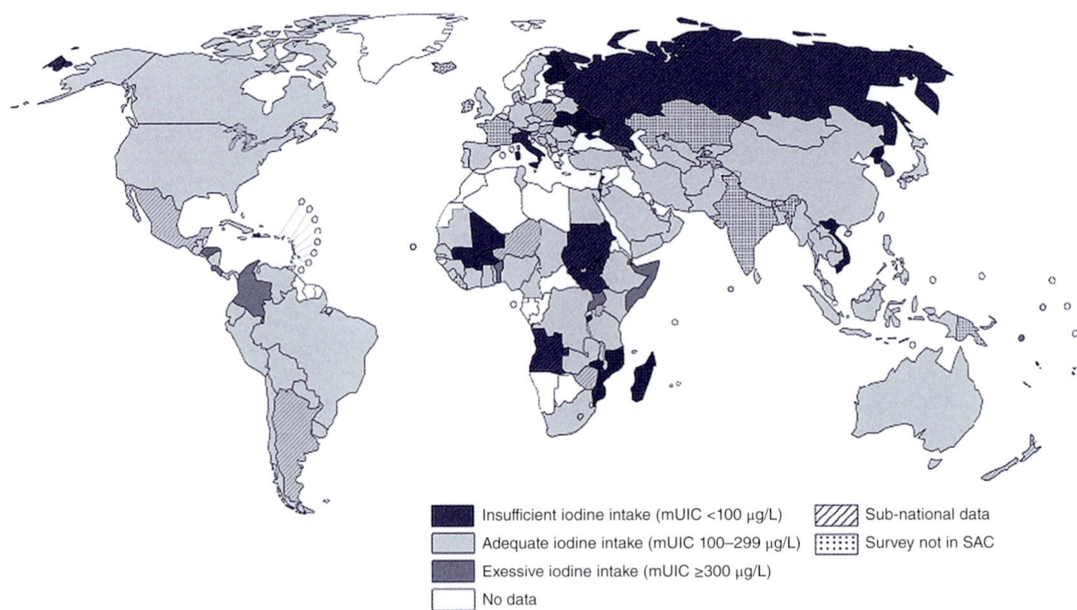

Figure 11.14 Global incidence of iodine nutrition in school-age children and adults based on median urinary iodine concentrations in 2017. Source: Iodine Global Network www.ign.org.

manifestations of IDDs, including mental deficiency, hypothyroidism and goitre. The iodisation of salt is the most recommended strategy to control iodine deficiency and also the most cost-effective means of improving child development and adult cognition within a population. Yet not all countries' food industries iodise salt for reasons that might conflict with the national public health advice on salt consumption. Furthermore, even in countries that have adopted USI, there is evidence that iodine deficiency remains a problem. The most recent evaluation of global monitoring data of urinary iodine concentrations from school-age children shows that 111 countries have sufficient iodine intake, with 30 countries still having mild-to-moderate deficiency.

Goitrogenic factors, including exposure to environmental endocrine disruptors, limiting bioavailability appear to aggravate iodine deficiency particularly in regions with low soil iodine concentrations. In addition, genetic variation, immunological factors, sex, age, and growth factors seem to modify expression of the conditions, producing a wide range of symptoms and severity of IDDs with similar iodine intakes.

Toxicity

A wide range of iodine intakes is tolerated by most individuals, and is owing to the ability of the thyroid to regulate total body iodine. Over 2 mg iodine/day for long periods should be regarded as excessive or potentially harmful to most people. Such high intakes are unlikely to arise from natural foods, except for diets that are very high in seafood and/or seaweed or comprising foods contaminated with iodine. In contrast to iodine-replete individuals, those with IDDs or previously exposed to iodine-deficient diets may react to sudden moderate increases in iodine intake, such as from iodised salt. Iodine-induced thyrotoxicosis (hyperthyroidism) and toxic nodular goitre may result from excess iodine exposure in these individuals. Hyperthyroidism is largely confined to those over 40 years of age and symptoms are rapid heart rate, trembling, excessive sweating, lack of sleep, and loss of weight and strength.

Individuals, who are sensitive to iodine, usually have mild skin symptoms, but very rarely fever, salivary gland enlargement, visual problems, and skin problems, and, in severe cases, cardiovascular collapse, convulsions, and death may occur. The occurrence of allergic symptoms, for example to iodine medications or antiseptics, however, is rare.

In iodine deficient populations, the introduction of iodine fortification has coincided with a rise in the incidence of thyroid disorders. There is also some concern that excessive iodine intakes can increase the presence of thyroid antibodies, which may increase the risk of autoimmune thyroid disease among susceptible individuals.

Genetics

Pendred's syndrome is an autosomal recessive inherited disorder with a frequency of 100 or less per 100 000. It is characterised by goitre and profound deafness in childhood and is caused by mutations in the *Pendrin* gene located on chromosome 7. The gene codes for pendrin, a transporter protein for chloride/ iodine transport across the thyroid apical membrane; this results in defective iodination of thyroglobulin. Mutations in another gene, the NIS gene, can occasionally cause defective iodide transport and goiter, whereas single nucleotide polymorphisms in the TSH receptor gene may predispose individuals to the hyperthyroidism of toxic multinodular goitre and Graves' disease. There is also some evidence that polymorphisms in genes encoding thyroid-specific selenoproteins, the iodothyronine deiodinases and the thioredoxin reductases, may influence iodine homeostasis. However, it remains unknown how important these genetic differences are at the population level.

Assessing status

The critical importance of iodine for the thyroid indicates that iodine status is assessed by thyroid function. A standard set of indicators (goitre rate by palpation or thyroid volume by ultrasound, median urinary iodine, serum TSH, and serum thyroglobulin (Tg)) is used to determine prevalence in countries with endemic deficiency. The goitre rate, which reflects long-term iodine status, can be assessed by palpating the thyroid in the neck. In populations with mild-to-moderate deficiency, measurement of thyroid volume by ultrasound is advised.

Measurement of serum thyroid hormones (TSH, T_4, and T_3) provides useful indicators of functional iodine status in the individual. However, serum TSH is not as sensitive a measure of deficiency in older children and adults as it is possible to have TSH and T_3 values within the reference range despite deficiency. In newborns, TSH is a more sensitive measure of status and is used in routine clinical practice to detect congenital hypothyroidism.

More recently, measurement of serum Tg has been advised as a functional measure of iodine status in children and pregnant women, and may be more sensitive than serum TSH, by reflecting status over a period of weeks to months. It is also possible to analyse Tg by dried blood spot sample collection, although there is a suggestion that co-measurement of Tg antibodies is warranted when assessing this biomarker.

Dietary intakes and requirements

Requirements in infancy and children up to 18 years of age range from 50 to 150 μg iodine/day. Adult requirements are estimated at 150 μg iodine/day, with the UK RNI at 140 μg/d. The EFSA, US Institute of Medicine and the World Health Organization recommend incremental intakes of 200, 220-290 and 250 μg/day for pregnancy and lactation. However, there is no established incremental intake recommended for pregnant and lactating women in the UK. The reason for increased iodine requirements in pregnancy are as a result of elevated oestrogen and human chorionic gonadotropin, thyroid hormone transfer to the fetus and increased glomerular filtration rate. Safe upper levels for iodine intakes in pregnancy are not well defined. Therefore, it is important that maternal hypothyroidism is routinely monitored in clinical practice.

The UL for adults is set at 600 μg/day (EU) and at 1.1 mg/day (USA).

Under normal circumstances, about 90% of iodine intake is from food, with about 10% from water. The concentration of iodine in most foods is low and, in general, reflects the iodine content of the soil, water, and fertilisers used in plant and animal production within the region of production. In most countries, other sources, such as iodised salts or foods, are required. Seafoods and seaweed concentrate iodine from seawater and are the richest available dietary sources. However, in many European populations, milk has become a major source of iodine, owing to the use of iodine-containing disinfectants in farming practice and the use of iodine-enriched cattle feed. Where milk and dairy products are commonly consumed, milk can provide as much as up to one third of the daily iodine intake. However, contributions from milk and dairy can be seasonal as a direct result of variations in farming practice.

Micronutrient interactions

From a public health viewpoint, the most important metabolic interaction of iodine with other micronutrients is with selenium. Adequate selenium status is essential for thyroid hormone metabolism and, therefore, normal growth development, by ensuring sufficient T_3 supply to extrathyroidal tissues. Most T_3 is formed from T_4 by the selenium-dependent deiodinases. Selenium is also a component of the antioxidants, thioredoxin reductase and glutathione peroxidase, which help prevent the accumulation of peroxides in the thyroid. Iodine and selenium deficiencies overlap in various parts of the world and concurrent deficiencies of both may contribute to the etiologies of Kashin–Beck disease in Russia, China, and Tibet, and myxedematous congenital hypothyroidism in Zaire. In addition, both nutrients are required for normal reproduction, normal gene expression, synthesis of xenobiotic and metabolising enzymes in the liver, and normal tolerance against cold stress. It is possible that hypothyroidism associated with suboptimal selenium status may explain some of the etiology of cardiovascular disease and certain cancers.

Hypothyroidism is associated with deficiencies of other trace elements, including zinc, iron, and copper, while there are close metabolic relationships at the molecular and transport levels between iodine and vitamin A. Conversely, deficiencies in these micronutrients can also impact thyroid function and potentially affect the efficacy of iodine prophylaxis

11.12 Manganese

Manganese is widely distributed in the biosphere: it constitutes approximately 0.085% of the Earth's crust, making it the twelfth most abundant element. Manganese is a component of numerous complex minerals, including pyroluosite, rhodochrosite, rhodanite, braunite, pyrochite, and manganite. Chemical forms of manganese in their natural deposits include oxides, sulphides, carbonates, and silicates. Anthropogenic sources of manganese are predominantly from the manufacturing of steel, alloys, and iron products. Manganese is also widely used as an oxidising agent, as a component of fertilisers and fungicides, and in dry cell batteries. The permanganate is a powerful oxidising agent and is used in quantitative analysis and medicine.

Manganese is a transition element. It can exist in 11 oxidation states from −3 to +7, with the most common valences being +2, +4, and +7. The +2 valence is the predominant form in biological systems, the +4 valence occurs in MnO_2, and the +7 valence is found in permanganate.

Absorption, transport, and tissue distribution

The total amount of manganese in the adult human is approximately 15 mg. Up to 25% of the total body stores of manganese may be located in the skeleton and may not be readily accessible for use in metabolic pathways. Relatively high concentrations have been reported in the liver, pancreas, intestine, and bone.

Intestinal absorption of manganese occurs throughout the length of the small intestine. Mucosal uptake appears to be mediated by two types of mucosal binding, one that is saturable with a finite capacity and one that is nonsaturable. Manganese absorption, probably as Mn^{2+}, is relatively inefficient, generally less than 5%, but there is some evidence of improvement at low intakes. High levels of dietary calcium, phosphorus, and phytate impair the intestinal uptake of the element but are probably of limited significance because, as yet, no well-documented case of human manganese deficiency has been reported.

Systemic homeostatic regulation of manganese is brought about primarily through hepatobiliary excretion rather than through regulation of absorption (e.g., the efficiency of manganese retention does not appear to be dose dependent within normal dietary levels). Manganese is taken up from blood by the liver and transported to extrahepatic tissues by transferrin and possibly α_2-macroglobulin and albumin. Manganese is excreted primarily in faeces. Urinary excretion of manganese is low and has not been found to be sensitive to dietary manganese intake.

Metabolic function and essentiality

Manganese is required as a catalytic cofactor for mitochondrial superoxide dismutase, arginase, and pyruvate carboxylase. It is also an activator of glycosyltransferases, phosphoenolpyruvate carboxylase, and glutamine synthetase.

Deficiency symptoms

Signs of manganese deficiency have been demonstrated in several animal species. Symptoms include impaired growth, skeletal abnormalities, depressed reproductive function, and defects in lipid and carbohydrate metabolism. Evidence of manganese deficiency in humans is poor. It has been suggested that manganese deficiency has never been observed in noninstitutionalised human populations because of the abundant supply of manganese in edible plant materials compared with the relatively low requirements of mammals. There is only one report of apparent human manganese deficiency. A male subject was fed a purified diet deficient in vitamin K, and was also accidentally deficient in manganese. Feeding this diet caused weight loss, dermatitis, growth retardation of hair and nails, reddening of black hair, and a decline in concentrations of blood lipids. Manganese deficiency may be more frequent in infants owing to the low concentration of manganese in human breast milk and varying concentrations in infant formulae.

Toxicity

Manganese toxicity of dietary origin has not been well documented. Toxicity has been observed only in workers exposed to high concentrations of manganese dust or fumes in air. For example, mine-workers in Chile exposed to manganese ore dust developed, possibly as a result of inhalation rather than ingestion, "manganic madness," manifested by psychosis, hallucinations, and extrapyramidal damage with features of parkinsonism.

Genetics

Mutations in the solute carrier (SLC) gene superfamily can lead to hypermanganesaemia with similar neurological symptoms and variants in some of these genes can impair the function of manganese-dependent enzymes. There is interest in polymorphisms in the MnSOD enzyme, which detoxifies reactive oxygen species in the mitochondria, and the role that these polymorphisms may play in the regulation of oxidative stress and the on-set of some chronic diseases, particularly cancer.

Assessing status

Progress in the field of manganese nutrition has been hampered because of the lack of a practical method for assessing manganese status. Blood manganese concentrations appear to reflect the body manganese status of rats fed deficient or adequate amounts of manganese, but consistent changes in blood or plasma manganese have not been observed in depleted or repleted human subjects. Researchers are actively investigating whether the activities of manganese-dependent enzymes, such as manganese-SOD in blood lymphocytes and blood arginase, may be of use in detecting low manganese intake; however, there is evidence that these enzymes can be influenced by certain disease states.

Requirements and dietary sources

Relatively high concentrations of manganese have been reported in cereals (20–30 mg/kg), brown bread (100–150 mg/kg), nuts (10–20 mg/kg), ginger (280 mg/kg), and tea (350–900 mg/kg dry tea). Concentrations of manganese in crops are dependent on soil factors such as pH, whereby increasing soil pH decreases plant uptake of manganese. Products of animal origin such as eggs, milk, fish, poultry, and red meat contain low amounts of manganese (Table 11.21) and dietary intakes may be declining partly because of nutrition transition in developing countries. Many multivitamin and mineral supplements for adults provide 2.5–5.0 mg of manganese.

There is currently no RDA set for dietary manganese; instead, there is an AI value [these values were established by the US Food and

Table 11.21 Dietary sources of manganese

Rich sources (>20 mg/kg)	Intermediate sources (1–5 mg/kg)	Poor sources (<1 mg/kg)
Nuts	Green leafy vegetables	Animal tissue
Wholegrain cereals	Dried fruits	Poultry
Dried legumes	Fresh fruits	Dairy products
Tea	Non-leafy vegetables	Seafood

Nutrition Board in 2001]: infants 0.003 mg (first 6 months), 0.6 mg (7–12 months), children 1.2 and 1.5 mg (1–3 and 4–8 years, respectively), teenage boys 1.9 and 2.2 mg (9–13 and 14–18 years, respectively), adult men 2.3 mg (19 years and older), teenage girls 1.6 mg (9–18 years), adult women 1.8 mg (19 years and older), pregnant women 2.0 mg, and lactating women 2.6 mg. The AI was set based on median intakes reported from the US Food and Drug Administration Total Diet Study.

In 2001, the US Food and Nutrition Board set the tolerable UL for manganese at 11 mg/day for adults (19 years and older). Elevated blood manganese concentrations and neurotoxicity were selected as the critical adverse effects on which to base their UL for manganese.

Micronutrient interactions

Iron–manganese interactions have been demonstrated whereby iron deficiency increased manganese absorption, and high amounts of dietary iron inhibit manganese absorption, possibly by competition for similar binding and absorption sites between non-haem iron and manganese.

11.13 Molybdenum

Molybdenum does not exist naturally in the pure metallic state but rather in association with other elements, or predominantly in solution as the molybdate anion. Insoluble molybdenum compounds include molybdenum dioxide and molybdenum disulfide. The metal has five oxidation states (2–6), of which +4 and +6 are the predominant species. Major molybdenum-containing ores are molybdenum sulphites and ferric molybdenum ores, usually produced as by-products of copper mining operations, while other molybdenum salts are by-products of uranium mining. Molybdenum is used mostly in metallurgical applications such as stainless steel and cast iron alloys, and in metal–ceramic composites. Molybdenum compounds have anticorrosive and lubricant properties and can act as chemical catalysts.

Molybdenum uptake into plants and hence into the food chain occurs mostly from alkaline or neutral soils. Water usually contains little molybdenum except near major mining operations.

Absorption, transport, and tissue distribution

Molybdenum is readily absorbed (40–100%) from foods and is widely distributed in cells and in the ECF. Some accumulation can occur in liver, kidneys, bones, and skin. The major excretory route of molybdenum after ingestion is the urine, with significant amounts also excreted in bile.

Metabolic functions and essentiality

Molybdenum functions as a cofactor for the iron- and flavin-containing enzymes that catalyze the hydroxylation of various substrates. The molybdenum cofactor in the enzymes aldehyde oxidase (oxidises and detoxifies purines and pyrimidines), xanthine oxidase/hydrogenase (production of uric acid from hypoxanthine and xanthine), and sulfite oxidase (conversion of sulfite to sulfate) has molybdenum incorporated as part of the molecule.

Deficiency symptoms

Although there is a clear biochemical basis for the essentiality of molybdenum, deficiency signs in humans and animals are difficult to induce. Naturally occurring deficiency, uncomplicated by molybdenum antagonists, is not known with certainty. In animal experiments, where large amounts of the molybdenum antagonist tungsten have been fed, deficiency signs are depressed food consumption and growth, impaired reproduction, and elevated copper concentrations in the liver and brain.

Toxicity

In humans high molybdenum intakes occur with industrial exposure or through food. It is associated with raised xanthine dehydrogenase activity, uricaemia, uricosuria and a higher incidence of gout. In areas with high geological molybdenum levels the human xanthine oxidase level is increased. Biochemical changes noted were hypoalbuminaemia, a rise in α-globulins, and raised serum bilirubin as sign of hepatotoxicity. It may be associated with oesophageal cancer.

Genetics

A rare unborn error of metabolism, resulting in the absence of the molybdenum pterin cofactor, may give some clue to the essentiality of molybdenum. These patients have severe neurological dysfunction, dislocated ocular lenses, mental retardation, and biochemical abnormalities, including increased urinary excretion of xanthine and sulfite and decreased urinary excretion of uric acid and sulfate.

Assessing status

Determining the body status of molybdenum is difficult. Homeostatic control of molybdenum ensures that plasma concentrations are not elevated, except after extremely high dietary intakes. Decreased urinary concentrations of sulphite, hypoxanthine, zorithine, and other sulphur metabolites, however, are generally indicative of impaired activities of the molybdoenzymes. Adult requirements for molybdenum have been estimated at about 45 μg/day (Institute of Medicine, USA, 2001). Average intakes tend to be considerably above this value. Milk, beans, bread, and cereals (especially the germ) are good sources of molybdenum, and water also contributes small amounts to the total dietary intakes.

In 2001, the US Food and Nutrition Board set the tolerable UL for molybdenum at 2 mg/day for adults (aged 19 years and older). Impaired reproduction and growth in animals were selected as the critical adverse effects on which to base their UL for molybdenum.

Micronutrient interactions

The major micronutrient interactions with molybdenum are those involving tungsten and copper. Molybdenum supplementation depletes body levels of the essential trace element, copper, and has been used as a chelating agent for conditions such as Wilson's disease, which cause elevated concentrations of copper in the body.

11.14 Fluoride

Fluorine, a gaseous halogen, occurs chiefly in its anionic form (as fluoride [F^-]) in rocks and soil as fluorspar and cryolite, but is widely distributed in other minerals. Fluoride is present in small but widely varying concentrations in practically all soils, water supplies, plants and animals, and is a constituent of all diets.

Absorption, transport and tissue distribution

Fluoride appears to be soluble and rapidly absorbed, and is distributed throughout the ECF in a manner similar to chloride. The concentrations of fluorine in blood, where it is bound to albumin, and tissues are small. The elimination of absorbed fluoride occurs almost exclusively via the kidneys. Fluoride is freely filtered through the glomerular capillaries and undergoes tubular reabsorption in varying degrees.

Fifty percent of orally ingested fluoride is absorbed from the gastrointestinal tract after approximately 30 minutes. In the absence of high dietary concentrations of calcium and certain other cations with which fluoride may form insoluble and poorly absorbed compounds, 80–90% is typically absorbed. Body fluid and tissue fluoride concentrations are proportional to the long-term level of intake; they are not homeostatically regulated. About 99% of the body's fluoride is found in calcified tissues (bone and teeth), to which it is strongly but not irreversibly bound.

In general, the bioavailability of fluoride is high, but it can be influenced to some extent by the vehicle with which it is ingested. When a soluble compound such as sodium fluoride is ingested with water, absorption is nearly complete. If it is ingested with milk, baby formula, or foods, especially those with high concentrations of calcium and certain other divalent or trivalent ions that form insoluble compounds, absorption may be reduced by 10–25%. Fluoride is absorbed passively from the stomach, but protein-bound organic fluoride is less readily absorbed.

The fractional retention (or balance) of fluoride at any age depends on the amount absorbed and the amount excreted. In healthy, young, or middle-aged adults, approximately 50% of absorbed fluoride is retained by uptake in calcified tissues and 50% is excreted in urine. In young children, as much as 80% can be retained owing to the increased uptake by the developing skeleton and teeth. In later life, it is likely that the fraction excreted is greater than the fraction retained. However, this possibility needs to be confirmed.

Metabolic function and essentiality

Although there is no known metabolic role in the body for fluorine, it is mainly associated with calcified tissue (bone and teeth). While the status of fluorine (fluoride) as an essential nutrient has been debated, the US Food and Nutrition Board in 1997 established a dietary reference intake for the ion that might suggest their willingness to consider fluorine to be a beneficial element for humans, if not an "essential nutrient." Likewise, and more recently, EFSA, in 2013, established AIs for fluoride, although stated that it is not an essential nutrient.

The function of fluoride appears to be in the crystalline structure of bones; fluoride forms calcium fluorapatite in teeth and bone. The incorporation of fluoride in these tissues is proportional to its total intake. There is an overall acceptance of a role for fluoride in the care of teeth. The cariostatic action (reduction in the risk of dental caries) of fluoride on erupted teeth of children and adults is owing to its effect in the metabolism of bacteria in dental plaque (i.e., reduced acid production) and on the dynamics of enamel demineralisation and remineralisation during an acidogenic challenge. The ingestion of fluoride during the pre-eruptive development of the teeth also has a cariostatic effect because of the uptake of fluoride by enamel crystallite and formation of fluorhydroxyapatite, which is less acid soluble than hydroxyapatite. When drinking water contains 1 mg/l there is a coincidental 50% reduction in tooth decay in children. Fluoride accretion in bone increases bone density by stimulating the formation of new bone, but excessive long-term intakes reduce bone strength and increase risk of fracture and skeletal fluorosis.

Deficiency symptoms

No signs of fluoride deficiency have been identified in humans. The lack of exposure to fluoride, or the ingestion of inadequate amounts of fluoride at any age, places the individual at increased risk for dental caries, even though tooth development *per se* will not be altered. Many studies conducted before the availability of fluoride-containing dental products demonstrated that dietary fluoride exposure is beneficial, owing to its ability to inhibit the development of dental caries in both children and adults. This was particularly evident in the past when the prevalence of dental caries in communities without water fluoridation was shown to be much higher than that in communities who had their water fluoridated. Both the intercommunity transport of foods and beverages and the use of fluoridated dental products have blurred the historical difference in the prevalence of dental caries between communities with and without water fluoridation. This is referred to as a halo or diffusion effect. The overall difference in caries prevalence between fluoridated and non-fluoridated area regions in the USA was reported to be 18% (data from a 1986–1987 national survey), whereas the majority of earlier studies reported differences of approximately 50%. Therefore, ingestion of adequate amounts of fluoride is of importance in the control of dental caries.

Toxicity

Fluorine, like other trace elements, is toxic when consumed in excessive amounts. The primary adverse effects associated with chronic, excessive fluoride intake are enamel and skeletal fluorosis. Enamel fluorosis is a dose-related effect caused by fluoride ingestion during the pre-eruptive development of the teeth. After the enamel has completed its pre-eruptive maturation, it is no longer susceptible. Inasmuch as enamel fluorosis is regarded as a cosmetic effect, it is the anterior teeth that are of most concern. The pre-eruptive maturation of the crowns of the anterior permanent teeth is finished and the risk of fluorosis is over by eight years of age. Therefore, fluoride intake up to the age of eight years is of most interest. Mild fluorosis (which is not readily apparent) has no effect on tooth function and may render the enamel more resistant to caries. In contrast, the moderate and severe forms of enamel fluorosis are generally characterised by aesthetically objectionable changes in tooth colour and surface irregularities.

Skeletal fluorosis has been regarded as having three stages. Stage 1 is characterised by occasional stiffness or pain in joints and some osteosclerosis of the pelvis and vertebrae, whereas the clinical signs in stages 2 and 3, which may be crippling, include dose-related calcification of ligaments, osteosclerosis, exostoses, and possibly osteoporosis of long bones, muscle wasting, and neurological defects owing to hypercalcification of vertebrae. The development of skeletal fluorosis and its severity are directly related to the level and duration of exposure. Most epidemiological research has indicated that an intake of at least 10 mg/ day for 10 or more years is needed to produce the clinical signs of the milder form of the condition. Crippling skeletal fluorosis is extremely rare. For example, only five cases have been confirmed in the USA since the mid-1960s.

Assessing status

A high proportion of the dietary intake of fluoride appears in urine. Urinary output in general reflects the dietary intake.

Requirements and dietary sources

Most foods have fluoride concentrations well below 0.05 mg/100 g. Exceptions to this observation include fluoridated water, beverages, and some infant formulae that are made or reconstituted with fluoridated water, teas, and some marine fish. Because of the ability of tea leaves to accumulate fluoride to concentrations exceeding 10 mg/100 g dry weight, brewed tea contains fluoride concentrations ranging from 1 to 6 mg/l depending on the amount of dry tea used, the water fluoride concentration and brewing time.

Intake from fluoridated dental products can add considerable fluoride, often approaching or exceeding intake from the diet, particularly in young children who have poor control of the swallowing reflex. The major contributors to non-dietary fluoride intake are toothpastes, mouth rinses, and dietary fluoride supplements.

In 1997 the US Food and Nutrition Board established AI values for fluoride: infants 0.01 mg (first 6 months), 0.5 mg (7–12 months), children and adolescents 0.7, 1.0, and 2.0 mg (1–3, 4–8, and 9–13 years, respectively), male adolescents and adults 3 and 4 mg (14–18 and 19 years and older, respectively), female adolescents and adults 3 mg (over 14 years, including pregnancy and lactation). The AI is the intake value of fluoride (from all sources) that reduces the occurrence of dental caries maximally in a group of individuals without causing unwanted side-effects. With fluoride, the data are strong on caries risk reduction but the evidence upon which to base an actual requirement is scant, thus driving the decision to adopt an AI as the reference value. More recently, EFSA in 2013 suggested that as fluoride is not an essential nutrient, and EAR could not be defined but rather setting AIs was more appropriate. The AI of fluoride from all sources for both children and adults can be set at 0.05 mg/kg body weight per day. Thus, for adolescents and adults the AIs from all sources range from 2.2 to 3.4 mg/day, dependent on sex and age-grouping.

Based largely on the data on the association of high fluoride intakes with risk of skeletal fluorosis in children (>8 years) and adults, the US Food and Nutrition Board has established a tolerable UL of fluoride of 10 mg/day for children (>8 years), adolescents, and adults, as well as pregnant and lactating women. EFSA set tolerable UL of fluoride of 5 mg/day for children (9–14 years) and 7 mg/day for those aged ≥15 years (including pregnancy and lactation).

Micronutrient interactions

The rate and extent of fluoride absorption from the gastrointestinal tract are reduced by the ingestion of foods particularly rich in calcium (such as milk or infant formulae).

11.15 Other elements

In addition to the essential elements discussed in this chapter, other elements in the periodic table may emerge as being essential for human nutrition. For 15 elements, aluminum, arsenic, boron, bromine, cadmium, chromium, fluorine, germanium, lead, lithium, nickel, rubidium, silicon, tin, and vanadium, specific biochemical reactions have not been defined and their suspected essentiality is based on circumstantial evidence from data emanating from animal models, from essential functions in lower forms of life, or from biochemical actions consistent with a biological role or beneficial action in humans. Two elements, fluorine and lithium, have beneficial actions when ingested in high (pharmacological) amounts. Lithium is used to treat bipolar disorder, and fluorine (as fluoride) is discussed in Section 11.14 because of its important beneficial actions in preventing dental caries in susceptible population groups. Some have indicated that the observed beneficial effects of chromium on rodent models of insulin resistance and diabetes are best interpreted in terms of a pharmacological role for chromium rather than a role based on essentiality. The EFSA has no longer proposed a Dietary Reference Value (DRV) for chromium owing to the general lack of effect of chromium in human studies. The estimated or suspected requirement of all of these elements (including the essential trace elements, iodine, selenium, and molybdenum) is usually less than 1 mg/day and they are defined as ultratrace elements. Cobalt is not included in the list of ultratrace elements because the only requirement for cobalt is as a constituent of preformed vitamin B_{12}.

These elements are not discussed at length in this chapter and the reader is referred to other reading material. For completeness, three tables, on absorption, transport, and storage characteristics (Table 11.22), excretion, retention, and possible biological roles of the ultratrace elements (Table 11.23), and human body content and food sources (Table 11.24) are included here.

11.16 Perspectives on the future

The preceding parts of this chapter have highlighted some issues in the area of minerals and trace elements for which we have an incomplete understanding. In the future, nutritional scientists, dieticians, and other health care professionals will have to:

- obtain a greater understanding of the molecular and cellular processes involved in the intestinal absorption and tissue uptake of certain minerals and trace elements
- identify functional markers of mineral and trace element status. These markers could be defined as a physiological/biochemical factor that (1) is related to function or effect of the nutrient in target tissue(s) and (2) is affected by dietary intake or stores of the nutrient (which may include markers of disease risk). Examples of such indicators or markers are those related to risk of chronic diseases, such as osteoporosis, coronary heart disease, hypertension or diabetes. However, for many nutrients there are as yet no functional indicators that respond to dietary intake and, in such cases, nutrient requirements are established using more traditional approaches, such as balance data. The lack of functional markers of mineral and trace element status is a significant disadvantage for studies relating their intake or status to health outcomes such as hypertension, cardiovascular disease, osteoporosis, diabetes, and other disorders. For example, widely used biochemical indicators of essential trace element status generally lack both the sensitivity and the specificity that are required to define optimal intake at various stages of the life cycle. A number of potential "sensors" of cellular copper, zinc, and manganese status have been proposed and merit further evaluation. The judicious application of methods in molecular biology (including genomics and proteomics) and noninvasive imaging techniques is likely to provide new breakthroughs and rapid advances in the nutrition and biology of trace elements.
- evaluate further the specific health risks associated with marginal deficiencies of various minerals and trace elements. There is a need to determine reliable relationships between mineral status and disease and then to demonstrate that the incidence or severity of specific diseases is reversible by repletion of mineral status. The development and validation of reliable assessment tools and functional markers of mineral status are the utmost priority for this field.
- define the adverse effects of acute and chronic high intakes of some minerals and trace elements. Interest in mineral fortification of foods is higher than ever before. Governments worldwide are increasingly tackling the common deficiencies of iron and iodine by adding these minerals to widely consumed staple foods such as cereal flours, sugar, or salt. The food industry in industrialised countries is manufacturing an increasing number of

Table 11.22 Absorption, transport and storage characteristics of the ultratrace elements

Element	Major mechanism(s) for homeostasis	Means of absorption	Percentage of ingested absorbed	Transport and storage vehicles
Aluminum	Absorption	Uncertain; some evidence for passive diffusion through the paracellular pathway; also, evidence for active absorption through processes shared with active processes of calcium; probably occurs in proximal duodenum; citrate combined with aluminum enhances absorption	<1%	Transferrin carries aluminum in plasma; bone a possible storage site
Arsenic	Urinary excretion; inorganic arsenic as mostly dimethylarsinic acid and organic arsenic as mostly arsenobetaine	Inorganic arsenate becomes sequestered in or on mucosal tissue, then absorption involves a simple movement down a concentration gradient; organic arsenic absorbed mainly by simple diffusion through lipid regions of the intestinal boundary	Soluble inorganic forms, >90%; slightly soluble inorganic forms, 20–30%; inorganic forms with foods, 60–75%; methylated forms, 45–90%	Before excretion inorganic arsenic is converted into monomethylarsonic acid and dimethylarsinic acid; arsenobetaine not biotransformed; arsenocholine transformed to arsenobetaine
Boron	Urinary excretion	Ingested boron is converted into $B(OH)_3$ and absorbed in this form, probably by passive diffusion	>90%	Boron transported through the body as undissociated $B(OH)_3$; bone a possible storage site
Cadmium	Absorption	May share a common absorption mechanism with other metals (e.g. zinc) but mechanism is less efficient for cadmium	5%	Incorporated into metallothionein which probably is both a storage and transport vehicle
Germanium	Urinary excretion	Has not been conclusively determined but probably is by passive diffusion	>90%	None identified
Lead	Absorption	Uncertain; thought to be by passive diffusion in small intestine but evidence has been presented for an active transport perhaps involving the system for calcium	Adults 5–15%, children 40–50%	Bone is a repository for lead
Lithium	Urinary excretion	Passive diffusion by paracellular transport via the tight junctions and pericellular spaces	Lithium chloride highly absorbed: >90%	Bone can serve as a store for lithium
Nickel	Both absorption and urinary excretion	Uncertain, evidence for both passive diffusion (perhaps as an amino acid or other low molecular weight complex) and energy-driven transport; occurs in the small intestine	<10% with food	Transported in blood principally bound to serum albumin with small amounts bound to L-histidine and α_2-macroglobulin; no organ accumulates physiological amounts of nickel
Rubidium	Excretion through kidney and intestine	Resembles potassium in its pattern of absorption; rubidium and potassium thought to share a transport system	Highly absorbed	None identified
Silicon	Both absorption and urinary excretion	Mechanisms involved in intestinal absorption have not been described	Food silicon near 50%; insoluble or poorly soluble silicates ~1%	Silicon in plasma believed to exist as undisassociated monomeric silicic acid
Tin	Absorption	Mechanisms involved in intestinal absorption have not been described	~3%; percentage increases when very low amounts are ingested	None identified; bone might be a repository
Vanadium	Absorption	Vanadate has been suggested to be absorbed through phosphate or other anion transport systems; vanadyl has been suggested to use iron transport systems; absorption occurs in the duodenum	<10%	Converted into vanadyltransferrin and vanadyl-ferritin; whether transferrin is the transport vehicle and ferritin is the storage vehicle for vanadium remains to be determined; bone is a repository for excess vanadium

Table 11.23 Excretion, retention, and possible biological roles of the ultratrace elements

Element	Organs of high content (typical concentration)	Major excretory route after ingestion	Molecules of biological importance	Possible biological role
Aluminum	Bone (1–12 μg/g) Lung (35 μg/g)	Urine; also significant amounts in bile	Aluminum binds to proteins, nucleotides and phospholipids; aluminum-bound transferrin apparently is a transport molecule	Enzyme activator
Arsenic	Hair (0.65 μg/g) Nails (0.35 μg/g) Skin (0.10 μg/g)	Urine	Methylation of inorganic oxyarsenic anions occurs in organisms ranging from microbial to mammalian; methylated end-products include arsenocholine, arsenobetaine, dimethylarsinic acid and methylarsonic acid; arsenite methyltransferase and monomethylarsonic acid methyltransferase use S-adenosylmethionine for the methyl donor	Metabolism of methionine, or involved in labile methyl metabolism; regulation of gene expression
Boron	Bone (1.6 μg/g) Fingernails (15 μg/g) Hair (1 μg/g) Teeth (5 μg/g)	Urine	Boron biochemistry essentially that of boric acid, which forms ester complexes with hydroxyl groups, preferably those adjacent and *ds*, in organic compounds; five naturally occurring boron esters (all antibiotics) synthesised by various bacteria have been characterised	Cell membrane function or stability such that it influences the response to hormone action, transmembrane signaling or transmembrane movement of regulatory cations or anions
Bromine	Hair (30 μg/g) Liver (40 μg/g) Lung (6.0 μg/g) Testis (5.0 μg/g)	Urine	Exists as Br– ion *in vivo*, binds to proteins and amino acids	Electrolyte balance
Cadmium	Kidney (14 μg/g) Liver (4 μg/g)	Urine and gastrointestinal tract	Metallothionein, a high sulfhydryl-containing protein involved in regulating cadmium distribution	Involved in metallathionein metabolism and utilisation
Germanium	Bone (9 μg/g) Liver (0.3 μg/g) Pancreas (0.2 μg/g) Testis (0.5 μg/g)	Urine	None identified	Role in immune function
Lead	Aorta (1–2 μg/g) Bone (25 μg/g) Kidney (1–2 μg/g) Liver (1–2 μg/g)	Urine; also significant amounts in bile	Plasma lead mostly bound to albumin; blood lead binds mostly to haemoglobin but some binds a low molecular weight protein in erythrocytes	Facilitates iron absorption and/or utilisation
Lithium	Adrenal gland (60 ng/g) Bone (100 ng/g) Lymph nodes (200 ng/g) Pituitary gland (135 ng/g)	Urine	None identified	Regulation of some endocrine function

Nickel	Adrenal glands (25 ng/g) Bone (33 ng/g) Kidney (10 ng/g) Thyroid (30 ng/g)	Urine as low molecular weight complexes	Binding of Ni^{2-} by various ligands including amino acids (especially histidine and cysteine), proteins (especially albumin) and a macroglobulin called nickeloplasmin important in transport and excretion; Ni^{2+} component of urease; Ni^{3+} essential for enzymic hydrogenation, desulfurisation and carboxylation reactions in mostly anaerobic microorganisms	Cofactor or structural component in specific metalloenzymes; role in a metabolic pathway involving vitamin B^{12} and folic acid; role similar to potassium; neurophysiological function
Rubidium	Brain (4 µg/g) Kidney (5 µg/g) Liver (6.5 µg/g) Testis (20 µg/g)	Urine; also significant amounts excreted through intestinal tract	None identified	Role similar to potassium; neurophysiological function
Silicon	Aorta (16 µg/g) Bone (18 µg/g) Skin (4 µg/g) Tendon (12 µg/g)	Urine	Silicic acid (SiOH4) is the form believed to exist in plasma; magnesium orthosilicate is probably the form of silicon in urine. The bound form of silicon has never been rigorously identified	Structural role in some mucopolysaccharides or collagen; role in the initiation of calcification and in collagen formation
Tin	Bone (0.8 µg/g) Kidney (0.2 µg/g) Liver (0.4 µg/g)	Urine; also significant amounts in bile	Sn^{2+} is absorbed and excreted more readily than Sn^{4+}	Role in some redox reactions
Vanadium	Bone (120 ng/g) Kidney (120 ng/g) Liver (120 ng/g) Spleen (120 ng/g) Testis (200 ng/g)	Urine; also significant amounts in bile	Vanadyl (VO^{2+}), vanaclate ($H_2VO^-_4$ or VO^-_3) and peroxovanadyl [V-OO]; VO^{2+} complexes with proteins, especially those associated with iron (e.g. transferrin, haemoglobin)	Lower forms of life have haloperoxiclases that require vanadium for activity; a similar role may exist in higher forms of life

Reproduced from Nielsen (1999) in Sadler *et al. Encyclopaedia of Human Nutrition,* copyright 1999 with permission of Elsevier.
None of the suggested biological functions or roles of any of the ultratrace elements has been conclusively or unequivocally identified in higher forms of life.

Table 11.24 Human body content and deficient, typical, and rich sources of intakes of ultratrace elements

Element	Apparent deficient intake (species)	Human body content	Typical human daily dietary intake	Rich sources
Aluminum	160 μg/kg (goat)	30–50 mg	2–10 mg	Baked goods prepared with chemical leavening agents (e.g. baking powder), processed cheese, grains, vegetables, herbs, tea, antacids, buffered analgesics
Arsenic	<25 μg/kg (chicks) <35 μg/kg (goat) <15 μg/kg (hamster) <30 μg/kg (rat)	1–2 mg	12–60 μg	Shellfish, fish, grain, cereal products
Boron	<0.3 mg/kg (chick) 0.25–0.35 mg/day (human) <0.3 mg/kg (rat)	10–20 mg	0.5–3.5 mg	Food and drink of plant origin, especially noncitrus fruits, leafy vegetables, nuts, pulses, legumes, wine, cider, beer
Bromine	0.8 mg/kg (goat)	200–350 mg	2–8 mg	Grain, nuts, fish
Cadmium	<5 μg/kg (goat) <4 μg/kg (rat)	5–20 mg	10–20 μg	Shellfish, grains, especially those grown on high-cadmium soils, leafy vegetables
Germanium	0.7 mg/kg (rat)	3 mg	0.4–3.4 mg	Wheat bran, vegetables, leguminous seeds
Lead	<32 μg/kg (pig) <45 μg/kg (rat)	Children less than 10 years old 2 mg, Adults 120 mg	15–100 μg	Seafood, plant foodstuffs grown under high lead conditions
Lithium	<1.5 mg/kg (goat) <15 μg/kg (rat)	350 μg	200–600 μg	Eggs, meat, processed meat, fish, milk, milk products, potatoes, vegetables (content varies with geological origin)
Nickel	<100 μg/kg (goat) <20 μg/kg (rat)	1–2 mg	70–260 μg	Chocolate, nuts, dried beans and peas, grains
Rubidium	180 μg/kg (goat)	360 mg	1–5 mg	Coffee, black tea, fruits and vegetables (especially asparagus), poultry, fish
Silicon	<20 mg kg (chick) <4.5 mg/kg (rat)	2–3 g	20–50 mg	Unrefined grains of high fiber content, cereal products
Tin	<20 μg/kg (rat)	7–14 mg	1–40 mg	Canned foods
Vanadium	<10 μg/kg (goat)	100 μg	10–30 μg	Shellfish, mushrooms, parsley, dill, seed, black pepper, some prepared foods

Reproduced from Nielsen (1999) in Sadler *et al. Encyclopaedia of Human Nutrition,* copyright 1999 with permission of Elsevier.

functional foods designed to provide the consumer with protection against diseases of major public health significance, such as osteoporosis, cancer, and heart disease, and fortified with minerals such as calcium, selenium, zinc, magnesium, and copper. The same minerals are added to dietetic products, including infant foods, foods for pregnant and lactating women, and enteral feeds for hospital patients, all designed to cover the nutritional requirements of specific consumers. Voluntary fortification practices have been shown to increase intake and improve status of important minerals in population groups and do not appear to contribute appreciably to risk of adverse effects.

- elucidate the impact of single nucleotide polymorphisms in the human genome on mineral and trace element dietary requirements. The key to future applications of the DNA polymorphisms will be to mine the human genome for DNA sequence information that can be used to define biovariation in nutrient absorption and use. More nutritional biology research is needed to correlate gene polymorphism with nutritional outcomes.
- Explore how sustainability policies will influence mineral and trace element intakes and status. Countries with identified micronutrient deficiencies would benefit from sustainable dietary diversification which could potentially be introduced through biofortification and agricultural diversification. In combination, improvements in education and the provision of nutritional knowledge are key to sustainably addressing malnutrition.

References

Aburto, N.J., Ziolkovska, A., Hooper, L. *et al.* (2013). Effect of lower sodium intake on health: systematic review and meta analyses. *BMJ*. **346**: f1326

Beal, T., Massiot, E., Arsenault, J.E. *et al.* (2017). Global trends in dietary micronutrient supplies and estimated prevalence of inadequate intakes. *PLoS ONE*. **12**(4), e0175554.

Bjorklund, G. (2015). Selenium as an antidote in the treatment of mercury intoxication. *Biometals* **28**, 605–614.

Bost M, Houdart S, Oberli M *et al.* (2016). Dietary copper and human health: Current evidence and unresolved issues. *Journal of Trace Elements in Medicine and Biology*. **35**, 107–115.

Combs, G.F. (2015). Biomarkers of selenium status. *Nutrients* **7**, 2209–2236

Committee on Medical Aspects of Food Policy. (1991). Report on Health and Social Subjects 41. Dietary Reference Values for Food Energy and Nutrients in the UK. London: HMSO, Department of Health, London.

Danzeisen, R., Araya, M., Harrison, B. *et al.* (2007). How reliable and robust are current biomarkers for copper status? *British Journal of Nutrition*. **98**, 676–683.

Day, K., Adamski, M.M., Dordevic, A.L. *et al.* (2015). *Genetic* variations as modifying factors to dietary zinc requirements – A systematic review. *Nutrients*. **9**, 148; doi:10.3390/nu9020148

Dhar, S.K. and St. Clair, D.K. (2012). Manganese superoxide dismutase regulation and cancer. *Free Radical Biology and Medicine*. **52**, 2209–2222.

European Food Safety Authority (2006). Tolerable upper intake levels for vitamins and minerals. European Food Safety Authority, Parma, Italy. http://www.efsa.europa.eu/sites/default/files/efsa_rep/blobserver_assets/ndatolerableuil.pdf.

EFSA NDA Panel (EFSA Panel on Dietetic Products, Nutrition and Allergies). (2015a). Scientific Opinion on Dietary Reference Values for calcium. *EFSA Journal*. **13**(5):4101, 82 pp. doi:10.2903/j.efsa.2015.4101

EFSA NDA Panel (EFSA Panel on Dietetic Products, Nutrition and Allergies). (2015b). Scientific Opinion on Dietary Reference Values for magnesium. *EFSA Journal*. **13**(7):4186, 63 pp. doi:10.2903/j.efsa.2015.4186

EFSA NDA Panel (EFSA Panel on Dietetic Products, Nutrition and Allergies). (2015c). Scientific Opinion on Dietary Reference Values for phosphorus. *EFSA Journal*. **13**(7):4185, 54 pp. doi:10.2903/j.efsa.2015.4185

EFSA NDA Panel (EFSA Panel on Dietetic Products, Nutrition and Allergies). (2015d). Scientific Opinion on Dietary Reference Values for iron. *EFSA Journal*. **13**(10):4254, 115 pp. doi:10.2903/j.efsa.2015.4254

EFSA NDA Panel (EFSA Panel on Dietetic Products, Nutrition and Allergies). (2014a). Scientific Opinion on Dietary Reference Values for zinc. *EFSA Journal*. **12**(10):3844, 76 pp. doi:10.2903/j.efsa.2014.3844

EFSA NDA Panel (EFSA Panel on Dietetic Products, Nutrition and Allergies). (2014b). Scientific Opinion on Dietary Reference Values for selenium. *EFSA Journal*. **12**(10):3846, 67 pp. doi:10.2903/j.efsa.2014.3846

EFSA NDA Panel (EFSA Panel on Dietetic Products, Nutrition and Allergies). (2015e). Scientific Opinion on Dietary Reference Values for calcium. *EFSA Journal*. **13**(5):4101, 82 pp. doi:10.2903/j.efsa.2015.4101

Fairweather-Tait, S.J., Collings, R., and Hurst, R. (2010). Selenium bioavailability: current knowledge and future research requirements. *American Journal of Clinical Nutrition*. **91** (suppl): 1484S–91S.

Finglas, P.M., Roe, M.A., Pinchen, H.M. *et al.* (2015). *McCance & Widdowson's The Composition of Foods*, 7e. Cambridge: Royal Society of Chemistry.

Freeland-Graves, J.H., Mousa, T.Y., and Kim, S. (2016). International variability in diet and requirements of manganese: Causes and consequences. *Journal of Trace Elements in Medicine and Biology*. **38**, 24–32.

Gibson, R.S., King, J.C., and Lowe, N. (2016). A review of dietary zinc recommendations. *Food and Nutrition Bulletin*. **37** (4), 443–460.

Hallberg, L., Sandstrom, B., Aggett, P.J. (1993). Iron, Zinc, and Other Trace Elements. In: (Eds) J.S. Garrow, W.P.T. James, and A. Ralph. *Human Nutrition and Dietetics*, 9e. London: Churchill Livingstone.

Harding, K.B., Pena-Rosas, J.P., Webster, A.C. *et al.* (2017). Iodine supplementation for women during the preconception, pregnancy and postpartum period (Review). *Cochrane Database of Systematic Reviews*. (3). DOI: 10.1002/14651858.cd011761.pub2

Holland, B., Welch, A.A., Unwin, I.D. *et al.* (Eds). (1995). *McCance & Widdowson's The Composition of Foods*, 5e. Royal Society of Chemistry and Ministry of Agriculture, Fisheries and Food. London: HMSO.

Institute of Medicine (USA). (1997). *Dietary Reference Intakes for Calcium, Phosphorus, Magnesium, Vitamin D, and Fluoride*. Washington, DC: National Academy Press.

Institute of Medicine (USA). (2001). *Dietary Reference Intakes for Vitamin A, Vitamin K, Arsenic, Boron, Chromium, Copper, Iodine, Iron, Manganese, Molybdenum, Nickel, Silicon, Vanadium, and Zinc*. Washington, DC: National Academy Press.

Institute of Medicine. (2011). *Dietary reference intakes for calcium and vitamin D*. Washington, DC: National Academy Press.

Maret, W. (2009). Molecular aspects of human cellular zinc homeostasis: redox control of zinc potentials and zinc signals. *Biometals*. **22**: 149–157.

Mills, C.F. (Ed.) (1989). *Zinc in Human Biology*. London: Springer-Verlag.

Nielsen, F. (1999). In: (Ed. M.J. Sadler, J.J. Strain, and B. Caballero) *Encyclopedia of Human Nutrition*. London: Academic Press.

Nicastro, H.L., Dunn, B.K. (2013). Selenium and prostate cancer prevention: Insights from the Selenium and Vitamin E Cancer Prevention Trial (SELECT). *Nutrients*. **5**, 1122–1148.

Pearce, E.N., Lazarus, J.H., Moreno-Reyes, R. *et al.* (2016). Consequences of iodine deficiency and excess in pregnant women: an overview of current knowns and unknowns. *American Journal of Clinical Nutrition*. **104** (suppl): 918S–23S.

Rayman, M.P. (2000). The importance of selenium to human health. *Lancet*. **356**: 233–241.

Ristic-Medic, D., Piskackova, Z., Hooper, L. *et al.* (2009). Methods of assessment of iodine status in humans: a systematic review. *American Journal of Clinical Nutrition*. **89**(suppl): 2052S–69S.

Reilly, C. (1996). *Selenium in Food and Health*. London: Blackie.

Reilly, C. (2006). *The Nutritional Trace Metals*. Oxford: Blackwell Publishing.

Sánchez-Castillo, C.P. and James, W.P.T. (1999). In: (Ed. M.J. Sadler, J.J. Strain, and B. Caballero) *Encyclopedia of Human Nutrition*. London: Academic Press.

Sanna, A., Firinu, D., Zavattari, P. *et al.* (2018). Zinc status and autoimmunity: a systematic review and meta-analysis. *Nutrients.* **10**, 68; doi:10.3390/nu10010068.

Steinbrenner, H., Speckmann, B., and Klotz, L.-O. (2016). Selenoproteins: Antioxidant selenoenzymes and beyond. *Archives of Biochemistry and Biophysics.* **595**, 113–119.

Strain, J.J., Benzie, I.F.F. (1999). In: (Ed. M.J. Sadler, J.J. Strain, and B. Caballero) *Encyclopedia of Human Nutrition*. London: Academic Press.

Tripathi, D.K., Singh, V., Gangwar, S. *et al.* (2015). Micronutrients and their diverse role in agricultural crops: advances and future perspectives. *Acta Physiologiae Plantarum.* **37**, 139.

Velasco, I., Bath, S.C., and Rayman, M.P. (2018). Iodine as essential nutrient during the first 1000 days of life. *Nutrients.* **10**, 290; doi:10.3390/nu10030290.

Vincent, J. (2014). Is chromium pharmacologically relevant? *Journal of Trace Elements in Medicine and Biology.* **28**, 397–405.

Vinceti, M., Filippini, T., Del Giovane, C. *et al.* (2018). Selenium for preventing cancer (Review). *Cochrane Database of Systematic Reviews.* (1). DOI: 10.1002/14651858.CD005195.pub4.

WHO. (2014). Comprehensive implementation plan on maternal, infant and young child nutrition (WHO/NMH/NHD/14.1). Geneva: World Health Organization.

WHO. (2015). *The global prevalence of anaemia in 2011.* Geneva: World Health Organization.

Zimmermann, M.B., Jooste, P.L., and Pandav, C.S. (2008). Iodine-deficiency disorders. *Lancet.* **372**, 1251–62.

Further reading

Bowman, B., Russel, R. (Eds). (2001). *Present Knowledge in Nutrition,* 8e. Washington, DC: ILSI Press.

Passmore, R., Eastwood, M.A. (Eds). (1986). *Davidsons and Passmore Human Nutrition and Dietetics*, 8e. London: Churchill Livingstone.

Optimal Nutrition Symposium. (1999). A series of papers. *Proceedings of the Nutrition Society*, **58**: 395–512.

Sadler, M.J., Strain, J.J., and Caballero, B. (Eds). (1999). *Encyclopedia of Human Nutrition*, Vol. 3, Parts 1–3. London: Academic Press.

Websites

Online Mendelian Genetics in Man (OMIM) website at the National Institute for Biotechnology Information: http://www. ncbi.nlm.nih.gov/Omim

12 Phytochemicals

Gary Williamson

Key messages

- Commonly-studied phytochemicals (polyphenols, carotenoids and glucosinolates) are derived from plants and consumed regularly in the diet.
- The pathways of absorption and metabolism are well established, and involve digestion of attached chemical groups, followed by absorption either in the small intestine or after catabolic reactions by gut microbiota.
- Phytochemicals act by specific mechanisms and regular consumption in foods reduces the risk of some chronic diseases: polyphenols against type 2 diabetes; polyphenols and carotenoids against cardiovascular disease; glucosinolates against colon cancer; carotenoids against age-related macular degeneration and prostate cancer.

12.1 Introduction to phytochemicals

What are phytochemicals?

The term "phytochemicals" literally means chemicals from plants, but sometimes implies naturally-occurring plant secondary metabolites, present in foods and beverages, which have possible biological activities and effects on health when consumed orally. Many different types are present in foods and beverages, but here the focus will be on the most abundant and well-studied, namely the polyphenols, carotenoids, and glucosinolates. In plants, phytochemicals protect against UV light, pests, infection, and oxidative stress. In foods, they contribute to nutrition, but can also confer colour and astringent/bitter sensory properties, and these factors influence nutrition via food preference and choice.

Why are phytochemicals not classed as vitamins?

Phytochemicals are not strictly classed as vitamins or nutrients as they are not stored in the body, but exert an effect via a regular and sustained mild pharmacological-type action. They are metabolised in the body by xenobiotic-metabolising enzymes, by the gut microbiota, or via pathways which are normally considered as primary metabolism. They are part of a healthy diet as they are present in fruits, vegetables, and products derived from them such as coffee, tea and cocoa. Normally they are consumed every day, and the amount in the diet is very much dependent on the specific foods eaten. There are no recommended intake values for phytochemicals as there are for vitamins, but there are many claims made throughout the world on their health benefits. There are

Introduction to Human Nutrition, Third Edition. Edited on behalf of The Nutrition Society by Susan A. Lanham-New, Thomas R. Hill, Alison M. Gallagher and Hester H. Vorster.

Companion website: www.wiley.com/go/lanham-new/humannutrition

some comparisons to vitamins, however. Although essential amounts of vitamin C are required to prevent the deficiency disease of scurvy, the benefits of taking larger quantities either in food or supplements is less well established (see Chapter 10 on vitamins). It is this type of action that phytochemicals display, where the biological effects of both above-deficiency amounts of vitamin C or of phytochemicals are to counteract the effects of stress in the widest sense. In this case, stress can be derived from, for example, ageing processes to biochemical changes arising from post-prandial metabolism of nutrients.

Phytochemicals not covered in this chapter

Phytochemicals consist of a wide range of compounds, but the three main classes which will be considered here are polyphenols, glucosinolates, and non-vitamin A precursor carotenoids (Fig. 12.1) as they are the most widely consumed in the Western diet. Other phytochemicals occurring in small amounts will not be covered here as they are only consumed in minor amounts from specific foods. Terpenoids are a diverse group of compounds which often have potent sensory properties, but are present only at low amounts in foods, although they can be present at high levels in herbal medicines. Diterpenes, such as cafestol and kahweol, are present in some types of coffee and in some situations may increase cholesterol levels, and carnosol is present in rosemary with claimed effects on health. Alkaloids are found in some plants and include drugs and toxins, but their level is low in regularly-consumed foods of good quality; for example, glycoalkaloids are toxic compounds mostly present in the parts of the potato which have turned green or have sprouted. Allyl sulphides are found in Allium vegetables and may have some health benefits, notably as reported for garlic. Saponins in beans and grains have a mild detergent like action and can lead to formation of weak foams, but any effects on health are not well-studied.

12.2 Nomenclature and chemical structures

Polyphenols

In the diet, polyphenols consists of three main sub-groups, the phenolic acids/derivatives, the broad flavonoid class, and the isoflavones (Fig. 12.1). It is often stated that there are many thousands of flavonoids made by plants, and while this is true chemically, the number which are present and relevant to health in commonly-consumed foods and beverages is much smaller. Chemically, flavonoids and isoflavones consist of a basic three-ring structure, where the B-ring is a benzene ring decorated with hydroxyl groups. Phenolic acids are single phenolic rings, and contain an aliphatic side chain with a terminal carboxyl group. Multiple phenolic acids can be linked together to form more tannin-like structures, such as ellagic acid or curcumin. Some common structures are shown in Figure 12.1.

The nomenclature of polyphenols is highly complicated, since they have been named historically in various ways mostly after the first species they were obtained from. For example, hesperidin was first isolated in the nineteenth century from citrus trees and was named after the word "hesperidium", which refers to fruit produced by citrus trees. Quercetin was also first reported in the nineteenth century, from oak trees of the genus Quercus. The orange-coloured pigment pelargonidin, an anthocyanin, was first isolated from Geranium flowers of the Genus Pelargonium. On the other hand, the word anthocyanin is derived not from its source, but from its properties: from the Greek for flower (ἄνθός) and blue (κυάνός). Chlorogenic acids were named in a way describing their properties, but only after a chemical treatment: the Greek χλωρός (green) and -γένος (derived from), which describes the green colour obtained after oxidation. The IUPAC name for chlorogenic acid, one of the more simple phenolic structures, is (1S,3R,4R,5R)-3-[[(2E)-3-(3,4-dihydroxyphenyl) prop-2-enoyl]oxy]-1,4,5-trihydroxycyclohexane-carboxylic acid, which is even less memorable and helpful! Since the common names have been around for a long time, they are unlikely to change, but they can add to confusion as there are some very similar names which refer to different compounds. Hesperidin is hesperetin-7-O-rhamnoglucoside, where the flavonoid moiety itself is called hesperetin and, when alone, is often referred to as an "aglycone" (literally without the attached sugar). Many of the flavonoids have a sugar or several sugars attached, which is how the plant tames

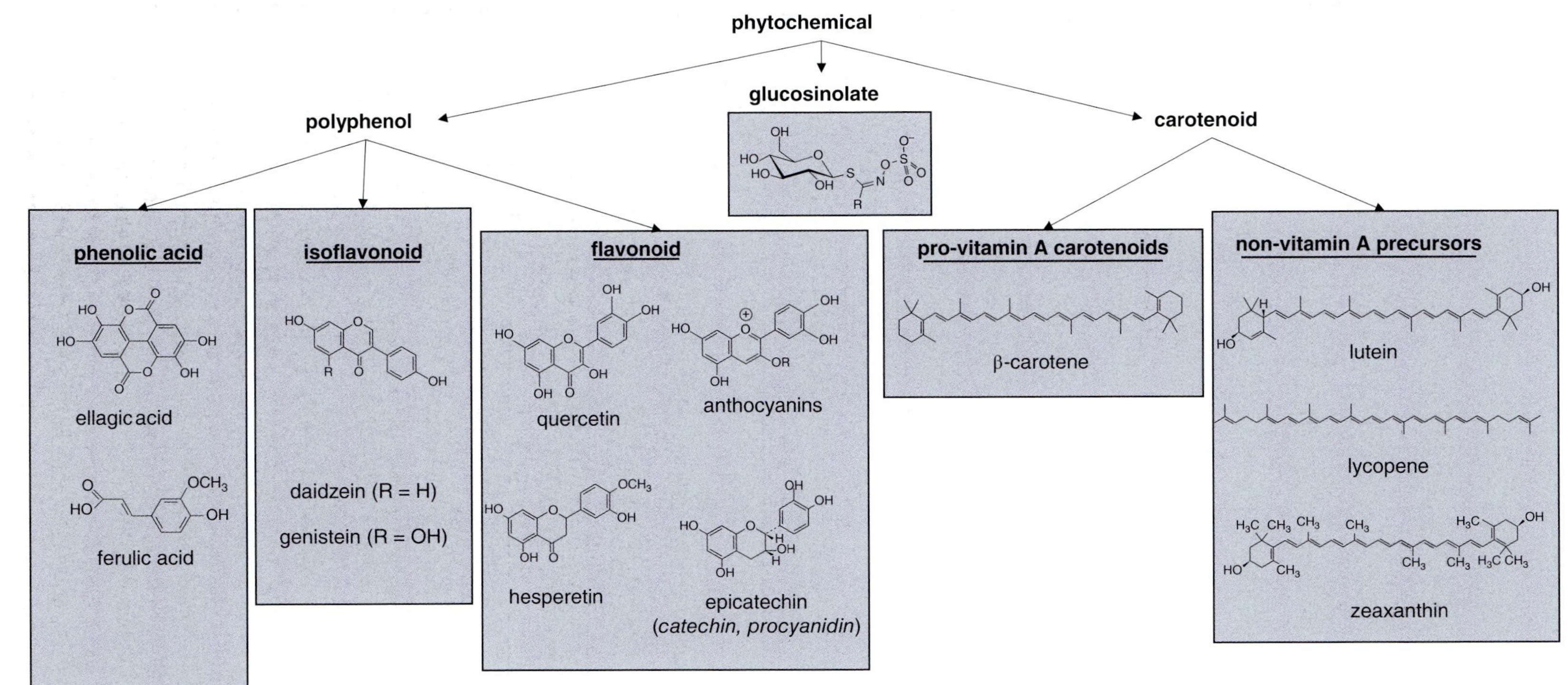

Figure 12.1 Phytochemical families and structures.

the flavonoids in planta. This also adds confusion to the nomenclature, since, for example, the word "rutin" is commonly used for quercetin-3-O-rhamnoglucoside, which is the quercetin moiety chemically attached via the carbon(3) position to two sugars, rhamnose and glucose. When linked to sugars or organic acids, polyphenols are mostly water soluble and unable to passively cross biological membranes. The aglycone forms are somewhat less water soluble and able to diffuse across membranes. Flavonoids such as epicatechins from tea are water soluble in their naturally-occurring aglycone forms and have a limited but significant ability to cross biological membranes.

Carotenoids

Carotenoids are a large class of hydrophobic molecules found in a range of plants, particularly in vegetables. They can be broadly divided into two types, xanthophylls, which contain oxygen atoms, and carotenes, which are purely hydrocarbons with no oxygen (Figure 12.1). A particularly notable point is that some carotenoids such as α and β-carotene can be converted to vitamin A, and this is covered in Chapter 10 on vitamins. Only aspects of carotenoids which are not related to pro-vitamin A activity will be covered in this Chapter. As indicated above for polyphenols, the naming of carotenoids has also not been systematic. The name zeaxanthin is derived from corn (Zea mays) and xanthos (Greek for yellow), whereas lutein is derived from the Latin word for yellow (luteus). Lycopene is derived from the Latin word for tomato (Lycopersicum) and carotene from the Latin for carrot (carota). Common examples of xanthophylls are zeaxanthin and lutein, and of carotenes are α and β-carotene; these are present in several fruits and vegetables, usually in low milligram amounts. Many other carotenoids exist but only the well-studied main representatives of the regular diet will be discussed here. Carotenoids are highly lipohillic; lycopene is insoluble in water, and zeaxanthin, although containing several hydroxyl groups, is also effectively insoluble in aqueous media. Chemically, naturally occurring carotenoids in planta are in the all-trans form, but are readily isomerised to cis isomers during processing and passage in the GI tract.

Glucosinolates

Naturally occurring glucosinolates are (Z)-cis-N-hydroximinosulfate esters, possessing a sulfur-linked β-D-glucopyranose moiety and an amino acid-derived side chain (Figure 12.1). There are over 100 known examples defined by the side chain. In the diet, they are restricted to Cruciferous vegetables, which includes the Brassica family. It should be noted that the glucosinolate content is often higher in seeds and young shoots compared to the mature plant. In the same way as polyphenols, the glucose moiety must be removed for the glucosinolate to be activated for plant defence. This occurs by the enzyme myrosinase, present in the plant, and activated during attack or damage e.g., by insects, or during chewing or food processing. Glucosinolate hydrolysis products exert antifungal, antimicrobial, and insecticidal properties, contributing to the defence mechanisms of the plant. The main glucosinolates in the diet can be classified by the nature and length of the side chain. Glucosinolates are quite water-soluble, even though the side chain may be aromatic (benzyl, substituted benzyl), heterocyclic (indolyl) or aliphatic (alkyl, alkenyl, hydroxyalkenyl or o-methylthioalkyl). In the latter class, sinigrin, glucoiberin, and glucoiberverin have 3 carbon side chains, glucoraphanin, progoitrin and gluconapin have 4 carbon side chains, and glucobrassicanapin has five carbon side chains. In the diet, glucosinolates are most commonly found distributed in Brassica rapa (turnip, Chinese cabbage), B. oleraceae (white cabbage, red cabbage, broccoli, cauliflower, kale, Brussels sprouts, kohlrabi) and B. napus (rapeseed and swede). Certain types are also abundant in watercress and mustard, where the glucosinolates hydrolysis products are responsible for the pungent taste of these plants.

12.3 Distribution of phytochemicals in foods and beverages

Contents in raw foods

The contents of some commonly consumed plants are shown in Figure 12.2. Many fruits contain tens or hundreds of milligrams of polyphenols per portion, whereas carotenoids are mostly found in the

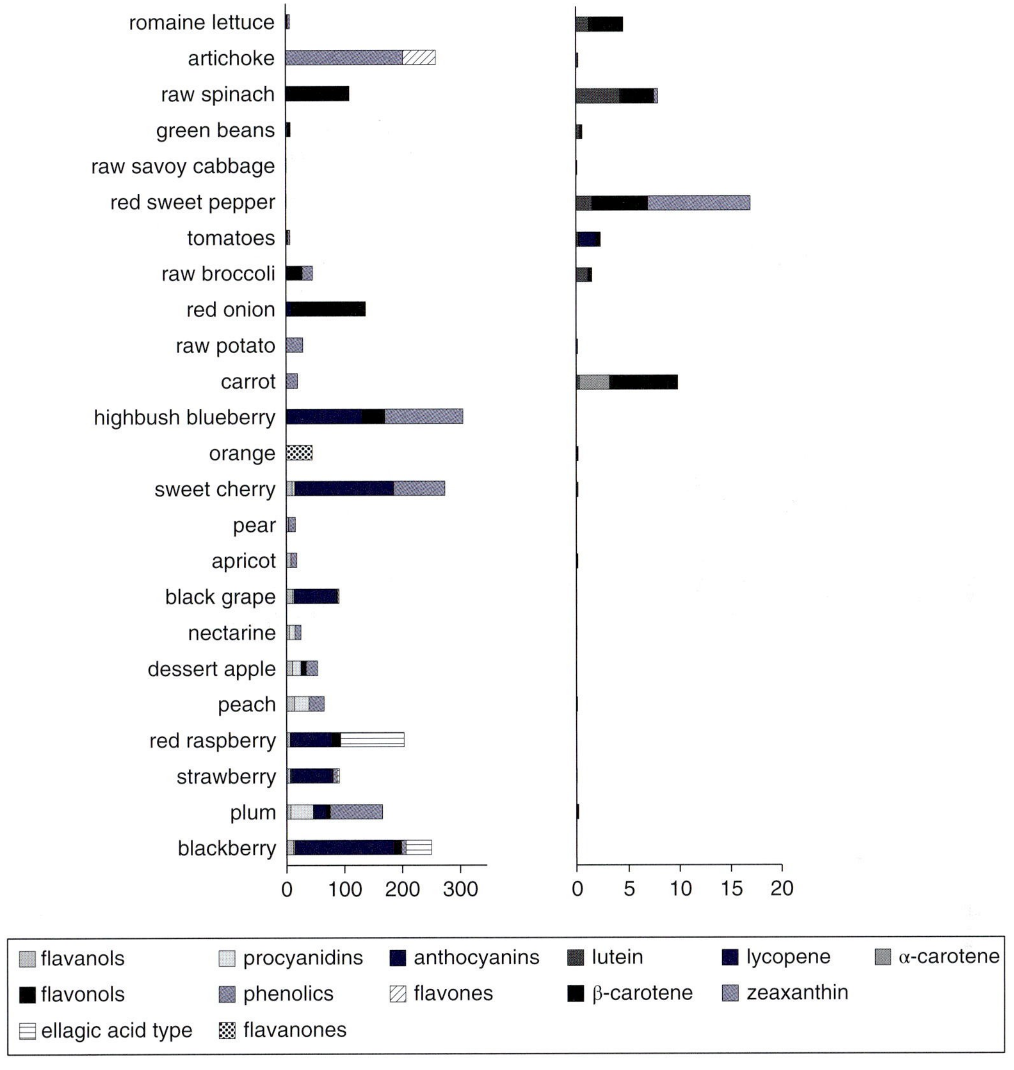

Figure 12.2 Distribution of polyphenols and carotenoids in foods.

very low milligram amounts. Glucosinolates are only found in Cruciferous vegetables, and the active components are breakdown products of glucosinolates which depend on several factors, and so it is not meaningful to give a general mg amount of active phytochemical in a portion of Cruciferous vegetable. Some vegetables, such as broccoli, contain substantial amounts of glucosinolates, polyphenols and carotenoids, but most are dominated by one class in an edible portion.

Although there are no recommended intake values as exist for vitamins, some claims have been allowed by governments around the world. However, as is evident from section 12.6, it is very difficult at present to define the amount of phytochemicals that should be consumed per day for optimal health. One way to begin to understand this is to calculate the type and amount of various phytochemical classes in a "five-a-day" diet. If the five-a-day portion of the diet consists, for example, of blackberries, blueberries, tomatoes, broccoli, and an apple, plus one coffee and tea per day, then it is possible to calculate the average phytochemical content in this diet (Figure 12.3), and similarly for strawberries, red onions, orange, carrot and spinach based on publically available databases. However, these diets also contain other components which may also influence health, such as fibre, vitamin C, minerals such as magnesium (e.g., ~20 mg/100 g

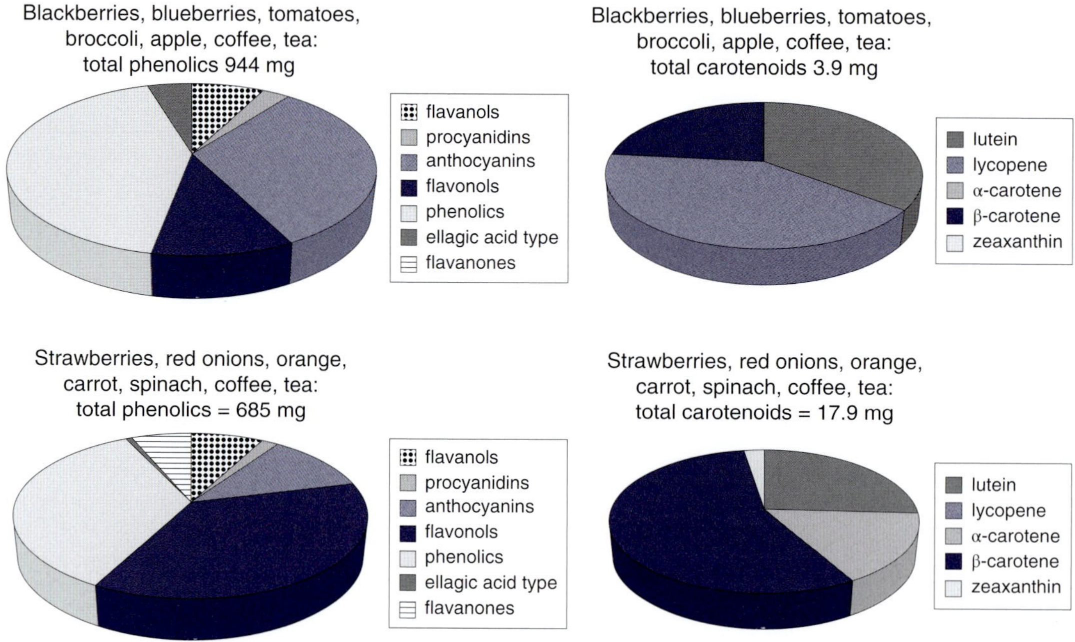

Figure 12.3 Distribution and content of polyphenols and carotenoids in diets.

broccoli and ~ 10 mg/100 g onion) and potassium (153 mg/100 g strawberries). The consequence of such complexity is that it is difficult to pinpoint the contribution of specific phytochemicals or nutrients to health benefits, unless there is an associated deficiency disease.

What happens to phytochemicals during processing?

Many fruits and vegetables are processed into commercially available products, and this affects the amount and quality of the phytochemicals in the food or beverage. For polyphenols and glucosinolates, in general, the harsher and more extensive the processing, the more will be degraded and lost. For glucosinolates, the cooking method is important as they can be easily lost, for example, into the cooking water during boiling. Chewing and processing of Brassica vegetables releases myrosinase which then converts glucosinolates into biologically active breakdown products such as sulphoraphane (from the parent glucoraphanin) or other isothiocyanates. Some polyphenols are unstable during processing: anthocyanins, for example, are very unstable, which is the reason why cooked berries lose some of their colour. On the other hand, hesperidin from oranges is quite stable, and is not lost during processing of citrus fruits. Obviously, if processing removes a part of the fruit which contains phytochemicals, then then this will be lost to the final product. Polyphenols can be readily lost during food manufacture. For example, raw unprocessed strawberries contain ~73 mg anthocyanins /100 g fruit, whereas they are mostly lost during processing into strawberry jam (<2 mg anthocyanins/100 g product); raw apples contain a high level of polyphenols (60 mg polyphenols including flavanols up to dimer, flavonols and phenolic acids/100 g fruit), fresh apple juice contains about 50% of this, but highly processed apple juice from concentrate contains less than 10% of the polyphenol content of the original apple. On the other hand, carotenoids may benefit from processing since they are highly fat soluble and require fat for absorption. Release of the carotenoid from the plant cell and into the lipid phase of the food improves the amount which is available for absorption in the gut, and so tomato ketchup is claimed to be a better source of lycopene than uncooked tomatoes.

12.4 Bioavailability: absorption and metabolism

A distinguishing feature of vitamins and minerals is that they have specific transporters, e.g., vitamin C is transported by SVCT1 and SVCT2 (see Chapter 10) which moves the compounds around the body at the molecular and cellular level. Although phytochemicals can be taken up and exported by transporters, these are not specific for phytochemicals and instead belong to families which metabolise xenobiotics. The specificity is defined by the transporter three-dimensional protein structure and not whether the compound in question is beneficial, toxic, or neutral. The body does not distinguish between drugs or phytochemicals which will confer a benefit compared to those that will not, and so will excrete everything that is chemically "foreign", even if it is potentially beneficial. Consequently the effects of drugs or phytochemicals are transient, even though some changes may be longer lasting. Phytochemical molecules, as for most conventional drugs, can be considered as just "travelling through", but may leave lasting effects and consequences.

Unlike minerals, where bioavailability can be calculated by "amount consumed" minus the "amount excreted", the situation with vitamins and phytochemicals is more complex. This is because any phytochemical (or vitamin) which is not absorbed in the small intestine will be transformed by the microbiota in the colon, and so will appear to be absorbed based on the above equation for minerals. Estimation of bioavailability of phytochemicals is complex and can involve several methods and calculations, all of which are comparative. Commonly used systems to estimate phytochemical bioavailability are measurement of post-prandial concentrations in blood over time, and measurement of the amount excreted in urine over 24–72 hours. In this way, it is possible to compare between phytochemicals and to estimate if a particular food or treatment can modify the bioavailability.

Ileostomist subjects have been very valuable for understanding phytochemical absorption. Since they lack a colon and its associated microbiota, then researchers have studied the intake of food and compared this to the outflow of waste from the small intestine into the collection pouch. In this way, the absorption of phytochemical in the small intestine can be calculated, provided that the stability of the compound in the gut lumen is accounted for.

Polyphenols

The pathway of absorption of polyphenols involves several well-defined steps. There are key factors that need to be taken into account in order to define the exact pathway for specific polyphenols. If the polyphenol has a chemical attachment, such as a sugar or organic acid, then this will have an enormous influence on the pathway of absorption, the amount that is absorbed, and where in the gastrointestinal tract that the compound is absorbed. Other factors that are important are the water-lipid solubility and the molecular size.

A good example is the flavonoid quercetin, since it is found in foods linked to a glucose, as in onions, or to both a glucose and a rhamnose, as in tea. The absorbable "unit" is the quercetin molecule itself, the aglycone. For this to be absorbed, the sugars must first be removed, which is akin to the digestive processes occurring in the gut. Lactose is a sugar which occurs in milk, and since it is a disaccharide of glucose linked to galactose, this molecule is too water soluble and too large to be absorbed. The first step in absorption is hydrolysis into glucose and galactose by the enzyme lactase, which is attached to the brush border membrane of the small intestine, facing into the lumen. It has access to the gut contents and so can access lactose. The same enzyme hydrolyses the bond between quercetin and glucose, and after this reaction on the surface of the small intestine enterocytes, the resulting quercetin is now lipid-soluble enough to pass through the enterocyte membrane by passive diffusion and enter the cell (Figure 12.4). On the other hand, because lactase cannot hydrolyse the sugar rhamnose, then quercetin with glucose and rhamnose attached is not a substrate for this enzyme. The molecule is too water-soluble and too large to be absorbed passively, there are no transporters for it, and so it will not be absorbed in the small intestine. This process is illustrated in Figure 12.4. This passage across the membrane into the enterocyte is a key process in absorption of most

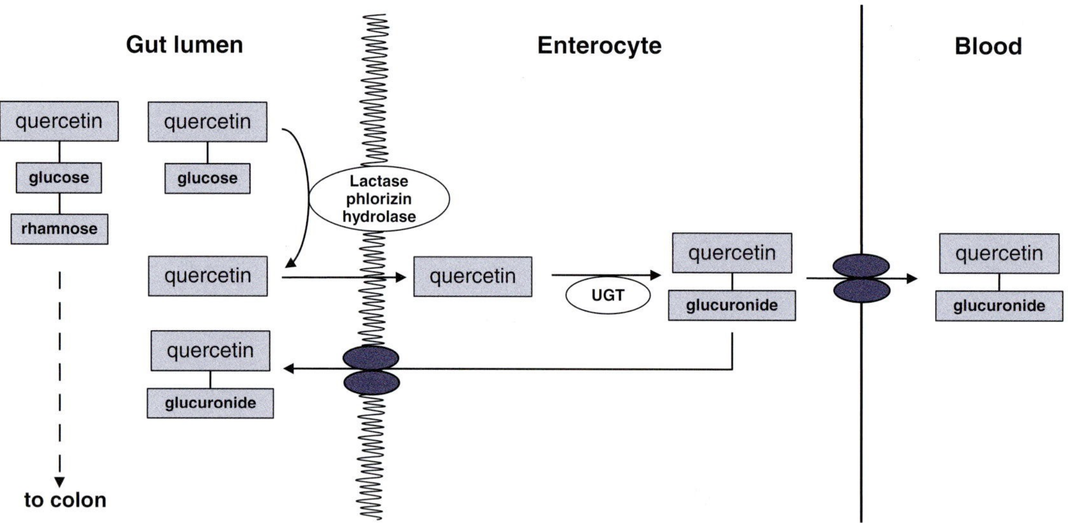

Figure 12.4 Polyphenol pathways of absorption using quercetin as an example.

phytochemicals, drugs and nutrients. Nutrients such as glucose or vitamin C have their own specific transporters, which take the molecules across the cell membrane. Many drugs and phytochemicals are sufficiently small and hydrophobic enough to diffuse across the membrane passively and so rely on a concentration gradient. The result of this first step in absorption is the presence of the compound of interest inside the enterocyte. Using ileostomist subjects, more than 70% of the phytochemicals present in apple were shown to be absorbed in the small intestine (Kahle *et al.*, 2005) and 65–80% of quercetin from onions was absorbed (Walle *et al.*, 2000). 25% and 40% of β-carotene and lutein respectively were absorbed from whole leaf spinach in vegetable oil and yogurt in ileostomist subjects (Faulks *et al.*, 2004).

Once inside the enterocyte, the polyphenol is then conjugated with another chemical group, either a glucuronic acid, through the action of the group of enzymes called uridine diphosphate glucuronosyl transferases (UGTs), a sulfate group (by sulfotransferases) and/or with a methyl group, via the action of catechol-O-methyl transferase (COMT). The resulting conjugate is then exported out of the cell, either into the blood, or back into the gut lumen, by different transporters located on the apical and basal membranes of enterocytes. The mechanism described applies to other polyphenols such as hesperidin and hesperetin-7-O-glucoside. Epicatechin and other flavonoids which are not glycosylated are also absorbed through the same pathway, but without the lactase step.

For some polyphenols which are not absorbed in the small intestine, the gut microbiota play an essential role in metabolism and absorption. Polyphenols such as rutin and hesperidin, which are not absorbed in the small intestine, are hydrolysed by the bacteria in the colon and the sugars are used as energy substrates for the microorganisms. The remaining aglycone is then either absorbed intact, or is broken down by the gut microbiota into smaller compounds or may be consumed entirely. The smaller compounds, which are shown in Figure 12.4, can then be absorbed by the colon, and enter the bloodstream. Following this, they are eventually conjugated by the liver and excreted in the urine. The concentration of these phenolics in the blood can reach much higher levels than the "parent" compound, and are also more persistent with longer half-lives. As a result of the absorptive steps, several polyphenol conjugates are found circulating in the blood including both the parent compounds and lower molecular weight compounds produced by microbial catabolism. The absorption of isoflavones follows a similar pattern, but a specific feature is that the gut microbiota can convert daidzein into equol. There is a clear difference in equol production between people, and some volunteers are classified as "equol producers". This may be an important metabolite but the relevance is uncertain as yet.

Glucosinolates

Glucosinolates are too large and too hydrophilic to be absorbed intact, and there are no transporters for glucosinolates in the gut. Glucosinolates which have not been broken down by the myrosinase enzyme present in the cruciferous vegetable can also reach the colon and be subject to breakdown by the gut microbiota (Angelino *et al.*, 2015). As for the plant enzyme, bacterial myrosinases break down the glucosinolate into a mixture of isothiocyanates, nitriles, thiocyanates and epithionitriles, depending on the chemical structure of the glucosinolates and the conditions, and these products are mostly consumed by the resident micro-organisms. One of the most studied isothiocyanates is sulphoraphane, derived from glucoraphanin. After consumption of broccoli, sulphoraphane is found in blood in the free form or conjugated to cysteine, cysteinylglycine, or glutathione. After consumption of broccoli soup, these metabolites appear early in the blood showing absorption in the small intestine, but with very little contribution from the gut microbiota (Al Janobi *et al.*, 2006). For sulforaphane, the driving force for transport into cells is the rapid conjugation with cellular thiols, especially glutathione.

Carotenoids

The essential first step in the gut lumen is solubilisation of the carotenoid in the lipid phase, and the most significant factor affecting absorption is the presence of fat. In some fruits and vegetables, such as mango and pumpkin, the carotenoids are present in the fruit in oil droplets, whereas in some plants they are associated with chloroplasts in a more crystalline form and so are less likely to become dissolved, and this affects the absorption. However, mild processing releases them into the food matrix and the absorption is then dependent on the fat content. The hydroxyl groups of xanthophylls are often attached to fatty acids, and these moieties need hydrolysing before absorption of the carotenoid, comparable to removal of the sugars from polyphenols, organic acids from phenolic acids, or the glucose from glucosinolates. The hydrolysis of fatty acids from xanthophylls occurs efficiently in the GI tract. Xanthophylls are more easily absorbed than carotenes, since they are more hydrophilic and easily incorporated into mixed micelles in the GI tract. Carotenoids are mostly absorbed passively, as they are hydrophobic in nature, but there are some suggestions of a limited contribution by specific transporters. The absorption of dietary carotenoids involves transfer of the carotenoid from the food matrix into micelles, followed by uptake by enterocytes by passive and active mechanisms such as SR-BI (scavenger receptor class B type I). ABCA1 expression and apoA1 acceptor activity have been suggested to contribute to the intestinal uptake of lutein and zeaxanthin, by an HDL-dependent pathway (Niesor *et al.*, 2014). After absorption across the enterocyte, carotenoids are packaged into chylomicrons and released into the lymphatic system, and then ultimately secreted into the plasma. Carotenoids are reprocessed by the liver and appear in the blood as VLDL particles. Carotenes are found mainly in LDL, whereas xanthophylls tend to be higher in HDL, and both classes are taken up into organs, especially into the liver and adipose tissue.

The bioavailability and/or serum concentration of β-carotene, lycopene, and lutein is markedly reduced in the presence of different types of dietary fibre, and differs substantially among high-carotenoid containing vegetables such as spinach, green beans and broccoli. The uptake of carotenoids is also dependent on the presence of other carotenoids (Marriage *et al.*, 2017). The lycopene level in plasma is dependent on the type of diet, and is on average 0.4 μM in North and Central Europe with up to 1.3 μM in Southern Italy, but typically less than 0.13 μM in North America (Muller *et al.*, 2016).

12.5 Bioavailability: Urinary excretion

Since phytochemicals are mostly not stored in the body, then a proportion of the parent compound, or most likely the metabolites and catabloites, appear in the urine after oral consumption. The amount in urine and the chemical nature of the metabolites is dependent on the original phytochemical. For glucosinolates, no intact parent compound is found in the urine, but the hydrolysis and breakdown products are found at fairly high levels. The hydrolysis product of glucoraphanin, sulphoraphane, is present in urine mostly as the N-acetylcysteine or cysteine conjugates within 24 hours after consumption of glucosinolate-rich food. Since the carotenoids are hydrophobic, very little intact carotenoid, if any, is found in the urine. For lycopene, ~ 20% of the dose appears in urine as catabolites (not intact lycopene), having been broken down at least partly through β-oxidation and microbial metabolism. For polyphenols, some intact parent compound is found in urine, together with conjugates with glucuronide or sulphate groups, as well as microbial metabolites and conjugates. For example, up to 5% of the dose of quercetin from onions appears in the urine, mostly as quercetin glucuronide conjugates (Mullen *et al.*, 2006). In addition, there are substantial amounts of catabolites from quercetin also found in the urine. No intact procyanidins or conjugates are found in the urine but when given in a labelled form, the microbial catabolites are absorbed into the blood and account for over 80% of the dose.

The amount of phytochemicals, metabolites, and breakdown products can be used to estimate the minimum amount absorbed, since any biomarker found in urine must have, by definition, been absorbed. Specific biomarkers can also be used as a biomarker of consumption in intervention and population studies. For example, urinary phloretin is correlated with apple consumption, naringenin for grapefruit, and hesperetin for oranges. For a given phytochemical, it can also indicate differences in absorption, metabolism and excretion between individuals when measured during intervention studies.

12.6 Biological effects

The information on phytochemicals in sections 12.1 to 12.5 is based on analytically verifiable evidence and accurate measurements of biomarkers. We can measure the level of phytochemicals in foods and of metabolites in biological fluids reliably by highly accurate and quantitative analytical techniques such as mass spectrometry, confirmed in many cases using authentic chemically synthesised standards. However, there is a larger degree of uncertainty associated with estimating and proving the effects of phytochemicals on health. In general, epidemiological studies can generate hypotheses, where consumption of phytochemical-rich fruits and vegetables is associated with an improved health outcome, such as less cardiovascular disease or type 2 diabetes. This can then be tested in intervention studies where the phytochemical-rich foods or diets, or even pure phytochemicals, are given to volunteers, sometimes with mildly impaired health, and surrogate biomarkers of a disease measured in order to indicate any protective effects of due to phytochemicals. However, these types of studies are expensive and require large numbers of volunteers in order to power the study for the subtle changes in biomarkers expected. For any effect measured in humans to be fully convincing, studies in vitro, or less commonly in a suitable animal model, must indicate credible mechanisms of action. For nutritional claims on phytochemicals, all of the evidence needs to be considered from all types of study in order for a claim to be considered substantiated. This means that proving the health benefits of phytochemicals is very difficult, especially as any effects are likely to be observed over an entire lifetime or at least several years. In addition, since phytochemicals are not deemed essential in that there are no official deficiency diseases, mostly their effect is to correct and restore the balance of a stressed system. Clearly the consequence of this is that some individuals within a study may respond to the phytochemical-rich diet or treatment, and some may not, giving nightmares to nutritional scientists in terms of powering a study and choosing the right at-risk populations.

Despite these limitations, there is a great potential to improve health by consumption of phytochemical-rich foods or even supplements, and so the biological activities of phytochemicals have been a subject of scientific interest for several decades. Phytochemicals are key compounds in fruits and vegetables, and also in many beverages derived from plants, and it has long been established that plant-based food are a key component of a healthy diet and associated with a reduced risk of chronic diseases according to epidemiological studies. Teasing out the individual roles of phytochemicals is, however, much more difficult. The free radical theory of ageing hypothesises that ageing processes are due to build-up of free radical-derived damaged macromolecules, and the theory still holds some validity. Because of this, it was originally thought that the protective effects of phytochemicals could be explained by general chemical antioxidant action and free radical scavenging activity. In the 1990s in particular, it was very easy and convenient to measure an antioxidant activity in the lab and, if a compound was a strong antioxidant, then it was claimed to be healthy. Measurement such as "ORAC", "TRAP" and "TEAC" were easy to use and allowed foods and compounds to be easily ranked by their "healthiness". However, in the last two decades, chemical antioxidant measurements as an indicator of health have been largely discredited because the mechanisms involved are much more complicated, the measure fails to take into account bioavailability and metabolism and the result includes multiple unrelated components.

The evidence for actions of phytochemicals is derived from epidemiology, which is based on phytochemical containing foods or diets, and on human intervention studies in both healthy and health-compromised individuals, backed up by studies on human cells in vitro and, to a lesser extent, on animal models. Animal models have several limitations, and it is important to understand that humans are one of the few mammal species who are, for example, unable to synthesise vitamin C, and unable to metabolise uric acid (lacking the enzyme uricase). Since animal models are often used in nutritional studies, it is important to correctly interpret the results based on metabolic differences between humans and other species.

There have been many studies reporting the action of phytochemical-rich food on biomarkers of health in both healthy and compromised individuals, many epidemiological studies on populations and many systematic reviews and meta-analyses. One of the issues is that most of the studies on humans are on phytochemical-rich foods, which also contain many other components including nutrients, minerals and vitamins, exerting their own effect. Broccoli, for example is high in carotenoids, flavonoids, and glucosinolates, as well as high in fibre and low in sugar. There have been far fewer studies on pure phytochemicals, and these studies have the disadvantage of being more like pharmaceutical studies. In addition, many of the health effects are only apparent when the organism is out of balance: quercetin, for example, reduced blood pressure, but only in hypertensive men, according to systematic review (Rangel-Huerta *et al.*, 2015). The same systematic review also indicated that consumption of isoflavones in soy led to an improvement in chronic inflammation and endothelial function, but only in post-menopausal women.

Since foods rich in phytochemicals are undoubtedly good for health, supplements containing phytochemicals have become commercially available alongside vitamin and mineral supplements. However, the health benefits of phytochemicals on their own, either as enriched extracts or pure chemicals, does not necessarily lead to the same effects as the equivalent phytochemical-rich food. An excessive consumption of green tea extracts has been reported to lead to liver toxicity in one individual who was obese and presumably had taken the supplements to enhance weight loss (Monliari *et al.*, 2006), but a systematic review suggested that a more moderate consumption of green tea could reduce the risk of liver disease (Jin *et al.*, 2008).

Effects of polyphenols

In the 1930s, an unknown plant constituent having "vitamin-like" qualities was investigated, originally called "vitamin P", since compounds in citrus acted in synergy with ascorbic acid against haemorrhagic symptoms and associated capillary fragility. A crystalline component, "citrin", affected the activity of vitamin C on micro-vessel permeability and eventually was found to be the flavonoids hesperidin and eriodictyol-O-glucoside. Although ultimately shown not to be a classic vitamin, several lines of research have indicated a beneficial effect of polyphenols. The history of polyphenol research is comprehensively presented in a review (Williamson *et al.*, 2018). Today, a substantial number of human intervention studies, supported by mechanistic and epidemiological evidence, have been published on the effects of polyphenols on health. These can be summarised. Flavanols and procyanidins, high in cocoa, protect against endothelial dysfunction. Consumption of flavanols in cocoa in intervention studies reduced blood pressure, improved endothelial dysfunction, decreased blood cholesterol, and decreased oxidative stress markers. Several meta-analyses and systematic reviews showed that flavanol-rich foods, either as pure epicatechin or in cocoa-based products, improved FMD as a cardiovascular benefit (Hooper *et al.*, 2012). The mechanism is through effects on metabolism of nitric oxide, and subsequent vasodilation. Similarly, flavanols, from green tea, reduced the risk of developing cardiovascular disease, since Cochrane analysis showed some evidence (weak to moderate) that tea over a 3-6 month period reduced pressure and lowered LDL cholesterol, but did not affect HDL cholesterol. There is good epidemiological evidence that coffee, both caffeinated and decaffeinated, and constituent phenolic acids, dose-dependently reduce the risk of developing type 2 diabetes. Tea consumption also reduces the risk of developing type 2 diabetes, but the effect is weaker than coffee.

One of the mechanisms of the action of polyphenols is to influence metabolism post-prandially, by slowing down carbohydrate and lipid digestion and so blunting unfavourable glucose spikes in the blood, and protecting the endothelial cells lining the blood vessels from stress derived from high concentrations of nutrients in the blood after a meal. Isoflavones help to attenuate oestrogen-deficient bone loss in post-menopausal women (Lambert, Hu and Jeppersen, 2017), through interactions with estrogen receptor (ER) α and ERβ. Isoflavone consumption is also associated with a reduced risk of colorectal cancer based on epidemiological studies in Asian populations (Yu *et al.*, 2016). Some individuals produce equol as a microbial colonic metabolite of daidzein, and it has been suggested, but not proven, that these equol producers obtain more benefit from soy consumption with regard to cardiovascular risk factors (Birru *et al.*, 2016).

Effects of glucosinolates

Glucosinolates were originally studied as anti-nutritional factors, owing to high consumption of oil seed rape by farm animals. Other glucosinolates, however, have been studied for their potential health effects, most notably glucoraphanin (as sulforaphane precursor) and gluconasturtiin (phenethylisothiocyanate). Several possible mechanisms have been reported, but the most established is induction of phase two enzymes by sulphoraphane. This is due to interaction with the stress response transcription factor nrf2 and related cellular proteins (Kerimi and Williamson, 2017). Phase two enzymes increase the rate of elimination of carcinogens and toxins, and hence their induction would reduce exposure to these types of compound. These experimental studies are complemented by epidemiological observations but there are very few intervention studies on the health effects of glucosinolates. Consumption of cruciferous vegetables reduced the risk of developing colon cancer, but this was dependent on the polymorphisms in glutathione S-transferase of affected individuals (Tse and Eslick, 2014).

Effects of carotenoids

Most information on the health effects of carotenoids is derived from epidemiological studies. There is strong epidemiological evidence to show a reduced risk of lung cancer by fruits and vegetables containing high levels of β-carotene, and this is believed to be true today. However, studies on β-carotene supplements showed that these could increase the risk of lung cancer in current smokers, and effectively stopped research into the beneficial effects of carotenoid supplements. Further studies showed that supplementation of β-carotene was associated with higher risk of cancer of lung and stomach in smokers and asbestos workers (Druesne-Pecollo *et al.*, 2010). A high concentration of lycopene in blood is associated with reductions in the risk of stroke and cardiovascular diseases according to a comprehensive meta-analysis (Cheng *et al.*, 2017). Intervention studies with high tomato intake showed reduction in LDL cholesterol, the inflammatory marker interleukin-6, and improvements in flow mediated dilation, while lycopene supplementation reduced systolic blood pressure. Higher dietary and circulating lycopene concentrations are inversely associated with risk of developing prostate cancer but not with a reduced risk of advanced prostate cancer (Rowles *et al.*, 2017). The xanthophyll lutein is a naturally occurring carotenoid that is synthesised by dark green leafy vegetables such as spinach and kale. A higher dietary intake, together with higher blood concentrations, of lutein, are associated with better cardiometabolic health, but with no effect on risk of diabetes (Leermakers *et al.*, 2016). Age-related macular degeneration (AMD) is the main cause of blindness in older people in industrialised countries, and affects the macula, which is the middle region of the retina responsible for central vision. In a meta-analysis, lutein and zeaxanthin were not significantly associated with a reduced risk of early AMD, but were protective against late AMD (Ma *et al.*, 2012).

References

Angelino, D., Dosz, E.B., Sun, J. *et al.* (2015). Myrosinase-dependent and -independent formation and control of isothiocyanate products of glucosinolate hydrolysis, *Front Plant Sci.* **6**, 831.

Al Janobi, A.A., Mithen, R.F., Gasper, A.V. *et al.* (2006). Quantitative measurement of sulforaphane, iberin and their mercapturic acid pathway metabolites in human plasma and urine using liquid chromatography-tandem electrospray ionisation mass spectrometry. *J Chromatogr B Analyt Technol Biomed Life Sci* **844**, 223–234.

Birru, R.L., Ahuja, V., Vishnu, A. *et al.* (2016). The impact of equol-producing status in modifying the effect of soya isoflavones on risk factors for CHD: a systematic review of randomised controlled trials, *J Nutr Sci*, **5**, e30.

Cheng, H.M., Koutsidis, G., Lodge, J.K. *et al.* (2019). Lycopene and tomato and risk of cardiovascular diseases: A systematic review and meta-analysis of epidemiological evidence, *Crit Rev Food Sci Nutr*, **59**, 141–158.

Druesne-Pecollo, N., Latino-Martel, P., Norat, T. *et al.* (2010). Beta-carotene supplementation and cancer risk: a systematic review and metaanalysis of randomized controlled trials, *Int J Cancer*, **127**, 172–184.

Faulks, R.M., Hart, D.J., Brett, G.M. *et al.* (2004). Kinetics of gastro-intestinal transit and carotenoid absorption and disposal in ileostomy volunteers fed spinach meals, *Eur J Nutr.* **43**, 15–22.

Hooper, L., Kay, C., Abdelhamid, A. *et al.* (2012). Effects of chocolate, cocoa, and flavan-3-ols on cardiovascular health: a systematic review and meta-analysis of randomized trials, *Am. J. Clin. Nutr.* **95**, 740–751.

Jin, X., Zheng, R.H., and Li, Y.M. (2008). Green tea consumption and liver disease: a systematic review, *Liver Int*, **28**, 990–996.

Kahle, K., Kraus, M., Scheppach, W. *et al.* (2005). Colonic availability of apple polyphenols - A study in ileostomy subjects, *Mol Nutr Food Res.* **49**, 1143–1150.

Kerimi, A. and Williamson, G. (2018). Differential impact of flavonoids on redox modulation, bioenergetics and cell signalling in normal and tumor cells: a comprehensive review, *Antioxid Redox Signal*, **29**, 1633–1659.

Lambert, M.N.T., Hu, L.M., and Jeppesen, P.B. (2017). A systematic review and meta-analysis of the effects of isoflavone formulations against estrogen-deficient bone resorption in peri- and postmenopausal women, *Am J Clin Nutr.* **106**, 801–811.

Leermakers, E.T., Darweesh, S.K., Baena, C.P. *et al.* (2016). The effects of lutein on cardiometabolic health across the life course: a systematic review and meta-analysis, *Am J Clin Nutr*, **103**, 481–494.

Marriage, B.J., Williams, J.A., Choe, Y.S. *et al.* (2017). Mono- and diglycerides improve lutein absorption in healthy adults: a randomised, double-blind, cross-over, single-dose study, *Br J Nutr*, **118**, 813–821.

Muller, L., Caris-Veyrat, C., Lowe, G. *et al.* (2016). Lycopene and Its Antioxidant Role in the Prevention of Cardiovascular Diseases-A Critical Review, *Crit Rev Food Sci Nutr* **56**, 1868–1879.

Mullen, W., Edwards, C.A., and Crozier, A. (2006). Absorption, excretion and metabolite profiling of methyl-, glucuronyl-, glucosyl- and sulpho-conjugates of quercetin in human plasma and urine after ingestion of onions, *Br J Nutr* **96**, 107–116.

Molinari, M., Watt, K.D., Kruszyna, T. *et al.* (2006). Acute liver failure induced by green tea extracts: case report and review of the literature, *Liver Transpl* **12**, 1892–1895.

Ma, L., Dou, H.L., Wu, Y.Q. *et al.* (2012). M. Lin, Lutein and zeaxanthin intake and the risk of age-related macular degeneration: a systematic review and meta-analysis, *Br J Nutr.* **107**, 350–359.

Niesor, E.J., Chaput, E., Mary, J.L. *et al.* (2014). Effect of compounds affecting ABCA1 expression and CETP activity on the HDL pathway involved in intestinal absorption of lutein and zeaxanthin, *Lipids*, **49**, 1233–1243.

Rangel-Huerta, O.D., Pastor-Villaescusa, B., Aguilera, C.M. *et al.* (2015). A systematic review of the efficacy of bioactive compounds in cardiovascular disease: Phenolic compounds, *Nutrients*, **7**, 5177–5216.

Rowles, J.L., 3rd, Ranard, K.M., Smith, J.W. *et al.* (2017). Increased dietary and circulating lycopene are associated with reduced prostate cancer risk: a systematic review and meta-analysis, *Prostate Cancer Prostatic Dis*, **20**, 361–377.

Tse, G. and Eslick, G.D. (2014). Cruciferous vegetables and risk of colorectal neoplasms: a systematic review and meta-analysis, *Nutr Cancer*, **66**, 128–139.

Walle, T., Otake, Y., Walle, U.K. *et al.* (2000). Quercetin glucosides are completely hydrolyzed in ileostomy patients before absorption, *J Nutr*, **130**, 2658–2661.

Williamson, G.K., Kay, C.D., and Crozier, A. (2018). The bioavailability, transport, and bioactivity of dietary flavonoids: A review from a historical perspective, *Comprehensive Reviews in Food Science and Food Safety*, **17**, 1054–1112.

Yu, Y., Jing, X., Li, H. *et al.* (2016). Soy isoflavone consumption and colorectal cancer risk: a systematic review and meta-analysis, *Sci Rep* **6**, 25939.

13
Physical Activity: Concepts, Assessment Methods and Public Health Considerations

Angela Carlin, Marie H. Murphy, and Alison M. Gallagher

Key messages

- Physical activity is defined as any bodily movement produced by the skeletal muscles that requires energy expenditure and can be described in terms of the type of physical activity performed, the duration of physical activity (time) and the intensity at which the activity is undertaken.
- The terms physical activity and exercise are often used interchangeably but exercise is a specific subset of physical activity undertaken with the aim of improving physical fitness. Physical fitness is defined as a set of attributes that people have or develop that determine their ability to perform physical activity.
- The intensity of activities be quantified in terms of Metabolic Equivalents (METs); 1 MET is the energy expenditure associated with resting metabolic rate (equivalent to consuming 3.5ml/kg/min of oxygen). All activities can be classified as a multiple of this energy expenditure rate.
- Sedentary behaviour is defined as any waking behaviour characterised by an energy expenditure ≤1.5 METs (in a seated or supine position) whereas physical inactivity refers to whether or not someone is engaged in sufficient levels of physical activity to meet current recommendations for health. Individuals can be classed as physically active yet still engage in significant amounts of sedentary behaviour.
- For children/adolescents, at least 60 minutes per day of moderate-to-vigorous intensity physical activity (MVPA) is recommended together with muscle and bone strengthening activities on at least three days per week.
- For adults, 150 minutes per week of MVPA or 75 minutes per week of vigorous intensity activity is recommended, together with muscle and bone strengthening activities on at least two days per week. Current guidelines for older adults (aged 65 years and above) are similar but include additional recommendations in relation to balance and coordination.
- Physical inactivity (i.e., failing to meet the recommended levels of physical activity for health) has been highlighted as the fourth leading risk factor for global mortality with levels of physical activity rising in many countries.
- It is important that measurement considers the type of physical activity being performed alongside the duration, intensity and frequency of the physical activity. At present no single assessment technique that is able to capture all the components of physical activity (i.e., the type, frequency, intensity, and duration of physical activity) and consideration of study characteristics, population characteristics, device characteristics and activity characteristics is needed when selecting physical activity assessment methods.
- Given the high levels of inactivity in society and the well-established negative effects of such inactivity on health, it is important that effective interventions are developed to change behaviours and increase physical activity at all stages across the lifecycle.

13.1 Introduction

Nutrition and physical activity have traditionally been considered separately as disciplines, however, with our increased understanding of the impact of diet and physical activity on health it is important that we consider the importance of both. Energy balance is achieved when the total energy expenditure of an individual equals his or her total energy intake from the diet. If intake

Introduction to Human Nutrition, Third Edition. Edited on behalf of The Nutrition Society by Susan A. Lanham-New, Thomas R. Hill, Alison M. Gallagher and Hester H. Vorster.

Companion website: www.wiley.com/go/lanham-new/humannutrition

exceeds expenditure the result is an increase in the storage of energy, primarily as body fat. If intake is below expenditure, body energy content or body fat decreases. An individual's energy expenditure is determined by three factors; resting metabolic rate, the thermic effect of feeding, and energy expenditure related to physical activity. Further detail on resting metabolic rate and the thermic effect of feeding is provided in Chapter 10 Energy Metabolism (IHN Chapter on Energy Metabolism). This chapter will introduce some key concepts (physical activity, physical fitness, intensity of physical activity and sedentary behaviour), consider current recommendations for physical activity, current levels of physical activity/inactivity, and the potential health benefits of increased physical activity. Approaches to the assessment of physical activity and efforts to promote physical activity within the population will also be introduced and considered.

Physical activity

Physical activity is defined as any bodily movement produced by the skeletal muscles that requires energy expenditure. The continuum of human movement is highlighted in Figure 13.1.

Physical activity is the component of energy expenditure with the greatest flexibility, and the means through which large increases in energy expenditure can be achieved. It is important to note there is a clear distinction between physical activity and energy expenditure; physical activity describes bodily movement, whereas energy expenditure results from bodily movement.

Physical activity encompasses all aspects of human movement, and is undertaken in different contexts or domains, including occupation, personal transport, domestic and recreational activities. Occupational physical activity refers to job-related activities undertaken outside the home while domestic activities include housework and gardening. Personal transport includes active travel from place to place, for example, walking or cycling while recreational activities refer to activities undertaken during leisure time, including exercise and sport participation.

The terms physical activity and exercise are often used interchangeably but exercise is a specific subset of physical activity with the aim of improving fitness or competence. Exercise is defined as physical activity which is planned, structured, repetitive, and purposive in that the objective is often improvement or maintenance of one or more components of physical fitness. Aerobic exercise involves a sustained period of rhythmic activity using large muscle groups that improves the function the cardiovascular system, for example, running or cycling. Exercise also encompasses resistance training (or weights training), which improves muscular strength and endurance by working against a force that "resists" the body's movement, and flexibility exercises such as stretching which maintain improve the range of motion around a joint.

Physical fitness

Physical fitness is defined as a set of attributes that people have or develop (through exercise) that enable them to perform physical activity. Physical fitness can encompass aspects of an individual's ability that are skill-related, for example, focusing on the performance of certain tasks that require an element of motor skill in addition to physical fitness. A number of components of physical fitness are health-related, for example, flexibility, muscular strength and endurance, and cardiorespiratory fitness. Cardiorespiratory fitness refers to the ability

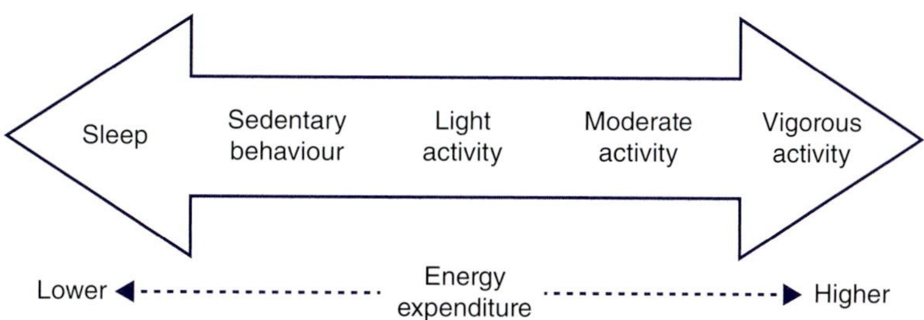

Figure 13.1 The continuum of human movement and energy expenditure.

of the circulatory, respiratory, and muscular systems to supply oxygen during sustained physical activity. The accurate measurement of cardiorespiratory fitness is important within a research context as it enables associations to be drawn between fitness and a number of health outcomes, irrespective of physical activity levels.

Oxygen uptake (VO_2) is a measure of an individual's ability to utilise oxygen to create the energy required for muscle contraction. This depends on the ability of the cardiovascular and muscular systems to take in oxygen and deliver it to the working tissues, and use it in the metabolism of fats, carbohydrates and protein.

Maximal oxygen uptake (VO_2 max) is the maximum amount of oxygen that an individual can utilise during intense or maximal exercise, and is measured as millilitres of oxygen used in one minute per kilogram of body weight (ml/kg/min) for weight bearing exercise (e.g., running) or in litres per minute for non-weight bearing exercise (e.g., cycling). The measurement of VO_2 max is regarded as the gold standard measurement of cardiorespiratory fitness. This direct method of assessing cardiorespiratory fitness requires an incremental maximal test i.e., it involves the participant exercising progressively harder to the point of exhaustion on a treadmill or cycle ergometer. The use of maximal fitness testing may not be suitable for certain clinical populations, where other factors aside from exertion may limit performance. This method of testing is also time and resource intensive, thus a range of field-based measurement tests and sub-maximal tests have been developed and are widely used within to predict VO_2 max and thereby assess cardiorespiratory fitness. Such methods include timed distance walks/runs, step tests, cycle ergometer tests, and graded treadmill tests.

Exercise intensity

Exercise intensity can be considered as a continuum from rest through to intense "all out" effort. The rate of muscular contraction, as well as the force required by muscle with each contraction determines the energy demands. These energy demands in turn determine the rate at which the body must resynthesise ATP. As the demand for energy increases the body increases its transport (cardiac output) and utilisation of oxygen (VO_2) to help meet this demand using the aerobic energy system. Exercise intensity is therefore often defined in terms of the heart rate response it induces or the oxygen uptake it requires, and may be described as light, moderate or vigorous. Accordingly, moderate intensity has been defined either as activity which requires 40 –50% of an individual's VO_2 reserve (i.e., the difference between maximal and resting oxygen consumption) or Heart Rate Reserve (the difference between maximal and resting heart rate) or 55–69% of Maximal Heart Rate (American College of Sports Medicine, 2017).

The intensity of activities undertaken can also be quantified in terms of the energy expended or Metabolic Equivalents (METs). Using this system, 1 MET is considered to be the energy expenditure that occurs while sitting quietly, in other words, resting metabolic rate, and equates to the amount of oxygen consumed at rest, equivalent to 3.5ml/kg/min. All other activities can be classified as a multiple of this energy expenditure rate with examples of MET values for various activities given in Table 13.1 (Ainsworth *et al.* 2011). A 4 MET activity (e.g. brisk walking) expends 4 times the energy used by the body at rest; thus if a person does a 4 MET activity for 30 minutes, he or she has done 4 × 30 = 120 MET-minutes (or 2.0 MET-hours) of physical activity. A person could also achieve 120 MET-minutes by doing an 8 MET activity (running) for 15 minutes. A compendium of physical activities has been developed to quantify the energy costs of physical activities

Table 13.1 Examples of metabolic equivalent (MET) values for various physical activities

Activity	MET
Lying quietly, watching television	1.0
Sitting, studying, light effort	1.3
Washing and waxing car	2.0
Cleaning, sweeping, slow, light effort	2.3
Walking the dog	3.0
Indoor bowling, bowling alley	3.8
Walking, 3.5 mph, level, brisk	4.3
Tennis	4.5–8.0
Mowing lawn, general	5.5
Cycling, leisure, 9.4 mph	5.8
Running, 4mph, 15 minute mile	6.0
Football, competitive	8.0

Source: Ainsworth et al. (2011).

(Ainsworth *et al.*, 2011). Activities are ranked in terms of their MET values, and the compendium can be used to quantify the intensities of activities undertaken; sedentary (1.0–1.5 METs), light intensity (1.6–2.9 METs), moderate (3.0–5.9 METs) and vigorous intensity (>6 METs). This method for categorising physical activity takes no account of fitness and therefore may overestimate the physiological demands of activity for a young fit individual while underestimating them for older adults or those with lower levels of fitness.

Sedentary behaviour

The term sedentary behaviour is increasingly used within the physical activity literature and has been defined as "any waking behaviour characterised by an energy expenditure ≤ 1.5 METs while in a sitting or reclining posture" (Sedentary Behaviour Research Network, 2012). Sedentary behaviour is therefore differentiated from physical inactivity, which refers to someone not engaging in sufficient levels of physical activity to meet current physical activity recommendations for health. Thus, individuals can be classed as physically active yet still engage in multiple sedentary behaviours.

Historical evidence shows us that our ancestors led a lifestyle characterised by being physically activity (hunters and gatherers), with evidence suggesting humans walked distances of up to 22 km (or 30 000 steps) daily (Cordain *et al.*, 1998). Given that the portion of our genome responsible for our basic anatomy and physiology has remained relatively unchanged over tens of thousands of years, the complex relationships that existed between energy intake and energy expenditure, particularly physical activity requirements, for our ancestors remain similar today, although physical activity is no longer a requirement for daily living (Cordain *et al.*, 1998). As society evolved through the agricultural and industrial revolutions, jobs and tasks that once required human movement were replaced with machines and technology. In modern society, labour saving technologies, motorised transport, and an increase in sedentary leisure activities, such as television viewing and smartphone use, have further reduced levels of physical activity.

13.2 Recommendations for physical activity

Physical activity guidelines provide recommendations on physical activity in terms of type, dose, intensity, and total amount of physical activity needed for the prevention of non-communicable diseases. The World Health Organisation's (WHO) report on "Global Recommendations for Physical Activity and Health" in 2010, providing national and regional policy makers with guidance on physical activity for health (WHO, 2010). Stemming from this, many countries have their own specific guidelines developed by Government health bodies.

Physical activity guidelines can act as an awareness tool, providing the general public with the levels of physical activity needed to achieve the associated health benefits. As outlined by the Department of Health (UK), the guidelines assist policy makers and healthcare professionals in their roles but also provide individuals with the opportunity to take ownership of their own lifestyle choices (Department of Health, 2011). The development of national guidelines also enables adherence to physical activity recommendations to be measured (physical activity surveillance), and trends in physical activity levels over time to be established.

Current recommendations

Physical activity guidelines are evidence based and are generated from extensive reviews of the scientific literature (e.g., Department of Health and Human Services, 2018). The "Global Recommendations for Physical Activity and Health" from the WHO (2010) address three age groups across the lifecycle; namely children and adolescents (aged 5–17 years), adults (aged 18–64 years) and older adults (aged 65 years and above). For children and adolescents, at least 60 minutes per day of moderate-to-vigorous intensity physical activity is recommended. In addition, vigorous intensity physical activities, including those that strengthen muscle and bone, should be incorporated on at least three days. For adults (aged 18–64 years), 150 minutes per week of moderate intensity aerobic activity or 75 minutes per week of vigorous intensity activity is recommended. The guidelines for older adults (aged 65 years and above) are similar but include additional recommendations in relation to poor mobility and health conditions. Older adults with poor mobility should perform activities to enhance balance and prevent falls on three or more days per week, while older adults who are unable to meet the recommendations should aim to be as physically active as their conditions allow.

Physical activity guidelines have evolved from their initial inception and are updated regularly, with the Department of Health currently reviewing the UK guidelines (previously updated in 2011). Updates to guidelines in other countries, for example, Canada and Australia have recently evolved to express physical activity in the context of 24-hour movement guidelines for pre-school and school-aged children.

"Steps per day" message

Although the physical activity guidelines summarised above prescribe physical activity in terms of intensity, frequency, and duration, such guidelines have been translated into step-based indices, for example, the "aim for 10 000 steps per day" health message. Despite a general consensus on physical activity guidelines across countries and health organisations, there is wide discrepancy in step-based recommendations and how these are communicated (Tudor-Locke *et al.*, 2011). The accumulation of daily steps to achieve the recommended levels of physical activity stems from Japanese walking clubs, with the origins of the "10 000 steps per day" message attributed to a Japanese marketing campaign in the run up to the 1964 Tokyo Olympic Games. Although steps per day guidelines are useful to describe volume of physical activity they cannot easily be used to describe intensity which is an important component of physical activity and one which influences the nature and extent of health benefits achieved by becoming active.

Normative data has shown that healthy adults accumulate between 4000–18 000 steps/day, with the above target of 10 000 steps/day regarded as an appropriate level of physical activity for this population (Tudor-Locke *et al.*, 2011). This target may be too low for children, and may be unattainable for older adults or those whose ability to be physically activity is impeded by disease or illness. In terms of communicating how many steps/day are enough for physical activity, the utilisation of a steps/day scale that takes account of different sub-groups and provides cadence recommendations which help individuals to select a walking speed which is likely to be to moderate-to-vigorous intensity may be useful in both research and practise (Tudor-Locke *et al.*, 2011).

13.3 Physical Activity and Health

Physical inactivity, i.e., failing to meet the recommended levels of physical activity for health has been highlighted as the fourth leading risk factor for global mortality, with over 5 million deaths worldwide attributed to physical inactivity. Physical inactivity levels are rising in many countries with major implications for the prevalence of non-communicable diseases and the general health of the population worldwide. Physical inactivity is estimated to be the main cause for approximately 21–25% of breast and colon cancers, 27% of diabetes and approximately 30% of ischaemic heart disease burden. A brief overview of the evidence for physical activity and health is provided below. For a more in-depth overview please consult the recommended reading (e.g., Warburton *et al.*, 2006; Physical Activity Guidelines Advisory Committee Scientific Report, 2018).

Cardiovascular Health

Early observations in the relationship between physical activity and health were first established in the seminal work of Jeremy Morris in the 1950s and Ralph Paffenbarger in the 1970s. Morris and colleagues investigated the incidence of deaths from coronary heart disease amongst London Transport workers and found that bus conductors, who climbed stairs regularly throughout the day, experienced less than half the incidence of heart attacks when compared with sedentary bus drivers, who spent the majority of their work shifts sitting (Morris *et al.*, 1953). Further occupational studies conducted in the USA confirmed the protective effect of occupational work on coronary heart disease, with Paffenbarger and Hale (1975) demonstrating that men who undertook light or moderate intensity exercise were twice as likely to die as their co-workers who engaged in heavy occupational labour.

More recent investigations have demonstrated even greater reductions in the risk of death from cardiovascular disease and have observed a 50% greater reduction in risk for individuals classed as being fit or active. Additionally, an increase in exercise capacity (physical fitness) of 1-MET unit has been associated with a reduced mortality of approximately 20%. There is now irrefutable epidemiological evidence that regular physical activity plays an important role in the primary and secondary prevention of cardiovascular disease. Furthermore, evidence has highlighted a dose response relationship, with those presenting with the highest levels of physical activity and physical fitness at the lowest risk of premature death. Whilst the body of epidemiological evidence supports the premise that exercise should be at least moderate intensity to elicit benefits for cardiovascular health, what constitutes optimal frequency intensity, duration, and type of activity is much less clear (Warburton *et al.*, 2006).

Diabetes

The incidence of type 2 diabetes has increased in many countries, with evidence suggesting a link between the increase in obesity rates and type 2 diabetes. Participation in both aerobic exercise and resistance training has been shown to reduce the risk of type 2 diabetes in adults (Warburton *et al.*, 2006). A key study in the early 1990s identified an inverse relationship between weekly energy expenditure and the risk of developing type 2 diabetes. Helmrich and colleagues found that each increase of 500 kcal/week in energy expenditure (walking, stair climbing, and sports) was associated with a 6% lower incidence of type 2 diabetes (Helmrich *et al.*, 1991). Moderately intense levels of physical activity and cardiovascular fitness have both been shown to be protective against the risk of type 2 diabetes in males. Furthermore, the benefits observed are found to be greatest in those already at increased risk of diabetes, for example, those with an increased BMI. Systematic reviews of lifestyle interventions have demonstrated that modest weight loss (achieved by a combination of diet and exercise approaches) could reduce the incidence of type 2 diabetes by around 40–60% over three to four years in at-risk individuals (Warburton *et al.*, 2006). There is still uncertainty as to the relative contributions of diet and exercise in such studies. Exercise interventions are thought to be effective in the management of type 2 diabetes, through improvements in glucose homeostasis. Further research is needed to determine the ideal type of exercise (for example, aerobic vs resistance training) and intensity levels of exercise for both the primary and secondary prevention of type 2 diabetes.

Cancer

Cancer is a major cause of morbidity and mortality worldwide. Research has shown that increasing levels of physical activity are associated with reductions in the risk of several site-specific cancers, in particular breast and colon cancer (Department of Health and Human Services, 2018). Epidemiological evidence has demonstrated that moderate intensity physical activity (>4.5 METs) was associated with a greater protective effect when compared to activities of lower intensity. Compared with inactive individuals, males and females who are physically active have a 30–40% reduction in the risk of developing colon cancer. For breast cancer, the reduction in risk is 20–30% for physically active women compared with their inactive counterparts. Although the available data are sparse, it appears that 30–60 minutes/day of moderate-to-vigorous intensity physical activity is needed to decrease risk of these site specific cancers. A dose-response relationship is also evident, with greater reductions in risk observed at higher levels of physical activity. Evidence on the optimal amount of physical activity for cancer prevention is less clear and warrants further investigation. Evidence has also shown a beneficial effect for exercise in individuals diagnosed with cancer. Further research in the form of RCTs is needed to determine the role of physical activity in the secondary prevention of cancers, and in particular, the role that physical activity can play in improving the health status of cancer patients.

Osteoporosis

Osteoporosis is a leading healthcare problem worldwide, characterised by low bone mass and micro-architectural deterioration of the bone tissue. Weight-bearing exercise, in particular resistance training, appears to have the greatest effects on bone mineral density. Evidence demonstrates that routine physical activity can increase bone mineral content during childhood and prevent the losses in bone mass associated with aging, particularly in post-menopausal women. Exercise training has also been shown to reduce both the risk and incidence of falls. The benefits of regular physical activity and structured exercise on bone health have been shown to outweigh the potential risks, especially in older adults. Further reading on the effects of sport/exercise on bone health is provided in Chapter 19 of the Sport and Exercise Nutrition textbook, (Bone Health, Sanborn *et al.*, 2011).

Obesity

Observational studies suggest that there is an association between increasing levels of physical inactivity and an increase in the prevalence of obesity, however there is a lack of robust evidence from intervention studies on the role of physical activity in the prevention of obesity. Evidence from longitudinal cohort studies has shown that individuals who report higher levels of physical activity are less likely to gain weight, with this relationship most pronounced when physical activity levels are above 150 minutes per week. Strong evidence also supports the significant relationship between physical activity and attenuated weight gain when activity is of a moderate-to-vigorous intensity; however, evidence for light intensity physical activity is insufficient. Although physical activity may play a role in energy balance, evidence suggests that a combination of diet and exercise is likely to be most effective for weight loss. Evidence also suggests that those who are physically active are more likely to maintain weight loss compared to those who are inactive.

Mental health

Physical activity has been associated with acute and chronic improvements in mental health and wellbeing, and may play an important role in the management of certain mental health diseases, including depression and anxiety. Evidence has shown that individuals with depression tend to be less physically active than those without depression. Increased aerobic training or strength training has also been associated with significant reductions in depressive symptoms, with evidence highlighting the beneficial role of regular exercise in mediating symptoms associated with anxiety disorders. Further research is needed to establish both the physiological and psychological mechanisms that explain the link between physical activity and mental health, and to evaluate the mental health benefits of physical activity across sub-groups of the population.

13.4 Physical activity levels

Trends in physical activity

The cost of physical inactivity to healthcare systems globally is estimated to be approximately £35 billion per year. Governments and other health agencies regularly monitor the physical activity levels of populations, to monitor adherence to physical activity recommendations and evaluate the potential impact of changes in policy and practice to improve physical activity. A lack of longitudinal population level data on physical activity, and in particular, data collected using standardised measurement tools, limits the identification of long-term trends.

Over time, an increase in leisure-time physical activity has been observed, while occupational related physical activity is declining. For younger people, the evidence is less clear but points to lower levels of physical activity during physical education within schools over time. Recent data from young people in 32 countries across Europe and the USA highlighted that although many countries were reporting either increased or stable levels of overall physical activity, the proportion of young people meeting the physical activity guidelines (60 minutes per day of moderate-to-vigorous physical activity) had declined in nine countries and remains low.

Prevalence of physical activity/inactivity

Much progress has been made on physical activity surveillance worldwide, particularly in adults, with approximately two thirds of WHO member states now collecting some level of surveillance data that can contribute to the global picture of participation levels and the risk of inactivity (Hallal *et al.*, 2012).

On a global scale, the most recent data released in 2012 estimates that one in four adults and three in four adolescents (aged 11–17 years) do not currently meet the recommended physical activity levels set by the WHO. A number of notable disparities exist in relation to the prevalence of physical inactivity. The frequency of physical inactivity varies across WHO regions, with 27·5% of people in Africa classified as inactive in Africa compared with 43·3% and 34.8% in the Americas and Europe respectively. Levels of physical activity decline with age across all WHO regions (Figure 13.2), with females more likely to be classed as inactive compared with males (33·9% vs 27·9%) at all ages. Within the UK, 39% of adults fail to meet the recommended guidelines, with women 36% more likely to be classed as physically inactive compared to men.

The Health Behaviour in School-aged Children (HBSC) survey is routinely conducted across 42 countries across the WHO European Region and North America (Inchley *et al.*, 2016). The survey collects self-report data on physical activity from boys and girls aged 11, 13, and 15 years. Data from the 2013/2014 survey highlighted that the proportion of children achieving at least 60 minutes per day of moderate-to-vigorous physical activity was less than 50% across all countries and regions. The prevalence of participation varied across countries, with Finland reporting the highest participation among 11 year olds (boys 47%; girls 34%) compared with lower countries such as Italy (boys 17%; girls 8%). This data highlights the potential influence of policy and guidelines variation across countries, with Finland's physical activity recommendations for children and youth exceeding the WHO guidelines.

The International Children's Accelerometry Database has collated accelerometer derived data on children's physical activity from 20 studies across 10 countries. Although physical activity levels differed across countries, the associations between demographic characteristics, such as age and gender, and physical activity were consistently observed (Cooper *et al.*, 2015). This data further supports the observation that boys tend to be physically active and less sedentary than girls during childhood and adolescence. An age related decline in physical activity was also observed from the age of five years, with each year associated with a cross-sectional

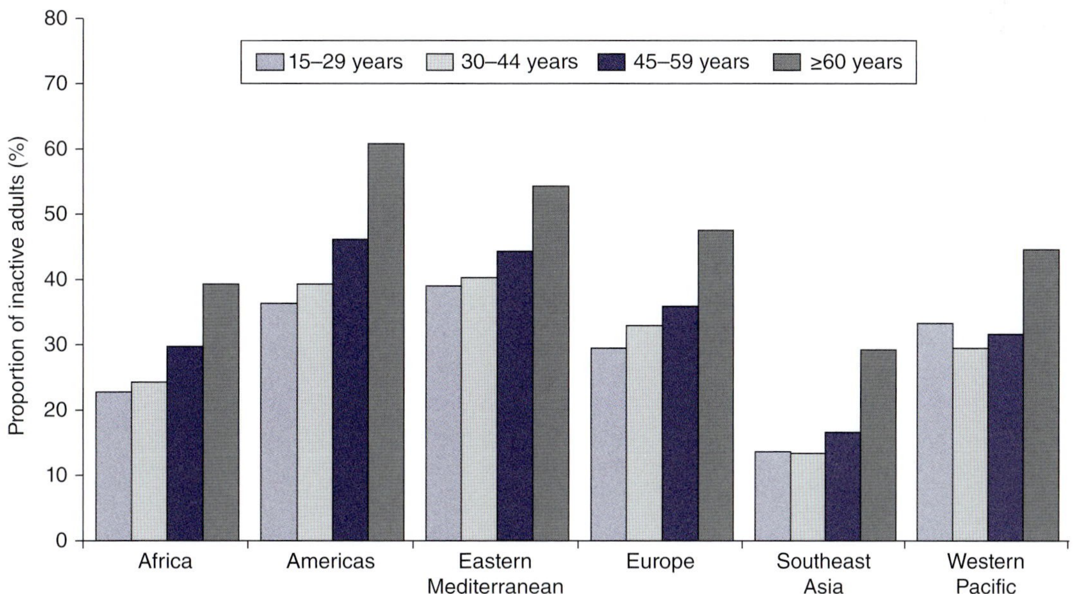

Figure 13.2 Physical inactivity* in age groups by WHO region (from Hallal et al., 2012).
* Physical inactivity defined as not meeting any of the following criteria: (a) 5 x 30 minutes of moderate-intensity activity per week; (b) 3 x 20 minutes of vigorous-intensity activity per week; (c) an equivalent combination achieving 600 MET-min per week.

decline of 4.2% in total physical activity (Cooper *et al.*, 2015). Data from both self-report and device measures also shows that physical inactivity is more prevalent among girls. As well as spending less time engaging in moderate-to-vigorous physical activity, girls are also less likely to be involved in sports, which is an important source of moderate-to-vigorous intensity physical activity during childhood, compared with their male counterparts.

Gaps in physical activity surveillance

Methods for assessing physical activity vary, with many large-scale surveys relying on the use of self-report measures, which are recognised as imprecise tools subject to memory recall challenges and social desirability bias. Despite progress made on global surveillance of physical activity, approximately one third of countries have no data highlighting a gap in surveillance data for low and middle-income countries in central Asia and Africa in particular. To date, there is also limited evidence on trends in physical activity over time (Hallal *et al.*, 2012). The development of measurement tools, in particular wearable devices, is promising for future surveillance.

13.5 Measurement of physical activity

The measurement of physical activity is important for a number of reasons; for example, it enables population level data on participation and adherence to the guidelines to be measured, allowing researchers to evaluate the relationships between levels of physical activity and associated health benefits. Measurement of physical activity is also important for the evaluation of interventions aimed at promoting physical activity. To effectively assess physical activity, it is important that measurement tools encompass the type of activity being performed alongside the duration, intensity and frequency of the activity. Recent advances in technology have accelerated the potential to objectively measure physical activity, particularly with increases in the development and ownership of smartphone applications and wearable technologies to capture our physical activity behaviours. The measurement tools used to assess physical activity can be divided into three main categories: primary or criterion methods, objective measures and subjective measures. A number of factors need to be considered when assessing physical activity, including the type of physical activity performed, the duration/amount of physical activity (time) and the intensity at which the activity is undertaken. Given the various dimensions of physical activity that need to be considered, there is no one tool or assessment technique that is able to capture all the components, i.e., the type, frequency, intensity and duration of physical activity. Selection of an appropriate tool for physical activity assessment is not a straightforward task and the researcher should aim to select a tool that will decrease the likelihood of measurement error and increase the precision of the physical activity assessment; Pettee-Gabriel and colleagues identified four domains which researchers should consider when choosing an appropriate measurement tool including study characteristics, population characteristics, instrument characteristics and activity characteristics (Figure 13.3).

An overview of methods for assessment of physical activity is provided below. Further detail on these methods can be found in Chapter 7 of the Public Health Nutrition textbook (Assessment of Physical Activity, Hansen and Ekelund, 2018).

Criterion methods

When assessing physical activity, proposed methods should be measured against a "gold standard" (criterion validity). Primary or criterion methods for assessing physical activity include the doubly-labelled water (DLW) technique, direct observation and direct or indirect calorimetry and are briefly described.

The doubly labelled water technique

DLW is regarded as the most reliable and valid measure of energy expenditure and enables researchers to measure physical activity in free-living conditions. DLW involves administering an oral dose of a radio-labelled isotope ($^2H_2{}^{18}O$) as drinking water and measuring the difference between the elimination rates of the isotopes over a period of time (one to three weeks). The difference in rate of elimination of ^2H and ^{18}O is equivalent to CO_2 production, therefore

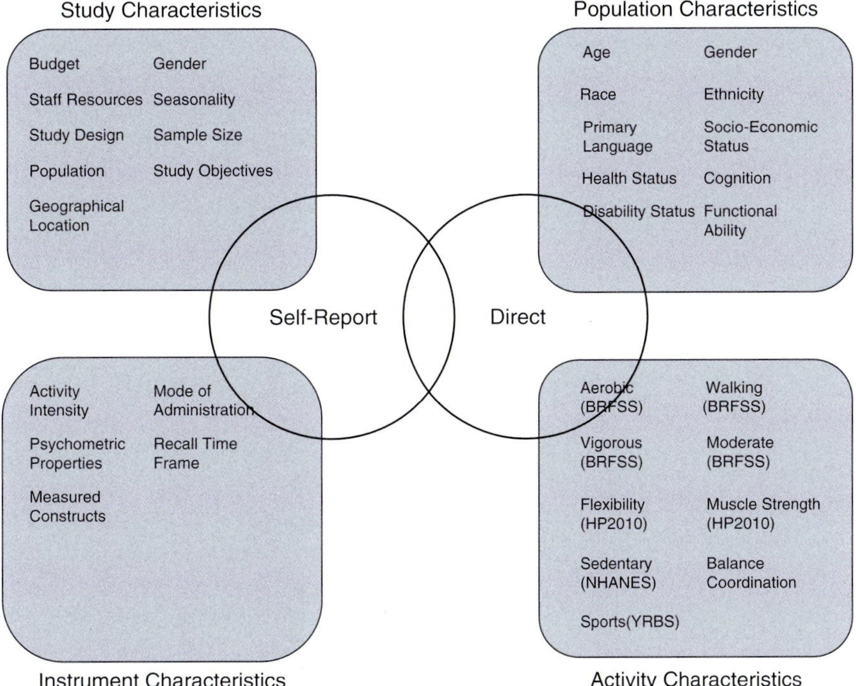

Figure 13.3 Methodological issues that impact physical activity and sedentary behaviour measures (Pettee-Gabriel et al., 2012). Activity characteristics as derived from a range of surveys: BRFSS, Behavioral Risk Factor Surveillance System; HP2010, Healthy People 2010 NHANES, National Health and Nutrition Examination Survey, YRBS, Youth Risk Behavioral Surveillance System.

providing an accurate measure of energy expenditure. DLW is a non-invasive method and can be applied across the population, from infants to adults. Although an accurate measure of energy expenditure, the application of DLW to larger populations may not be suitable due to the high cost and logistics involved during the measurement period. The accuracy of DLW as an estimate of energy expenditure also depends on participants providing a detailed dietary record of the entire measurement period, which can be burdensome for participants, and for children and adolescents in particular. Furthermore, using this method to assess physical activity does not provide information in relation to the intensity or duration of activities performed, and cannot capture qualitative data in relation to energy expenditure.

Direct observation

Direct observation involves watching and recording any physical activity related behaviours over a set period of time. Observing physical activity in a small geographical location, for example, a school playground or workplace can provide detailed information on physical activity behaviours, including the type, amount, and context (when, where, and with whom) in which physical activity is undertaken. Direct observation is used to assess physical activity more commonly in children than adults and may be advantageous for researchers working with children, particularly younger children who may not be able to accurately recall their movements. Although the methodology involved with this measurement tool can be burdensome and costly for researchers, direct observation is advantageous over other methods in that it can provide additional information on factors that may be influencing the observing physical activity behaviours, for example, the influences of other people, the environment and availability of equipment and other resources.

Calorimetry

Measuring energy expenditure by direct calorimetry entails measurement of the heat produced by a participant enclosed within a chamber. Indirect calorimetry involves the measurement of energy expenditure from consumption of O_2

and production of CO_2 using gas analysis equipment. Indirect calorimetry may entail the use of whole-body room calorimeters or computerised metabolic cart systems comprising of gas analysers to measure the volume and content of expired air. Although not widely used to measure physical activity due to portability and cost of equipment, indirect calorimetry provides a useful instrument for the validation of other tools used to assess physical activity for example, heart rate monitors and motion sensors (i.e., pedometers, accelerometers).

Objective methods

Heart rate monitoring

Heart rate monitoring enables the researcher to assess patterns of physical activity over time, and in particular to determine exercise intensity over time. An individual's heart rate will increase in proportion to an increase in exercise intensity. As a result, cut-points can be used to determine time spent in different exercise intensities (i.e., light, moderate or vigorous) based on a % of the individual's maximal heart rate.

The linear relationship between heart rate and consumption of oxygen enables researchers to estimate energy expenditure; however, one of its main limitations is that it may not accurately estimate energy expenditure when activities are performed at a low intensity. In addition, other factors aside from physical activity, such as environmental and psychological stressors can influence heart rate over the course of the day and reduce the accuracy of heart rate monitoring.

Physical activity monitors

Given that physical activity is defined as any type of bodily movement, the use of motion sensors, including pedometers and accelerometers, to directly capture this movement can be used to estimate physical activity. These devices provide an objective measure of movement that can be analysed in its raw format (for example, steps) or converted into estimates of physical activity.

Pedometers are relatively cheap, waist worn devices that can be used for the measurement of steps taken or distance walked over a period of time. Pedometers are readily used within physical activity research, both as an instrument for measuring physical activity and as an intervention tool. Studies have shown pedometers to be a valid and reliable measure of steps taken, which can be translated into an indicator of total volume of physical activity. Research has also highlighted the benefits of utilising pedometers to promote physical activity, with pedometer users demonstrating significant increases in physical activity levels, and significant decreases in BMI and blood pressure. Whether these health benefits can be maintained in the longer term is less certain at present. Pedometers are a good measure of walking and given that most physical activity movement captured is customary daily activity as opposed to structured physical activity, which is intermittent in nature, they represent the best solution for low-cost, objective monitoring of physical activity. A major limitation when using pedometers to measure physical activity is their inability to provide information on the type, duration and intensity of activities performed and their inability to detect motion such as cycling and activities where there is little or no vertical displacement (e.g., some resistance exercises).

As the field of physical activity measurement advances with developments in technology, accelerometers are increasingly used to measure physical activity within research. Accelerometers are a more sophisticated electronic model of capturing movement compared with the traditional pedometer. The accelerometer measures accelerations produced by the body over time (i.e., changes in velocity) which are converted into "counts", providing a readable measure of movement that is collected in defined time sampling periods set by the researcher. Accelerometers capture changes in velocity along one, two or three axes. Triaxial accelerometers (i.e., multidirectional) may be more suitable for assessing physical activity in children and adolescents than uniaxial measurements, given the sporadic nature of physical activity, particularly amongst young children. Accelerometers have been shown to provide a valid and reliable measure of physical activity. Accelerometers have distinct advantages over the other assessment methods mentioned previously, as this method of data collection enables a number of components of physical activity to be measured, for example, the intensity, duration and frequency, which can be measured over a set period of time (days or weeks).

The use of accelerometers is not without its limitations. The wearing of accelerometers may not be practical during certain organised or contact sports, most are not waterproof therefore cannot be worn during aquatic activities. Accelerometers are unsuitable for capturing certain types of physical activity, for example, cycling, and accelerometers cannot account for the increased energy costs associated with performing certain activities under different circumstances, for example walking on flat ground compared with walking up a hill. Although accelerometers provide an objective measure of physical activity, the researcher needs to make a series of decisions during data acquisition and processing which may impact upon the objectivity of the data collected. A protocol needs to be developed which includes placement of the device, sampling frequency and days of wear. Following data collection, further decisions then need to be taken in relation to defining valid wear time, removing periods of non-wear, and deciding what cut-points to use quantify physical activity intensity and the current lack of consensus within the literature on a standardised protocol, which may inhibit comparisons across studies. For further detail please refer to Chapter 7, Assessment of Physical Activity, PHN textbook.

Subjective methods

Subjective measures of physical activity include questionnaires (either self- or interviewer-administered), physical activity diaries and other proxy measures.

Questionnaires

Self-report methods, for example, questionnaires, are advantageous for large-scale population surveys, due to their low-cost and convenient administration. Questionnaires are the most commonly utilised method of physical activity assessment although the data captured across questionnaires varies, including how the data is obtained (for example, computer based questionnaires, interviews or pen and paper assessment), what is measured (for example, mode, duration or frequency), the quality of the data (for example, measures of intensity, distinguishing between types of physical activity) and how data is reported (for example, as computed activity scores, time spent in physical activity or energy expenditure) (Sylvia *et al.*, 2014).

Although widely applied, the use of questionnaires to assess physical activity is not without its limitations, some of which are more pronounced when these tools are applied to subgroups (i.e., children and adolescents), for example, inaccurate recall. Questionnaires have been shown to be less robust at measuring light or moderate physical activity, and may be influenced by other external factors such as social desirability bias, i.e., when participants deliberately over-report data to present themselves in a more positive light to the researcher. Despite these limitations, questionnaires represent a useful assessment tool for physical activity, particularly at the group level (Sylvia *et al.*, 2014).

Activity diaries

Physical activity diaries require participants to record their physical activity in real time, with diaries often broken up into specific time segments, for example, every 15 minutes. Diaries have an advantage over questionnaires in that they can provide the researcher with much more detailed information on the context in which activity is undertaken, although this can be burdensome for the participant. Traditionally, paper diaries have been used; however, smartphone applications and computer-based diaries are more commonly employed now. Similar to the limitations with questionnaires, activity diaries are also reliant on the ability of participants to accurately recall their physical activity and may also be susceptible to reporting bias. As a result, the use of diaries is limited within children and adolescent populations, partly due to the burden the place upon participants having to recall and record daily physical activity.

Emerging role of technology

Developments in technology have altered how researchers measure physical activity, with the use of motion sensors such as accelerometers now widely used within physical activity research. Alongside this, the development and availability of commercial fitness trackers and smartwatches has escalated. Such technology enables individuals to monitor and receive feedback on their individual physical activity and other health-related indices, for example, sleep duration and estimated energy expenditure.

The increased ownership of these devices may also present opportunities for researchers given the wealth of physical activity data generated by such devices. The wide array of fitness trackers and smartwatches available means the technology utilised by these devices also varies greatly, which may have implications for physical activity assessment. Although a wide range of devices exist, the evidence highlights that only a minority of brands are used frequently within research, with even fewer devices fully validated (Henriksen *et al.*, 2018). Furthermore, as the landscape of wearable devices is constantly changing, researchers need to give careful consideration when selecting these devices for projects, as devices currently considered relevant may change over time (Henrisksen *et al.*, 2018).

13.6 Physical activity promotion

Given the high levels of inactivity in society and the well-established negative effects of such inactivity on health, it is important that effective interventions are developed to change behaviours and increase physical activity at all stages across the lifecycle. The promotion of physical activity for health is not a new phenomenon. The idea that being physically active can improve health and longevity of life has been noted throughout history, with evidence dating back to Ancient Greece; "*Eating alone will not keep a man well; he must also take exercise. For food and exercise, while possessing opposite qualities, yet work together to produce health*" (Hippocrates, 400 BC).

The WHO's global action plan published in 2018 aims to reduce physical inactivity in adults and adolescents by 15% by 2030 (WHO, 2018). This action plan outlines a set of 20 policy areas, focusing on creating active systems, active people, active societies, and active environments.

Physical activity is a health behaviour and much research has sought to gain an understanding of the factors that determine physical activity behaviour (i.e., determinants). These determinants may include biological, behavioural, psychological, socio-cultural, built environmental, economic and policy determinants. Identifying key determinants of physical activity behaviour across different stages of the lifecycle can enhance the development of future behaviour change interventions.

The development of effective interventions to promote physical activity is a public health priority for researchers and practitioners. Promoting physical activity may vary in relation to target groups or populations (see Biddle *et al.*, 2012). Traditionally, interventions to promote physical activity were targeted at the individual level, but this has changed drastically over the past 10–15 years, with interventions that only focus on the individual level, for example, providing education on physical activity, viewed as ineffective.

It is now increasingly recognised that in order to achieve effective and sustainable changes in physical activity behaviour, strategies for behaviour change must include interventions targeted across a range of levels. The socio-ecological model, for example, has been applied to physical activity behaviour and examines behaviours at multiple levels (i.e., the individual, interpersonal, organisational, community and public policy level) and how the interrelationships between these levels influences behaviours. In addition to targeting the different levels of behaviour, researchers and practitioners working in physical activity behaviour change should utilise appropriate behaviour change theories and techniques to inform intervention design.

Promoting physical activity in sub-groups of the population

Children and adolescents

This sub-group of the population have been extensively studied, particularly in relation to the correlates of physical activity participation amongst this age group (Biddle *et al.*, 2012). Given that children and adolescents spend more time in school than in any other setting, aside from the home, schools are often considered an ideal environment for the promotion of physical activity and other health-related behaviours at a population level. Evidence from interventions to promote physical activity in this age group show that school-based interventions have the potential to increase physical activity in the short-term, however, less is known about the longer-term effects of such interventions on physical activity. Interventions that target the school setting alongside either the family or community level appear to be most successful in adolescents. Further research is needed, particularly in reporting the process evaluation findings of such interventions, to fully understand the reasons behind effectiveness or lack of effect. Furthermore, policy level approaches such as legislating that all children must have 2 hours of physical education per week, and implementation of no car zones near schools together with improvements to cycling and walking infrastructure also have potentially beneficial effects on the physical activity of children and adolescents.

Adults

Physical activity promotion strategies amongst adults include providing information, advice and counselling, physical activity programmes, and social networking and infrastructure. The use of interventions to increase knowledge and awareness, for example, through mass media campaigns has been shown to have little impact on physical activity behaviours. Counselling and structured, professionally led exercise programmes may be effective at promoting physical activity in this population. The workplace setting has been cited as having great potential for health promotion, with growing evidence indicating that that interventions delivered within the workplace can positively influence physical activity behaviour in adults.

Elderly

Promoting physical activity amongst older adults may be more challenging, given that barriers to physical activity participation in this age group may be influenced by the risk of, or actual, functional impairment and/or physical disabilities that may stem from existing co-morbidities. Regular participation in physical activity should be strongly advocated for this population as the best means to promote independence and increase quality of life. Guidance from the National Institute for Health and Clinical Excellence has identified a number of key components that should be integrated within physical activity programmes targeted at older adults, including exercise counselling and instruction, structured classes and group based activities and home-based physical activities such as walking.

13.7 Perspectives on the future

The purpose of this chapter was to introduce key concepts of physical activity, exercise, physical fitness, and sedentary behaviour and to consider approaches for the assessment of physical activity. Many within the general population do not meet current recommendations for physical activity, warranting efforts to promote physical activity and reduce sedentary behaviours in these individuals/groups; however, more work is needed to effectively evaluate current efforts to promote physical activity within the population and to develop tools to monitor physical activity at a population level. Finally, as the links between diet and physical activity and their combined effect on health are better understood, there is an increasing need to adopt a more holistic approach which targets the multiple determinants of health behaviour when developing and implementing public health interventions.

References

Ainsworth, B.E., Haskell, W.L.,Herrmann, S.D. *et al.* (2011). Compendium of Physical Activities: a second update of codes and MET values. *Medicine and Science in Sports and Exercise.* **43**(8):1575–1581. Available at: https://sites.google.com/site/compendiumofphysicalactivities/ [Last accessed on 01/08/18].

American College of Sports Medicine. (2017). *ACSM's Guidelines for Exercise Testing and Prescription,* 10e, Philadelphia, USA.

Biddle, S.J.H., Brehm, W., Verheijden, M. *et al.* (2012). Population physical activity behaviour change: A review for the European College of Sport Science. *European Journal of Sport Science,* **12**(4):367–383.

Buttriss, J.L., Welch, A.A., Kearney, J.M. & Lanham-New, S.A. (Eds.) (2019). Introduction to Human Nutrition, 3rd Edition. Wiley-Blackwell, Chichester. The Nutrition Society.

Cooper, A.R., Goodman, A., Page, A.S. *et al.* (2015). Objectively measured physical activity and sedentary time in youth: the International children's accelerometry database (ICAD). *The International Journal of Behavioral Nutrition and Physical Activity,* **12**:113.

Cordain, L., Gotshall, R.W., Eaton, S.B. *et al.* (1988). Physical activity, energy expenditure and fitness: an evolutionary perspective. *International Journal of Sports Medicine,* **19**(5):328–35.

Department of Health. (2011). *Start Active, Stay Active: A report on physical activity from the four home countries' Chief Medical Officers.* https://assets.publishing.service.gov.uk/government/uploads/system/uploads/

attachment_data/file/216370/dh_128210.pdf [Last accessed 08/08/2018].

Department of Health and Human Services. (2018). Physical Activity Guidelines Advisory Committee Scientific Report https://health.gov/paguidelines/second-edition/report/pdf/PAG_Advisory_Committee_Report.pdf [Last accessed on 01/08/18].

Hallal, P.C., Andersen, L.B., Bull, F.C. *et al.* (2012). Lancet Physical Activity Series Working Group. (2012) Global physical activity levels: surveillance progress, pitfalls, and prospects. *Lancet.* **380**(9838):247–257.

Helmrich, S.P., Ragland, D.R., Leung, R.W. *et al.* (1991). Physical activity and reduced occurrence of non-insulin-dependent diabetes mellitus. *New England Journal of Medicine*, **325**(3):147–52.

Henriksen, A., Haugen Mikalsen, M., Woldaregay, A.Z. *et al.* (2018). Using fitness trackers and smartwatches to measure physical activity in research: analysis of consumer wrist-worn wearables. *Journal of Medical Internet Research*, **20**(3):e110.

Inchley, J., Currie, D., Young, T. *et al.* (Eds.) (2016). Growing up unequal: gender and socioeconomic differences in young people's health and well-being. Health Behaviour in School-aged Children (HBSC) study: international report from the 2013/2014 survey. *Health Policy for Children and Adolescents,* No. 7. Copenhagen: WHO Regional Office for Europe.

Lanham-New, S.A., Stear, S.J., Shirreffs, S.M. & Collins, A.L. (Eds.) (2011). Sport and Exercise Nutrition. Wiley-Blackwell, Chichester. The Nutrition Society.

Morris, J.N., Heady, J.A., Raffle, P.A. *et al.* (1953). Coronary heart-disease and physical activity of work. *Lancet*, **265**(6796):1111–1120.

Paffenbarger, R.S. and Hale, W.E. (1975). Work activity and coronary heart mortality. *New England Journal of Medicine*, **292**(11):545–50.

Pettee Gabriel, K.K., Morrow, J.R. Jr., and Woolsey, A.L. (2012). Framework for physical activity as a complex and multidimensional behavior. *Journal of Physical Activity and Health.* **9**(Suppl 1):S11–S18.

Sedentary Behaviour Research Network. (2012). Standardized use of the terms "sedentary" and "sedentary behaviours". *Applied Physiology, Nutrition, and Metabolism.* **37**:540–542.

Sylvia, L.G., Bernstein, E.E., Hubbard, J.L. *et al.* (2014). Practical guide to measuring physical activity. *Journal of the Academy of Nutrition and Dietetics*, **114**(2):199–208

Tudor-Locke, C., Craig, C.L., Brown, W.J. *et al.* (2011). How many steps/day are enough? For adults. *The International Journal of Behavioral Nutrition and Physical Activity*, **8**:79.

Warburton, D.E., Nicol, C.W., and Bredin, S.S. (2006). Health benefits of physical activity: the evidence. *Canadian Medical Association Journal.* **174**(6):801–9.

World Health Organisation. (2010). *Global recommendations on physical activity for health.* Geneva: World Health Organization. Available at: http://www.who.int/dietphysicalactivity/publications/9789241599979/en/ [Last accessed 01/08/18].

World Health Organisation. (2018). *Global action plan on physical activity 2018–2030: more active people for a healthier world.* Geneva: World Health Organization. Available at: http://www.who.int/ncds/prevention/physical-activity/global-action-plan-2018-2030/en/ [Last accessed 01/08/18].

14 Nutrition Research Methodology

J. Alfredo Martínez, Estefania Toledo, and Miguel A. Martínez-González

Key messages

- This chapter identifies critical aspects and factors involved in nutritionally orientated investigations as well as valuable measurements in research procedures.
- It describes how to select methods and techniques as well as in vitro and animal models to assess causal relationships in the field of nutrition.
- It defines indicators and markers of dietary intake and metabolism in human studies.
- It helps to choose methods to investigate the causal relationships between diet and disease.

14.1 Introduction

Research is a meticulous process to discover new, or collate old, facts by the scientific study of a subject or through a critical investigation. In this context, nutrition research involves advances in knowledge concerning not only nutrient functions and the short- or long-term influences of food and nutrient consumption on health, but also involves assessments of food composition, dietary intake, and food and nutrient utilisation by the organism, as well as field studies.

The design of any investigation requires the selection of the research topic accompanied by the formulation of both the hypotheses and the aims, the preparation of a research protocol with appropriate and detailed methods and, eventually, the execution of the study under controlled conditions and the analysis of the findings leading to a further hypothesis. These stages of a typical research program are commonly followed by the interpretation of the results and subsequent theory formulation. Other important aspects concerning the study design are the selection of appropriate statistical analyses as well as the definition of the ethical commitments.

This chapter begins with a review of some of the important issues in statistical analysis and experimental design. The ensuing sections look at *in vitro* techniques, animal models, and finally human studies. The primary purpose is to provide the foundations in nutrition research methods to allow a more critical review of the many studies that, from time to time, an investigator will need to consider in the course of their study and career.

14.2 Statistical analysis and experimental design

In all areas of research, statistical analysis of results and data plays a pivotal role. This section is intended to give some basic concepts of statistics as it relates to research methodology.

Introduction to Human Nutrition, Third Edition. Edited on behalf of The Nutrition Society by Susan A. Lanham-New, Thomas R. Hill, Alison M. Gallagher and Hester H. Vorster.

Companion website: www.wiley.com/go/lanham-new/humannutrition

Validity

Validity describes the degree to which the inference drawn from a study is warranted when account is taken of the study methods, the representativeness of the study sample and the nature of its source population. Validity can be divided into internal validity and external validity. Internal validity refers to the subjects actually sampled. External validity refers to the extension of the findings from the sample to a target population.

Accuracy

Accuracy is a term used to describe the extent to which a measurement is close to the true value, and it is commonly estimated as the difference between the reported result and the actual value (Figure 14.1).

Reliability

Reliability or reproducibility refers to the consistency or repeatability of a measurement. Reliability does not imply validity. A reliable measure is obtaining the same results consistently, but not necessarily estimating its true value. A measure is said to have a high reliability when it produces similar results under consistent conditions. If a measurement error occurs in two separate measurements with exactly the same magnitude and direction, this measurement may be fully reliable but invalid. The kappa inter-rate agreement statistic (for categorical variables) and the intra-class correlation coefficient are frequently used to assess reliability. Other statistics used to assess consistency or reliability include the Cronbach's alpha that assesses internal consistency of the items included in a multi-item score, the coefficient of variation across repeated measurements, the Lin's concordance correlation coefficient and Passing-Blablok's non-parametric regression analysis.

Precision

Precision is described as the quality of being sharply defined or stated; thus, sometimes precision is indicated by the number of significant digits in the measurement (Figure 14.1).

In a more restricted statistical sense, precision refers to the reduction in random error. It can be improved either by increasing the sample size of a study or by using a design with higher efficiency. For example, a better balance in the allocation of exposed and unexposed subjects, or a closer matching in a case–control study usually obtains a higher precision without increasing the size of the study.

Sensitivity and specificity

Measures of sensitivity and specificity relate to the validity of a value. Sensitivity is the proportion of subjects with the condition who are correctly classified as having the condition. Specificity is the proportion of persons without the condition who are correctly classified as being free of the condition by the test or criteria. Sensitivity reflects the proportion of affected individuals who test positive, while specificity refers to the proportion of non-affected individuals who test negative (Table 14.1).

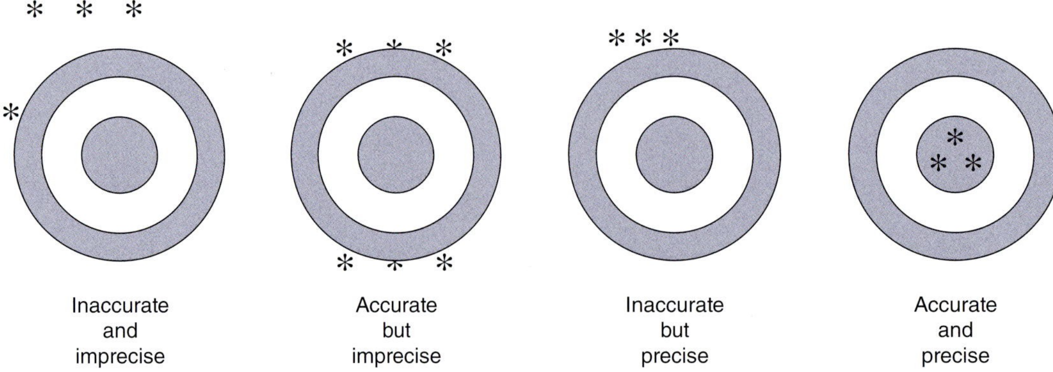

Figure 14.1 Accuracy and precision.

Table 14.1 Estimation of sensitivity and specificity

	True condition or outcome present	True condition or outcome absent
Test +	*A*	*B*
Test –	*C*	*D*
	Sensitivity = A/(A+C)	Specificity = D(/D+B)

Data description

Statistics may have either a descriptive or an inferential role in nutrition research. Descriptive statistical methods are a powerful tool to summarise large amounts of data. These descriptive purposes are served either by calculating statistical indices, such as the mean, median, and standard deviation, or by using graphical procedures, such as histograms, box plots, and scatter plots. Some errors in the data collection are most easily detected graphically with the histogram plot or with the box plot chart (box-and-whisker plot). These two graphs are useful for describing the distribution of a quantitative variable. Nominal variables, such as sex, and ordinal variables, such as educational level, can be presented simply tabulated as proportions within categories (for nominal variables) or ranks (for ordinal variables). Continuous variables, such as age and weight, are customarily presented by summary statistics describing the data distribution. These summary statistics include measures of central tendency (mean, median) and measures of spread (variance, standard deviation, coefficient of variation). The standard deviation describes the "spread" or variation around the sample mean.

Hypothesis testing

The first step in hypothesis testing is formulating a hypothesis called the null hypothesis. This null hypothesis can often be stated as the negation of the research hypothesis that the investigator is looking for or the absence of association. For example, if we are interested in showing that, in the European adult population, a lower amount and intensity of physical activity during leisure time has contributed to a higher prevalence of overweight and obesity, the research hypothesis might be that there is a difference between sedentary and active adults with respect to their body mass index (BMI). The negation of this research hypothesis is called the null hypothesis. This null hypothesis simply holds that the difference in BMI between sedentary and active individuals is zero. In a second step, the probability that the result could have been obtained if the null hypothesis were true in the population from which the sample has been extracted is calculated. This probability is usually called the *p*-value. Consequently, a *p*-value is the probability under a specified statistical model that a statistical summary of the data (e.g., the sample mean difference between two compared groups) would be equal to or more extreme than its observed value given that the null hypothesis was true. The maximum value or a *p*-value is 1 and the minimum is 0. The *p*-value is a conditional probability:

$$p\text{-Value} = \text{prob}\,(\text{differences} \geq \text{observed differences found} \,|\, \text{null hypothesis}\,(\text{H}_0)\,\text{was true})$$

where the vertical bar (|) means "conditional to." In a more concise mathematical expression:

$$p\text{-Value} = \text{prob}\left(\text{difference} \geq \text{data} \,|\, \text{H}_0\right)$$

The above condition is that the null hypothesis was true in the population that gave origin to the sample. The *p*-value *by no means* expresses the probability that the null hypothesis is true. This is a frequent and unfortunate mistake in the interpretation of *p*-values.

An example of hypothesis testing is shown in Box 14.1. Hypothesis testing helps in deciding whether or not the null hypothesis can be rejected. A low *p*-value indicates that the data are not likely to be compatible with the null hypothesis. A large *p*-value indicates that the data are compatible with the null hypothesis. Many authors accept that a *p*-value lower than 0.05 provides enough evidence to reject the null hypothesis. The use of such a cut-off for *p* leads to treating the analysis as a decision-making process. Two possible errors can be made when making such a decision (Table 14.2).

A type I error consists of rejecting the null hypothesis, when the null hypothesis is in fact true. Conversely, a type II error occurs if the null hypothesis is accepted when the null hypothesis is in fact not true. The probabilities of type I and type II errors are called alpha (α) and beta (β), respectively.

Box 14.1 Example of hypothesis testing

Among a representative sample of 7097 European men, the authors found that each 10-unit increase in the leisure-time physical activity was associated with -0.074 kg/m^2 in BMI. Physical activity was measured in units of MET-hours/week (1 MET-hour is the energy expenditure during 1 resting hour).

What is the probability of finding, in such a sample, a BMI 0.074 kg/m^2 lower (or still lower) for those whose energy expenditure is 10 MET-hours higher, if there was no actual difference in BMI according to physical activity? This probability is the *p*-value; the smaller the *p*-value is, the stronger is the evidence to reject the null hypothesis.

In this example, the *p*-value was 0.001, i.e., chance would explain a finding like this, or an even more extreme one under the null hypothesis, in only 1 out of 1000 replications of the study. The conclusion is that we reject the null hypothesis (population difference in BMI = 0) and (provisionally) accept the hypothesis that states that lower physical activity during leisure time is associated with a higher BMI. We call the latter hypothesis the alternative hypothesis.

Table 14.2 Right and wrong decisions in hypothesis testing

		Truth (population)	
		Null hypothesis	Alternative hypothesis
Decision	Null hypothesis	Right decision (probability $= 1 - \alpha$)	Type II error (probability $= \beta$)
	Alternative hypothesis	Type I error (probability $= \alpha$)	Right decision (power $= 1 - \beta$)

Some important cautions are needed when interpreting the *p*-values. Though a *p*-value can be useful, *p*-values have been frequently misused and misinterpreted. Some scientific journals discourage the use of *p*-values and prefer the reporting of estimates of effect size together with their confidence intervals. Some scientists and statisticians are recommending the complete abandonment of *p*-values or setting a stricter cut-off point of 0.005 instead of 0.05 for the alpha error (the threshold for deciding that a finding is "statistically significant"). The statement released in 2016 by the American Statistical Association proposed to maintain the use of *p*-values, with the following cautions or principles:

- *P*-values can indicate how incompatible the data are with a specified statistical model.
- *P*-values do not measure the probability that the studied hypothesis is true, or the probability that the data were produced by random chance alone.
- Scientific conclusions or policy decisions should not be based only on whether a *p*-value passes a specific threshold.
- A *p*-value, or statistical significance, does not measure the size of an effect or the importance of a result.
- By itself, a *p*-value does not provide a good measure of evidence regarding a model or hypothesis.
- Conducting multiple analyses of the data and reporting only those with certain *p*-values (typically those passing a significance threshold) renders the reported *p*-values essentially uninterpretable.

For scientific inference, *p*-values alone will be always less useful than estimates of effect size along with their confidence intervals, because the estimation of the magnitude of the association is more important than the erroneous dichotomous use of *p*-values. The estimation of confidence intervals provides an assessment about the range of credible values for the association. This is more meaningfully presented as a confidence interval, which expresses, with a certain degree of confidence, usually 95%, the range from the smallest to the largest value that is plausible for the true population value, assuming that only random variation has created discrepancies between the true value in the population and the value observed in the sample of analysed data. A common error is to dichotomize these confidence intervals according to whether or not they include the null value. This mistake would be even more directly against the 2016 recommendation by the American Statistical Association, because this will be equivalent to transforming the confidence intervals into dichotomous *p*-values to make decisions based on this dichotomy or "bright-line" rule.

Power calculations

The power of a study is the probability of obtaining a statistically significant result when a true effect of a specified size truly exists. The power of a study is not a single value, but a range of values, depending on the assumption about the size of the effect. The plot of power against size of effect is called a power curve. The calculations of sample size are based in the principles of hypothesis testing. Thus, the power of a study to detect an effect of a specified size is the complementary of beta (1 − β). The smaller a study is, the lower is its power. Calculation of the optimum sample size is often viewed as a rather difficult task, but it is an important issue because a reasonable certainty that the study will be large enough to provide a precise answer is needed before starting the process of data collection (Box 14.2).

The necessary sample size for a study can be estimated taking into account at least three inputs:

- the expected proportion in each group or the expected between-group difference and, consequently, the expected magnitude of the true effect
- the beta error (or alternatively, the power) that is required
- the alpha error.

Box 14.2 Example of sample size calculation

Let us suppose that we want to compare the proportion of subjects who develop a given outcome depending on whether they have been assigned to diet A or diet B. We expect that 5% of subjects in the group assigned to diet A and 25% of those assigned to diet B will develop the outcome of interest. We are willing to accept a type I error with a 5% probability and a type II error with a 10% probability. A simplified equation* for sample size (n) calculation would be:

$$n=\frac{(z_{\alpha/2}+z_{\beta})^2 2pq}{(p_A-p_B)^2}$$

$$n=\frac{(1.96+1.28)^2 2\times0.15\times0.85}{(0.05-0.25)^2}$$

$$n=65$$

where $z_{\alpha/2}$ and z_{β} are the values of the normal distribution corresponding to alpha 0.05 ($z_{\alpha/2}$ = 1.96) and beta 0.10 (z_{β} = 1.28), P_A and P_B are the expected proportions in each group, p is the average of both proportions ((0.05+0.25)/2 = 0.15) and $q = 1 - p$. Therefore, in this example:

$$z_{\alpha/2=0.05\,(\text{two tailed})}=1.96$$
$$z_{\beta=0.10\,(\text{one tailed})}=1.28$$
$$p_A=0.05\,(q_1=0.95)$$
$$p_B=0.25\,(q_2=0.75)$$

These values are substituted in the equation and thus the required sample size for each group is obtained (65). Therefore, we shall need 130 participants, 65 in each group.

*When the outcome is a quantitative variable, sample means (x_A and x_B) replace proportions in the denominator, while the product terms p_Aq_A and p_Bq_B are replaced by the respective variances (s^2) of the two groups in the numerator:

$$n=\frac{(z_{\alpha/2}+z_{\beta})^2\left[s_A^2+s_B^2\right]}{(\bar{x}_A-\bar{x}_B)^2}$$

Options for statistical approaches to data analysis

Different statistical procedures are used for describing or analysing data in nutritional epidemiology (Table 14.3). The criteria for selecting the appropriate procedure are based on the nature of the variable considered as the outcome or dependent variable. Three main types of dependent variable can be considered: quantitative (normal), qualitative (very often dichotomous), and survival or time-to-event variables.

Within bivariate comparisons, some modalities deserve further insights (Table 14.4).

The validity of most standard tests depends on the assumptions that:

- the data follow a normal distribution
- the variability within groups (if these are compared) is similar.

Tests of this type are termed parametric and are to some degree sensitive to violations of these assumptions. Alternatively, nonparametric or distribution-free tests, which do not depend on the normal distribution, can be used. Nonparametric tests are also useful for data collected as ordinal variables because they are based on ranking of the values. Relative to their parametric counterparts, nonparametric tests have the advantage of ease, but the disadvantage of less statistical power if a normal distribution could be assumed. Another additional disadvantage is that nonparametric tests do not provide confidence intervals for the parameters to be estimated.

A common problem in nutrition literature is multiple significance testing. Some methods to consider in these instances are analysis of variance together with multiple-comparison methods specially designed to make several pairwise comparisons, such as the least significant difference method, the Bonferroni and Scheffé procedures, and the Duncan test.

The false discovery rate (FDR) is the proportion of rejected null hypotheses that should have not been rejected. For example, if an investigator conducted 200 studies, and she or he rejected the null hypothesis (i.e., she obtained a discovery) in 100 studies, but 20 of these discoveries were not true, her FDR would be 20%. Please do not confuse this with the alpha error (Table 14.5).

Table 14.3 Common statistical methods used in nutritional epidemiology

Dependent variable ("outcome")	Univariate description	Bivariate comparisons	Multivariable analysis (Katz, 2006)
Quantitative (normal) 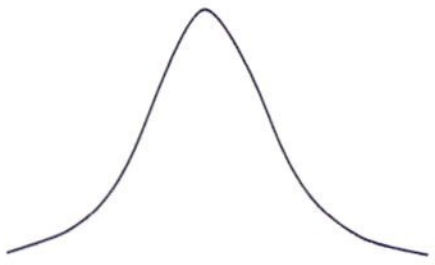	Mean, standard deviation	*t*-Tests (two groups) Analysis of variance (more than two groups) Regression and correlation (two quantitative variables)	Multiple regression
Qualitative (dichotomous) 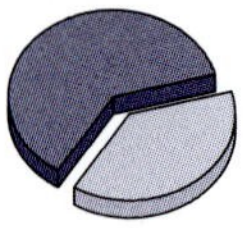	Proportion, odds	Chi-squared McNemar paired test Fisher's exact test Cross-tables Odds ratio Relative risk	Multiple logistic regression Conditional logistic regression (matched data)
Survival or time-to-event 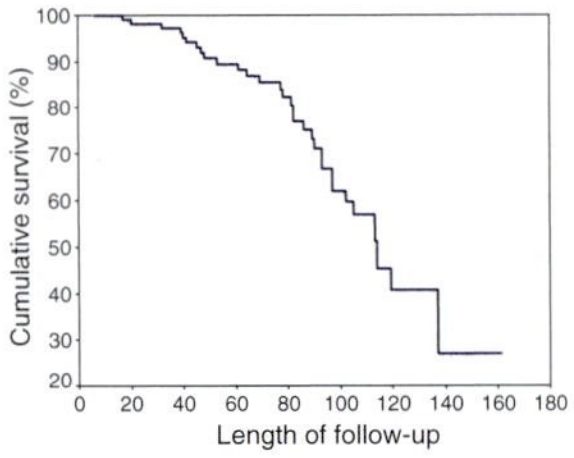	Kaplan–Meier (product-limit) estimates and plots	Log-rank test (Mantel–Haenszel)	Proportional hazards model (Cox regression)

Table 14.4 Common statistical methods for comparison of means

	Two samples		More than two samples	
	Parametric	Nonparametric	Parametric	Nonparametric
Independent samples	Student's *t*-test Welch test (unequal variances) Satterthwaite test (unequal variances)	Mann–Whitney U-test	Analysis of variance Bonferroni, Scheffé, Tamhane, Dunnet, Sidak, or Tukey post-hoc tests General linear models ANCOVA (analysis of covariance)	Kruskal–Wallis test
Paired or related samples	Paired t-test	Wilcoxon test	Analysis of variance for repeated measurements Generalised estimating equations	Friedman's test

Table 14.5 Explanation of the false discovery rate (FDR) based on 200 studies conducted by a researcher

		Truth (population)	
		Null hypothesis was true	Alternative hypothesis was true
Decision	Null hypothesis	95 true null studies	5 false null studies
	Alternative hypothesis: discovery	20 false discoveries	80 true discoveries

Alpha error = 20 / (20+95) = 0.17.
FDR = 20 / (20+80) = 0.20.

Recently, methods based on the FDR instead of the alpha eror have been demonstrated to be more efficient for controlling for multiple testing. FDR-controlling procedures provide less stringent control of Type I errors compared to family-wise error rate controlling procedures (such as the Bonferroni or Scheffé corrections), which control the probability of at least one Type I error (based on the alpha error). Thus, FDR-controlling procedures have greater power and efficiency, at the cost of increased numbers of Type I errors. These methods included the methods proposed by Benjamini–Hochberg,

Benjamini–Hochberg–Yekutieli, Holm, Sidak and Simes. They are implemented in statistical software such as the R package p.adjust and the downloadable command qvalue in Stata.

Repeated-measurement analysis of variance, mixed-models for analyses of variance and generalised estimating equations can also be used for replicate measurements of a continuous variable. The use of generalised estimating equations is more powerful and efficient when the design includes repeated measurements of the outcome variable along time.

Correlation is the statistical method to use when studying the association between two continuous variables. The degree of association is usually measured by Pearson's correlation coefficient. This calculation leads to a quantity that can take any value from −1 to +1. The correlation coefficient is positive if higher values of one variable are related to higher values of the other and it is negative when one variable tends to be lower while the other tends to be higher. The correlation coefficient is a measure of the scatter of the points when the two variables are plotted. The greater the spread of the points, the lower the correlation coefficient. Correlation involves an estimate of the symmetry between the two quantitative variables and does not attempt to describe their relationship. The nonparametric counterpart of Pearson's correlation coefficient is the Spearman rank correlation. It is the only nonparametric method that allows confidence intervals to be estimated.

To describe the relationship between two continuous variables, the mathematical model most often used is the straight line. This simplest model is known as simple linear regression analysis. Regression analysis is commonly used not only to quantify the association between two variables, but also to make predictions based on the linear relationship. Nowadays, nutritional epidemiologists frequently use the statistical methods of multivariable analysis (Table 14.3). These methods usually provide a more accurate view of the relationship between dietary and non-dietary exposures and the occurrence of a disease or other outcome, while adjusting simultaneously for many variables and smoothing out the irregularities that very small subgroups can introduce into alternative adjustment procedures such as stratified analysis (Katz, 2006).

Most multivariable methods are based on the concept of simple linear regression. An explanation of the variation in a quantitative dependent variable (outcome) by several independent variables (exposures or predictors) is the basis of a multiple-regression model. However, in many studies the dependent variable or outcome is quite often dichotomous (diseased/non-diseased) instead of quantitative and can also be explained by several independent factors (dietary and non-dietary exposures). In this case, the statistical multivariate method that must be applied is multiple logistic regression. In follow-up studies, the time to the occurrence of disease is also taken into account. More weight can be given to earlier cases than to later cases. The multivariate method most appropriate in this setting is the proportional hazards model (Cox regression) using a time-to-event variable as the outcome (Table 14.3).

14.3 *In vitro* studies

Scientific research involves studies across a reductionist spectrum. As studies become more reductionist, more confounding factors are stripped away. *In vitro* studies represent part of the reductionist approach in nutrition research. The range of techniques used is large.

- Chemical analysis studies provide data on nutrient and non-nutrient content of foods.
- Digestibility techniques, in which a substrate is exposed to enzymes capable of digesting the substrate, help to refine the gross chemical analytical data to predict nutritional potential.
- Intact organs such as the liver of experimental animals can be used in studies such as perfused organ studies. In such studies, the investigator can control the composition of material entering an isolated organ and examine the output. Sections of organs can also be used, such as the everted gut sac technique. A small section of the intestine is turned inside out and placed in a solution containing some test material. Uptake of the test material into the gut can be readily measured.
- Another approach is the construction of mechanical models that mimic an organ, usually the gut (in nutrition research). Many

of these models successfully predict what is observed *in vivo* and have advantages such as cost and flexibility in altering the experimental conditions with great precision. System biology is a recently launched platform to integrate metabolic pathways using computational biology.

The application of molecular biology techniques to tissue and cell culture systems has provided researchers with powerful strategies to evaluate and establish metabolic pathways and regulatory roles of nutrient and non-nutrient components of food. Thus, Northern, Southern, and Western blotting techniques to quantitate specific RNA, DNA, and proteins in tissues in response to nutrients are common tools in the nutrition laboratory. The influence of some nutrients or nutritional conditions on ribosomal dynamics as well as on cell hyperplasia or hypertrophy processes has been estimated through RNA, DNA, or protein/ DNA values, respectively.

Furthermore, molecular biological approaches have allowed numerous *in vitro* discoveries that have aided our understanding of the genetic basis of nutrient functions and metabolic states *in vivo*. The polymerase chain reaction (PCR) can be used for DNA and/or messenger RNA (mRNA) amplification to determine the genetic background and/or gene expression in very small cellular samples. Transfection studies allow the insertion of DNA into cells to examine nutrient function. Thus, cell lines that usually lack the expression of a particular gene can be transfected with DNA containing the gene promoter, as well as all or part of the transfected gene of interest, to study the interactions of various nutrients with the expression of a particular gene. Conversely, knockout cell lines allow us to investigate the consequences of losing a specific gene. In either case, nutrient function at the cell level and the cell–gene level may be studied and provide definitive results. Gene regulation by nutrients has been assessed in different isolated cells and tissues using appropriate indicators and markers of gene expression RNA levels.

The integration of biochemical and molecular technologies into nutrition research allows the potential for an integrated systems biology perspective examining the interactions among DNA, RNA protein, and metabolites. Following the completion of the human genome sequence, new findings about individual genes functions and their involvement in body homeostasis is emerging (see the Nutrition Research Methodolgy textbook, Chapter 13). Thus, technologies to achieve a simultaneous assessment of thousands of gene polymorphisms, the quantitation of mRNA levels of a large number of genes (transcriptomics) as well as proteins (proteomics), or metabolites (metabolomics) is rapidly progressing. Advances in DNA and RNA microarray-based tools as well in the application of classic two-dimensional gel electrophoresis, various Liquid chromatography-mass spectrometry (LC-MS) techniques, image scanning, or antibody arrays contribute to unravelling the intimate mechanisms involved in nutritional processes. Epigenetics studies constitute a rising methodology to be applied in nutritional research as well as metabolomics and metagenomics.

14.4 Animal models in nutrition research

Whole animal systems have been used in measuring the utilisation, function, and fate of nutrients. Thus, a part of our knowledge regarding nutrition concepts stems from animal experiments, which are often extrapolated to humans and referred to as animal models. There are many reasons for choosing an animal study over a human study. We can and do subject animals to experimental conditions that it would ethically not be allowed to apply to humans. For example, to study the manner in which a nutrient influences the scale and histopathology of atherosclerosis, animal studies are needed. Just as studies with humans are governed by the rules of ethics committees, so too are studies with animals. These rules involve the regulation of facilities, accommodation and animal care, competence, alternatives to animal experimentation, anaesthesia and euthanasia procedures, registration, supply of animals, and the involvement of an ethical committee.

In general, the use of animals as models for human nutrition research can be examined from three aspects:

- the animal model
- the experimental diet and its delivery
- the experimental techniques available.

The animal model

Many species have been used in the study of nutrition. Many are pure-bred strains such as the Wistar rat, the Charles River mouse, or the New Zealand white rabbit. Some animal models have been specially selected to exhibit particular traits, making them very useful models for research. The Wattanable rabbit has defective low-density lipoprotein (LDL) receptor function, making this animal model very useful for studying the role of diet in influencing LDL receptor-mediated arterial disease. The ob/ob mouse develops gross obesity because of an alteration in a genetic profile affecting leptin functions. A rise in the use of transgenic animal models that have been produced through advanced molecular genetic techniques. In such models, specific genes can be inserted or deleted to fulfil specific functions. For example, the peroxisome proliferator-activated receptor-alpha (PPAR-α) is not expressed in one knockout mouse model, giving rise to fat accumulation. Another example of a transgenic mouse presents an overexpression of the Cu/Zn-superoxide dismutase enzyme.

The experimental diet and convenient delivery

The nature of the diet and the mode of delivery are centrally important in understanding the role of animal models in human nutrition issues. There are several types of diets offered to laboratory animals.

Commercially available diets made to internationally accepted nutritional norms are often referred to as chow diets or laboratory chow. For the vast majority of laboratory animals in studies where nutrient intake is not the central area of interest, such chow diets are used. However, when nutrition is the area of research, special diets will almost always have to be formulated. The type of diet that needs to be formulated will depend on the nature of the research question.

Terms such as semipurified, purified, and chemically defined diets are often used but frequently it is difficult to know exactly which type of term fits different formulations. The least refined experimental diet uses ingredients such as barley, soybean, and wheat. An example is given in Table 14.6, taken from a study of rapeseed glucosinolates on the iodine status of piglets. The purpose of the study was to assess the effects of glucosinolate derived from ground rapeseed. A direct comparison between the ground rapeseed and the control is not possible because the ground rapeseed contains twice as much fat as the controls. Thus, the rapeseed oil diet is included because it contains no glucosinolate, but the same amount of fat as the control diet. The ingredients used in these diets contain usually several nutrients. Thus, the main staple ingredient, barley, contains protein, carbohydrate, and fat as well as fibre and micronutrients. That can create problems when there is a need to examine the effects of specific nutrients, such as fatty acids. The fatty acids naturally present in barley cannot be ignored. In the case of the rapeseed oil diet in Table 14.6, 40 g of the 56 g of fat per kilogram of diet comes from the rapeseed oil, but 16 g (or 28.6%) comes from barley lipid.

Table 14.6 An example of less refined experimental diets to test the effects of rapeseed-derived glucosinolate

	Control (g/kg)	Rapeseed oil (g/kg)	Ground rapeseed (g/kg)
Soybean meal[a]	220	240	195
Rapeseed oil	5	40	–
Ground rapeseed	–	–	100
Barley	755	700	685
Mineral/vitamin	20	20	20
Total	1000	1000	1000
Energy (MJ/kg)[b]	12.6	13.3	13.0
Protein (g/kg)	183	177	182
Fat (g/kg)	29	56	58
Glucosinolate (mmol/kg)	0	0	1.9

[a] Solvent-extracted soybean meal.
[b] Metabolisable energy.
From Schone *et al.* (2001). Reproduced with permission.

To deal with this, more refined diets are used. An example of such a diet is given in Table 14.7. In this instance, the authors were examining how different dietary fats influence blood cholesterol in normal mice and in transgenic mice not expressing the gene for the cholesteryl ester transfer protein (CETP), which is a key protein in lipid metabolism. In this instance, the ingredients are almost all pure. Thus, casein is pure protein and nothing else. Similarly, sucrose is pure carbohydrate and cellulose is pure fibre. The diets differ only in the source of fat. The high-fat

Table 14.7 An example of more refined experimental diets to examine the cholesterolemic effects of fats in transgenic CETP mice

	Control diet		Low-fat diet		High-fat	
	(g/100 g)	(g/MJ)	(g/100 g)	(g/MJ)	diet (g/100 g)	(g/MJ)
Casein	20	12	19	12	24	12
L-Cystine	0.03	0.18	0.28	0.18	0.36	0.18
Maize starch	40	24	48	31	13	6
Dextrinised starch	13	8	12	8	16	8
Sucrose	10	6	9	6	12	6
Cellulose	5	3	5	3	6	3
Soybean oil	7	4	0	0	0	0
Safflower oil	0	0	2	1.2	2.4	1.2
Experimental oil[a]	0	0	0	0	22	11
Mineral mix	3.5	2.1	3.3	2.1	4.2	2.1
Vitamin mix	1	0.6	0.9	0.6	1.2	0.6
Energy (%)						
Total fat	16.9		5.7		48.6	
Sugar	10.1		10.9		10.5	
Starch	54.1		22.3		22.1	
Protein	20.2		20.9		20.7	
MJ/kg	16.7		15.9		20.1	

[a] Three different experimental oils were used (butter, safflower, high oleic safflower) for three different high-fat diets varying in types of fatty acids.
From Chang and Snook (2001). Reproduced with permission.

diet obviously has more fat and thus more energy per kilogram of diet. It is thus critically important to note that as the energy density goes up, most other things must also go up to ensure a common concentration, not on a weight-for-weight basis but on a weight-for-energy basis. A simple illustration is the level of the mineral mix used: 2.5 g/100 g in the control diet, 3.2 g/100 g in the low-fat diet and 4.2 g/100 g in the high-fat diet. But when considered on a weight-for-energy basis, all five diets contain 2.0 g/MJ. The only changes are in fat and in maize starch, which always vary in opposite directions.

Variations in diet composition are often the key for the design of nutrition experiments. In this context, different feeding regimens can be applied to laboratory animals depending on scientific criteria. In *ad libitum* feeding the animals have free access to food; in controlled feeding animals are offered a limited amount of food (restricted feeding) or receive as much food as can be fed to them (forced feeding). A specific form of restricted feeding is pair-feeding, which involves the measurement of food consumed by some animals to match or equalise the intake of a test group on the following day. There are many reasons why pair feeding is critically important. An experiment may seek to examine how a new protein source, rich in some nutrient of interest, influences some aspect of metabolism. Let us consider a compound in the protein source that may reduce blood LDL cholesterol. A control diet is constructed based on casein. In the experimental diets, this casein is replaced on an isonitrogenous basis with the test protein source. Otherwise the diets are identical. After several weeks of *ad libitum* feeding a blood sample is taken and the results show that blood cholesterol rose with the experimental diet. Then the researcher begins to look at other data and observes that growth rates in the control rats were far higher than in the experimental group because the latter had a much lower food intake. Quite simply, the new protein source was unpalatable. The experiment will now have to be carried out as a pair-fed study. The food intake of rats given the experimental diet will be measured each day. On the following day, the control rats will be rationed to that amount. Food intakes and probably growth rates are identical. Only the protein source differs. Now the researcher can truly reach conclusions as to the effect of the new protein source on LDL cholesterol metabolism. The intake or supply of nutrients may be administered orally, intravenously, intraperitoneally, or by means of some specific tools (gavage, stereotaxis, etc.).

The experimental techniques available

The outcome or variables of interest to be assessed condition the experimental techniques to be applied, which may include growth curves, nutrient and energy balance, nutrient utilisation and signalling, etc., using cellular, molecular or other strategies.

Another approach to investigate nutritional processes is to overexpress, inactivate, or manipulate specific genes playing a role in body metabolism (Campión *et al.*, 2004). These technologies allow the study of the regulation and function of different genes. The current standard methods for manipulating genes in nutrition research depend on the method of introducing/blocking genes. Thus, genetic manipulation can be sustained for generations by creating germline transmission. In this way, there are examples of transgenic animals, overexpressing or knocking out genes, but still controlling this gene manipulation in a spatial or temporal manner. However, when the aim is not to transfer genetic information to subsequent generations, the most usual method is gene transfer to somatic cells. Different viral and non-viral vectors are used for the *in vivo* gene transfer, allowing a transient or permanent overexpression of the gene of interest. The RNAi (interference) approach allows the creation of new *in vivo* models by transient ablation of gene expression by degrading target mRNA. Moreover, by inserting RNAi encoding sequences in the genome, permanent silencing of the target gene can be obtained. Undoubtedly, new models of investigation will be developed, combining the different genetic manipulation techniques to achieve the creation of new models to understand the function and the regulation of metabolism, nutritional, and disease-related genes. Indeed, research concerning inhibiting/activating the expression of different genes (transgenic/ knockout animals), gene transfer, and RNAi application is allowing us to specifically investigate functions and metabolism of regulatory processes.

14.5 Human studies

In human nutrition, the ultimate court where hypotheses are both generated and tested are people. Nutritional epidemiology, through observational studies, demonstrates possible links between diet, physical activity, and disease (Willett, 2012). It is not the only way in which such possible links are generated but observational studies are critically important in modern nutrition. Experimental human nutrition takes the hypothesis and through several experiments tries to understand the nature of the link between nutrients and the metabolic basis of the disease. Once there is a reasonable body of evidence that particular nutritional conditions are related to the risk of disease, experimental nutritional epidemiology examines how population level interventions actually influence the incidence of disease (see Section 14.6). Accordingly, experimental human nutrition and experimental nutrition epidemiology both involve hypothesis testing. However, the former is more often intended to understand mechanisms and generally involves small numbers. The latter, in contrast, uses very large numbers to examine the public health impact of a nutrition intervention that, under the controlled conditions of the laboratory, showed promise.

The ultimate goal is to set public health recommendations that may improve population's health. Currently, there is growing interest in personalised nutrition. It aims to tailor recommendations to specific personal traits, conditions or goals. But the biological processes underpinning these recommendations are extremely complex. Thus, in the context of precision nutrition, a systems biology-based approach is needed to better understand the interplay between different biological mechanisms (van Ommen, 2017).

Human nutrition experimentation

The use of experimental animals for nutrition research offers many possible solutions to experimental problems. However, the definitive experiments, where possible, should be carried out in humans. Studies involving humans are more difficult to conduct for two major reasons. First, humans vary enormously compared with laboratory animals. They vary genetically and they also vary greatly in their lifestyle, background diet, health, physical activity, literacy, and in many other ways. Second, it is far more difficult to manipulate human diets since we do not eat purified or semi-purified diets.

Experimental diets in human nutrition intervention studies

In the 1950s, an epidemiological study across seven countries presented data to suggest that the main determinant of plasma cholesterol was the balance of saturated, monounsaturated, and polyunsaturated fatty acids (MUFAs and PUFAs). To test this hypothesis, a series of studies was carried out on human volunteers using "formula diets." Dried skimmed milk powder, the test oil, and water were blended to form a test milk with specific fatty acid compositions. The volunteers lived almost exclusively on these formulae. Although this type of study is simple to conduct, it does not represent the true conditions under which normal humans live. At the other end of the spectrum of options for manipulating human diets is that of issuing advice that the subjects verify with a food record. It is difficult to prove that subjects actually ate what they say they have eaten. Sometimes, adherence to dietary advice can be ascertained using tissue samples (blood, saliva, hair, fat) and biomarkers. For example, adherence to advice to increase oily fish intake can be monitored using platelet phospholipid fatty acids. In addition, there is interest in identifying novel biomarkers of food intake based on new food metabolomics techniques. These new techniques may allow to ascertain thousands of metabolites in a single determination and be, thus, applied in intervention and observational studies.

In between these two extremes of formula feeds and dietary advice lies an array of options in which convenience is generally negatively correlated with scientific exactitude. In the case of minerals and vitamins, it is feasible simply to give out pills for the volunteers to take and measure compliance by counting unconsumed pills and perhaps using biomarkers. When it comes to macronutrients this is not generally possible. Whereas asking someone to take a mineral supplement should not alter their eating habits, asking someone to consume one litre of milk a day or a bowl of rice bran per day will alter other aspects of the diets of the volunteers. It will not then be possible to attribute definitively an event to the intervention (1 l/day of milk or 1 bowl/day of rice bran). The event could have been caused by possible displacement of some other foods by the intervention. The only option in human intervention experiments is to prepare foods for volunteers to eat, which differ only in the test nutrient. If the objective is to examine the effect of MUFAs relative to saturated fatty acids (SFAs) on blood lipids, then fat-containing foods can be prepared that are identical except for the source of fat. The more foods and dishes that can be prepared in this way, the more successful the experiment will be.

The final dilemma is whether the test foods will be consumed. A volunteer may share the test foods, which are almost always supplied free of charge, with friends or family. To be sure of consumption, volunteers may be asked to consume the test meal in some supervised space, usually a metabolic suite. This, however, is a very costly option. Nutritional intervention studies with different macronutrient distribution of food content within energy-restricted diets are common in nutrition research (Abete *et al.*, 2006).

Study designs in human nutrition

The randomised clinical trial is the most powerful design to demonstrate cause–effect relationships. It is unique in representing a completely experimental approach in humans. The major strength of randomised trials is that they are able to control most biases and confounding even when confounding factors cannot be measured. The CONSORT statement has established the CONsolidated Standards Of Reporting Trials (http://www.consort-statement.org/). The CONSORT guidelines comprise a checklist and a flow diagram offering a standard way for reporting the research and assessing its quality. The major methodological issues to be considered and reported in a randomised trial include the following aspects: enrolment, allocation, follow-up, and inclusion in analysis of participants, sample size, proceedings for the randomisation, blinding of the allocation, blinded assessment of the outcome, comparability of groups regarding major prognostic variables, ascertainment and measurement of end-points, statistical analyses, subgroup analyses, results description, ancillary analyses, adverse events, interpretations, generalisability, and overall quality of the reported evidence.

As the researcher designs the options for altering the intake of nutrient under investigation, so too the design of the study requires careful thought. The metabolic effect of the nutrient in question may be influenced by age, sex, and other variables, such as high levels of alcohol intake or physical activity, smoking, health status, prescribed drug use, and family history. On an experiment-by-experiment basis, the researcher must decide which attributes will exclude a volunteer (exclusion criteria).

The volunteers recruited can now be assigned to the various treatments. When the numbers are small, randomly assigning subjects to the treatments may lead to imbalances that could confound conclusions. For example, if one has 45 volunteers for three treatments, it could be that the 15 assigned to treatment A include the five heaviest subjects and the five lightest subjects. Another treatment may include predominantly men. In such instances, a minimisation scheme can be used. Minimisation is a technique in which individuals are allocated to treatment groups, ensuring a balance by minimising the differences between groups in the distribution of important characteristics (age, weight, physical activity). To apply minimisation, during the recruitment process the investigators must keep an ongoing analysis of differences between groups in the major variables that may affect the result and adapt the allocation probabilities for the new individuals to the group that leads to a more balanced distribution of these characteristics. Another option is stratified randomisation in which strata are identified and subjects are randomly allocated within each stratum. While stratification and minimisation are potentially very useful, it is impractical to stratify individuals for many variables at the same time or to try to minimise every conceivable variable that may affect the result. To a considerable extent, the need to balance groups becomes less important when all subjects are rotated through all treatments (crossover designs). For this to happen, the number of experimental periods must equal the number of treatments. For any given period, all treatments must be represented. An important factor to consider in this type of design is whether or not a washout period is needed between treatments, and its duration.

Consider the situation above if the study was to examine the effect of fish oil (treatment A) versus olive oil (treatment B) on lymphocyte function. If it is deemed necessary that 20 days are needed to alter the membrane phospholipids of lymphocytes, then it is likely that 30 days will be needed to return to baseline. If it is necessary that each treatment should commence at baseline, then a washout period, where volunteers resume their normal routine, is needed.

A final consideration is the occasion when it is not possible to balance all confounding factors. Take as an example a study to examine the effect of supplemental calcium on bone mineral density in premenopausal women. The treatment group will receive a supplement of 1000 mg of calcium as a tablet and the control will receive a placebo tablet. What factors might one wish to balance in such a study? Among the possibilities are age, parity, use of oral contraceptives, intake of coffee, smoking, and physical activity. To balance these factors adequately is impossible. However, if they are recorded, then, when the data are being evaluated on a statistical basis, they can be included to ascertain their effect on the measured outcome, bone mineral density. To accomplish this aim, multivariate methods such as multiple regression or logistic regression should be used (see Section 14.2).

14.6 Epidemiological designs

Epidemiology is a health-related science dealing with the distribution and determinants of health and illness in populations. Nutritional epidemiology integrates the knowledge derived from nutrition research, to examine diet–disease relationships at the level of free-living populations. Nutritional epidemiology provides scientific evidence to understand the role of nutrition in the cause and prevention of disease.

The comparison and choice of different epidemiological study designs depends on exposure measures, outcome measures, costs, and expected length of follow-up. The selection of a study method is often influenced by

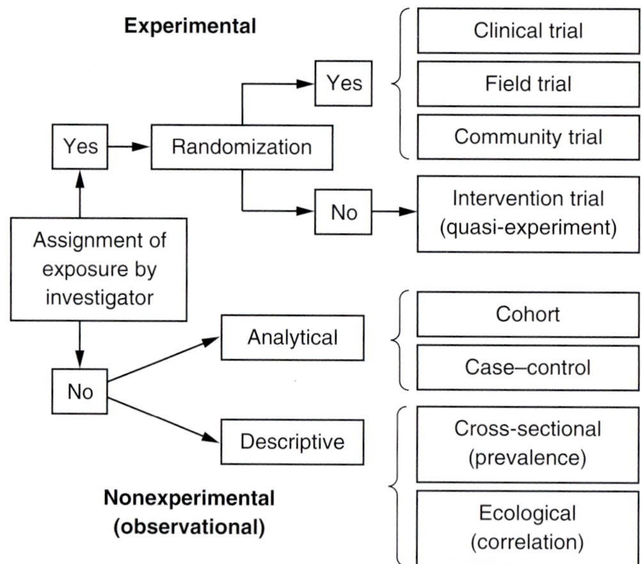

Figure 14.2 Classification of epidemiological designs.

pragmatic issues such as feasibility, as well as by ethical questions.

Epidemiological studies can be divided into two broad categories (Figure 14.2): experimental and nonexperimental (observational) studies. In a wide sense, an experiment is a set of observations, conducted under controlled circumstances, in which the scientist manipulates the conditions to ascertain the effect of such manipulation on the observations. Observational studies can be further divided into descriptive and analytical studies. Contrarily to experimental studies, in observational studies, the scientist does not allocate the exposure to the study participants.

Experimental studies in nutritional epidemiology

It is necessary to consider that in biological experimentation, it is not possible for the scientist to completely control all of the relevant circumstances, and the manipulation will consist in increasing at most the degree of variation in the factor that the scientist is investigating. The ideal will be to obtain two almost identical sets of circumstances where all factors are the same with the only difference in the factor to be studied. If a strong variation is then introduced in the latter factors, all of the observed differences between the two sets that occurred thereafter would be causally attributed to the single factor that the investigator had manipulated.

Experimental epidemiological designs are those in which the investigator assigns the exposure to each subject. In these studies, the treatment (or exposure) is assigned with the aim of attaining maximum comparability between treated and untreated groups regarding all other characteristics of the subjects apart from the treatment or exposure of interest. In epidemiological research, the best way to achieve identical sets of circumstances is to assign subjects randomly to exposure (treatment) or control groups. This process is called randomisation. All randomised studies are experimental designs.

Exposure, from an epidemiological point of view, describes lifestyle or environmental factors that may be relevant to health. Outcome is another generic term used to describe the health-related events or variables that are being studied in relation to the effect of an exposure. In nutritional epidemiology, the primary exposure of interest is dietary intake, whereas outcome measures usually involve disease occurrence or nutritional status indicators (anthropometry, clinical signs of disease/health status, biological or physiological measures or dietary habits).

It is also possible to design experimental studies assigning whole population groups to different exposures. These studies are called community trials. For example, if a whole town is assigned to receive an educational program about healthy eating and another neighbouring town is assigned to control (no educational program), this would be a community trial; when randomisation is used, it is termed "cluster randomisation." However, when the number of randomised units is scarce–even though each unit may be large–there would be no guarantee that the groups to be compared would be identical. Conversely, if the randomisation has been done on an individual basis and the whole sample is large enough, a random scheme will usually accomplish its objective of distributing the participants in groups that are essentially homogeneous in all measured and unmeasured factors. This balance makes groups directly comparable and ensures the validity of causal inferences extracted from a randomised design (individual randomisation).

In general, experimental studies with individual randomisation provide the strongest evidence for the effect of an exposure on an outcome. Experimental studies are the inferentially strongest designs to demonstrate causality, but they may raise substantial ethical problems because the scheme of random assignment is used to help not the subject, but the experiment. Subjects are exposed only to meet the needs of the protocol of the study and not the individual needs of the participant. Therefore, randomised experiments with humans can only be conducted under strict ethical conditions (see Boxes 14.3 and 14.4). It is not permissible to carry out experimental studies where the exposure is potentially harmful. Therefore, under these conditions, nonexperimental (observational) study designs must be applied. The design options in nutritional epidemiology must take into account the setting, uses, advantages, and limitations (Table 14.8).

Experimental designs in epidemiology

Experimental epidemiologists try to conduct controlled studies, and, in these studies, it is the investigator who assigns the exposure. Human studies, however, unlike animal studies, involve aspects that the investigator cannot control. This is particularly so when they are carried out on a free-living population. Two study designs

Box 14.3 Sample ethics form for completion prior to research

The proposal respects the fundamental ethical principles including human rights and will deal only with individuals adequately informed and willing to participate. Also, all research data partners will obtain national authorisation from an institutional review board or equivalent body before any intervention with subjects. The study does not involve any genetic manipulation.

- Requested specifications:
  - Human embryos or fetus — No Yes
  - Use of human embryonic or fetal tissue — No Yes
  - Use of other human tissue — No Yes
  - Research on persons — No Yes
  - If yes, further specify if it involves:
    - children — No Yes
    - persons unable to consent — No Yes
    - pregnant women — No Yes
    - healthy volunteers — No Yes
  - Use of nonhuman primates — No Yes
  - Use of transgenic animals — No Yes
  - Use of other animals — No Yes
  - Genetic modification of animals — No Yes
  - Genetic modification of plants — No Yes
- Other specifications:
  - The regulations, concerning human and medical research, will be respected with precise reference to the recommendations of the Helsinki (1964), Tokyo (1975), Venice (1983), Hong Kong (1989), Somerset West (1996), Edinburgh (2000), Washington DC (2002), Tokyo (2004), Seoul (2008) and Fortaleza (2013) committees, as well as other country specific regulations.

Box 14.4 Sample of an informed consent form

This form will cover the following aspects:

I .... (name)
I have read the volunteer's information
I have felt free to make questions concerning the study
I have received enough information
I have talked to the following personnel responsible (names . . .)
I understand that my participation is on a voluntary basis
I understand that I can withdraw from the study:
1 If I wish
2 Without further explanations
Therefore, I freely confirm my availability to be involved in the trial

Date
Signature

In addition, all the partners agree with the following statement
In implementing the proposed research I shall adhere most strictly to all national and international ethical and safety provisions applicable in the countries where the research is carried out.
I shall conform in particular to the relevant safety regulations concerning the deliberate release into the environment of genetically modified organisms.

Table 14.8 Design options in nutritional epidemiology

Design	Setting	Uses	Advantages	Limitations
Clinical trial	Secondary prevention (diseased participants)	Treatment–outcome association	Strongest evidence for causality Highest internal validity Very low potential for bias	Low external validity Ethical problems High cost
Field trial	Primary prevention (healthy participants)	Exposure–onset of disease association	Strong evidence for causality High internal validity Low potential for bias	Very large sample and long follow-up Low external validity Highest costs
Community trial	Group randomisation (towns, work-sites, schools)	Evaluation of community interventions or educational activities	If multiple, and small groups are randomised, it has the advantages of an experimental design	Low internal validity if the number of randomised units is low
Quasi-experiment	Intervention study (not randomised)	Evaluation of community interventions or educational activities	High feasibility More applicable Investigator controls exposure	Difficulties in finding comparable groups High potential for bias Underlying trends may alter results
Cohort	Participants are initially classified as exposed or nonexposed and followed up in time to monitor the incidence of the outcome. Retrospective or historical cohort studies are conducted using previously collected information (files)	The most powerful observational tool in nutritional epidemiology to study diet–health associations	Very low potential for bias Ability to study rare exposures, complex dietary patterns and multiple outcomes of a single exposure Allows direct estimation of risks and rates Minimal ethical problems	Large sample and very long follow-up No ability to study rare outcomes Bias by low follow-up (attrition) Requires collaborative participants High costs
Case–control	Exposure is compared between subjects with and without the outcome. Nested case–control studies are conducted within an ongoing cohort using the data of cohort members who develop the disease (cases) and a sample of non-diseased members (controls)	Practical analytical tool in nutritional epidemiology to study diet–health associations	Ability to study rare outcomes Ability to study multiple potential causes of a single outcome No problems with losses to follow-up Minimal ethical problems Low cost	Potential for biased recall of exposure and biased participation of controls Inability to study rare exposures and multiple outcomes of a single exposure Inability to estimate risks and rates
Cross-sectional	Past exposure and outcome are simultaneously assessed in a representative sample of the population	Estimation of the prevalence of a disease or an exposure Population assessment in health planning Monitoring trends if it is periodically repeated	Highest external validity Relatively low costs Minimal ethical problems A wide spectrum of information about diet and health can be collected	Difficult to assess the temporal sequence: very low ability for causal inference Potential for biased participation and response bias
Ecological	The unit of analysis is not the individual but a community. Exposure and/or disease are not measured at the individual level	Generation of new hypothesis and contextual or multilevel analysis	Ability for assessing exposures at the community level Relatively low costs Minimal ethical problems	Very low internal validity ("ecological fallacy")

dominate this area of epidemiology: randomised controlled trials and crossover studies. In these studies, subjects are randomly assigned to either an exposed or a non-exposed group, commonly referred to as the treatment group and the placebo group, respectively. The placebo is a substance that is indistinguishable from the treatment and enables both subjects and investigators to be blinded to the treatment. Changes in indicators of health or disease status are compared between the two groups at the end of the experiment to identify the effect of the exposure.

Crossover designs in epidemiology operate on the same principles as the repeated-measures designs common to basic science research. All study subjects receive the treatment and the placebo for equal periods, with a washout period in between, and the order of treatment or placebo administration is selected at random for each study subject. Crossover designs are appropriate only for studies of treatments that have no long-term effects, a feature that limits their utility in nutritional epidemiology.

In general, experimental epidemiological study designs are well suited to the identification of causal relationships between specific exposures and indicators of health or disease status. Application of these methods is limited, however, by the difficulty in controlling exposures and by the enormous expense associated with population-based intervention trials aimed at modifying risk or chronic diseases. It is perhaps more feasible to apply experimental study designs to contrast the effects of pharmacological doses of specific nutrients or food components, the exposures of which can be more easily controlled. This approach has been increasingly selected from the 1990s to assess the effects of specific micronutrients (β-carotene, α-tocopherol, folic acid, and other minerals and vitamins) using large-scale randomised trials.

When only one micronutrient is compared with a placebo, the study is called a single trial, whereas multiple or factorial trials involve designs where several micronutrients are compared with a placebo. In a 2 × 2 factorial design, two treatments are evaluated simultaneously by forming four groups (treatment A, treatment B, both treatments, and placebo).

Experimental studies keep the highest internal validity among epidemiological designs. However, they may lack generalisation (i.e., they may have low external validity) and their applicability to free-living populations may be poor insofar as the dietary intake patterns do not correspond to isolated nutrients but to the combination of more complex food items. Moreover, the induction time needed to appraise the effect of a postulated cause may last longer than the observation period of a randomised trial, thus precluding the ability of the trial to ascertain the causal relationship.

Quasi-experimental studies are those in which the assignment of exposure is controlled by the investigator, but subjects are not randomly allocated. They are sometimes called intervention trials (Figure 14.2).

Some randomised trials are referred to as primary prevention trials and others as secondary prevention trials. Primary prevention trials are those conducted among healthy individuals with the aim of preventing the onset of disease. For example, in the Women's Health Initiative (Howard *et al.*, 2006) more than 48 000 healthy postmenopausal women were randomly assigned to receive either a low-fat diet or placebo to prevent the onset of cardiovascular disease (CVD). All participants were free of this disease at the start of the study and they were followed up for several years to assess the incidence of fatal and nonfatal coronary heart disease, fatal and nonfatal stroke, and CVD (composite of both). This is an example of a primary prevention trial. Primary prevention trials are also called field trials.

Secondary prevention trials are conducted among patients who already suffer from a particular disease and they are randomly assigned to treatment or placebo groups to prevent adverse outcomes. For example, to study the benefits of a Mediterranean-style diet, in the Lyon Diet Heart Study, patients were randomised to two different dietary patterns after suffering a myocardial infarction (de Lorgeril *et al.*, 1999). The outcome was not the onset of disease but the incidence of a new infarction or cardiac death during the follow-up period.

Nonexperimental (observational) epidemiological studies

When experiments are not feasible or are unethical, other nonexperimental designs are used. In nonexperimental (observational) studies the investigator has no control over the exposure, because the participants freely determines being exposed or not. In nonexperimental studies the investigator may take advantage of "natural experiments," where exposure only appears in some defined groups. An example of this would be an "experiment" where dietary intake is culturally determined, such as in Indonesia, where white rice is consumed rather than brown rice, and beriberi is common as a result of vitamin B_1 deficiency.

Nonexperimental (observational) designs can be further classified into four main subtypes:

- cross-sectional studies
- case–control studies
- cohort studies
- ecological studies.

Among observational studies, the main differences between study designs relies on the time when exposure and outcome are measured. The initiative "STrengthening the Reporting of OBservational studies in Epidemiology (STROBE)" – www. strobe-statement.org – provides a check-list to assess the methodological quality of the three major epidemiological designs: cohort studies, case–control studies, and cross-sectional studies (Von Elm and Egger, 2004).

Cross-sectional (prevalence) studies

Cross-sectional or prevalence studies measure both exposure and outcome in the present and simultaneously. Cross-sectional surveys provide a snapshot of descriptive epidemiological data on nutrition, identifying nutritional needs in the population and informing health promotion and disease prevention programs at a single point in time. Several countries conduct regular cross-sectional surveys on representative samples of their populations focusing on dietary habits and frequencies of illness. Dietary factors can then be correlated with prevalence of illness, which may be helpful for national nutrition policy.

Case–control studies

In case–control studies, outcome is measured in the present, and past exposure is ascertained. Usually the dietary and lifestyle patterns of patients with a disease (cases) are compared with those of age- and sex-matched people without disease (controls).

Subjects are identified and recruited on the basis of the presence or absence of the disease or the health outcome variable of interest. Ideally, the controls are randomly selected from the same study base as the cases, and identical inclusion and exclusion criteria are applied to each group. The presence of specific dietary exposures or other factors of etiological interest in subjects is generally established using interviews, questionnaires, or medical record reviews. Within the general framework for case–control studies, there are several options for study design and control selection.

For example, controls may be matched with cases at an individual level on the basis of age, sex, or other variables believed to affect disease risk. Matching eliminates variability between cases and controls with respect to the matching variables and thus leads to a higher efficiency in the analysis. Case–control studies are by far the most logistically feasible of the analytical study designs in epidemiology, but their application to questions of interest to nutritionists is limited by the particular nature of diet–disease relationships.

The insight to be gained from a comparison of dietary exposures between cases and controls is limited by the possibility that the dietary patterns of subjects changed since the time when diet was most important to the disease initiation process. Case–control studies attempt to overcome this limitation by measuring past diet using food frequency or diet history methods. One concern is that recall of past diet by cases may be influenced by their present disease status. For example, patients who have had a heart attack may attach an unfair level of importance to their intake of specific foods, based on misinformation.

A primary factor in choosing between a case–control design and a cohort design is whether the exposure or the outcome is rare. If the outcome is rare, case–control studies are preferable, because a cohort would need a very large sample to observe a sufficient number of events. If the exposure is rare, cohort studies are preferable.

A nested case–control design consists of selecting as cases only those members of a previously defined cohort who develop the disease during their follow-up period. A random sample or a matched sample of non-cases is also selected from the cohort to make up the control series as the comparison group.

Cohort studies

In cohort studies exposure is evaluated in the present and outcome ascertained in the future.

Cohort studies are most commonly longitudinal or prospective, with subjects being followed forward in time over some predefined period to assess disease onset. They may also be retrospective (historical cohorts), with groups identified on the basis of exposure sometime in the past and then followed from that time to the present to establish presence or absence of the outcome. The feasibility of retrospective cohorts depends on the availability of good-quality data from pre-existing files. The research costs associated with cohort study designs mean that such studies are less common than other approaches. Nevertheless, a substantial effort to develop large cohort studies in nutritional epidemiology has been made since the early 1980s. Cohort studies can assess multiple outcomes, whereas case–control studies are restricted to assessing one outcome, but may be able to assess many different exposures. If an absolute measure of the effect of the exposure on the outcome is required, the only design that is appropriate is a cohort study, as case–control studies cannot be used to estimate incidence.

For example, to ascertain the relationship between olive oil consumption and coronary heart disease, a case–control study would compare the previous consumption of olive oil between cases of myocardial infarction and healthy controls. A cohort study would start with a roster of healthy individuals whose baseline diet would be recorded. They would then be followed up over several years to compare the occurrence of new cases of myocardial infarction between those consuming different levels of olive oil as recorded when they were healthy at baseline.

Ecological studies

Epidemiological studies can be classified according to whether measurements of exposure and outcome are made on populations or individuals. Observational investigations in which the unit of observation and analysis is not the individual but a whole community or population are called ecological studies. In ecological studies, measures of exposure routinely collected and aggregated at the household, local, district, regional, national, or international level are compared with outcome measures aggregated at the same level. An example of an ecological study would be plotting the mortality rates for colon cancer in several countries against the average intakes of saturated fat in these same countries and calculating the correlation between the two variables.

Studies considering the individual (instead of the population) as the unit of observation are always preferable because in an individually based study it is possible to relate exposure and outcome measures more directly, preventing many flaws that are likely to invalidate the findings of ecological studies. One of these flaws is known as the "ecological fallacy" and it is the bias resulting because an association observed between variables on an aggregated level does not necessarily represent the association that exists at an individual level.

Ecological studies measure diet less accurately because they use the average population intake as the exposure value for all individuals in the groups that are compared, leading to a high potential for biased ascertainment of diet–disease associations. Ecological studies, also termed correlation studies, may compare indicators of diet and health or disease within a single population over time to look for secular trends, or to compare the disease incidence rates and dietary intake patterns of migrant groups with those of comparable populations in the original and new country. Ecological comparisons have been important in hypothesising diet and disease associations. Nevertheless, they are not able to establish causal relationships.

Definition of outcomes and end-points

Epidemiological outcomes must be clearly defined at the outset of a study. For example, a study of diet and CVD may specify that the outcome (CVD) is verified by specific clinical tests such as cardiac enzyme level or electrocardiographic changes. Taking the word of the patient or the doctor may not sufficient. Two main measures of the frequency for an outcome are used in epidemiology: prevalence and incidence.

Prevalence

The prevalence of an outcome is the proportion of subjects in a population who have that outcome at a given point in time. The numerator of prevalence is the number of existing cases and the denominator is the whole population:

$$\text{Prevalence} = \frac{\text{Existing cases}}{\text{Total population}}$$

Incidence

The incidence of an outcome is the proportion of new cases that occur in a population during a period of observation. The numerator of incidence is the number of new cases developing during the follow-up period, while the denominator is the total population at risk at the beginning of the follow-up time:

$$\text{Incidence} = \frac{\text{New cases}}{\text{Population inititally at risk}}$$

When calculated this way, incidence is a proportion. However, incidence can also be expressed as a rate (velocity or density), when the time during which each person is observed (i.e., person-time of observation) is included in the denominator. Then it is called incidence rate or incidence density and it is expressed as the number of new cases per person-time of observation.

Other epidemiological methods

Epidemiological studies have also been conducted to assess: consumer attitudes to and beliefs about food, nutrition, physical activity patterns, and health to provide policy-makers, researchers and the food industry with data to promote health messages concerning the relation between food or nutrient intake and chronic diseases. These surveys seek information about influences on food choice, health determinants, criteria about perceptions of healthy eating, regular sources of nutritional information, expected benefits and barriers to healthy diet implementation, in order to identify consumers' knowledge, attitudes, and beliefs concerning food and health interactions and to promote more focused nutrition education messages. Design and validation of questionnaires for physical activity assessment, depression, quality of life, etc, are emerging as useful instruments not only for nutrition research but also for nutrition status evaluation (Taberna, 2019).

Meta-analysis and pooled analysis

The role of meta-analysis for systematically combining the results of published randomised trials has become routine, but its place in observational epidemiology has been controversial despite widespread use in social sciences. Some have argued that the aggregation of data from randomised trials is appropriate because statistical power is increased without concern for validity since the comparison groups have been randomised, but that in observational epidemiology the issue of validity is determined largely by confounding and bias rather than limitations of statistical power. Thus, the greater statistical precision obtained by the combination of data may be misleading because the findings may still be invalid. An alternative to combining published epidemiological data is to pool and analyse the primary data from all available studies on a topic that meets specified criteria. Ideally, this should involve the active collaboration of the original investigators, who are fully familiar with the data and its limitations. This kind of study conducted with a combination of the original data from several studies, is the basis of pooled analysis or pooling projects. In a pooled analysis, the range of dietary factors that can be addressed may be considerably greater than in the separate analyses, because any one study will have few subjects in the extremes of intake and, sometimes, the studies will vary in distribution of dietary factors. The advantages of pooled analyses in nutritional epidemiology are so substantial that they are becoming common practice for important issues, such as alcoholic intake and breast cancer, body size and breast cancer, or alcohol beverages and coronary heart disease.

Analysis of epidemiological data requires careful consideration of the criteria for acceptable data quality, but also of the presentation of categorised or continuous independent variables and the application of empirical scores. The study of subgroup analysis and interactions and error correction are other issues of interest. Other limitations are the requirement of the sample to be considered as representative, compliance, inaccuracies of information in retrospective studies, and confounding effects by factors that are simultaneously associated with both the exposure and the outcome.

14.7 Perspectives on the future

Future nutrition research will develop new methods for studying those processes whereby cells, tissues and the whole body obtain and utilise substances contained in the diet to maintain their structure and function in a healthy manner. Particular emphasis will be paid to molecular and cellular based strategies devised to understand better the genetic basis of nutritional outcomes.

It can also be anticipated that many ongoing large cohort studies with tens of thousands of participants will provide valuable information on the role of nutrition in disease prevention, and also on nutritional management of a large number of diseases by dietary means, and gene–nutrient and gene–environment interactions. Moreover, pooling of data from several cohort studies may provide a very powerful tool to assess the benefits of a healthy diet. An increasing interest in a dietary pattern approach instead of a single nutrient approach will be seen in nutritional epidemiology in the forthcoming decades. In addition, large primary prevention trials using the approach of assessing the effect of an overall dietary pattern (Estruch *et al.*, 2018; Howard *et al.*, 2006) are growing nowadays and their results will be on the rise during the next decade (Martinez-Gonzalez, 2004).

Nutritional epidemiology will also adopt a wider, multidisciplinary approach, with more studies concerning the impact of factors affecting social determinants of eating patterns, food supplies, and nutrient utilisation on health to facilitate the decisions of policy-makers, food industry managers, investigators, and consumers Furthermore, omics technologies are emerging as important tools for precise nutrition implementation.

References

Abete, I., Parra, M.D., Zulet, M.D. *et al.* (2006). Different dietary strategies of weight loss in obesity: role of energy and macronutrient content. *Nutr Res Rev.* **19**: 5–12.

Brouwer-Brolsma, E.M., Brennan, L., Drevon, C.A. *et al.* (2017). Combining traditional dietary assessment methods with novel metabolomics techniques: present efforts by the Food Biomarker Alliance. *Proc Nutr Soc.* **76**: 619–627.

Campión, J., Milagro, F.I., and Martinez, J.A. (2004). Genetic manipulation in nutrition, metabolism, and obesity research. *Nutr Rev.* **62**(8): 321–330. Review.

Chang, C.K. and Snook, J.T. (2001). The cholesterolaemic effects of dietary fats in cholesteryl ester transfer protein transgenic mice. *British Journal of Nutrition.* **85**: 643–648.

Estruch, R., Ros, E., Salas-Salvadó, J. *et al.* (2018). Primary prevention of cardiovascular disease with a Mediterranean diet supplemented with extra-virgin olive oil or nuts. *N Engl J Med.* 378:e34.

Howard, B.V., Van Horn, L., Hsia, J. *et al.* (2006). Low-fat dietary pattern and risk of cardiovascular disease. *JAMA.* **295**: 655–666.

Katz, M.H. (2006). *Multivariable Analysis: a Practical Guide for Clinicians*, 2e. Cambridge: Cambridge University Press.

Lorgeril de, M., Salen, P., Martin, J.L. *et al.* (1999). Mediterranean diet, traditional risk factors, and the rate of cardiovascular complications after myocardial infarction: final report of the Lyon Diet Heart Study. *Circulation.* **99**: 779–785.

Martínez-González, M.A. and Estruch, R. (2004). Mediterranean diet, antioxidants, and cancer: the need for randomised trials. *European Journal of Cancer Prevention.* **13**: 327–335.

Schone, F., Leiterer, M., Hartung, H. *et al.* (2001). Rapeseed glucosinolates and iodine in sows affect the milk iodine concentration and the iodine status of piglets. *British Journal of Nutrition.* **85**: 659–670.

Taberna, D.J., Navas-Carretero, S., and Martinez, J.A. (2019). Current nutritional status assessment tools for metabolic care and clinical nutrition. Curr Opin Clin Nutr Metab Care. Epub ahead of print.

van Ommen, B., van den Broek, T., de Hoogh, I. *et al.* (2017). Systems biology of personalized nutrition. *Nutr Rev.* **75**: 579–599.

Von Elm, M. and Egger, M. (2012). The scandal of poor epidemiological research. *BMJ.* **329**: 868–869.

Willett, W. (2012). *Nutritional Epidemiology*, 3e. New York: Oxford University Press.

Further reading

Armitage, P. and Colton, T. (2007). Encyclopaedia of Biostatistics, 2e. New York: John Wiley and Sons.

Breslow, N.E. (2000). Statistics. *Epidemiologic Reviews.* **22**: 126– 130.

Corthésy-Theulaz, I., den Dunnen, J.T., Ferre, P. *et al.* (2005). Nutrigenomics: the impact of biomics technology on nutrition research. *Annals of Nutrition & Metabolism.* **49**: 355–365.

Fernandez-Jarne, J., Martínez, E., Prado, M. *et al.* (2002). Risk of non-fatal myocardial infarction negatively associated with olive oil consumption: a case-control study in Spain. *International Journal of Epidemiology.* **31**: 474–480.

Kussmann, M., Raymond, F., and Affolter, M. (2006). OMICS – driven biomarker discovery in nutrition and health. *Journal of Biotechnology.* **124**: 758–787.

Leedy, P.D. (1980). *Practical Research: Planning and Designs*, Vol. 2. New York: Macmillan.

Rosner, B. (2015). *Fundamentals of Biostatistics*, 8e. Boston: Cengage Learning.

Scheweigert, F.J. (2007). Nutritional proteomics: methods and concepts for research in nutritional science. *Annals of Nutrition & Metabolism.* **51**: 99–107.

15 Food Safety: A Public Health Issue of Growing Importance

Catherine M. Burgess, Cristina Arroyo, Declan J. Bolton, Martin Danaher, Lisa O'Connor, Patrick J. O'Mahony, and Christina Tlustos

Key messages

After reading this chapter the student should have an understanding of:

- factors contributing to food safety issues
- types and sources of contamination in foods
- food-borne bacterial pathogens
- food-borne viruses
- food-borne parasites
- transmissible spongiform encephalopathies and food
- chemical contamination of food
- allergens in food
- food safety control programs
- emerging food safety concerns

15.1 Introduction

In recent years the reported incidence of food-borne diseases has continued to increase worldwide, with a number of extremely serious outbreaks occurring on every continent. In addition, various high-profile food safety issues, including shiga-toxin producing *Escherichia coli* (e.g. E. coli O157 and O104), melamine, bovine spongiform encephalopathy (BSE), dioxins, acrylamide, *Listeria monocytogenes* and the red colorant Sudan Red 1 have presented themselves to consumers, industry and regulators alike.

People most vulnerable to food poisoning are generally the very young and people whose natural defence barriers have been affected by aging, disease and/or medication. In a nutritional context, food-borne illness is often associated with malnutrition. To convey positive public health nutritional messages, nutritionists should understand the scientific basis of "food scares" that affect attitudes to food, nutrition, and health. This chapter aims to highlight the reasons for concern about the safety of food, the types and sources of biological, chemical and physical contaminants and allergens which may be present in foods, and possible control and prevention strategies.

15.2 Factors contributing to food safety concerns

Although it is difficult to determine the global incidence of food-borne disease with accuracy, the World Health Organization (WHO) recently published a study on the global disease burden of 22 food-borne diseases of bacterial, protozoal, and viral origin and estimated that two billion cases and over one million deaths occurred in 2010 (Kirk *et al.*, 2015). In the USA alone it has been reported that 31 microbial pathogens cause 9.4 million episodes of food-borne illness and 1351 deaths each year (Scallan *et al.*, 2011). The

Introduction to Human Nutrition, Third Edition. Edited on behalf of The Nutrition Society by Susan A. Lanham-New, Thomas R. Hill, Alison M. Gallagher and Hester H. Vorster.

Companion website: www.wiley.com/go/lanham-new/humannutrition

WHO study included three chemical hazards (aflatoxin, cassava cyanide, and dioxin), however limited conclusions were drawn because health effects of chemical hazards may not be observed for years following exposure (e.g., aflatoxin and liver cancer; lead and cardiovascular disease; Havelaar *et al.*, 2015).

Changing food supply system

The increasing incidence of food-borne diseases is due to a number of factors, including the globalisation of the food supply chain, changes in food production on the farm, new systems of food processing, longer distribution chains, new food preparation, storage methods and consumer trends. Changing lifestyles have led to a far greater reliance on convenience foods that are prepared outside the home, and which may have a longer preparation to consumption time. In addition, the food chain has become longer and more complex, giving increased opportunities for food contamination. International trade in foods has expanded dramatically, where trade in agricultural goods has almost tripled from 2000 to 2016 from US$570 billion to US$1.6 trillion (FAO, 2018). Globalisation of food trade presents a major challenge to food safety control authorities, in that food can become contaminated in one country and cause outbreaks of food-borne illness in another. It is not unusual for an average meal to contain ingredients from many countries that have been produced and processed under different standards of food safety. Food-borne zoonoses (i.e., diseases that can be transmitted between humans and animals either through direct or indirect contact) have most commonly been associated with foods of animal origin, including meat and dairy. However, in recent years, coupled with changes in dietary patterns and globalisation of the food supply, there has been an increase in the number of outbreaks associated with fresh produce as a result of direct and indirect contamination of the produce.

Acute and chronic effects of food-borne illness

Food-borne diseases are classified as either infections or intoxications. Food-borne infections are caused when viable pathogenic microorganisms are ingested, and these can then multiply in the human body. Intoxications are caused when microbial toxins or naturally occurring toxins (e.g., of animal origin such as saxitoxins produced by shellfish or of plant origin such as cyanide produced by some fruit trees) are consumed in foods contaminated with those. Illnesses that relate to the consumption of foods that are contaminated with naturally occurring toxins or microorganisms or their toxins are collectively referred to as food poisoning.

The health consequences of food-borne illness caused by microorganisms are varied and depend on factors such as the type of disease, the virulence of the pathogen and the individual's susceptibility. Symptoms are often mild and self-limiting in healthy individuals and people recover within a few days from acute health effects. Acute symptoms include diarrhoea, stomach pain and cramps, vomiting, fever, and jaundice. However, in some cases microorganisms or their products are directly or indirectly associated with long-term health effects such as reactive arthritis and rheumatoid syndromes, endocarditis, Reiter syndrome, Guillain–Barré syndrome, renal disease, cardiac and neurological disorders, and nutritional and other malabsorptive disorders. It is generally accepted that chronic, secondary after-effect illnesses may occur in 2–3% of cases of food-borne infections and that the long-term consequences to human health may be greater than the acute disease (Lindsay, 1997).

Vulnerable groups

Vulnerable groups tend to be more susceptible to food-borne infections and generally suffer more severe illness, because their immune systems are in some way impaired. The immune system of infants and young children is immature. In pregnant women, increased levels of progesterone lead to the downregulation of cell-mediated immunity, increasing the susceptibility of both mother and fetus to infection by intracellular pathogens (Smith, 1999). In older people, a general decline in the body's immune response occurs with age, as does a decrease in stomach acid production. Immune responses in older people are also adversely affected if that person is malnourished through poor diet. Furthermore, age-related loss of sensory abilities, such as sight and taste, and even chewing and swallowing (dysphagia) difficulties can lead to problems in choosing and preparing food. An ageing population is one factor influencing the increase in the prevalence of food-borne disease. This trend is likely to continue with the number of people aged 65 or over projected to triple to nearly 1.5 billion by 2050 (WHO, 2011). Other groups for whom their immune system may be suppressed, making them more susceptible to food-borne infection, include cancer patients, transplant patients receiving immunosuppressant drugs, and patients with acquired immunodeficiency syndrome (AIDS). In non-industrialised countries, political unrest, war, and famine lead to increased malnutrition and can expose poorer populations to increased risk of food-borne disease. For vulnerable groups, the risk of food poisoning is much greater with particular types of foods. For this reason national food safety authorities often recommend safer food options (FSAI, 2018).

Improved surveillance

Improved surveillance systems lead to an increase in the reported incidence of food-borne disease. Using information technology, many countries have developed enhanced surveillance systems to gain a better picture of the true incidence of food-borne disease. International outbreaks are more readily detectable with the use of electronic databases for sharing molecular typing data (such as PulseNet International) and rapid alert systems (such as the International Food Safety Authorities Network (INFOSAN)), websites, or list servers. In recent years significant advances have been made in the area of DNA (deoxyribonucleic acid) sequencing technology with the advent of next generation sequencing (NGS), with a concomitant decrease in cost. This has enabled the rapid sequencing of outbreak strains, facilitating traceback investigations with greater accuracy and the identification of outbreaks which may go unnoticed otherwise. Whole genome sequencing, one of the most popular uses of NGS, provides the highest degree of subtyping resolution and accordingly, has been introduced into regulatory laboratories worldwide. A landscape paper by the WHO on the use of whole genome sequencing for food-borne disease surveillance outlines the public impact of its use, as well as potential barriers for implementation in low- and middle-income countries (WHO, 2018). However, even with these enhanced surveillance and typing capabilities, it is unlikely that statistics reflect the true incidence of food-borne disease worldwide.

Economic consequences of food-borne illness

As well as morbidity and mortality associated with food-borne diseases, there are direct economic costs incurred. In the USA a state by state analysis indicated the national cost of food-borne illness to be in the region of $55.5 to 93.2 billion annually (Scharff, 2015). The *E. coli* O104 outbreak which occurred in Europe in 2011 was estimated to have resulted in economic losses worth over two billion dollars. A recent study by Tam and O'Brien (2016) reported that *Campylobacter* and Norovirus cost the United Kingdom £50 million and £81 million per annum respectively.

However, the true estimates of food-borne disease and the likely economic costs are unknown. In industrialised countries only a small proportion of cases of food-borne diseases is reported, and even fewer are investigated. Very few non-industrialised countries have established food-borne disease reporting systems, and in those that have, only a small fraction of cases is reported.

15.3 Physical hazards

Physical hazards include solid materials that are not meant to be in a particular food such as glass, rubber and metal fragments, jewellery, dirt, and stones. They can be the result of accidents or errors but are usually associated with poor quality control and low standards of production, processing and handling. Although such contaminants are generally non-toxic, they can result in choking incidents or internal lacerations.

15.4 Biological hazards

Food-borne bacterial pathogens

There are many types of bacterial food-borne pathogens. The characteristics of food-borne

Table 15.1 Characteristics of food-borne bacterial intoxications

Bacteria	Comment	Food-borne illness (a) Onset (b) Duration	Food-borne illness (a) Symptoms (b) Infectious dose	(a) Min. temp (b) Opt. temp (c) Min. pH[a] (d) Min. A_w[b]	Forms spores	Heat resistance	(a) Gram stain (b) Aerobic/ anaerobic	(a) Source (b) Associated foods[b]
Bacillus cereus (Emetic)	Vegetative cells (i.e. cells that are actively growing rather than forming spores) are inactivated by normal cooking temperatures; however, spores are quite heat resistant. Emetic illness is caused by consumption of heat-stable emetic toxin produced by cells growing to high numbers in food. This is most likely to happen when cooked foods are not served while hot or not cooled rapidly	(a) 1–5 h (b) 6–24 h	(a) Nausea and vomiting (b) >10^5 cells (12–32 μg toxin/kg)	(a) 4°C (b) 30–35°C (c) 4.3 (d) 0.93	Yes	Heat-sensitive, but can form heat-resistant spores Emetic toxin: extremely heat resistant	(a) Gram positive (b)Facultative anaerobe	(a) Soil, dust and vegetation (b) Cooked rice, cereals and cereal-based products, herbs and spices
Clostridium botulinum Group I (proteolytic) Group II (nonproteolytic)	Food-borne botulism is caused when food becomes contaminated with spores from the environment, which are not destroyed by initial cooking or processing. If the food is packaged anaerobically and provides a suitable environment for growth, spores will germinate, leading to toxin production. The toxin is heat sensitive, so further heat treatment of the food would prevent illness. The so called "botulinum cook" (heat treatment to 121°C for 3 min or equivalent) is used for low acid canned food products to destroy these spores	(a) 12–36 h but may take days (b) Variable (from days to months)	(a) Blurred and/or double vision, dryness of the mouth followed by difficulties swallowing and finally breathing. Vomiting and mild diarrhoea may occur in the early stages (b) 0.005–0.5 μg toxin	Group I (a) 10°C (b) 30–40°C (c) 4.3 (d) 0.94 Group II (a) 3.3°C (b) 25–37°C (c) 5.0 (d) 0.97	Yes	Toxin: destroyed by 5 min at 85°C	(a) Gram positive (b) Obligate anaerobe	(a) Soil, sediment, intestinal tract of fish and mammals (b) Canned foods, smoked and salted fish, honey
Staphylococcus aureus	Food handlers play a major role in transmission. *S. aureus* is carried in nose/ throat of ~40% of healthy individuals and can be easily transferred to food via the hands. Most implicated foods have been ready-to-eat foods that have been contaminated by poor handling practices and stored at incorrect temperatures, allowing *S. aureus* to grow to levels (>10^5 cells/g) that will produce sufficient heat-stable staphylococcal toxin	(a) 1–6 h (b) 1–2 days	(a) Severe nausea, vomiting, abdominal pain and diarrhoea (b) <1.0 μg toxin (>10^5 cells/g needed to produce sufficient toxin)	Under aerobic conditions: (a) 7°C (b) 40–45°C (c) 4.0 (d) 0.83	No	Toxin: heat resistant	(a) Gram Positive (b) Facultative anaerobe	(a) Exposed skin lesions, nose, throat and hands (b) Generally foods of animal origin that have been physically handled and have not received a subsequent bactericidal treatment

[a] Under otherwise optimal conditions; limits will vary according to strain, temperature, type of acid (in the case of pH), solute (in the case of A_w), and other factors.
[b] Not an exhaustive list.
Min., minimum; Opt., optimal; A_w, water activity (based on a saturated NaCl solution).

Table 15.2 Characteristics of food-borne bacterial infections

Bacteria	Comment	Food-borne illness (a) Onset (b) Duration	Food-borne illness (a) Symptoms (b) Infectious dose	(a) Min. temp (b) Opt. temp (c) Min. pH[a] (d) Min. A_w	Heat resistance	(a) Gram stain (b) Aerobic/ anaerobic	(a) Source (b) Associated foods[b]
Bacillus cereus (diarrhoeal)	Vegetative cells are inactivated by normal cooking temperatures; however, spores are quite heat resistant. The diarrhoeal enterotoxin is produced when spores germinate in the small intestine after consumption of contaminated food	(a) 8–16 h (b) 12–14 h	(a) Abdominal pain and diarrhoea (b) >10^5 cells	(a) 4°C (b) 30–35°C (c) 4.3 (d) 0.93	Heat-sensitive, but forms heat-resistant spores (D_{121} = 0.03–2.35 min)	(a) Gram positive (b) Facultative anaerobe	(a) Soil and dust (b) Meat, milk, vegetables, fish and soups
Clostridium perfringens	Illness results from consumption of food containing high numbers of cells (>10^6/g) followed by enterotoxin production in the large intestine. When contaminated food is cooked, sporulation is induced. As the food cools, the spores germinate and vegetative cells continue to multiply, unless the food is cooled quickly and stored under refrigerated conditions.	(a) 12–18 h (can be 8–22 h) (b) 24 h	(a) Diarrhoea and severe abdominal pain (b) >10^6 cells/g	(a) 10°C (b) 43–45°C (c) 5.5 (d) 0.93	Heat-sensitive, but forms heat-resistant spores	(a) Gram positive (b) Obligate anaerobe	(a) Soil and animal faeces (b) Meat, poultry, gravy, dried and precooked foods
Clostridium difficile	*Clostridium difficile* causes infectious diarrhoea in humans. Traditionally occurs in patients over 65 years old and is associated with healthcare facilities and patients undergoing antibiotic treatment where the treatment allows proliferation of *C. difficile* in the colon. However, the incidence of non-healthcare, community acquired *C. difficile* infections is increasing and food-borne sources are suspected. These bacteria produce enterotoxins, (*Clostridium difficile* toxin A and *Clostridiun difficile* toxin B), which produce inflammation and diarrhoea in infected patients.	(a) 5–10 days after the start of a course of antibiotic and 2–3 days after exposure	Symptoms include watery diarrhoea, fever, nausea, and abdominal pain, but in susceptible patients complications may occur including pseudomembranous colitis, perforation of the colon and sepsis.	(a) 25°C (b) 30–37°C (c) 5.0 (d) 0.95	Heat sensitive but forms heat resistant spores	(a) Gram positive (b) Obligate anaerobe	May be part of the normal gut microflora but may also be food-borne.
Campylobacter	C. *jejuni* is one of the most common causes of bacterial food poisoning in many industrialised countries. Although campylobacters are fragile organisms, and do not survive or multiply very well on foods, the low infectious dose means that a small level of contamination may result in illness. Compared with other food-borne bacteria with low infectious doses, relatively few outbreaks have been identified.	(a) 2–5 days (b) 1–7 days	(a) Moderate to severe diarrhoea, sometimes bloody diarrhoea. Severe abdominal pain. Vomiting is rare. Complications are uncommon, but include bacteremia, reactive arthritis and Guillain–Barré syndrome (b) 500 cells	(a) 32°C (b) 42–43°C (c) 4.9 (d) 0.98	Heat-sensitive	(a) Gram negative (b) Fastidious microaerophile	(a) Chickens, birds, cattle, flies, and water (b) Undercooked chicken, raw milk, beef, pork, lamb, shellfish, and water

Verotoxigenic *Escherichia coli* (VTEC). Also referred to Shiga toxin producing *Escherichia coli* (STEC)	VTEC/STEC is of considerable concern due to the severity of illness. The organism is easily killed by cooking, but the low infective dose means that foods must be cooked thoroughly and protected from cross-contamination. Most cases are associated with 6 serogroups; O157, O26, O103, O111, O145 and O104.	(a) 1–6 days (b) 4–6 days	(a) Severe abdominal cramps, bloody diarrhoea (hemorrhagic colitis), approx. 5% (mostly children) develop hemolytic uremic syndrome (HUS) (b) 10–100 cells	(a) 7°C (b) 37°C (c) 3.6 (d) 0.95	Heat-sensitive	(a) Gram negative (b) Facultative anaerobe	(a) Cattle, sheep, pigs, deer (b) Undercooked beef burgers, raw milk, salad vegetables, and unpasteurised apple juice
Listeria monocytogenes	*L. monocytogenes* causes serious illness in individuals with impaired cell-mediated immunity. Highly susceptible individuals include pregnant women, neonates, older people and immunocompromised individuals. The organism is also reported to cause febrile gastroenteritis (FG) in healthy persons. Foods associated with transmission tend to be processed, ready-to-eat foods, with long shelf-lives (>5 days) stored at refrigeration temperatures.	(a) Up to 10 weeks for invasive disease (FG: 20–27 h) (b) Days to weeks (FG: self-limiting, usually 1–3 days)	(a) Flu-like symptoms, meningitis and/or septicemia. While pregnant women may experience a mild flu-like illness, infection may result in miscarriage, stillbirth or birth of a severely ill infant. (FG: fever, watery diarrhoea, nausea, headache and pains in joints and muscles) (b) Unknown	(a) 0°C (b) 30–37°C (c) 4.3 (d) 0.92	Heat-sensitive relative to spores but considered to be one of the most heat resistant vegetative cells	(a) Gram positive (b) Facultative anaerobe	(a) Soil, improperly made silage (b) Fresh soft cheeses, raw milk, deli meats, pâté, hot dogs, raw vegetables, ice cream, and seafood
Salmonella	Although there are over. 2400 different *Salmonella* serotypes only a small number account for most human infections, with *S.* Typhimurium and *S.* Enteritidis predominating. Undercooked food from infected food animals is most commonly implicated. Egg-associated salmonellosis is an important public health problem.	(a) Usually 12–36 h, but may be 6–72 h (b) 2–5 days	(a) Fever, abdominal pain, diarrhoea, nausea and sometimes vomiting. Can be fatal in older people or those with weakened immune system (b) ~10^6 cells	(a) 7°C (b) 35–37°C (c) 4.0 (d) 0.93	Heat-sensitive, although some serotypes are reported to be very heat resistant in certain foods which provide a protective effect (e.g., chocolate)	(a) Gram negative (b) Facultative anaerobe	(a) Water, soil, animal faeces, raw poultry, raw meats, and raw seafood (b) Raw meats, poultry, eggs, raw milk and other dairy products, raw fruits and vegetables (e.g., alfalfa sprouts and melons)

(*Continued*)

Table 15.2 (Continued)

Bacteria	Comment	Food-borne illness (a) Onset (b) Duration	Food-borne illness (a) Symptoms (b) Infectious dose	(a) Min. temp (b) Opt. temp (c) Min. pH[a] (d) Min. A_w	Heat resistance	(a) Gram stain (b) Aerobic/anaerobic	(a) Source (b) Associated foods[b]
Vibrio cholerae serogroup non-01	*Vibrio cholerae* non-01 is related to *V.* cholerae 01 (the organism that causes Asiatic or epidemic cholera), but causes a disease reported to be less severe than cholera. It has been generally believed that water was the main vehicle for transmission, but an increasing number of cases have been associated with food.	(a) 1–3 days (b) Diarrhoea lasts 6–7 days	(a) Diarrhoea, abdominal cramps, fever, some vomiting, and nausea (b) >10^6 cells	(a) 10°C (b) 37°C (c) 5.0 (d) 0.97	Heat-sensitive	(a) Gram negative (b) Facultative anaerobe	(a) Costal waters, raw oysters (b) Shellfish
Vibrio parahaemolyticus	*V. parahaemolyticus* can be considered to be the leading cause of seafood-borne bacterial gastroenteritis. It is frequently isolated from fish from both marine and brackish-water environments.	(a) 12–24 h (b) <7 days	(a) Diarrhoea, abdominal cramps, nausea, vomiting, headache, fever, chills (b) >10^6 cells	(a) 5°C (b) 37°C (c) 4.8 (d) 0.94	Heat-sensitive	(a) Gram negative (b) Facultative anaerobe	(a) Costal and estuarine waters, raw shellfish (b) Fish and raw shellfish
Vibrio vulnificus	*V. vulnificus* is considered to be one of the most invasive and rapidly lethal of human pathogens. Infection starts with a gastrointestinal illness, and rapidly progresses to a septicemic condition. It is mostly associated with the consumption of raw oysters. Human infections are rare, but those at most risk either have underlying illnesses (e.g. liver disease) or are immunocompromised.	(a) 16 h (b) Days to weeks	(a) Wound infections, gastroenteritis, primarily septicemia (b) Unknown in healthy individuals but in predisposed <100 cells	(a) 8°C (b) 37°C (c) 5 (d) 0.96	Heat-sensitive	(a) Gram negative (b) Facultative anaerobe	(a) Coastal waters, sediment, plankton, shellfish (b) Oysters, clams, crabs
Yersinia enterocolitica	*Y. enterocolitica* is psychrotrophic and known to be quite resistant to freezing, surviving in frozen food for extended periods. The organism is present in a wide range of animals, especially pigs. Milk and pork have been implicated in outbreaks, especially in countries where pork is eaten raw or undercooked.	(a) 3–7 days (b) 1–3 weeks	(a) Diarrhoea, abdominal pain and fever. Intestinal pain, especially in young adults, may be confused with appendicitis (b) Unknown	(a) −1.3°C (b) 25–37°C (c) 4.1 (d) 0.94	Heat-sensitive	(a) Gram negative (b) Facultative anaerobe	(a) Wide range of animals (e.g., pigs, dogs, cats) and water (b) Undercooked pork, raw milk and water

[a] Under otherwise optimal conditions; limits will vary according to strain, temperature, type of acid (in the case of pH), solute (in the case of A_w) and other factors.
[b] Not an exhaustive list.
Heat-sensitive: cells destroyed by typical cooking temperatures; Min.: minimum; Opt.: optimal; A_w: water activity (based on a saturated NaCl solution).
Based on data from ICMSF (1996), Jay *et al.*, (2005) and FSAI (2019).

bacterial intoxications and infections are summarised in Tables 15.1 and 15.2, respectively.

Food-borne viruses

Food may be contaminated with a variety of viruses capable of infecting humans, with symptoms ranging from mild diarrhoea to more severe outcomes including gastroenteritis, hepatitis, myocarditis, respiratory disease or hemorrhagic fever. The most common viruses in food include norovirus (NoV), hepatitis A virus (HAV) and hepatitis E virus (HEV). Most cases involve infection via the faecal-oral route. Infected patients shed high numbers of virus particles which may be as high as 10^{10} per gram of faeces and 10^{7} in vomit (Teunis *et al.*, 2015; Hall *et al.*, 2014). Indeed, shedding peaks immediately before the onset of symptoms. Although many different products may be contaminated, the majority of cases are associated with bivalve molluscan shellfish and fruit. Although less common, humans may also be infected through ingestion of animal products infected with a zoonotic virus. HEV cases have been documented, for example, after consumption of pig, wild boar or deer products produced from infected animals (Ruggeri *et al.*, 2013; Van der Poel, 2014).

Hepatitis A virus

HAV is a member of the picornaviruses. It is still the most common cause of acute hepatitis worldwide and one of the more severe food-borne diseases. The illness results from immune destruction of infected liver cells, and a few weeks of debility are common (Table 15.3). Although considered to be associated with developing countries, HAV has reemerged in developed countries. Infected children under six years of age are often asymptomatic. Thereafter the severity increases becoming very severe in the over sixties. Human strains are found in three genotypes (I, II and III) and seven sub-genotypes (IA, IB, IC, IIA, IIB, IIIA and IIIB). Genotypes IA and IB are especially common worldwide. Genotype IIIA is also very common in South Asia, but is spreading rapidly, which is of major public health concern as this genotype is associated with a more severe form of the disease. The virus can be shed in faeces for up to 14 days before the onset of illness. It is therefore possible for an infected food handler with poor personal hygiene (handwashing, in particular) to contaminate food during this period. The virus may be shed in the faeces for one to two weeks after onset of symptoms.

Food becomes contaminated with this virus via infected persons or via faecally contaminated water, as is usual with shellfish. Examples of other foods implicated in hepatitis A outbreaks are oysters, raw mussels, drinking water, bakery products and frozen berries. HAV has been shown to be more heat resistant than most enteric viruses and is also quite resistant to

Table 15.3 Characteristics of the illnesses caused by hepatitis A and norovirus

	Hepatitis A (picornavirus)	Norovirus (calicivirus)
Properties	Particles are featureless spheres 28 nm in diameter, single-stranded RNA coated with protein	Particles are spheres 25–35 nm in diameter, single-stranded RNA coated with protein that has characteristic cupped surface depressions
Infection	Infection via intestine to liver, incubation period 15–20 days (mean 18 days)	Infection of intestinal lining, incubation period 24–48 h
Illness	Illness from immune destruction of infected liver cells: fever, malaise, anorexia, nausea, abdominal discomfort, often followed by jaundice; severity tends to increase with age: ranges from unapparent infection to weeks of debility, occasionally with permanent sequelae	Nausea, vomiting, diarrhoea, etc., lasting for 24–48 h
Shedding	Shedding of virus peaks during the second half of the incubation period (10–14 days), usually ends by 7 days after onset of jaundice	During illness (in vomitus and faeces), possibly 7 days after onset
Diagnosis	Based on detection of IgM class antibody. Hepatitis A virus in the patient's blood serum (kits available)	Detection of virus in stool by ELISA or PCR, or by antibody against the virus in patient's blood serum
Immunity	Immunity is durable (possibly lifelong) after infection	Apparently transient

RNA, Ribonucleic acid; ELISA, enzyme-linked immunosorbent assay; IgM, immunoglobulin M; PCR, polymerase chain reaction.

drying. The virus is susceptible to chlorination treatment, however, and water-borne HAV outbreaks have been linked to untreated water.

Hepatitis E virus

Traditionally associated with developing countries, HEV is now found in many developed countries and a link with undercooked pork meat and liver may be responsible for some of this increase. HEV virus belongs to the family *Hepeviridae*. Although the route of transmission is not fully understood, HEV can be transmitted by blood transfusion but may also be zoonotic, mainly via pig products but HEV has also been isolated from a range of mammals as well as poultry and fish (Smith *et al.*, 2014). Originally associated with acute self-limiting hepatitis, it is now known to persist in immune compromised patients, who may have no symptoms while developing liver cirrhosis. Other manifestations include aplastic anemia, acute thyroiditis, glomerulonephritis and neurological disorders (Kamar *et al.*, 2014, 2015). Approximately 5-10% of cases develop neurological illnesses including Guillain-Barré syndrome and neuralgic amyotrophy.

Noroviruses

Norovirus was the first enteric virus reported to be food-borne, and is one of the most common causes of food-borne disease. It was formerly known as Norwalk-like virus (NLV) or small round structured virus (SRSV). Noroviruses are a very diverse group of viruses belonging to the family *Caliciviridae*. Although there are an estimated 40 genotypes, only three genogroups (GI, II and IV) have been associated with human disease. The most common route of infection is person-to-person spread although this may also be acquired though the consumption of contaminated food (most notably raw oysters contaminated during production or any food contaminated by a food handler). The incidence of norovirus infection is expected to increase driven by changing population demographics, specifically more elderly and immune compromised persons in healthcare settings, and the challenge of producing food in an uncontaminated environment.

Astroviruses

First discovered in 1975, astroviruses are 28-35 nm in diameter and appear as small, round viruses that have surface projections resembling a five- or six-pointed star (Greek *astron*, star). They have been isolated from humans, other mammals, and avian species. With an incubation period of three to four days, these viruses destroy the intestinal epithelium and the main symptoms are diarrhoea, nausea, fever, malaise and abdominal pain. Vomiting may also occur but is less common than with other viral infections such as norovirus. These symptoms may persist for 7–14 days. The very young (<1 year), elderly and immune compromised are most at risk of astrovirus infection. Large astrovirus outbreaks have been reported, typically in crèches, schools, hospital wards, and nursing homes, but in many cases, there is no well-defined mode of transmission.

Rotaviruses

Rotaviruses are the single most important cause of infantile gastroenteritis worldwide, causing approximately one third of deaths of children from diarrhoea globally. Indeed, by the age of 5 nearly every child in the world has been infected with rotavirus. The rotavirus genome consists of 11 segments of double-stranded RNA surrounded by a double-shelled viral capsid. When examined by electron microscopy, the double-shelled particles resemble a wheel-like structure morphologically (Latin *rota*, wheel). There are nine species of the virus (A to I) with rotavirus A being responsible for more than 90% of human infections. The incubation period of the illness is one to three days. Transmission is usually via the faecal–oral route and once ingested, the virus damages the cells lining the small intestine. The resultant gastroenteritis is characterised by fever, vomiting, and diarrhoea. Although the majority of rotavirus infections involve infants, outbreaks of food-borne, and water-borne disease affecting all age groups have been reported, albeit infrequently.

Other viruses

Picornaviruses other than hepatitis A can also be transmitted by the food-borne route. Polioviruses are transmitted by food, but virulent strains of this agent are now extremely rare. Coxsackie virus and echovirus have been associated with food-borne outbreaks, but data are limited.

Food-borne parasites

Food-borne parasitic diseases are a major public health problem affecting millions of people, predominantly in non-industrialised countries. The incidence of parasitic disease associated with the consumption of foods of animal origin has declined in industrialised countries in recent years, where improvements in animal husbandry and meat inspection have led to considerable safety and quality gains. The situation in non-industrialised countries is very different, in that these diseases are associated with poor standards of sanitation and hygiene, low educational standards, and extreme poverty.

Parasites are organisms that live off other living organisms, known as hosts. They may be transmitted from animals to humans, from humans to humans, or from humans to animals. Food-borne parasitic disease occurs when the infective stages of parasites are eaten in raw or partially cooked protein foods, or in raw vegetables and fruits that are inadequately washed before consumption. These organisms then live and reproduce within the tissues and organs of infected human and animal hosts, and are often excreted in faeces. The parasites involved in food-borne disease usually have complex life cycles involving one or two intermediate hosts (Figure 15.1). The food-borne parasites known to cause disease in humans are broadly classified as helminths (multicellular worms) and protozoa (single-celled microscopic organisms). These include the major helminthic groups of trematodes, nematodes, and cestodes, and some of the emerging protozoan pathogens, such as cryptosporidia and cyclospora. The illnesses they can cause range from mild discomfort to debilitating illness and possibly death.

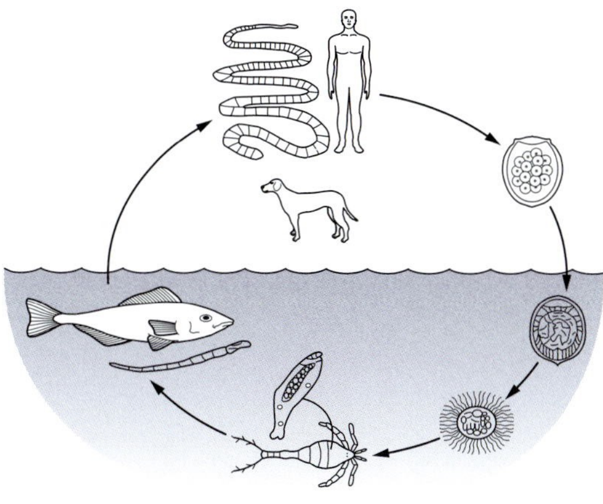

Figure 15.1 Life cycle of *Diphyllobothrium latum.*

These infections occur endemically in some 20 countries, where it is estimated that over 40 million people worldwide, mainly in eastern and southern Asia, are affected. Of major concern are the fish-borne trematode infections. The trematode species concerned all have similar life cycles involving two intermediate hosts. The definitive host is man and other mammals. Food-borne infection takes place through the consumption of raw, undercooked, or otherwise underprocessed freshwater fish or crustaceans containing the infective stages (metacercariae) of these parasites. Table 15.4 summarises the distribution, the principal reservoirs, and freshwater fish or crustaceans involved in the transmission of these parasites in the food chain. The most important parasites with respect to the numbers of people affected are species of the genera *Clonorchis, Opisthorchis,* and *Paragonimus.* The diseases caused by food-borne trematodes include cholangiocarcinoma, gallstones, severe liver disease, and gastrointestinal problems.

Nematodes

The food-borne roundworms of primary importance in humans belong to the phylum Nematoda and are known as nematodes. Undercooked or raw fishery products and pork meat are the usual foods involved.

Where fishery products are the food vector, the definitive hosts of roundworms causing disease in humans are piscivorous marine mammals such as seals. Marine invertebrates and fish are the two intermediate hosts and humans are infected when they consume raw or minimally processed products. Fish are the secondary hosts and are infected when they consume the invertebrate primary host or fish that are already infected. There are many species of nematodes and a very large number of species of fish, worldwide, that are known to act as intermediate hosts. The most common species of nematode causing disease in humans is *Anisakis simplex*, sometimes referred to as the herringworm. The other species involved in anisakiasis in North America, Europe, and Japan is *Pseudo-terranova decipiens* (the codworm or sealworm).

Table 15.4 Food-borne trematode infections

Parasite	Distribution	Principal reservoirs (other than humans)	Food involved in transmission to humans	Disease
Liver flukes *Clonorchis sinensis*	Widespread in China, Taiwan, Macao, Japan, Korea and Vietnam. Migrants to other countries found to be infected; cases in Hawaii attributed to consumption of fish imported from China	Dogs, cats, and many other species of fish-eating mammals	Many species (c. 110) of freshwater fish, mainly Cyprinidae, e.g., carp, roach and dace, most important being *Pseudorasbora parva*. Metacercariae in fish muscles	The liver flukes, *Opisthorchis viverrini, O. felineus* and *Clonorchis sinensis*, are biologically similar, food-borne trematodes that chronically infect the bile ducts and, more rarely, the pancreatic duct and gallbladder of humans and other mammals
Opisthorchis felineus	Commonwealth of Independent States (CIS), eastern and central Europe	Cats, dogs, and other mammals that eat fish or fish waste	Freshwater fish of family Cyprinidae. Metacercariae in muscle and subcutaneous tissue	
Opisthorchis viverrini	Laos and north-eastern Thailand (Mekong River basin)	Dogs, cats, fishing cats (*Felis viverrina*), and other mammals that feed on fish and fish waste	Species of freshwater fish including *Puntius orphoides* and *Hampala dispar* Metacercariae in fish muscles	
Fasciola hepatica	Europe, the Middle East, the Far East, Africa, Australia, USA	Sheep, cattle		Inflammation of the bile ducts which eventually leads to fibrosis
Intestinal flukes *Heterophyes heterophyes*	Mediterranean basin, especially Egypt and eastern Asia	Dogs, cats, jackals, foxes, pelicans, hawks, and black kite	Brackish water and freshwater fish, especially mullet (*Mugil* spp.), tilapia, and others. In Japan, species of fish genera *Acanthogobius* and *Glossogobius* also involved. Metacercariae in muscle and skin	The parasite can irritate the lining of the small intestine, resulting in diarrhoea and abdominal pain. In some instances, the lining of the small intestine breaks down, and the eggs produced by the parasite enter the bloodstream. Once in the bloodstream the eggs can be carried to other organs where they can cause significant pathology, especially in the liver, heart, and brain
Metagonimus yokogawai and related species	Eastern and southern Asia	Dogs, cats, pigs, and fish-eating birds	Freshwater fish, e.g., sweetfish (*Plecoglossus altivelis*), dace (*Tribolodon hakonensis*), trout, and whitebait. Metacercariae in gills, fin, or tail	Similar to *Heterophyes heterophyes*
Nanophyetus spp.	Eastern Siberia (mountain tributaries of Amur River) and parts of Sakhalin peninsula, north-western USA	Dogs, cats, rats, and badgers	Salmonid and other fish. Metacercariae in muscles, fins, and kidneys	Nanophyetiasis. Diarrhoea, usually accompanied by increased numbers of circulating eosinophils, abdominal discomfort and nausea. Sometimes asymptomatic
Spelotrema brevicaeca	Philippines	Sea birds	Crustaceans, amphipods, isopods, and brachyures	
Haplorchis spp.	Eastern and southern Asia	Cats, dogs, and fish-eating birds	Fish, frogs, and toads. Metacercariae in muscle	
Fasciolopsis buski	Oriental countries	Pigs	Uncooked contaminated water plants such as water cress	Most infections are light and asymptomatic. Heavy infections show symptoms of diarrhoea, abdominal pain, fever, ascites, anasarca, and intestinal obstruction
Lung fluke *Paragonimus westermani* and related species in Asia, Africa and the Americas	Siberia, west Africa (Nigeria, Cameroon), the Americas (Ecuador to USA), Japan, Korea, Thailand, Laos, China	Domestic and wild carnivora that feed on crustaceans	Freshwater and brackish water crabs (*Eriocheir, Potamon, Parathelphusa*), crayfish and shrimps. Metacercariae in muscles, gills, liver (hepatopancreas), and cardia region. Wild boar meat suspected as a source of infection	Paragonimiasis

Based on data from Abdussalam et al., 1995. Food safety measures for the control of food-borne trematode infections. *Food Control*, 6, 71–79; copyright with permission from Elsevier.

Nematodes are commonly present in fish caught in the wild, most frequently in the liver and belly cavity, but can also occur in the flesh. Anisakiasis is an uncommon disease because the parasite is killed by heating (55°C for 1 min), and by freezing (−20°C for 24 hours). There is a risk of illness from fishery products consumed raw, for example sushi, or after only mild processing, such as salting at low concentrations or smoking. Many countries now require that fish used for these mildly processed products be frozen before processing or before sale.

Trichinella spiralis is the cause of trichinosis in humans. This most commonly results from the consumption of contaminated raw or undercooked pork or pork products. Since the mid–1980s outbreaks have been associated with raw and undercooked horsemeat. Isolated cases have been reported from the consumption of bear meat and ground beef in the USA. The incidence of trichinosis can be controlled by avoiding feeding infected waste foods to pigs or by fully cooking pig swill. Freezing pork products (−15°C for 20 days) or thorough cooking (78°C at the thermal centre) before human consumption will destroy trichinella larvae.

Cestodes

Cestodes are tapeworms and the species of major concern associated with consumption of fish is the fish tapeworm, *Diphyllobothrium latum*. Humans are one of the definitive hosts, along with other fish-eating mammals. Freshwater copepods and fish are the intermediate hosts (Figure 15.1). The plerocercoid is present in the flesh of the fish and infects humans following the consumption of raw or minimally processed fish. The recorded epidemiology of *D. latum* shows it to be prevalent in many countries worldwide. The incidence is relatively high in Scandinavia and the Baltic region of Europe. Diphyllobothriasis in humans can be prevented by cooking or freezing fish before consumption. Infections with tapeworms are also associated with eating undercooked or raw pork and beef.

Taenia saginata (the beef tapeworm) and *Taenia solium* (the pork tapeworm) are unique among parasites in that they have no vascular, respiratory, or digestive systems. Humans are their definitive hosts and they rely solely on the human body for all their nourishment. Infections can be prevented by sanitary disposal and treatment of human waste and by thorough cooking and freezing of contaminated pork and beef.

Protozoa

The protozoal human parasites are unicellular organisms that colonise the intestinal epithelium and form cysts. These are excreted and may survive for long periods in the environment. There are five genera of concern in foods: *Giardia*, *Entamoeba*, *Toxoplasma*, *Cyclospora*, and *Cryptosporidium*. Table 15.5 summarises the distribution, principal reservoirs and route of transmission of these parasites in the food chain.

Toxoplasma gondii

There is only one species in the Toxoplasma genus, *T. gondii*, a non-flagellated apicomplexan parasite with three distinct infectious stages; the tachyzoites, the bradyzoites and the sporozoites. This obligate intracellular parasite has a complex life cycle with a wide variety of hosts. However, sexual replication can only occur in cats (Tenter *et al.*, 2000). *T. gondii* has a high prevalence in a range of warm-blooded animals including humans, especially immunosuppressed individuals. Cook *et al.* (2000) identified a range of risk factors associated with acquiring *T. gondii* infection. These included the consumption of meat especially if undercooked or raw, contact with the soil (e.g., gardening), and travel outside of Europe, USA or Canada. However, a large number of cases remain unexplained.

Transmissible spongiform encephalopathies and food

Transmissible spongiform encephalopathies (TSEs) are fatal degenerative brain diseases which include bovine spongiform encephalopathy (BSE) in cattle, scrapie in sheep, chronic wasting disease in deer and elk, and transmissible mink encephalopathy (Greenlee and Greenlee, 2015). Human forms of this disease include classic Creutzfeldt-Jakob disease (CJD), variant CJD, kuru, familial fatal insomnia, Gerstmann-Sträussler-Scheinker disease, and sporadic fatal insomnia.

TSEs are caused by a transmissible prion protein naturally present in the animal nervous tissue that can turn into a pathological form (PrPsc). The associated illness is characterised by the appearance in the brain of vacuoles – clear holes that give the brain a sponge-like appearance – from

Table 15.5 Food-borne protozoa

Occurrence	Transmission	Definitive host	Incubation	Infective dose	Pathogenesis
Giardia intestinalis worldwide	Food-borne, water-borne, person–person	Humans, domestic, and wild animals	3–25 days	Low (~10 cysts)	Chronic diarrhoea, malabsorption, weight loss
Entamoeba histolytica worldwide	Food-borne, water-borne, person–person (food handlers)	Humans	2–4 weeks	Very low (~1 cyst)	Amebiasis, abdominal pain, fever, diarrhoea, ulceration of the colon (severe cases)
Toxoplasma gondii worldwide	Food-borne (raw or inadequately cooked infected meat, inadequately washed fruit and vegetables), water-borne, faecal–oral (infected cats)	Humans, cats, several mammals	5–23 days	~1–30 cysts	Mostly asymptomatic. In severe cases: hepatitis, pneumonia, blindness, severe neurological disorders. Can also be transmitted transplacentally resulting in a spontaneous abortion, a stillborn, or mental/physical retardation
Cyclospora cayetanensis worldwide	Food-borne, water-borne	Humans	Several days to weeks	Not known, probably very low	Often asymptomatic. Abdominal cramps, vomiting, weight loss, diarrhoea
Cryptosporidium parvum worldwide	Food-borne, water-borne, animal–person, faecal–oral	Humans, domestic, and wild animals	Difficult to define, in most cases 3–7 days, occasionally longer	Very low (~1 cyst)	Often asymptomatic. Abdominal cramps, vomiting, weight loss, diarrhoea

which the conditions derive their name. Prions are relatively resistant to proteases, high temperatures, UV radiation, and disinfectants.

Bovine spongiform encephalopathy

BSE, sometimes referred to as "mad cow disease", was first identified in the UK in 1986. The incubation period is between 2 and 10 years. Affected animals may display changes in temperament, such as nervousness or aggression, abnormal posture, lack of coordination, and difficulty in standing, decreased milk production, or loss of body weight despite continued appetite. Most cattle with BSE show a gradual development of symptoms over a period of several weeks or even months, although some can deteriorate very rapidly. While the original source of the agent responsible for BSE remains unknown, currently the most plausible explanation is that a novel TSE appeared in the UK cattle population in the 1970s and subsequently spread as a consequence of intensive farming due to feedstuff containing animal meat and bone contaminated with PrPsc. Thus in 2001 the EU banned the use of animal proteins in livestock feed. Since then, approximately 114 million cattle and 8.4 million small ruminants have been tested in the EU. In 2015, 1.4 million bovine animals were tested and only five were positive. In the same year, 3 19 638 sheep and 1 35 857 goats were tested with 641 and 1052 scrapie cases detected in each animal species respectively (EFSA, 2016).

Creutzfeldt–Jakob disease and new variant CJD

CJD is a fatal disease of humans, first described in the 1920s and found worldwide. CJD is predominantly a sporadic disease, but about 14% of cases are familial (inherited) and associated with genetic mutations. Less than 1% are iatrogenic (i.e., accidentally transmitted from person to person as a result of medical or surgical procedures). Classically, sporadic CJD occurs in those over 65 years of age and presents as a rapidly progressive dementia with myoclonus (shock-like contractions of isolated muscles), usually fatal within six months. Surveillance of CJD was reinstituted in the UK in 1990 to evaluate any changes in the pattern of the disease that might be attributable to BSE. The overall incidence of CJD rose in the UK in the 1990s, although a portion of this increase was due to improved ascertainment of CJD in older people as a result of the reinstitution of surveillance.

New variant CJD, also referred to as variant CJD (vCJD), was first diagnosed in the UK in the mid-1990s. In contrast to the traditional forms of CJD, vCJD has affected younger patients (average age 29 years) and has a longer duration of illness (approximately 14 months). Early in the illness, patients usually experience behavioural changes, which most commonly take the form of depression or, less often, a schizophrenia-like disorder. Neurological signs such as unsteadiness, difficulty walking, and involuntary movements develop as the illness progresses and, by the time of death, patients become completely immobile and mute.

The link between BSE and vCJD

A geographical association exists whereby the majority of BSE cases occurred in the UK and the majority of vCJD cases were also reported there. The emergence of BSE preceded vCJD, indicating a temporal association. Studies of stored human brain tissue internationally have not identified the histopathological changes characteristic of vCJD before the BSE epidemic. Incubation period and pathological lesion studies in mice and molecular typing studies demonstrate that vCJD is similar to BSE but different from other TSEs. It is now widely accepted that vCJD was transmitted to humans through the consumption of contaminated food.

15.5 Chemicals affecting food safety

Chemicals may be present in food owing to their natural occurrence in soil (e.g., cadmium, lead) or from fungal contamination (e.g., aflatoxins, ochratoxin), from plant toxins present in weeds (e.g. tropane alkaloids), from algal contamination [e.g., amnesic shellfish poisoning (ASP), diarrhoetic shellfish poisoning (DSP), azaspiracid shellfish poisoning (AZP), paralytic shellfish poisoning (PSP)], from industrial or other pollution [e.g., lead, mercury, polychlorinated biphenyls (PCBs), dioxins], from agricultural and veterinary practices (e.g., pesticides, fertilizers, veterinary medicines, illegal growth promotors, sanitizing chemicals) or from food processing and packaging techniques [e.g. acrylamide, polycyclic aromatic hydrocarbons (PAHs), 3-monochloropropane-1,2-diol (3-MCPD), bisphenol A diglycidyl ether (BADGE)] (Box 15.1).

In Europe, toxicological assessments for the majority of these substances is carried out by the European Food Safety Authority (EFSA) and Member States' competent authorities. EFSA was set up in 2002 following several food incidents in the 1990s, and provides independent scientific advice underpinning European Union food safety

Box 15.1 Principal groups of chemicals affecting food safety

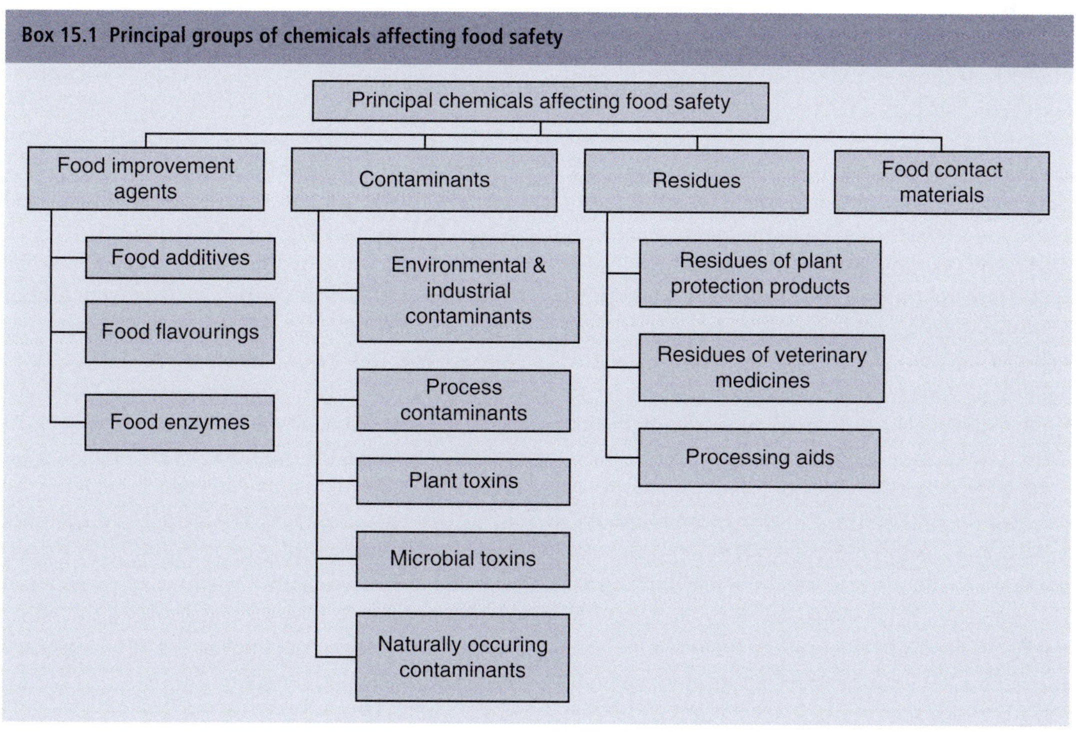

policies and legislation. On an international basis expert groups such as the Joint Expert Committee on Food Additives and Contaminants (JECFA) or Joint Meeting on Pesticide Residues (JMPR), both jointly organised by the WHO and FAO, carry out risk assessments. These expert groups advise on acceptable or tolerable levels of intake of these substances.

Health-based guidance values (HBGVs)

Health-based guidance values provide quantitative information on the level of oral exposure that would pose no appreciable risk to the consumer, on the basis of scientific evidence available at the time. Different types of HBGVs exist and are reflective of the type of exposure (intentional, residual or adventitious) and the timeframe of exposure (acute or chronic). The acceptable daily intake (ADI) is used for chemicals intentionally added to foodstuffs, such as food improvement agents and residues of plant protection products or veterinary medicines present in food.

The tolerable daily intake (TDI) represents permissible daily human exposure to those contaminants unavoidably associated with the consumption of otherwise wholesome and nutritious foods. The term tolerable signifies permissibility rather than acceptability for the intake of contaminants that have no necessary function in food, in contrast to those of permitted pesticides or food additives. For cumulative toxicants, such as cadmium and mercury, the tolerable intakes are expressed on a weekly basis (TWI) to allow for daily variations in intake levels, the real concern being long-term exposure to the contaminant.

One of the most difficult issues in food safety is to advise on the potential risks to human health for substances found in food which are both genotoxic (damaging DNA, the genetic material of cells) and carcinogenic (leading to cancer). For these substances, it is generally assumed that even a small dose can have an effect.

As a result, a different approach, "the margin of exposure" (MoE) approach, which can be used to assess the risks to human health of exposure to a substance in the absence of a tolerable daily intake or similar guidance value, has been endorsed by the EFSA Scientific Committee (EFSA, 2005) and the WHO/FAO Joint Expert Committee on Food Additives (WHO/ FAO, 2005). The margin of exposure is defined as the reference point on the dose -response curve (usually based on animal experiments in the absence of human data) divided by the estimated intake by humans. It enables the comparison of the risks posed by different genotoxic and carcinogenic substances. Differences in potency of the substances concerned and consumption patterns in the population are considered when applying the MoE approach. For substances that are both genotoxic and carcinogenic, the EFSA Scientific Committee considered an MoE of 10000 or higher of low concern from a public health point of view and might be reasonably considered as a low priority for risk management actions if it is based on the BMDL10 (lower confidence limit of the benchmark dose) from an animal carcinogenicity study, (EFSA Scientific Committee, 2005, 2012) However, the magnitude of an MoE only provides an indication of the level of concern and does not quantify the risk. The MoE can also be calculated for substances with threshold effects, for which a HBGV could not be set. In these cases, the acceptable margin will depend on the choice of appropriate uncertainty factors.

Setting health-based guidance values (HGBVs)

Traditionally HBGVs have been based on a reference point (often referred to as point of departure) derived from long term animal studies. In calculating a HBGV such as the ADI, a "safety factor" (often referred to as uncertainty factor) is applied to the no-observed-adverse-effect level (NOAEL) to provide a conservative margin of safety on account of the inherent uncertainties in extrapolating animal toxicity data to potential effects in humans and for variation within the human species (Box 15.2). Both JECFA and EFSA traditionally use a safety factor of 100 (10 × 10) in setting ADI values based on long-term animal studies. It is intended to provide an adequate margin of safety for the consumer by assuming that the human being is 10 times more sensitive than the test animal and that the difference in sensitivity within the human population is in a 10-fold range. However, different safety factors may apply depending on the substance and test species in question.

Box 15.2 Levels of intake of a chemical

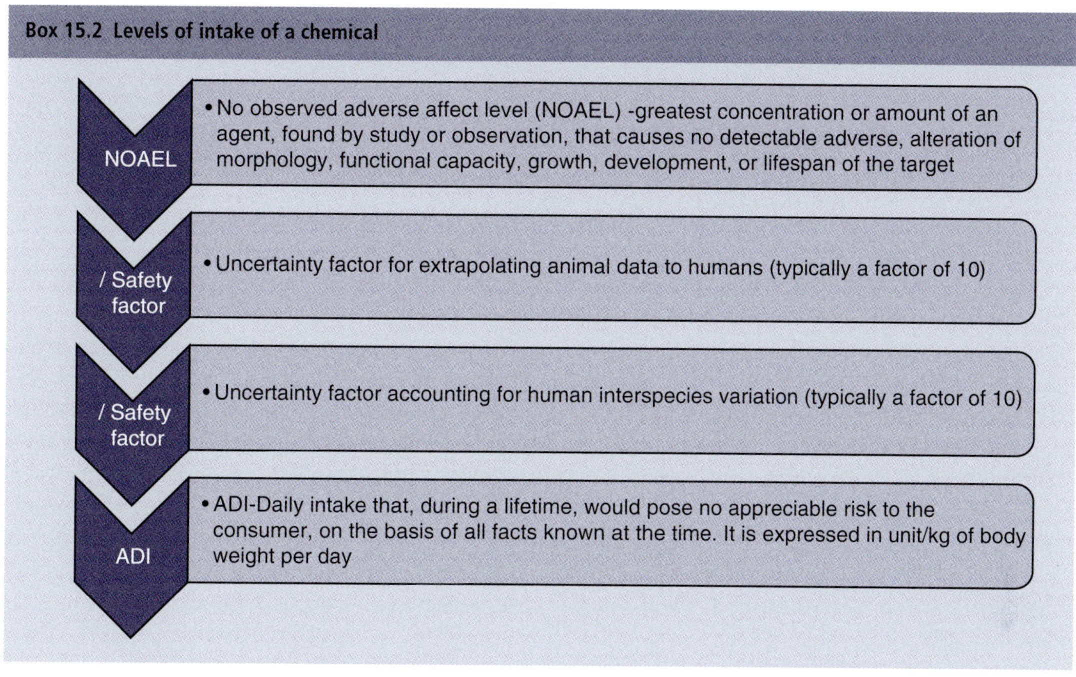

NOAEL
• No observed adverse affect level (NOAEL) -greatest concentration or amount of an agent, found by study or observation, that causes no detectable adverse, alteration of morphology, functional capacity, growth, development, or lifespan of the target
/ Safety factor
• Uncertainty factor for extrapolating animal data to humans (typically a factor of 10)
/ Safety factor
• Uncertainty factor accounting for human interspecies variation (typically a factor of 10)
ADI
• ADI-Daily intake that, during a lifetime, would pose no appreciable risk to the consumer, on the basis of all facts known at the time. It is expressed in unit/kg of body weight per day

In recent years a new approach to identifying the reference point has emerged and is considered superior to the above described "NOAEL approach". The "Benchmark Dose (BMD) approach" can be applied both for threshold and non-threshold effects, and utilises all of the dose -response data to estimate the shape of the overall dose -response relationship for a particular endpoint. The BMD is derived from the benchmark response (BMR), which reflects a measurable change in response derived from the dose-response curve (EFSA Scientific Committee, 2017). Different BMRs are recommended depending on the type of data used, but typically for carcinogens a BMR of 10% extra risk is used. The BMDL is the BMD's lower confidence bound and is typically used as the reference point. The BMDL can be used to derive HBGVs through application of uncertainty factors (as is done in the NOAEL approach), or where setting of a HBGV is not possible, the MoE approach can be applied.

Setting maximum levels for food commodities

The derivation of maximum levels for various chemicals in food are calculated by taking the above-mentioned HBGVs into consideration. Depending on the substance, different principles may apply. Residues such as pesticides and residues of veterinary medicines in foodstuffs are limited by setting a maximum residue limit (MRL). Additives are regulated by setting maximum limits or by applying the "quantum satis" principle (the least amount required to exert the desired technological function and in accordance with good manufacturing practice).

For contaminants, maximum levels/limits are established for those foods that provide a significant contribution to the total dietary exposure. However, as a general principle the levels in all foods should always be kept as low as reasonably achievable (i.e. the ALARA principle).

In Europe, food improvement agents, pesticides, veterinary medicines, and a wide range of contaminants are regulated by EU legislation in the form of directives or regulations that are transposed into national legislation by each member state.

Pesticide residues

Pesticides are chemicals or biological products used to control harmful or undesired organisms and plants, or to regulate the growth of plants crop protection agents. They are classified into the groups shown in Box 15.3.

Box 15.3 Classification of pesticides

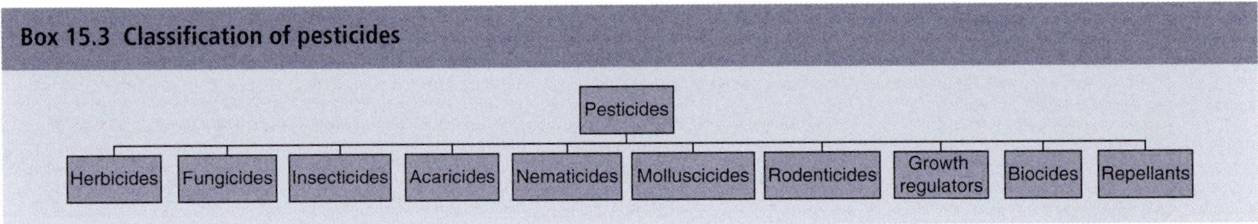

Most pesticides are toxic substances that are highly selective, especially those developed since the early 1980s, and only have an effect on those pests or plants to which they are applied. The most common application of pesticides is in the form of plant protection products (PPPs). Plant protection products protect crops or desirable or useful plants and are primarily used in the agricultural sector but also in forestry, horticulture, amenity areas and in residential gardens. Unlike other environmental contaminants, PPPs are applied under controlled conditions that should conform to "good agricultural practice" (GAP). This defines the effective use of PPPs, up to the maximum permissible level (maximum residue level (MRL)), applied in a manner that ensures the smallest amount of residue in the foodstuff.

Pesticides can also be toxic to humans since certain biochemical pathways are relatively conserved across species, as are some enzymes and hormones. In the context of food safety, exposure to pesticides is classified as acute or chronic. An acute intoxication usually has an immediate effect on the body, whereas a chronic effect may reveal itself over the lifespan. The severity depends on the dose and the toxicity of the pesticide compound or breakdown product. Toxic effects that have been identified include enzyme inhibition, endocrine disruption, and carcinogenic action, depending on the compound in question.

In the case of acute toxicity rather than chronic toxicity, the level of exposure is considered in relation to the acute reference dose (ARfD). ARfD values are measures of the maximum level of intake at one meal, or consumption over a day. This is the maximum intake level, which is judged to result in no adverse toxicological effect following such exposure. The ARfD value includes a safety factor to ensure that older people, infants and children, and those under stress due to illness are protected.

In the EU the marketing and use of PPPs and their residues are highly regulated. Plant protection products cannot be placed on the market or used without prior authorisation.

In Europe the control of pesticides is based on Council Directive 91/414/EEC. Under this legislation, pesticides must be evaluated for safety based on dossiers prepared by their manufacturers. If a pesticide is accepted it is placed on a positive list with an MRL assigned to it.

In the case of a limited number of highly toxic pesticides, for which the ADI is necessarily based on acute toxicity rather than chronic toxicity, the level of exposure is considered in relation to the acute reference dose (ARfD). ARfD values are measures of the maximum level of intake at one meal, or consumption over a day. This is the maximum intake level, which is judged to result in no adverse toxicological effect following such exposure. The ARfD value includes a safety factor to ensure that older people, infants and children, and those under stress due to illness are protected.

Residues of Veterinary Medicinal Products

Veterinary medicines include antibacterial compounds, antiparasitic medicines, tranquilizers/sedatives, hormones, and nonsteroidal anti-inflammatory preparations. As animal husbandry practices have intensified over the past few decades, antibacterial substances have been increasingly used as growth promoters to increase feed conversion efficiency, and for prophylaxis and therapy to prevent outbreaks and treat disease. Similarly, hormones are administered in some to increase growth rate and meat yield.

The use of growth promoting agents is banned within the EU. However, some veterinary medicines containing hormones are approved in the EU for therapeutic use and reproductive purposes in non-food producing animals. Table 15.6 shows the main types of antibacterial and hormonal compounds.

Table 15.6 Main types of veterinary medicines

Growth Promoting Agents
Stilbenes
Thyrostat
Steroids
Resorcylic lactones
β-Agonists
Veterinary medicines
Prohibited substances: Chloramphenicol, Chlorpromazine, Colchicine, Dapsone, Dimetridazole, Metronidazole, Nitrofurans (including furazolidone), Nitromidazoles
Antibacterial compounds: Aminoglycosides, β-Lactams, Macrolides, Cefalosporins, Penicillins, Phenicols, Sulfonamides, Tetracyclines, Quinolones.
Anthelmintic medicines
Anticoccidials
Antiparasitic agents: e.g., carbamates and pyrethroids
Sedatives and Tranquillisers
Non-steroidal anti-inflammatory medicines (NSAIDS)
Corticosteroids

Veterinary medicines are metabolised in the animal and are excreted in the milk, urine and faeces over time as the detoxification process continues. Hence, residue traces of medicines or their metabolites can be found in major organs, muscles, and body fluids. In general, antibacterial medicines are normally found in greatest concentration in the kidney, lesser concentrations in the liver and lowest concentrations in the muscle tissue, whereas hormones tend to concentrate in the liver.

The excessive use of antibacterial compounds in animal husbandry has raised concerns about the development of resistant bacteria and the effect that this may have on the usefulness of antibiotics in human medicine. There have also been concerns about the risk of allergic reactions in humans to antibacterial residues in food of animal origin. The use of hormones has raised issues surrounding the effects of hormone residues in foods of animal origin on human metabolism.

Environmental and industrial contaminants

These contaminants are of environmental origin or are by-products of industrial processes.

Polyhalogenated hydrocarbons (PHHs) are a category of environmental contaminants that includes toxaphene, dioxins, and polychlorinated biphenyls (PCBs). Certain polyhalogenated

Table 15.7 Metals in the food chain

Metal	Main food sources
Lead	Shellfish, finfish, kidney, liver
Cadmium	Shellfish, kidney, cereals, vegetables
Mercury	Finfish
Arsenic	Rice, seaweed, seafood

hydrocarbons are manufactured for use in plastics, paints, transformers, and herbicides; although their use is now either banned or severely restricted. In most industrialised nations the compounds have become ubiquitous in the environment. Hence, contamination of the food chain is inevitable, and it has been estimated that in Western industrialised countries 90% of human exposure is through ingestion of contaminated foods of animal origin.

Foods that are rich sources of fats and oils tend to accumulate PHHs because the compounds are lipophilic and bioaccumulate in lipid-rich tissues and fluids. Oily fish from areas such as the Baltic Sea, where levels of PHHs in the water are high, may contain elevated levels of these contaminants. Similarly, cows that graze on polluted pasture can accumulate unacceptable concentrations of PHHs in their milk. A recent incident in Belgium introduced PCBs and dioxins into the food chain via contaminated animal feed resulting from the accidental incorporation of industrial oil into the feed ration. The biological half-life of PHHs can range from a matter of months to 20 years in human adipose tissue. Hence, they are persistent and accumulate in the body. Exposure to PHHs can result in a variety of toxic effects that can be carcinogenic, including dermal toxicity, immunotoxicity, reproductive effects, and endocrine disruption.

Metals, metalloids, and their compounds have long been associated with food poisoning, with lead and mercury probably the best documented hazards. Metals are released into the environment as a result of natural geological action, and also as a result of man-made pollution from industrial processes.

Metals have an affinity for biological tissue and organic compounds, and hence they are often easily absorbed into the body and can often accumulate in organs and fat deposits. Table 15.7 shows some of the main metals linked with food-borne toxicity.

Lead toxicity has many symptoms, but the main issue relates to its effects on the nervous system of children. Here, lead interferes with the transmission of nervous signals around the body. This can manifest itself in a reduced intelligence quotient (IQ) and coordination problems. In adults, exposure to lead can result in hypertension and other blood effects such as anaemia. Cadmium is most often accumulated from occupational exposure or smoking and is known to affect the respiratory system. However, food exposure tends to be at a low level over longer periods. In this regard, cadmium bioaccumulates in the kidney and can cause renal damage. Mercury and its compounds also bioaccumulate in the body, where they are most frequently associated with neural effects and renal damage. In particular, methylmercury is highly toxic to the nervous system, and the developing brain is thought to be the most sensitive target organ for methylmercury toxicity.

Arsenic is most often an occupational hazard, but it can also be ingested with food and is responsible for acute and chronic poisoning. The toxicity of arsenic depends on its oxidation state and the type of complex that it forms with organic molecules in the body. In particular, inorganic arsenic is highly toxic. Chronic effects include gastroenteritis, nephritis, and liver damage. Arsenic is also considered to be a carcinogen. Other metals are also known contaminants and their toxic effects are diverse. Although this is not an exhaustive list, these metals include aluminum, copper, tin, zinc, nickel, and chromium.

Process contaminants

These types of contaminant occur during the processing and production of foods, and include acrylamide, PAHs, chloropropanols, and their esters, glycidol fatty acid esters (GE), furan and nitrosamines.

Acrylamide is a reactive unsaturated amide that has found several industrial uses. In 2002, it was discovered to occur in a variety of fried and baked foods, in particular carbohydrate-rich foods that had been subjected to high-temperature cooking/processing. Acrylamide has been shown to be neurotoxic in humans. It has been shown to induce tumours in laboratory rats and has been classified as a probable human carcinogen, and as such, several international bodies have concluded that dietary exposure should be as low as reasonably achievable. The most significant pathway of formation of acrylamide in foods has been shown to arise from the reaction of reducing sugars with asparagines via the Maillard reaction at temperatures above *c.* 120°C. Acrylamide has been found in a wide range of heat-treated foods; it is found in both foods processed by manufacturers and foods that are cooked in the home. Acrylamide has been found to be most prevalent in fried potato products (such as French fries and potato chips), cereals, bakery wares, and coffee.

PAHs are a group of over 100 different chemicals that are formed during certain technological processes and are common environmental contaminants. They are formed during incomplete combustion of coal and oil. They are also formed during barbecuing or grilling meat. Human exposure usually results from air pollution and from cigarette smoke. Foods most likely to be contaminated by PAHs are grilled or charred meats and smoked meats and fishery products. PAHs are toxins that have been documented by EFSA and the WHO as genotoxic, immunotoxic, and carcinogenic. Long-term exposure to foods containing PAHs can lead to serious health risks.

The chloropropanols 3-MCPD and 2-MCPD, and their fatty acid esters and GE are formed during the refining process of vegetable oils. 3-MCPD and 2-MCPD are also by-products in soy sauce and in hydrolysed vegetable protein produced through acid hydrolysis. 3-MCPD can cause organ damage (particularly to the kidney) and is a suspected carcinogen, whilst for GE genotoxic carcinogenicity has been confirmed.

Furans are another class of thermal processing contaminants and can be formed from a variety of natural components present in food. Grain and grain-based products as well as coffee are the main contributors to exposure. Furans exert liver toxicity and are carcinogens, a genotoxic mode of action is suspected but has yet to be confirmed.

Microbial toxins

Food poisoning can occur as a result of the ingestion of food containing preformed toxins that originate from bacterial growth, fungal growth, or algal growth. In the case of bacteria, the toxin is absorbed into the bloodstream via the intestine and illness results from intoxication rather than infection. In the case of fungi, several species are involved in the production of toxic substances during growth on foodstuffs. These toxins are known as mycotoxins. Algal toxins are usually associated with seafood, most notably molluscan shellfish.

Bacterial toxins

Three bacteria are most commonly associated with preformed toxin production: *Clostridium botulinum*, *Staphylococcus aureus* and *Bacillus cereus* (see Table 15.1).

Fungal toxins (mycotoxins)

Mycotoxins are secondary metabolites of molds that can induce acute and chronic symptoms, such as carcinogenic, mutagenic, and oestrogenic effects in humans and animals. Acute toxicity due to mycotoxins is associated with liver and kidney damage. Chronic toxicity resulting from the exposure of low levels of mycotoxins in the human diet is a major food safety concern. In non-industrialised countries mycotoxins have been reported to be responsible for increased morbidity and mortality in children owing to suppression of their immune systems and greater susceptibility to disease.

The term modified (including "masked" and "hidden) mycotoxin refers to substances whereby the chemical structure of the mycotoxin has been altered through biological or chemical mechanisms. It refers to e.g. metabolites of the parent mycotoxin formed in the plant or mycotoxins modified by living organisms other than plants. Further processing of the plants can also lead to modified mycotoxins. It also includes mycotoxins which are strongly bound to constituents in the (plant) matrix, as is the case for fumonisins, and which makes it difficult to analytically detect them (giving rise to the term "hidden").

EFSA have recently evaluated the risks to human and animal health related to modified forms of the Fusarium toxins deoxynivalenol, zearalenone, nivalenol, T-2 and HT-2 toxins and fumonisins. These modified forms of the mycotoxins have been shown to have a similar and in some cases, greater toxicity than their parent compound (EFSA Contam Panel, 2014, 2016, 2017, 2018).

The principal fungi that are associated with mycotoxin production are the genera *Aspergillus*, *Penicillium*, and *Fusarium*. *Aspergillus* and *Penicillium* are sometimes referred to as storage fungi as they can grow at low water activity levels and are associated with the post-harvest spoilage of stored food commodities such as cereals, nuts, and spices. *Fusarium* species are plant pathogens and can infect plants in the field and produce mycotoxins preharvest. Table 15.8 provides an overview of the most important mycotoxins.

Marine biotoxins

Fish and fishery products are nutritious foods and are desirable components of a healthy diet. Food-borne illnesses resulting from the consumption of seafood are associated with both finfish and molluscan shellfish. The major risk of acute illness is associated with the consumption of shellfish, particularly bivalve molluscs. The consumption of these toxic shellfish by humans can cause illness, with symptoms ranging from mild diarrhoea and vomiting to memory loss, paralysis, and death. These toxins have been responsible for incidents of wide-scale death of sea-life and are increasingly responsible for human intoxication.

Various seafood poisoning syndromes are associated with toxic marine algae and these include paralytic shellfish poisoning (PSP), amnesic shellfish poisoning (ASP), diarrhoetic shellfish poisoning (DSP), neurotoxic shellfish poisoning, and azaspiracid shellfish poisoning (AZP). There are also different types of food poisoning associated with finfish and these include ciguatera poisoning, scombroid, or histamine poisoning, and puffer fish poisoning. Consumption of raw molluscan shellfish poses well-known risks of food poisoning, but intoxication from finfish is not so well known. Most of the algal toxins associated with seafood poisoning are heat stable and are not inactivated by cooking. It is also not possible visually to distinguish toxic from nontoxic fish. Many countries rely on biotoxin monitoring programs to protect public health and close harvesting areas when toxin algal blooms or toxic shellfish are detected. In non-industrialised countries, particularly in rural areas, monitoring for harmful algal blooms does not routinely occur and deaths due to red-tide toxins commonly occur. Table 15.9

Table 15.8 Mycotoxins in the food supply

Mycotoxin	Producing fungi	Main foods affected	Toxicity
Aflatoxins	*Aspergillus flavus and A. parasiticus*	Nuts, cereals, dried fruit, herbs and spices, milk (aflatoxin M1)	Carcinogenic, hepatotoxic
Ochratoxin A	*Aspergillus ochraceus, Penicillium verrucosum, and other Aspergillus and Penicillium* spp.	Coffee, dried fruit, cereals, beans, pulses, wine, beer, grape juice; kidney, liver and blood from animals fed with contaminated feed	Nephrotoxic, immunotoxic
Patulin	*Aspergillus clavatus, also several species of Penicillium, Aspergillus, and Byssochlamys*	Fruits and grains, predominantly apples and apple products	Cytotoxic
Trichothecenes (nivalenol, deoxynivalenol, T2-toxin, etc.)	*Fusarium* spp.	Wheat, maize, barley, oats, rye, malt, beer, bread	Dermotoxic, enterotoxic, hemotoxic, immunotoxic
Fumonisins	*Fusarium spp.*	Cereals, mainly corn	Carcinogenic, cytotoxic, hepatotoxic
Sterigmatocystin	*Aspergillus versicolor, A. nidulans, and other Aspergillus spp.*	Cereals, green coffee, herbs and spices, raw meat products	Hepatotoxic and nephrotoxic, carcinogenic
Citrinin	Penicillium spp., Aspergillus spp.	Cereals	Nephrotoxic
Zearalenone	*Fusarium graminearum*	Maize, barley, oats, wheat, rice, sorghum, bread	Estrogenic effects, feed refusal, vomiting
Moniliformin	*Fusarium spp.*	Cereals, maize	Nephrotoxic, causes necrosis of the heart muscle
Alternaria toxins	*Alternaria spp.*	Wheat, sorghum, barley, oilseed, fruit and vegetables	Potential mutagens, carcinogens, fetotoxic an teratogenic
Ergot Alkaloids	*Claviceps* spp., particularly *C. purpurea*	Cereals, mainly rye	Effects on cardiovascular and central nervous system

provides an overview of the most important types of fish poisoning.

Naturally occurring plant toxins

Certain plants contain naturally occurring compounds that are toxic to humans or that reduce the bioavailability of nutrients in foods. Seeds or parts of certain plants have been found as impurities in important agricultural crops. Examples of naturally occurring toxins are listed in Table 15.10. Some species of mushroom also contain toxic compounds, for instance agaritine. Some cereal-based diets have restricted bioavailability of nutrients as a result of the presence of antinutritional factors such as phytate and tannins or polyphenols.

Food processing methods have evolved that reduce human exposure to both natural toxins and antinutritional compounds. For instance, cassava is a staple food of over 500 million people worldwide. Certain bitter varieties of cassava contain high levels of linamarin, a cyanogenic glycoside. The consumption of these varieties has been associated with health defects such as goiter and paralysis of the legs. Traditional processing of cassava in Africa that involves grating, soaking roots in water, and lactic acid fermentation completely removes the cyanide.

Adequate cooking of legume seeds such as kidney beans and disposal of the cooking water will remove the natural toxins present in these food products.

Antinutritional factors are those components of plants that interfere with metabolic processes and can lead to deficiencies of key nutrients in the diet. These are generally classified as enzyme inhibitors and mineral binding agents. Enzyme inhibitors are polypeptides and proteins that inhibit the activities of digestive enzymes, and

Table 15.9 Types of fish poisoning

Poisoning	Implicated foods	Associated toxin	Symptoms	Occurrence
Paralytic shellfish poisoning	Mussels, oysters, clams or scallops that have fed on toxigenic dinoflagellates (*Gonyaulax* spp.)	Saxitoxins	Neurotoxic; symptoms include numbness, tingling and burning of the lips, staggering, drowsiness, and in severe cases respiratory paralysis	Worldwide
Amnesic shellfish poisoning	Mussels and clams that have recently fed on a marine diatom *Nitzchia pungens*, viscera of crabs and anchovies	Domoic acid	Vomiting, cramps, diarrhoea, disorientation, and difficulty in breathing	USA, Canada, and Europe
Diarrhoetic shellfish poisoning	Toxic mussels, clams, and scallops that have fed on marine dinoflagellates (*Dinophysis spp.*)	Okadaic acid and associated toxins	Abdominal pain, nausea, vomiting, and severe diarrhoea	Europe, Japan, Chile, New Zealand, and Canada
Neurotoxic shellfish poisoning	Shellfish that have fed on the dinoflagellate *Gymnodinidum breve*	Brevitoxins	Nausea, diarrhoea, tingling and burning of the lips, tongue, and throat	Florida coast and Gulf of Mexico
Azaspiracid shellfish poisoning	Mussels, oysters, clams, scallops, and razor fish	Azaspiracid	Nausea, vomiting, severe diarrhoea, and stomach cramps	Europe, South America, Africa, Canada
Ciguatera fish poisoning	Flesh of toxic reef fish from tropical areas feeding on dinoflagellates (*Gambierdiscus toxicus*) and their toxins. Common species are amberjack, barracuda, moray eel, groupers, trevally, Spanish mackerel, and snapper	Ciguatera	Gastrointestinal (diarrhoea, vomiting, abdominal pain, nausea); neurological (paresthesia of the extremities, circumoral paresthesia, temperature reversal, ataxia, arthralgia, malign headache, severe pruritus, vertigo, and stiffness, convulsions, delirium, hallucinations, photophobia, transient blindness, salivation, perspiration, watery eyes, metallic taste in mouth, blurred vision, hiccups, exacerbation of acne, dysuria); cardiovascular (dyspnoea, bradycardia, hypotension, tachycardia)	Tropical reef waters, particularly in the island states of the South Pacific
Scombroid or histamine poisoning	Consumption of scombroid and scombroid- like marine fish species that have not been chilled immediately after capture. Commonly involved are members of the Scombridae family, e.g., tuna and mackerel, and a few nonscombrid relatives, e.g., bluefish, dolphin fish, and amberjack	Scombroid or histamine.	Initial symptoms are that of an allergic response with facial flushing and sweating, burning–peppery taste sensations around the mouth and throat, dizziness, nausea, and headache. A facial rash can develop as well as mild diarrhoea and abdominal cramps. Severe cases may blur vision and cause respiratory stress and swelling of the tongue. Symptoms usually last for approximately 4–6 h and rarely exceed 1–2 days	Worldwide
Puffer fish poisoning	Consumption of fish species belonging to the Tetraodontidea family, particularly those species caught in waters of the Indo-Pacific Ocean regions	Tetrodotoxin	Symptoms of puffer fish poisoning are similar to paralytic shellfish poisoning as the actions of both toxins are similar. Mild poisoning results in tingling and numbness of the lips, tongue, and fingers, and in severe cases death by asphyxiation due to respiratory paralysis	Most frequent in Japan, where puffer fish (called fugu in Japan) are eaten as a delicacy, Indo-Pacific Ocean region

Table 15.10 Examples of naturally occurring plant toxins

Compound	Plant genus/species/ family	Common name
Cyanogenic Glycosides:		
Amygdalin, Prunasin	*Prunus spp.*	Apricot and bitter almond kernels
Linamarin	*Manihot escaleatum*	Cassava
Dhurrin	*Sorghum spp.*	Sorghum
Glycoalkaloids:		
Solanin	*Solanium tuberosiem*	Potatoes
Pyrrolizidine alkaloids:		
Acetyllycopsaimine	*Symphytum spp.*	Comfrey
Senecionine	*Senccio jacobaea*	Ragwort
Glucosinolates:		
Sinigrin	*Brassica spp.*	Cabbage, Broccoli, Brussels sprouts
Tropane Alkaloids		
Atropine	*Datura*	Thorn apple/Jimson weed
	Atropa belladonna	Deadly nightshade
	Hyoscamus	Henbane
Opium alkaloids		
Morphine, Thebaine, Codeine, Nosapine, Papaverine	*Papaver somniferum L.*	Seeds of Poppy
Other		
Erucic acid	*Brassicaceae spp.*	Rape seed, mustard seed, seeds from cabbages, turnips
Tetrahydrocannabinol	*Cannabis sativa*	Hemp

most are thermolabile and are reduced by cooking. For example, trypsin inhibitors may cause poor protein digestion and a shortage of sulfur-containing amino acids in the diet. Lectins are proteins that occur in beans that alter the absorption of nutrients in the intestinal wall. Cooking beans will inactivate lectins. Tannins (polyphenols) occur in cereals, specifically in the seed coat. These form complexes with proteins and inhibition of digestive enzymes. Phytate is a natural component in plants and on digestion forms insoluble complexes with metal ions in the body. The result is reduced bioavailability of essential minerals such as iron. In addition, a range of natural plant toxins can cause allergic reactions in humans, but there is a general lack of knowledge about their properties and modes of action.

Food additives

Food additives are added to foods for a specific technological purpose during manufacture or storage and become an integral part of that foodstuff. Additives can be natural or synthetic and are usually categorised by their function (Table 15.11). For example, preservatives prevent the growth of bacteria, gelling agents maintain the structure of some foods during storage, and emulsifiers maintain the stability of fat structures. Without additives it would not be possible to manufacture many of the foods available today, especially convenience foods and low-fat foods.

Table 15.11 Categories of food additives according to their functional class

Acidity regulators	Foaming agents
Acids	Gelling agents
Anti-caking agents	Glazing agents
Anti-foaming agents	Humectants
Antioxidants	Modified starches
Bulking agents	Packaging gases
Carriers	Preservatives
Colours	Propellants
Contrast enhancers	Raising agents
Emulsifiers	Sequestrants
Emulsifying salts	Stabilisers
Firming agents	Sweeteners
Flavour enhancers	Thickeners
Flour treatment agents	

Source: Regulation (EC) No 1333/2008 of the European Parliament and of the Council of 16 December 2008 on food additives

Safety considerations involving additives have centered on allergic reactions and food intolerances. Studies have been conducted into allergies and they often find that the actual prevalence rate is much lower than the perceived prevalence rate.

At the EU and international level, additives are controlled by means of safety evaluation and the development of a positive list. To ensure transparency and choice, all additives that are used in prepackaged food should be labeled with their function and their name or approval number (E number). However, there are some exemptions specifically applying to additives that are in a foodstuff as a result of carry-over from an ingredient.

15.6 Food allergies and intolerances

Many foods can cause a hypersensitive reaction in susceptible consumers who are allergic to, or intolerant of a particular food or ingredient. Food allergy and intolerance can be associated with a wide variety of symptoms that occur within minutes to hours following exposure. A typical allergic reaction to food occurs when a person's immune system over-reacts in response to the ingestion of a specific constituent, usually a protein or a peptide, in that food. The symptoms of such allergic reactions can range from mild (e.g. rash, itching, hives) to severe (e.g., anaphylaxis), which can have potentially life-threatening consequences without swift medical intervention. Indeed, food allergy is the leading cause of non-drug-related anaphylaxis (Kurowski and Boxer, 2008). The foods most commonly associated with allergies in Europe, North America, Asia and Australia are peanuts, tree nuts, milk, egg, sesame seeds, fish, and crustaceans (Cianferoni and Muraro, 2012, Huang *et al.*, 2012). Children are particularly sensitive to eggs and milk but generally grow out of such allergies (Kurowski and Boxer, 2008). Food intolerance is different to a food allergy in that the immune system is not involved. For example, lactose intolerance is the reduced ability of the body to digest lactose (a type of sugar naturally found in milk) due to a deficiency of the enzyme lactase in the small intestine. Sulphur dioxide and sulphites, which can occur naturally in some foods or may be added as preservatives, can cause adverse reactions in certain people, especially those with asthma. However, its pathogenesis has not been clearly documented and given the nature of the molecule, an immune-mediated reaction to sulphites is unlikely (EFSA, 2014). Another common adverse reaction to food that is not classified as a food allergy or intolerance is coeliac disease, an auto-immune disorder caused by the consumption of gluten, a protein found naturally in cereals such as wheat, rye and barley and crossbreeds of these grains. Box 15.4 shows a broad classification of the adverse reactions to food.

As there is no cure yet, the generally accepted way of managing a food allergy or intolerance is the exclusion of the offending food(s) or

Box 15.4 Adverse reactions to food (adapted from EFSA, 2014). Ig-E, immunoglobulin type E

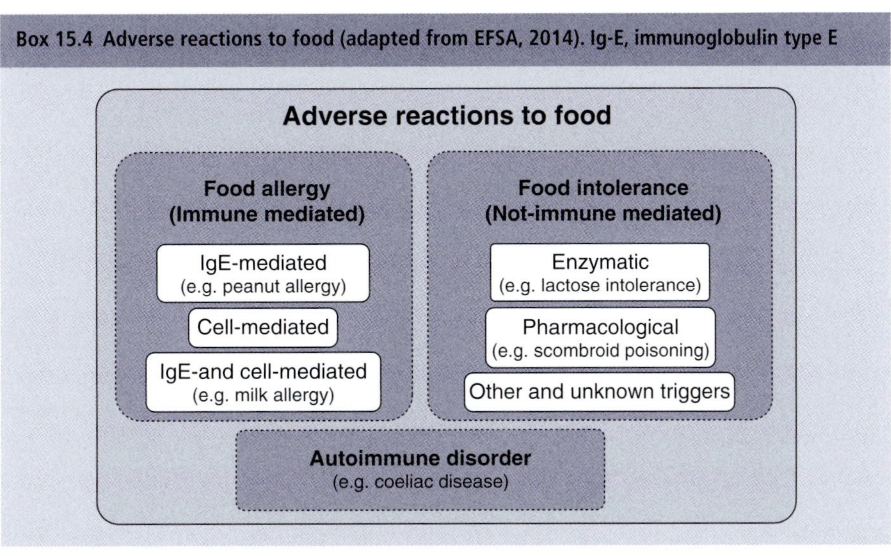

ingredient(s) from the diet (Lack, 2008; Burks *et al.*, 2011). People at risk of severe reaction to food are trained to recognise the initial onset of symptoms and to implement the appropriate response (e.g., application of a prefilled adrenalin auto-injector) in the event of accidental exposure (Davis and Kelso, 2018). In order to safeguard their health, people with food allergies or intolerances require accurate food information. Allergen labelling rules in various countries require food manufacturers to declare allergens when they are deliberately used in a product. Declaring the use of 14 food allergens in the manufacture or preparation of food in the EU is a legal requirement under the Food Information for Consumers legislation (Regulation (EU) No 1169/2011). The 14 regulated food allergens include cereals containing gluten, crustaceans, eggs, fish, peanuts, soybeans, milk, nuts (eight types), celery, mustard, sesame seeds, sulphur dioxide and sulphites, lupin and molluscs (Table 15.12). As explained earlier, cereals containing gluten and sulphites are not considered classical food allergens but are nevertheless included in the list for the purpose of regulatory clarity. For prepacked food, allergen declaration is facilitated by highlighting the allergens in the list of ingredients. However, it can be more complex for non-prepacked foods which are those sold without packaging, packed on the premises at the consumer's request or prepacked for direct sale from the premises where packed. Voluntary statements such as 'may contain (*allergen*)…' or 'prepared in premises that use (*allergen*)…' can provide a useful warning to vulnerable consumers when used judiciously. However, such precautionary statements relate to the risk of cross-contamination with food allergens rather than their deliberate use in the preparation or production of food (FSAI, 2015).

Research is ongoing at an international level to establish the minimum eliciting doses for the most common and serious of the food allergens (Taylor *et al.*, 2018) while prevalence data is also being collated by many jurisdictions in an attempt to understand what foods pose the biggest allergenic risk. The detection and quantification of food allergens in food is a critical tool enabling the food industry and regulators to manage the risk posed by the inadvertent and undeclared presence of allergens in food. Enzyme Linked Immunosorbent Assay (ELISA) is currently the preferred analytical method for most routine food allergen analysis, although it has limitations in certain situations due to the type of food matrix, poor sensitivity at low levels of the target allergenic protein and the potential for cross-reactivity with non-target proteins. Alternative detection and quantification methods include DNA analysis which has benefits over ELISA but also has some limitations. Mass spectrometry is also a promising technique currently under development (EFSA, 2014).

15.7 Food safety control programs

Each nation has a responsibility to ensure that its citizens enjoy safe and wholesome food. Governments aim to identify major food safety issues that can then be controlled through the development and implementation of targeted food safety control programs and monitoring and surveillance programs. This can be achieved either through legislation, or the use of standards or codes of practice. At the international level, the WHO and the FAO have worked since the 1960s on developing food standards that aim to protect the health of consumers and facilitate international trade of foods and animal feeding stuffs. This work is carried out by the Codex Alimentarius Commission (CAC), an intergovernmental body managed by the FAO and WHO. Food safety standards developed by the CAC serve as the baseline for harmonisation of global food standards, codes of practice, guidelines, and recommendations. Harmonisation of standards and recognition that different national food safety controls are equivalent are enshrined in the international agreements of the World Trade Organization.

The purpose of food safety legislation is to protect consumers' health and interests by providing controls throughout the food chain. The overhaul of EU food safety legislation clearly places the primary responsibility for food safety with the food business operator. It also recognises that food safety must start at primary production (i.e., the farmer) and places increased importance on the safety of animal feed. This concept of food safety control from "farm-to-fork" or "gate-to-plate" has been endorsed internationally, but implemented differently in different countries.

Table 15.12 Fourteen substances or products causing allergies or intolerances subject to declaration according to European legislation (Regulation (EU) No 1169/2011)

Category	Exceptions	Examples of food products (adapted from EFSA, 2014)
Celery and products thereof		Both the root and the stalks can be found raw in salads, dried as a spice and cooked in sauces and soups
Cereals containing gluten and products thereof	- Wheat based glucose syrups including dextrose - Wheat based maltodextrins - Glucose syrups based on barley - Cereals used for making alcoholic distillates including ethyl alcohol of agricultural origin	Wheat (such as spelt and khorasan wheat), rye, barley, oats[1] and their hybridised strains. These can be found in bread, biscuits, cakes, pasta, pizza, sauces, stock cubes, sausages, burgers, etc.
Crustaceans and products thereof		Shrimps, prawns, langoustines, lobsters, crabs and crayfishes. These can be found in seafood chowders, soups, fish cakes, pies, stock cubes, etc.
Eggs[2] and products thereof		Egg can be found in pasta, pizza, baked products, desserts, mayonnaise, burgers, etc.
Fish and products thereof	- Fish gelatine used as a carrier for vitamin or carotenoid preparations - Fish gelatine or Isinglass used as fining agent in beer and wine	Carp, cod, herring, perch, salmon, swordfish, tilapia, tuna, etc. These can be found in seafood chowders, soups, fish cakes, pies, stir-fry mixes, surimi, stock cubes, etc.
Lupin and products thereof		Lupin-derived drinks (lupin milks) and lupin seed flour which can be found in bread, biscuits, pasta, sauces, etc.
Milk[3] and products thereof (e.g. lactose)	- Whey used for making alcoholic distillates including ethyl alcohol of agricultural origin - Lactitol	Milk can be found in dairy products including milk powder, buttermilk, cream, cheese, yoghurt and ice cream, as well as in soups, meat and fish dishes, desserts, drinks, etc.
Molluscs and products thereof		Snails, clams, oysters, cockles, mussels, scallops, squids, octopuses, cuttlefishes. These can be found in seafood chowders, soups, fish cakes, pies, stock cubes, etc.
Mustard and products thereof		Mustard can be found in meat dishes such as hot-dogs and burgers, spices mixes, stock cubes, sauces, salad dressings, etc.
Nuts[4] and products thereof	Nuts used for making alcoholic distillates including ethyl alcohol of agricultural origin	Almonds, hazelnuts, walnuts, cashews, pecan nuts, Brazil nuts, pistachio nuts, and macadamia/Queensland nuts. These can be found in bread, breakfast cereals, cereal bars, biscuits, cakes, pasta, pizza, sauces, salad dressings, spreads, sweets, desserts, chocolates, stock cubes, stuffing, sausages, burgers, etc.
Peanuts and products thereof		Can be found raw, crushed or ground as 'butter', roasted or salted as snack and incorporated into a wide variety of foods including breakfast cereals, cereal bars, sauces, salad dressings, spreads, sweets, desserts, chocolates, etc.
Sesame seeds and products thereof		Sesame seeds can be found in bakery products, fast-foods, processed meat, vegetarian and ethnic dishes, etc.
Soybeans and products thereof	- Fully refined soybean oil and fat - Natural mixed tocopherols (E306), natural D-alpha tocopherol, natural D-alpha tocopherol acetate, natural D-alpha tocopherol succinate from soybean sources - Vegetable oils derived phytosterols and phytosterol esters from soybean sources - Plant stanol ester produced from vegetable oil sterols from soybean sources	Soy oil, soy flour, soymilk, soy drinks, soy flakes and fermented soybean products such as soy sauce, miso, okara, tempeh and tofu. These can also be found in a wide variety of processed foods such as meat products, sausages, bakery products, chocolate and breakfast cereals

(*Continued*)

Table 15.12 (Continued)

Category	Exceptions	Examples of food products (adapted from EFSA, 2014)
Sulphur dioxide and sulphites (when present at levels exceeding 10 mg/kg or 10 mg/L in the final product, expressed as total SO_2)		Sulphites occur naturally in some foods as a consequence of fermentation (e.g. wine) or may be added to fruits, vegetables, meats and alcoholic drinks as preservatives

[1] Oats are technically gluten-free as they do not naturally contain gluten. However, oats have avenin, a protein similar to gluten.
[2] It is understood that refers to eggs from all farmed avian species.
[3] It is understood that refers to milk from all farmed mammalian species.
[4] Nuts include a wide variety of fruits and seeds of various species contained within a hard shell.

The traditional "inspection and detection" aspects of food safety control are now being replaced with strategies for prevention of hazards occurring in the first place. In many countries, food businesses are now legally obliged to adopt the principles of HACCP (hazard analysis and critical control point) in order to identify which biological, chemical, physical or allergenic hazards are likely to occur in their process, so that they can implement control measures to prevent them happening.

15.8 Emerging food safety issues

The emergence of new food-borne pathogens is one factor leading to increased concern about food safety. During the twentieth century improvements in sewage treatment, milk pasteurisation, water treatments, and better controls on animal disease led to the control of food-borne and water-borne diseases such as typhoid, tuberculosis, and brucellosis. However, new food-borne pathogens have emerged. Food-borne organisms such as *E. coli* O157, *Campylobacter jejuni*, and *Salmonella* Enteritidis phage type 4 were virtually unknown in the 1970s, but have come to prominence as virulent pathogens associated with foods of animal origin. In recent times monophasic *Salmonella* Typhimurium has emerged as the dominant clone in many pig production systems. *Cyclospora cayetanensis* emerged as a food-borne pathogen in 1995, when it was associated with outbreaks of illness traced to raspberries imported into the USA from Guatemala. *Cryptosporidium parvum* emerged as a pathogen of worldwide significance during the 1990s and has been linked to contaminated drinking water and to a range of foods including salads, unpasteurised milk, and apple juice. The *E. coli* O104 outbreak in Europe in 2011 demonstrated clearly how emergent pathogens can come to the fore without warning. Pathogens such as *Listeria monocytogenes* can grow at refrigeration temperatures and have increased in importance with the expansion of the cold chain for food distribution. An EFSA opinion also identified a likely factor for the increased incidence rates of L. monocytogenes is the increased proportion of susceptible people in the age groups over 45 (EFSA, 2018). In addition, changing consumer practices (such as an increased preference for raw foods) has resulted in recent outbreaks, e.g. the multistate EU listeriosis outbreak reported to be linked to frozen corn and other frozen vegetables in 2018. This outbreak highlighted that consumers do not always follow manufacturers' instructions to cook food. *Cronobacter sakazakii* has been implicated in outbreaks of infection associated with powdered infant formula. Many of these emerging pathogens are of animal origin and do not usually cause serious illness in the animal host.

Another concern is that a proportion of food-borne illness is caused by pathogens that have not yet been identified, and therefore cannot be diagnosed. In the USA, it has been estimated that unknown food-borne agents caused 65% of the estimated 5,200 annual deaths from food-borne disease (Mead, 1999; Frenzen, 2004). This is of concern since many of today's commonly recognised food-borne pathogens were not recognised as causes of food-borne illness 40 years ago. In this regard, *Mycobacterium avium* sub-species *paratuberculosis* (MAP) is an organism of potential concern. MAP is the causative agent of Johne's disease in cattle, but it has been proposed that MAP is also the causative agent of Crohn's disease in humans, and that it may be transmitted via contaminated foods (including pasteurised milk) and water (McNees *et al.*, 2015).

The emergence of antibiotic-resistant food-borne pathogens that are associated with the inappropriate use of antibiotics in human medicine and animal husbandry is of particular concern. The European Centre for Disease Prevention and Control (ECDC) and the European Food Safety Authority (EFSA) published a joint European Union summary report on antimicrobial resistance in zoonotic and indicator bacteria from humans, animals and food and recently have reported resistance to critically important antimicrobials for clinical use in poultry isolates, albeit at low levels, as well as resistance to carbapenems (EFSA and ECDC 2018). Fluoroquinolone resistance is commonly observed in *Campylobacter*. An increasing focus is now placed on the role of the food chain in the dissemination of antimicrobial resistance and the importance of taking a One Health approach, incorporating surveillance of resistance of isolates from animals, food and humans, as well as the environment.

Additionally, chemical risks to food, such as pesticide residues, acrylamide, endocrine disrupting chemicals and the use of food additives, continue to concern consumers.

15.9 Perspectives on the future

As our society changes, so do the hazards involved in food-borne disease. Changes in food production systems and the globalisation of the food supply, as well as changes in the food we are eating, and where this food is prepared, expose us to an ever-changing spectrum of contamination. The global nature of our food supply poses greater risks to consumer health from the mass production and distribution of foods and increased risk for food contamination. For example, new food development has led to changing vectors for the spread of disease. Inappropriate use of antibiotics in human medicine and animal husbandry has led to the emergence of antibiotic-resistant food-borne pathogens. If not addressed, it has been estimated that by 2050 global deaths from resistant microorganisms will exceed current deaths from cancer (O'Neill, 2016).

Food safety and nutrition are inextricably linked because food-borne infections are one of the most important underlying factors of malnutrition, especially in poorer countries. Repeated episodes of food-borne infections can, over a period of time, lead to malnutrition, with serious health consequences. A safe food supply is essential for proper nutrition, basic health and well-being.

Maintaining a safe food supply is not difficult; however, it requires attention to detail at all stages of the food chain from agricultural inputs through farms, processing, the distribution network to retailers and catering outlets to consumers. There can be no gaps in the continuum from farm to fork if consumer protection is to be optimum. To ensure consumer protection, food standards have to be based on sound science and the principles of risk analysis. At the national level, food safety controls must be well coordinated and based on proportionate food legislation. The food industry must also recognise its primary responsibility for producing safe food and for ensuring that foods placed on the market meet the highest standards of food safety and hygiene. A multisectoral effort on the part of regulatory authorities, food industries and consumers alike are required to prevent food-borne diseases.

Acknowledgement

This chapter has been revised and updated by Catherine M. Burgess, Declan J. Bolton, Martin Danaher, Cristina Arroyo, Patrick J. O'Mahony, Lisa O' Connor, and Christina Tlustos based on the previous edition's chapter by Alan Reilly, Christina Tlustos, Judith O'Connor, and Lisa O'Connor.

References

Abdussalam, M., Käferstein, F.K., and Mott, K. (1995). Food safety measures for the control of food borne trematode infections. *Food Control*. **6**: 71–79.

Burks, A.W., Jones, S.M., Boyce, J.A. *et al.* (2011). NIAID-sponsored 2010 guidelines for managing food allergy: applications in the pediatric population. *Pediatrics*, **128**(5), 955–965.

Cianferoni, A. and Muraro, A. (2012). Food-induced anaphylaxis. *Immunol Allergy Clin North Am*, **32**(1), 165–195.

Cook, A.J., Gilbert, R.E., Buffolano, W. *et al.* (2000). Sources of toxoplasma infection in pregnant women: European multicentre case-control study. European Research Network on Congenital Toxoplasmosis. *BMJ*, **321**(7254), 142–147.

Davis, C.M., Kelso, J.M. (2018). Food Allergy Management. *Immunol Allergy Clin North Am.* **38**(1), 53–64.

EFSA. (2016). The European Union summary report on data of thesurveillance of ruminants for the presence of transmissiblespongiform encephalopathies (TSEs) in 2015. *EFSA Journal.* **14**(12):4643.

EFSA. (2014). Scientific Opinion on the evaluation of allergenic foods and food ingredients for labelling purposes. *EFSA Journal* **12**(11), 3894.

EFSA BIOHAZ Panel (EFSA Panel on Biological Hazards), Ricci A, Allende A, Bolton D, Chemaly M, Davies R, Fernández Escámez PS, Girones R, Herman L, Koutsoumanis K, Nørrung B, Robertson L, Ru G, Sanaa M, Simmons M, Skandamis P, Snary E, Speybroeck N, Ter Kuile B, Threlfall J, Wahlström H, Takkinen J, Wagner M, Arcella D, Da Silva Felicio MT, Georgiadis M, Messens W and Lindqvist R, 2018. Scientific Opinion on the Listeria monocytogenes contamination of ready-to-eat foods and the risk for human health in the EU. EFSA Journal 2018;16(1):5134, 173 pp.

EFSA CONTAM Panel (EFSA Panel on Contaminants in the Food Chain) (2014) Scientific Opinion on the risks for human and animal health related to the presence of modified forms of certain mycotoxins in food and feed. EFSA Journal 2014;12(12):3916, 107 pp. doi:10.2903/j.efsa.2014.3916

EFSA CONTAM Panel (EFSA Panel on Contaminants in the Food Chain) (2016) Scientific opinion on the appropriateness to set a group health-based guidance value for zearalenone and its modified forms. EFSA Journal 2016;14(4):4425

EFSA CONTAM Panel (EFSA Panel on Contaminants in the Food Chain), Knutsen HK, Alexander J, Barreg ard L, Bignami M, Brueschweiler B, Ceccatelli S, Cottrill B, Dinovi M, Grasl-Kraupp B, Hogstrand C, Hoogenboom LR, Nebbia CS, Oswald IP, Petersen A, Rose M, Roudot A-C, Schwerdtle T, Vleminckx C, Vollmer G, Wallace H, De Saeger S, Eriksen GS, Farmer P, Fremy J-M, Gong YY, Meyer K, Naegeli H, Parent-Massin D, Rietjens I, van Egmond H, Altieri A, Eskola M, Gergelova P, Ramos Bordajandi L, Benkova B, Doerr B, Gkrillas A, Gustavsson N, van Manen M and Edler L. (2017). Scientific Opinion on the risks to human and animal health related to the presence of deoxynivalenol and its acetylated and modified forms in food and feed. EFSA Journal 2017;15(9):4718, 345 pp.

EFSA CONTAM Panel (EFSA Panel on Contaminants in the Food Chain), Knutsen H-K, Alexander J, Barregard L, Bignami M, Brueschweiler B, Ceccatelli S, Cottrill B, Dinovi M, Edler L, Grasl - Kraupp B, Hogstrand C, Hoogenboom LR, Nebbia CS, Petersen A, Rose M, Roudot A-C, Schwerdtle T, Vleminckx C, Vollmer G, Wallace H, Dall'Asta C, Eriksen G-S, Taranu I, Altieri A, Roldan-Torres R and Oswald IP (2018) Scientific opinion on the risks for animal health related to the presence of fumonisins, their modified forms and hidden forms in feed. EFSA Journal 2018;16(5):5242

EFSA. Scientific Committee (2005) Opinion of the Scientific Committee on a request from EFSA related to a harmonised approach for risk assessment of substances which are both genotoxic and carcinogenic. *EFSA Journal* **282**: 1–31.

EFSA Scientific Committee (2012). Statement on the applicability of the Margin of Exposure approach for the safety assessment of impurities which are both genotoxic and carcinogenic in substances added to food/feed. EFSA Journal 2012;10(3):2578.

EFSA Scientific Committee, Hardy A, Benford D, Halldorsson T, Jeger MJ, Knutsen KH, More S, Mortensen A, Naegeli H, Noteborn H, Ockleford C, Ricci A, Rychen G, Silano V, Solecki R, Turck D, Aerts M, Bodin L, Davis A, Edler L, Gundert-Remy U, Sand S, Slob W, Bottex B, Abrahantes JC, Marques DC, Kass G and Schlatter JR (2017). Update: Guidance on the use of the benchmark dose approach in risk assessment. EFSA Journal 2017;15(1):4658.

EFSA and ECDC (2018). The European Union summary report on antimicrobial resistance in zoonotic and indicator bacteria from humans, animals and food in 2016. *EFSA Journal* **16**(2):5182, 270 pp.

FAO/WHO. (1978). *Evaluation of certain food additives and contaminants. 22nd Report of the Joint FAO/WHO Expert Committee on Food Additives.* WHO Technical Report Series No. 631. WHO, Geneva. 14–15.

Frenzen, P.D. (2004). Deaths due to unknown foodborne agents. *Emerging Infectious Diseases.* **10**: 1536–1543.

FAO. (2018). The State of Agricultural Commodity Markets 2018. Agricultural trade, climate change and food security. Rome.

FSAI. (2015). *Allergen information for non-prepacked food.* Retrieved from https://www.fsai.ie/resources_publications.html

FSAI (2018). Reduce the Risk of Food Poisoning: Information for People who are Particularly Vulnerable. www.fsai.ie

FSAI (2019). Guidance Note No 18 Validation of Product Shelf-life. (Revision 4). ISBN: 1-904465-33-1

Greenlee, J.J. and Greenlee, M.H.W. (2015). The Transmissible Spongiform Encephalopathies of Livestock. *ILAR J.* **56**(1):7–25.

Hall, A.J., Wikswo, M.E., Pringle, K. *et al.* (2014). Vital signs: foodborne norovirus outbreaks - United States, 2009-2012. *MMWR Morb Mortal Wkly Rep.* **63**(22), 491–495.

Havelaar, A.H., Kirk, M.D., Torgerson, P.R. *et al.* (2015). World Health Organization Global Estimates and Regional Comparisons of the Burden of Foodborne Disease in 2010. *PLoS Medicine.* **12**(12), e1001923. doi:10.1371/journal.pmed.1001923

Huang, F., Chawla, K., Jarvinen, K.M. *et al.* (2012). Anaphylaxis in a New York City pediatric emergency department: triggers, treatments, and outcomes. *J Allergy Clin Immunol.* **129**(1), 162–168 e161-163.

ICMSF (1996). In: Roberts, T.A., Baird-Parker, A.C & Tompkin, A.C. (Eds), Microorganisms in Foods 5 - Characteristics of Microbial Pathogens. London: Blackie Academic & Professional.

Jay, J.M., Loessner, M.J. & Golden, D.A. (2005). Intrinsic and Extrinsic Parameters of Foods that Affect Microbial Growth. In: Jay, J.M., Loessner, M.J., Golden, D.A. (Eds), Modern Food Microbiology, 7th Edition, (pp. 39 - 60). New York: Springer Science & Business Med Inc

Kamar, N., Abravanel, F., Lhomme, S. *et al.* (2015). Hepatitis E virus: chronic infection, extra-hepatic manifestations, and treatment. *Clin Res Hepatol Gastroenterol.* **39**(1), 20–27.

Kamar, N., Dalton, H.R., Abravanel, F. *et al.* (2014). Hepatitis E virus infection. *Clin Microbiol Rev.* **27**(1), 116–138.

Kirk, M.D., Pires, S.M., Black, R.E. *et al.* (2015). World Health Organization Estimates of the Global and

Regional Disease Burden of 22 Foodborne Bacterial, Protozoal, and Viral Diseases, 2010: A Data Synthesis. *PLoS Med.* **12**(12), e1001921.

Kurowski, K. and Boxer, R.W. (2008). Food allergies: detection and management. *Am Fam Physician.* **77**(12), 1678–1686.

Lack, G. (2008). Clinical practice. Food allergy. *N Engl J Med.* **359**(12), 1252–1260.

Lindsay, J.A. (1997). Chronic Sequelae of Foodborne Disease. *Emerg Infect Dis.* **3**(4), 443–452.

McNees, A.L., Markesich, D., Zayyani, N.R. *et al.* (2015). Mycobacterium paratuberculosis as a cause of Crohn's disease. *Expert Rev Gastroenterol Hepatol.* **9**(12):1523–34.

Mead, P.S., Slutsker, L., Dietz, V. *et al.* (1999). Food-related illness and death in the United Sates. *Emerg Infect Dis* **5**: 607– 625.

O'Neill, J. (2016). *Tackling drug-resistant Infections globally: final report and recommendations.* The review on antimicrobial resistance chaired by Jim O'Neill supported by the Wellcome Trust and UK Government.

Ruggeri, F.M., Di Bartolo, I., Ponterio, E. *et al.* (2013). Zoonotic transmission of hepatitis E virus in industrialized countries. *New Microbiol.* **36**(4), 331–344.

Scallan, E., Hoekstra, R.M., Angulo, F.J. *et al.* (2011). Foodborne illness acquired in the United States--major pathogens. *Emerg Infect Dis.* **17**(1), 7–15.

Scharff, R.L. (2015). State estimates for the annual cost of foodborne illness. *J Food Prot.* **78**(6), 1064–1071.

Smith, D.B., Simmonds, P., Jameel, S. *et al.* (2014). Consensus proposals for classification of the family Hepeviridae. *J Gen Virol.* **95**(Pt 10), 2223–2232.

Smith, J.L. (1999). Foodborne infections during pregnancy. *J Food Prot.* **62**: 818–829.

Tam, C.C., O'Brien, S.J. (2016). Economic Cost of *Campylobacter*, Norovirus and Rotavirus Disease in the United Kingdom. *PLoS One.* **11**(2), e0138526.

Taylor, S.B., Christensen, G., Grinter, K. *et al.* (2018). The Allergen Bureau VITAL Program. *J AOAC Int.* **101**(1), 77–82.

Tenter, A.M., Heckeroth, A.R., Weiss, and L.M. (2000). *Toxoplasma gondii*: from animals to humans. *Int J Parasitol.* **30**(12–13), 1217–1258.

Teunis, P.F., Sukhrie, F.H., Vennema H *et al.* (2015). Shedding of norovirus in symptomatic and asymptomatic infections. *Epidemiol Infect.* **143**(8), 1710–1717.

Van der Poel, W.H. (2014). Food and environmental routes of Hepatitis E virus transmission. *Curr Opin Virol.* **4**, 91–96.

WHO. Global Health and Aging. (2011). Retrieved from https://www.who.int/ageing/publications/global_health.pdf

WHO. (2018). Whole genome sequencing for foodborne disease surveillance: landscape paper. Geneva: World Health Organization. Licence: CC BY-NC-SA 3.0 IGO.

16
Food and Nutrition: Policy and Regulatory Issues

Aideen McKevitt, James Gallagher, and Cassandra H. Ellis

Key messages

- The human food supply is highly regulated and while in the past there was an emphasis on food safety, there is now a rapidly expanding regulatory base covering nutrition.
- Any policy decision in the nutrition regulatory framework needs to be evidence based and informed by relevant data on prevailing food and nutrient intake patterns. These metrics are compared with agreed standards for optimal food and nutrient intake and on the basis of any discrepancy, public health nutrition programmes encompassing regulatory issues are initiated.
- Public health nutrition programmes can be supply driven or demand driven. In the supply-driven option, the government takes the decision centrally to alter some properties of foods, the most common approach being mandatory food fortification. In demand-driven approaches, efforts are made to create a demand for a new food-purchasing pattern through a nutrition communication process.
- Nutrition communication should always be evidence-based and built on studies of consumers attitudes and beliefs. A number of tools are commonly used to communicate nutrition and health messages including nutritional labelling and nutrition claims.
- Based on consumer intake data, a wide range of policies and programmes can be used to improve the food environment and encourage healthier dietary patterns.
- Globalisation of the food supply has been accompanied by evolving governance issues that have produced a regulatory environment at national and global level led by large international agencies in order to facilitate trade and to establish and retain the confidence of consumers in the food supply chain.

16.1 Introduction

Few areas of our lives are more regulated than the food supply and within that regulatory framework, three distinct divisions are evident: food chemicals, food microbial hazards, and nutrition. In the past, food safety tended to dominate but in recent times, the regulatory environment for nutrition has begun to receive increasing attention given that (a) the role of diet in noncommunicable chronic disease has been so extensively accepted and woven into policy; and (b) food producers have made efforts to develop innovative products to help reduce the burden of disease risk. This chapter will provide a brief insight into the present direction of food and nutrition regulation as it relates to dietary choices, and outline the global and national organisations involved in these decisions.

16.2 Reference points in human nutrition

Chapter 2 in this textbook outlines the many options that are available for measuring food intake and converting those data into nutrient intakes. Such data are fundamental to the development of nutrition-related regulatory policy. Prevailing dietary habits, as measured through

Introduction to Human Nutrition, Third Edition. Edited on behalf of The Nutrition Society by Susan A. Lanham-New, Thomas R. Hill, Alison M. Gallagher and Hester H. Vorster.

Companion website: www.wiley.com/go/lanham-new/humannutrition

dietary surveys, represent the first reference point for nutrition policy. The second set of reference points are those targets set out by expert committees that aim to move populations toward healthier diets. Chapter 4 of this textbook describes the basic principles involved in setting out target values for the assessment of dietary intakes, primarily for micronutrients. These are defined using variable terms across the globe but, generally, all definitions employ the term "reference" and hence they can be classified as reference nutritional data. Such data were historically developed to ensure the adequacy of the human diet. However, as our knowledge of diet and chronic disease has evolved, a second set of reference nutrition values had to be developed, this time to minimize the risk of chronic disease (discussed in detail in chapter 17).

The whole purpose of devising these two sets of metrics – nutrient intakes and nutrient reference values – is to first measure where we are in relation to our nutritional well-being, and then to set targets to move the population toward a healthier diet. There is however, a very slight antagonism between the establishment of an ideal pattern of nutrient intake and developing public health nutrition programmes to achieve that goal. The reason is that the former does so in isolation from the real world of everyday eating. Its focus is on experimental studies that, for example, help delineate the optimal balance of dietary fatty acids to minimise plasma cholesterol. That optimal may be significantly different from prevailing dietary habits and to attempt to bridge the gap too fast might produce a public health nutrition programme that is unrealistic. Thus, nutritionists can look at prevailing intakes against ideal intakes and then set out interim attainable targets in realistic public health nutrition programmes that can be implemented over a defined and reasonable period of time. In summary, it is not possible to develop a meaningful nutrition regulatory framework without access to both nutrient intake data and dietary reference data.

16.3 Exploration of dietary patterns to inform policy

With a given set of population nutrient intake data and a given set of nutritional reference values, it is possible to divide the population into those closest to some nutritional ideal and those furthest from such an achievement. These two contrasting groups can now be laid against one another and a wide range of data, listed in Box 16.1, can be examined.

Box 16.1

Nutrients
Foods
Eating habits
Anthropometry
Socioeconomic data
Physical activity
Education
Others

Based on these comparisons and using appropriate statistical techniques, it is possible to begin to discern the reasons why one group are near optimum intake, and why another are far from optimum. These reasons now feed into policy advice and begin to form the nucleus of a nutrition regulatory structure that may help the population improve their diet. Given that the focus of this text is nutrition, it would be worthwhile to single out food patterns for a more critical analysis. The following is a hypothetical finding in relation to three foods that appear to be important in determining the nutritional adequacy of "achievers" and "non-achievers" of some nutrient goal.

Look at Table 16.1. At first glance C seems unimportant and A and B seem to be important and going in opposite directions. These are very typical data that emerge from such analyses and they hide two very important statistics that should always be sought in studies of this nature. The first missing statistic is "% consumers" and the second is the "intake among consumers only." Now reconsider the above data with these additional statistics and look at Table 16.2.

Now everything has changed with the five consumers converting population average intakes into consumer-only intakes. For any programme

Table 16.1 Achievers and non-achievers of nutrient goals

	Achievers	Non-achievers
	(g/day population average)	
Food A	100	40
Food B	20	60
Food C	50	50

Table 16.2 Achievers and non-achievers of nutrient goals with consumer-only intakes

	Achievers	Non-achievers	Achievers	Non-achievers	Achievers	Non-achievers
	g/day population average		% consumers		Consumer-only intake	
Food A	100	40	20	80	500	50
Food B	20	60	50	50	40	120
Food C	50	50	100	30	50	150

in public health nutrition, three important strategies which are often lost are (a) strategies to increase or decrease the five people eating a target food, (b) strategies to alter the frequency with which a target food is consumed, and (c) the portion size when the food is eaten. Thus, were we to look solely at population averages, food C was of no interest. Now it is of interest if not intriguing: "achievers" universally eat this food while only 30% of "non-achievers" partake of it, and, among the small group of "non-achievers" who do eat the food, they eat it at a much higher level (which might be the same amount more frequently or a higher amount less frequently).

16.4 Options to change food and nutrient intakes

Once the above analysis is complete and peer reviewed, definite directions in the consumption of nutrients and foods become apparent. In this section we focus on some of the options but the reader should always bear in mind that all options are possible and none is exclusive. Broadly speaking we can think of two contrasting options: "supply-driven" nutrition policy and "demand-driven" nutrition policy.

Supply-driven nutrition policy takes the food supply and in some way modifies it so that individuals consuming a habitual diet will have their nutrient intake altered without having to make any major changes in food choice. Mandatory fortification of foods with micronutrients is by far the best example of supply-driven food nutrition policy. There are certain essential prerequisites to the development of a successful supply-driven fortification programme. These are shown in Box 16.2.

Let us now consider these factors for a typical fortification process, the mandatory addition of folic acid to flour in the USA to reduce the incidence of the neural tube birth defect, spina bifida (Box 16.3).

Box 16.2

- a There is unequivocal evidence that the lack of a particular nutrient very strongly predisposes to some serious condition.
- b The evidence is based on properly conducted human nutrition intervention trials.
- c The effect of the nutrient in question on the problem to be solved is not dependent on other conditions being met.
- d There are no adverse effects from the fortification strategy.
- e The scale of the problem is a true public health issue.

Box 16.3

- a+b There is certainly unambiguous evidence from randomized controlled trials involving high-risk women who had a previous spina bifida baby that folic acid significantly reduces the risk of a second event.
- c The effect is independent of any other factor from age, smoking, weight, and ethnicity, and so on.
- d There is some concern that fortifying with folic acid might cause some B_{12} deficiency to go undiagnosed but the scale of that problem is not enough to halt the fortification programme.
- e This problem is a truly important public health issue.

Let us contrast the data in Box 16.3 with the evidence linking saturated fatty acids (SFAs) to plasma cholesterol shown in Box 16.4.

From the data in Boxes 16.3 and 16.4 it is easy to defend the folic acid option but less easy to defend the SFA option for supply-driven policy. It should be borne in mind that a supply-driven policy effectively takes away from the individual the right to choose in this regard and thus there are always social and sometimes ethical dimensions to this approach.

Demand-driven nutrition policy is based on educating the consumer to demand newer and healthier types of foods from the food supply. This is a chicken-and-egg situation. Consumers may want something that is not within the scope

Box 16.4

a+b There is certainly strong evidence that elevated levels of SFAs can raise plasma LDL cholesterol. However, within the category SFAs, some individual fatty acids are more potent than others and these are not uniquely found in one single dietary source of fat.

c The effect of SFAs is to some extent also dependent on the simultaneous intakes of trans unsaturated fatty acids and different forms of unsaturated fatty acids.

d+e There are no adverse effects known and the problem is not truly important.

of industry to produce either for economic or technical reasons. Equally many companies have developed food products with very obvious health benefits which were market failures because the consumer saw no benefit. The success of this area is thus very market driven. Industry made spreadable fats low in SFAs, which consumers liked. They developed immune-boosting probiotics, cholesterol-lowering phytosterols, high-fibre ready-to-eat cereals and cereal bars, juices with various antioxidants, low-fat milks, n-3 PUFA-enriched eggs, and so on. For demand-driven food supply to work, we need to invoke a major new area of public health nutrition – communication.

16.5 Nutrition communication

One of the great attractions of nutritional science is the breadth of topics to be covered, from molecular biology, through to public health to communication. The greatest mistake of a nutrition nutrition regulatory policy initiative is for scientists to think they understand consumer beliefs. The only way that this can be understood is to study what consumers feel and believe before we can expect them (a) to listen to our communication, (b) believe it, (c) understand it, or (d) care about it. The present section assumes that this a given. In terms of nutrition communication, there are three very important areas to consider: nutrition labelling, nutrition claims, and nutrition profiling.

Nutrition labelling

In most countries, packaged foods bear a label listing particular nutrients in particular ways. The number of nutrients listed can vary either because of prevailing food policy, or manufacturer preference but there are basic requirements which must be adhered to. In 1990, the European Union passed a directive to guide "clearly visible" nutritional labelling. The directive was superseded in 2014 by regulation (EU) No 1169/2011 making labelling mandatory on packaged foods, effective December 2016. This legislation standardised labelling by combining two previous directives on labelling and advertising including, improved legibility, clearer presentation of allergens, and mandatory nutrition information for the majority of prepacked processed foods.

This EU regulation only considers back of pack labelling, and whilst thorough, may not influence consumer choices at point of purchase. Front of pack (FOP) labels were initially designed to support consumers to make better choices at-a-glance. Initially, these varied greatly between manufacturers with studies reporting that this may impede consumer comprehension. The use of FOP nutritional information remains voluntary in the UK, but where present, the information must be standardised and report information per 100g/ml and per portion (Department of Health, 2016).

Outside of the UK, other countries have created FOP labels to quickly and simply inform consumers of the nutritional profile of a product to encourage healthier choices. Figure 16.1 gives an overview of these systems and provides a timeline of global activity in this area.

Out of home dining

Out of home dining is another area which has received consideration for nutritional labelling. In the UK, one fifth of calories consumed by men, and one quarter by women, are consumed outside of the home so can have a significant impact on dietary patterns. This pattern is even higher in the USA leading researchers, industry, and policy makers to consider how to help consumers make informed choices.

New York City was the first to implement calorie menu labelling in chain restaurants in 2010, this became national policy in 2016. Following suit, the UK now has voluntary menu labelling for energy, although if a restaurant chooses to display information, then it must meet the legal requirement that the information is not

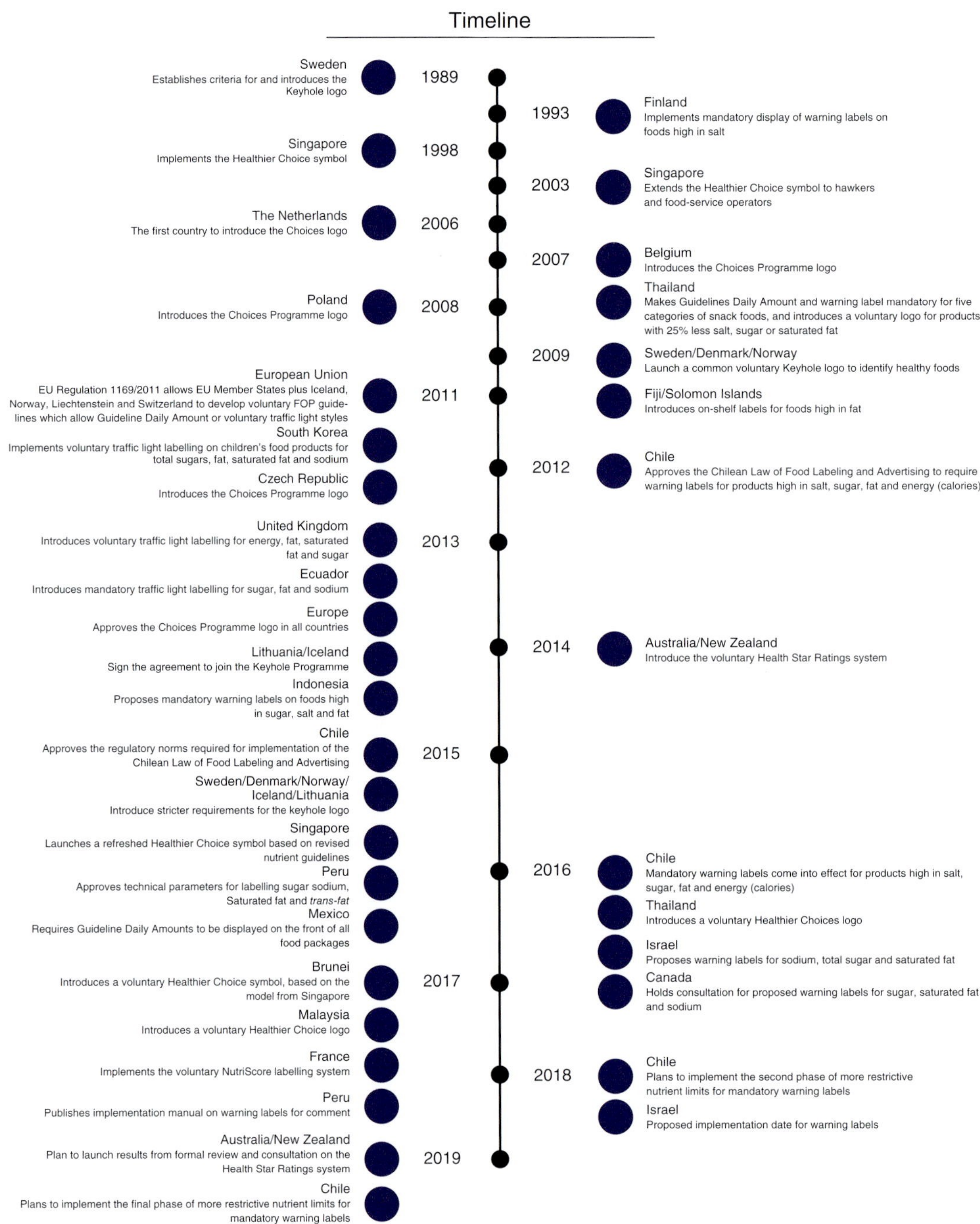

Timeline
Sweden
Establishes criteria for and introduces the Keyhole logo
1989
1993
Finland
Implements mandatory display of warning labels on foods high in salt
Singapore
Implements the Healthier Choice symbol
1998
2003
Singapore
Extends the Healthier Choice symbol to hawkers and food-service operators
The Netherlands
The first country to introduce the Choices logo
2006
2007
Belgium
Introduces the Choices Programme logo
Thailand
Makes Guidelines Daily Amount and warning label mandatory for five categories of snack foods, and introduces a voluntary logo for products with 25% less salt, sugar or saturated fat
Poland
Introduces the Choices Programme logo
2008
2009
Sweden/Denmark/Norway
Launch a common voluntary Keyhole logo to identify healthy foods
Fiji/Solomon Islands
Introduces on-shelf labels for foods high in fat
European Union
EU Regulation 1169/2011 allows EU Member States plus Iceland, Norway, Liechtenstein and Switzerland to develop voluntary FOP guidelines which allow Guideline Daily Amount or voluntary traffic light styles
2011
South Korea
Implements voluntary traffic light labelling on children's food products for total sugars, fat, saturated fat and sodium
Czech Republic
Introduces the Choices Programme logo
2012
Chile
Approves the Chilean Law of Food Labeling and Advertising to require warning labels for products high in salt, sugar, fat and energy (calories)
United Kingdom
Introduces voluntary traffic light labelling for energy, fat, saturated fat and sugar
2013
Ecuador
Introduces mandatory traffic light labelling for sugar, fat and sodium
Europe
Approves the Choices Programme logo in all countries
Lithuania/Iceland
Sign the agreement to join the Keyhole Programme
2014
Australia/New Zealand
Introduce the voluntary Health Star Ratings system
Indonesia
Proposes mandatory warning labels on foods high in sugar, salt and fat
Chile
Approves the regulatory norms required for implementation of the Chilean Law of Food Labeling and Advertising
2015
Sweden/Denmark/Norway/Iceland/Lithuania
Introduce stricter requirements for the keyhole logo
Singapore
Launches a refreshed Healthier Choice symbol based on revised nutrient guidelines
Peru
Approves technical parameters for labelling sugar sodium, Saturated fat and *trans-fat*
2016
Chile
Mandatory warning labels come into effect for products high in salt, sugar, fat and energy (calories)
Mexico
Requires Guideline Daily Amounts to be displayed on the front of all food packages
Thailand
Introduces a voluntary Healthier Choices logo
Israel
Proposes warning labels for sodium, total sugar and saturated fat
Brunei
Introduces a voluntary Healthier Choice symbol, based on the model from Singapore
2017
Canada
Holds consultation for proposed warning labels for sugar, saturated fat and sodium
Malaysia
Introduces a voluntary Healthier Choice logo
France
Implements the voluntary NutriScore labelling system
2018
Chile
Plans to implement the second phase of more restrictive nutrient limits for mandatory warning labels
Peru
Publishes implementation manual on warning labels for comment
Israel
Proposed implementation date for warning labels
Australia/New Zealand
Plan to launch results from formal review and consultation on the Health Star Ratings system
2019
Chile
Plans to implement the final phase of more restrictive nutrient limits for mandatory warning labels

Figure 16.1 Timeline of front-of-package (FOP) nutrition labelling globally. Source: Kanter, R., Vanderlee, L., & Vandevijvere, S. (2018). Front-of-package nutrition labelling policy: Global progress and future directions. Public Health Nutrition, 21(8), 1399–1408.

misleading. Through the Childhood Obesity Plan, consideration is being given to introduce legislation to mandate consistent calorie labelling in restaurants, cafes and takeaways in England. Consultation was carried out 2018. Updates can be found at: https://www.gov.uk/government/consultations/. To date there is no EU directive on out of home calorie labelling. Countries throughout Europe and beyond continue to evaluate the evidence.

Box 16.5 Conditions which must be fulfilled to make a nutrition claim

In order to make a claim, the following conditions must be fulfilled:

- The substances for which a claim is made, must be shown to have beneficial nutritional or physiological effects established by **generally accepted scientific principles**
- The beneficial nutrient or substance for which the claim is made, is present in the final product in a **significant quantity**
  - the nutrient or substance for which the claim is made is in a form that is **'available for use by the body'** (bioavailable)
  - the claimed beneficial effect has to be provided by a **'reasonable quantity of the consumed product'**. This means that an adequate amount of the active nutrient or substance has to be present in a reasonable amount of the food product
  - if the claimed beneficial effect is due to the absence or reduction of a nutrient or substance, then the nutrient or substance should be absent or reduced to the extent that produces the nutritional or physiological effect claimed
- The average consumer should understand the beneficial effects expressed in the claim
- The claim refers to the food ready for consumption according to the manufacturer's instructions
- The claim complies with the specific conditions for nutrition claims and health claims

Source: Information on Nutrition and Health Claims, Food Standards Agency Ireland.

Nutrition and Health Claims

Health claims, that is a claim which relates to the nutritional benefit of food, is highly regulated. In the USA, health claims must meet the Significant Scientific Agreement (SSA) standard. Legislation on permitted claims in the EU differs from that of the USA. According to EU Regulation (EC) no. 1924/2006, a claim consists of any message or representation, not mandatory under community or national legislation, including pictorial, graphic, or symbolic representation, in any form, which states, suggests or implies that a food has a particular characteristic (Box 16.5). A nutrition claim means any claim which states, suggests or implies that a food has particular beneficial nutritional properties. Examples include: low fat, with no added sugars, source of fibre, high in (name of vitamin/s) and/or (name of minerals). A health claim is any statement which suggests or implies that a relationship exists between a food category, a food, or one of its constituents and health. General health claims relate to the effect of a substance on a body function. Examples include: Vitamin D is needed for normal growth and development of bone in children; Calcium is needed for the maintenance of normal teeth. A reduction of disease risk claim suggests or implies that the consumption of a food category, a food, or one of its constituents, significantly reduces a risk factor in the development of human disease. Example: plant sterols have been shown to reduce blood cholesterol. High cholesterol is a risk factor in the development of coronary heart disease. Scientific rigour must increase as one goes up from nutrition claims to health claims and needs to be accompanied by significant supporting evidence from human dietary intervention studies. The EC holds a register of all nutrition and health claims. In 2018, of the 2327 claims listed, just 261 were authorised, quantifying the complexity of nutrition claims and the robust evidence required before companies can make them. Different parts of the globe are taking various approaches to these issues. A paper by Hieke *et al.* (2016) gives a comprehensive overview of nutrition claims and health symbols since the introduction of Regulation (EC) No 1924/2006.

As with many aspects of labelling communication, if companies are to innovate and develop new foods with enhanced nutritional properties or functions, they need to invest in research and development. If their research shows clear evidence of an effect in reducing a risk factor in development of a disease, they need to be able to make that claim and to prevent others who have not done this research from simply adopting that claim. This approach is perfectly understandable but it does cause problems for smaller companies and for industrial sectors in less developed countries for which such high stakes are unthinkable. The terms and conditions for the use of such claims has led to a third area in nutrition communication – nutrition profiling.

Nutrition profiling

As discussed above, certain nutritional standards are required before nutrition and health claims can be made. One way to determine these standards is through nutrient profiling, "the science of classifying or ranking foods according to their nutritional composition for reasons related to preventing disease and promoting health" (WHO, 2010). Whilst nutrient profiling will not cover all aspects of nutrition, diet and health it is a helpful tool to use alongside interventions aimed at improving diets in a region or country. This is commonly known as the Jelly Bean Rule – that is, if you added zinc to jelly beans, would one support the promotion of jelly bean consumption on the grounds that increased zinc intake may assist in minimizing poor immune function. The idea is that if the food supply needs zinc to be added, then a more suitable vehicle needs to be found. In principle this is not complex. In the real world it is an intellectual minefield.

Depending on the aim, there are different approaches in operation. One, seeks to take a single set of criteria and apply that universally to all foods. This has been the approach of what is called the UK Traffic Light System. Nutrients are classified into three types, which can be described as good (green), bad (red), or neither (orange). Inevitably, the application of such a simple system to something as complex as food leads to exceptions. Walnuts might get a red color because of their high fat content, and yet walnuts have been shown, along with other nuts, to be protective against heart disease. Maybe walnuts are now exceptionally excluded from a red sign, but the objectivity of the simple approach becomes gradually replaced with the subjectivity of exceptions.

Another approach is to take each food category separately and devise nutritional standards for each category then assign a labelling scheme to help consumers identify healthier option. An example of this is the Swedish Keyhole Method. For breads, certain standards are set and breads that meet these standards carry the keyhole symbol, which consumers recognise as a mark of nutritional quality. The advantage of this system is that the standards are not universal meaning consumers are comparing soups against soups, not against mayonnaise. Globally, different countries use different systems with no one system classified as perfect.

Advertising

Nutrient profiling goes beyond labelling and health claims and can be used to inform marketing and advertising policy. Using the UK Department of Health nutrient profiling system to define foods which are high in fat, salt, and sugar (HFSS), restrictions on food and drink advertising have been made to those under 16 years old in the UK. In 2007, restrictions were limited to television advertising. By 2017, the restrictions were extended to include print, cinema, online, and on social media (ASA, 2017), reflecting changes in how children interact with media.

On a global scale, in 2007 The World Health Assembly endorsed Resolution WHA 60.23 on the "Prevention and Control of Noncommunicable Diseases: Implementation of the Global Strategy". This resolution called for "the development of a set of recommendations on marketing of foods and non-alcoholic beverages to children" to reduce the impact of HFSS foods. Supporting the recommendations, the World Health Organization (WHO) published a framework to support development. To date, implementation of the WHO tools for the development of policy at a national and regional level has varied (Garde & Xuereb, 2017). A comprehensive overview of global policy implementation on restrictions to broadcast media, non-broadcast media and any media can be found on the WHO website.

16.6 Food environment

Public Health Nutrition 2nd edition provides a comprehensive chapter on "Obesogenic neighbourhood food environments" including the role of town planning and GIS technology. This section will give a brief overview of how the evidence translates to public health policy.

The relationship with dietary choices and the food environment is complicated, as identified by the Foresight Report (2007). Global policy makers continue to review policies to alter the food environment to enable individuals to make healthier choices with different countries implementing a variety of strategies (Table 16.3). Due to increased prevalence of out of home dining occasions, many countries have attempted to tackle this, as part of a suite of policies, to reduce obesity. A recent review concluded that "the food environment is an important factor to consider when contemplating the reasons for out-of-home food consumption and is a potential target for change" (Janesen *et al.*, 2018).

Table 16.3 National and international policy to improve the food environment

Locations	Actions
Australia	• Ban of fast food advertisements between 06·00 and 21·00 hour • Ban on takeaway outlets opening within 400 metres of schools or leisure centres • Taxes on high-fat fast foods and sugar-sweetened beverages
Europe	EU Action Plan on Childhood Obesity 2014–2020 • Promoting healthier environments, especially in schools and pre-schools • Make the healthy option the easy option • Restrict marketing to children • Inform and empower families
France	• Restrictions on vending machines in schools • Marketing restrictions only on HFSS foods/drinks • Mandatory food and nutrition education as part of curriculum
Scotland	Aim to tackle fast food outlets through: • Better quality food in schools • Activities to stop children seeking takeaways during lunch hours • Better education on healthy diet • Work with retailers to improve the offering
UK	Childhood obesity: a plan for action • Soft Drinks Industry Levy (April 2018), • Voluntary 20% sugar reduction target by 2020 (5% in first year), • Voluntary 20% calorie reduction by 2024 in everyday foods consumed by children, • Reduce the marketing and promotion of HFSS products

Fiscal policy

Fiscal policies, in the form of food taxation, to encourage healthier diets continue to be discussed. Some countries have chosen to implemented fat taxes (i.e., Denmark, although this was later repelled), but the more popular form of taxation is on sugar sweetened beverages (SSB). Whilst the format for these taxes vary, there remains a common goal, to decrease intake of free sugars. Figure 16.2 provides a timeline of implementation since January 2017 and the scope of taxation.

Mexico was the first country to implement a nationwide SSB tax in 2014 in response to increasing obesity and diabetes levels. Reports looking at efficacy show a decrease of 7.3% per capita in sugar sweetened beverage sales, and 5.2% increase in plain water sales since the tax was implemented (Colchero *et al.*, 2016). In the UK, the Soft Drinks Industry Levy was applied in April 2018 as in incentive to the food industry to reduce the amount of sugars in soft drinks. At the time of writing, it is too soon to measure efficacy although early indications suggest approximately half of all drinks that would otherwise have been within scope of the levy have reduced sugar content up to 50% (Child Obesity Plan part 2, 2018).

Energy drinks

In addition to concern about sugar sweetened beverages, energy drinks are also of concern due to high caffeine content. Globally, countries have taken a variety of measures to minimise the harmful effects of energy drink consumption. These include restrictions on marketing, clear labelling, taxation, and limiting the retail outlets where productions may be sold, i.e., pharmacies (Breda *et al.*, 2014). In the UK, industry led sales restrictions to under 16 years came into effect in supermarkets in March 2018. The UK carried out consultation on restriction of sales of energy drinks to under-16s which closed in November 2018. Updates can be found here: https://www.gov.uk/government/consultations/

16.7 Global food and nutrition regulation

Globalisation is one of the driving forces shaping the world economy. Food as a commodity and a product is not insulated or exempt from the effects of this phenomenon. Continuing technological advances in the area of food production and food processing have led to unprecedented levels of productivity. The pace of globalisation of trade in food products has accelerated accordingly. Although not without its critics, globalisation of trade in food products arguably benefits consumers in terms of quality, affordability, and a more reliable supply of increasingly safe food. Increasingly sophisticated and well-managed supply chains also provide a diversity of products, which can contribute to improved nutrition and health. However, globalisation of trade in food products brings with it a host of new and ever-evolving challenges and policy issues that require regulation and coordination at the national, regional, and global level. This multi-layered regulatory environment must function

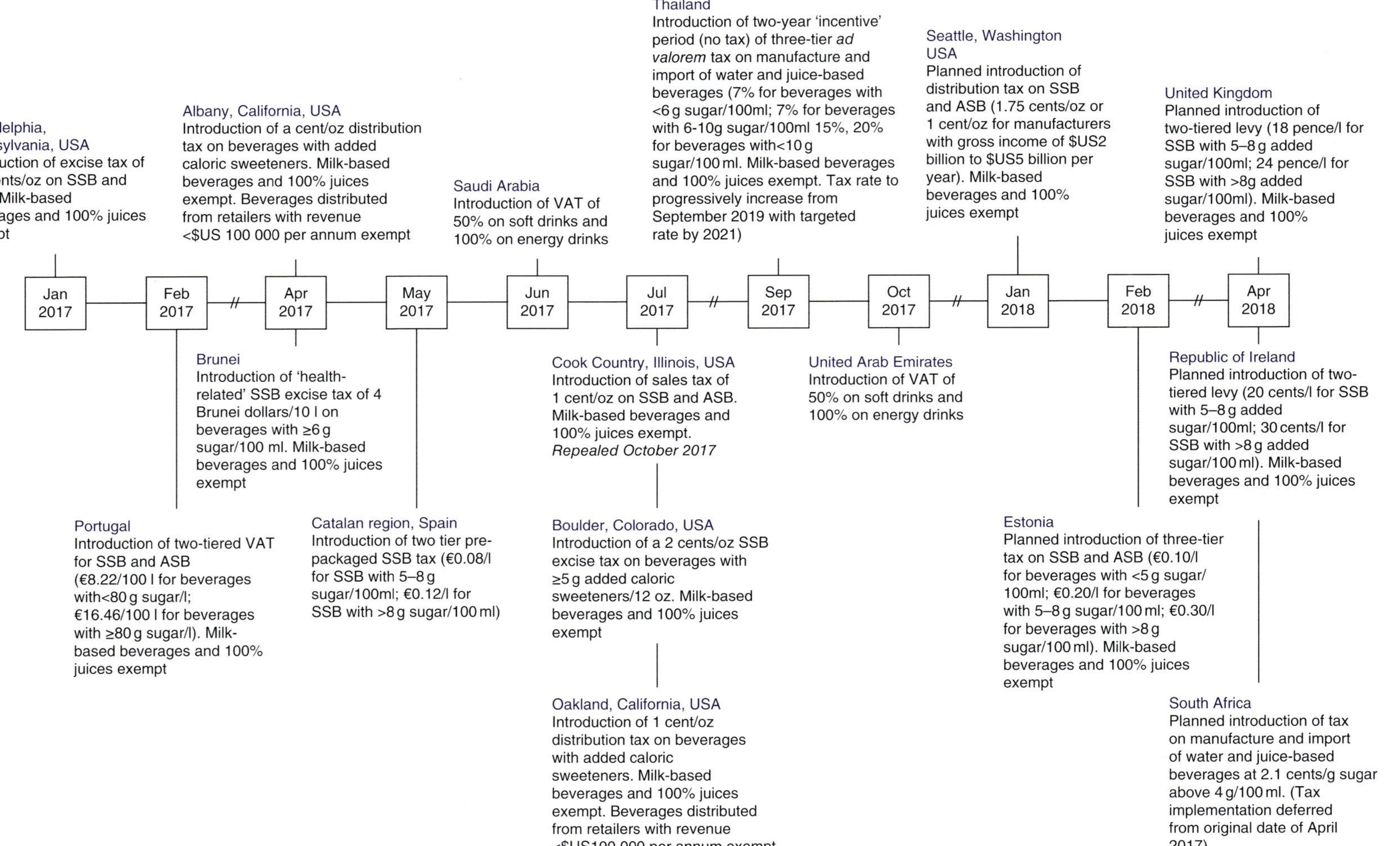
Philadelphia, Pennsylvania, USA
Introduction of excise tax of 1.5 cents/oz on SSB and ASB. Milk-based beverages and 100% juices exempt
Albany, California, USA
Introduction of a cent/oz distribution tax on beverages with added caloric sweeteners. Milk-based beverages and 100% juices exempt. Beverages distributed from retailers with revenue <$US 100 000 per annum exempt
Saudi Arabia
Introduction of VAT of 50% on soft drinks and 100% on energy drinks
Thailand
Introduction of two-year 'incentive' period (no tax) of three-tier *ad valorem* tax on manufacture and import of water and juice-based beverages (7% for beverages with <6 g sugar/100ml; 7% for beverages with 6-10g sugar/100ml 15%, 20% for beverages with<10 g sugar/100 ml. Milk-based beverages and 100% juices exempt. Tax rate to progressively increase from September 2019 with targeted rate by 2021)
Seattle, Washington USA
Planned introduction of distribution tax on SSB and ASB (1.75 cents/oz or 1 cent/oz for manufacturers with gross income of $US2 billion to $US5 billion per year). Milk-based beverages and 100% juices exempt
United Kingdom
Planned introduction of two-tiered levy (18 pence/l for SSB with 5–8 g added sugar/100ml; 24 pence/l for SSB with >8g added sugar/100ml). Milk-based beverages and 100% juices exempt
Jan 2017
Feb 2017
Apr 2017
May 2017
Jun 2017
Jul 2017
Sep 2017
Oct 2017
Jan 2018
Feb 2018
Apr 2018
Brunei
Introduction of 'health-related' SSB excise tax of 4 Brunei dollars/10 l on beverages with ≥6 g sugar/100 ml. Milk-based beverages and 100% juices exempt
Cook Country, Illinois, USA
Introduction of sales tax of 1 cent/oz on SSB and ASB. Milk-based beverages and 100% juices exempt.
Repealed October 2017
United Arab Emirates
Introduction of VAT of 50% on soft drinks and 100% on energy drinks
Republic of Ireland
Planned introduction of two-tiered levy (20 cents/l for SSB with 5–8 g added sugar/100ml; 30 cents/l for SSB with >8 g added sugar/100 ml). Milk-based beverages and 100% juices exempt
Portugal
Introduction of two-tiered VAT for SSB and ASB (€8.22/100 l for beverages with<80 g sugar/l; €16.46/100 l for beverages with ≥80 g sugar/l). Milk-based beverages and 100% juices exempt
Catalan region, Spain
Introduction of two tier pre-packaged SSB tax (€0.08/l for SSB with 5–8 g sugar/100ml; €0.12/l for SSB with >8 g sugar/100 ml)
Boulder, Colorado, USA
Introduction of a 2 cents/oz SSB excise tax on beverages with ≥5 g added caloric sweeteners/12 oz. Milk-based beverages and 100% juices exempt
Estonia
Planned introduction of three-tier tax on SSB and ASB (€0.10/l for beverages with <5 g sugar/100ml; €0.20/l for beverages with 5–8 g sugar/100 ml; €0.30/l for beverages with >8 g sugar/100 ml). Milk-based beverages and 100% juices exempt
Oakland, California, USA
Introduction of 1 cent/oz distribution tax on beverages with added caloric sweeteners. Milk-based beverages and 100% juices exempt. Beverages distributed from retailers with revenue <$US100 000 per annum exempt
South Africa
Planned introduction of tax on manufacture and import of water and juice-based beverages at 2.1 cents/g sugar above 4 g/100 ml. (Tax implementation deferred from original date of April 2017)

Figure 16.2 Timeline of notable international progress of sugar-sweetened beverage (SSB) taxation, 2017–18. (VAT, Value Added Tax; ASB, artificially sweetened beverage). Source: Backholer, K., Blake, M., & Vandevijvere, S. (2016). Have we reached a tipping point for sugar-sweetened beverage taxes? Public Health Nutrition, 19(17), 3057–3061

effectively in order to not only facilitate trade in food as a commodity, but to also retain the confidence of the consumer in the safety and integrity of increasingly globalised food supply chains.

Food and nutrition regulation spans the entire food chain, as demonstrated, for example, by the "Farm to Fork" principle set out in European Union food safety legislation.

In terms of primary production, regulation operates to control the various processes making up the farming and harvesting of plants as well as the raising and slaughter of animals. These primary products can then be subjected to any number of different forms of processing, where another range of regulations apply. For example, what is permitted to be added to the food, what must be in a food (nutrition), what must not be in a food (pesticides) and the physical and biological environment in which the food is processed. Once processed into a product to be offered to consumers, further regulations apply to packaging, labelling, nutrition and health claims, sales, and advertising. The distance that food and feed are now transported also potentially creates conditions more conducive to contamination of the supply chain, so methods of storage and transport are also subject to regulation. Modern food and nutrition regulation must address these activities on a global scale, where issues such as food sources from new areas with differing climates, growing and harvesting techniques, and public health infrastructure are constantly changing. In addition, there are very many national approaches to food regulation reflecting different perceptions about the value of new technology, different degrees of protection given by governments to food producers, and even different interpretations of the science involved in the regulatory process. The implication of globalisation for food regulation therefore requires both international cooperation among national food regulators and the effective balancing of gains from trade between states with regulatory differences.

United Nations agencies

In 1945 in the aftermath of World War II, the United Nations (UN) was established with the aim of preventing another such conflict. A body making up part of the UN, the Food and Agriculture Organization (FAO), was also established at this time and was originally created in order to address the food shortages that beset post-War Europe. Promoting global food security, defined as existing "when all people at all times have access to sufficient, safe, nutritious food to maintain a healthy and active life" remains the key focus of the work of the FAO. However, its activities expanded over the course of time to include sustainable management and utilization of natural resources.

The FAO is driven by five stated strategic objectives:

- Help eliminate hunger, food insecurity and malnutrition;
- Make agriculture, forestry, and fisheries more sustainable;
- Reduce rural poverty;
- Enable inclusive and efficient agricultural and food systems; and,
- Increase the resilience of livelihoods to threats and crises.

These objectives are realised through the implementation of action plans, the devising of agreements, codes and standards in coordination with UN member states; the collection, analysis and sharing of data on agriculture; and the facilitation of policy dialogue at global, regional and State levels. The FAO regularly publishes the results of its findings on a range of issues relating to its various activities.

A sister organisation to the FAO, the World Health Organization (WHO) is the agency tasked with coordinating and directing health policy within the UN. Established in 1948, its objective is the attainment by all peoples of the highest possible levels of health, with one of its most notable successes being the eradication of smallpox, which was declared eradicated globally in 1980 on foot of a worldwide immunization campaign led by the WHO.

In terms of public health as it relates to food, the WHO is involved in the formulation of guidance on good dietary practice, with many WHO reports having an influence on the formulation of national policies and guidelines. While the WHO has traditionally focused on nutritional deficiency and associated morbidity and mortality, the issue of malnutrition characterised by obesity and the long-term implications of unbalanced dietary and lifestyle practices that result in chronic diseases such as cardiovascular disease, cancer, and diabetes has assumed increasing importance in recent years. Using prevention of obesity as an example, the WHO has issued a series of guidelines, including those on free sugars intake for adults and children, which was published in 2015.

Since 2007, all WHO members (numbering 194 as of 2016) have been bound by the revised International Health Regulations (IHR), a suite of rules designed to assist the international community to prevent and respond to public health risks, such as food-borne illnesses, that have the potential to spread across large parts of the globe. While the IHR apply to public health emergencies generally (notable recent examples would include H1N1 influenza pandemic in 2009, the Ebola Virus outbreak in West Africa in 2014–15, and the emergence of Zika virus in Latin America and the Caribbean in 2015–2016), there are specific references to food-related issues contained in their terms. The IHR also designate the FAO as the competent inter-governmental organisation with which the WHO must co-operate and coordinate its activities.

As sister organisations, the WHO and FAO also share responsibility for the operation of the Codex Alimentarius Commission (described in further detail below). They also jointly operate the International Food Safety Authorities Network (INFOSAN), which is designed to facilitate communication and coordination between food safety authorities in UN Member States in order to improve responses to food safety emergencies. For example, in 2011, INFOSAN was engaged after the Great East Japan earthquake and tsunami, and provided an assessment of the potential risks of contamination of the food supply by the nuclear fallout from the damaged Fukushima Daiichi power plant. This network, which originated out of the Codex Alimentarius Principles and Guidelines for the Exchange of Information in Food Control Emergency Situations, and which has been in existence since 2004, has over 180 Member States, each having a designated contact point with the INFOSAN secretariat, depending on the nature of the emergency. INFOSAN can be alerted to a potential emergency through a reference from one of these national contact points, its own monitoring programmes (in conjunction with the WHO Alert and Response Operations Programme) or by working with the Global Outbreak Alert and Response Network as well as the Global Early Warning System for Major Animal Diseases (including zoonotic diseases).

The General Agreement on Tariffs and Trade (GATT)

GATT was signed by 23 nations in Geneva on 30 October 1947, and took effect on 1 January 1948. According to its preamble, its purpose was the "substantial reduction of tariffs and other trade barriers and the elimination of preferences, on a reciprocal and mutually advantageous basis." Participating countries subsequently agreed to lengthy "rounds" of negotiations to develop rules for "non-tariff barriers" to trade. The current Doha Round has been ongoing since 2001 with 159 countries taking part.

GATT, along with the World Trade Organization agreements (described below), contain the general principles of international trade law that oblige Members to act on the basis of:

- "Most favoured nation": where members should, where possible, treat their trade relations and conditions with all other Members in the same way that they treat the most favourable of these, and,
- "National treatment"; where Members should provide the same advantage for traders from other States as they provide to their own.

In both cases there is a general exemption in the case of trading blocs such as the EU. This has the effect that the treatment and advantages that EU member states afford to one another do not have to extend to all WTO members.

World Trade Organization (WTO) agreements

The completion of the Uruguay Round took place from 1986 to 1994 and led to the formation of the WTO on 1 January 1995, with the 75 existing GATT members and the European Communities as founding members. The other 52 GATT members rejoined the WTO in the following two years (the last being Congo in 1997). Since the founding of the WTO, 21 new non-GATT members have joined and 29 are currently negotiating membership. There are a total of 164 member countries in the WTO, with Liberia and Afghanistan being the newest members as of 2016.

The Uruguay Round WTO Agreements (which began at Punta del Este, Uruguay) for the first time incorporated agriculture and food under its rules. There are a number of WTO agreements that are relevant to food regulation:

Agriculture

The WTO Agreement on Agriculture is designed to facilitate market access for agricultural products amongst Member States by calling for Members to limit the use of direct and direct export subsidies for certain agricultural products and to reduce tariffs on international trade in food in order to reduce protectionism and increase competition.

Up until the conclusion of the Uruguay Round, Contracting Parties to GATT had difficulty reaching agreement on the use of tariffs, quotas and subsidies in the food sector. As a means of achieving compromise, the WTO Agreement on Agriculture contains a "Peace Clause" at Article 13, which provides that States should refrain from raising disputes on subsidies and similar issues for a period of nine years, as well as exercising "due restraint" on actions relating to such support measures indefinitely.

It has been noted that one of the key criticisms of the WTO Agreement on Agriculture is that it is incomprehensible in places, and is consequently difficult to implement properly.

Technical Barriers to Trade (TBT)

The WTO Agreement on Technical Barriers to Trade covers all products, including agricultural products. The TBT agreement seeks to ensure that technical regulations and product standards including packaging, marking and labelling requirements, and analytical procedures for assessing conformity with technical regulations and standards do not create unnecessary obstacles to trade. The importance of standards developed by the Codex Alimentarius Commission (CAC) is also recognised as part of the Technical Regulations and Standards provisions contained in Article 2 of the TBT Agreement. So, although Codex Alimentarius standards are not enshrined in international law, WTO endorsement of these standards through agreements such as TBT (and SPS) has effectively made them mandatory, and Codex standards are the benchmarks standards against which national measures and regulations are evaluated.

Most significantly for the liberalization for international trade in food, the TBT makes it clear that internationally set standards should be deemed to be the norm where they already exist or where their completion is imminent. This means that if a national standard is equivalent to a set international standard, then it benefits from a presumption of compliance with TBT requirements. The Codex standards, that exist in the form of a suite of codes and guidelines, are recognised as the relevant international standards for this purpose.

Sanitary and Phytosanitary Measures (SPS)

The SPS Agreement allows governments to take scientifically justified sanitary and phytosanitary measures to protect human health. The agreement commits members to base these measures on internationally established guidelines and risk assessment procedures. The SPS Agreement has chosen the standards guidelines and recommendations set out by the Codex Alimentarius Commission (see below) for food additives, veterinary drug and pesticide residues, contaminants, methods of analysis and sampling, and codes and guidelines of hygienic practice. Because of the general rule that existing international standards on safety or risk minimisation should be deemed the norm, compliance with the standards of other international bodies such as the World Organisation for Animal Health (formerly the International Office for Epizootics) or the FAO-run International Plant Protection Convention, is usually deemed to be compliant with SPS requirements also.

A national standard that provides a greater level of protection than Codex Alimentarius rules, for example, is considered to be a trade barrier unless the WTO decides that the stricter national standard is based on a risk assessment that demonstrates that the Codex standard, guideline, or recommendation provides insufficient protection or that the country maintaining the stricter standard has another scientific justification.

SPS has become an increasingly important agreement for EU Member States given the increased use of a precautionary approach to food safety regulation since 2000, and the fact that SPS measures, unless scientifically justified, are deemed as an impediment to international trade. This becomes particularly important because EU measures are subject to the Dispute Settlement Body of the WTO, where another Member raises a complaint. Well known examples of this include the *Hormones Dispute*, where the United States and Canada claimed that the EU had failed to comply with its obligations by introducing of a directive banning the use of hormones in meat production, and the *GMO Dispute*, which dealt with a complaint by the US, Australia, Argentina, Brazil, Canada, India, Mexico, and New Zealand against the EU arising from a *de facto* moratorium on genetically modified products.

Trade-Related Aspects of Intellectual Property (TRIPs)

Articles 22 to 24 of TRIPs are of particular relevance in the area of food regulation, applying as they do to "Geographical Indications", defined in TRIPs as being those indicators which "identify a good as originating in the territory of a Member … where a given quality, reputation or other characteristic of the good is essentially attributable to its geographical origin." Article 23 of TRIPs provides additional protections for such indications used for wines and spirits.

An EU system for the registration of protected geographical indications and protected designations of origin in 1992 also became the subject of complaints brought under Articles 22 and 24 of TRIPs by the USA and Australia, the *Geographical Indications Dispute*. The Dispute Settlement Body Panel found that although the EU's system was designed to fulfill a legitimate objective, it had failed to provide for national treatment in that it had provided a privileged status for applicants within its own member states, owing to the problems faced by applicants from third countries gaining recognition under the EU system. As an example of the effect that the WTO agreements can have on national and EU food law, the EU amended the system by adopting two new regulations in 2006 which recognised the significance of TRIPs for the content and application of EU food laws.

Codex Alimentarius

In the 1950s food regulators, traders, consumers, and experts were looking increasingly to the FAO and WHO for leadership about the plethora of food regulations that were impeding trade and that for the most part were not providing adequate protection for consumers.

In 1961, the 11th FAO Conference, on foot of a resolution of the Council of Codex Alimentarius Europaeus proposing that its work on food standards be taken over by FAO and WHO, established the Codex Alimentarius Commission (CAC) and requested endorsement by the WHO of a joint FAO/WHO Food Standards Programme. In 1962, the joint FAO/WHO Food Standards Conference requested the CAC to implement a joint FAO/WHO food standards programme and create the Codex Alimentarius. The inaugural meeting of the CAC took place in Rome in 1963, where the Sixteenth World Health Assembly (the governing body of the WHO, composed of representatives from each member state) approved the establishment of the Joint FAO/WHO Food Standards Programme and adopted the statutes of the Codex Alimentarius Commission (CAC).

The CAC is the pre-eminent global food standards organisation and has had an important impact on food producers, processors, and consumers. The principal aims of Codex are to protect consumers' health; ensure fair practices in the food trade through the development of science-based food quality and safety standards, guidelines, and recommendations; and to promote coordination of all food standards work undertaken by governmental and international organisations. These aims are pursued on the basis that harmonisation of food standards facilitates trade between countries, with said international trade benefitting from a form of guarantee that food that is traded will be safe and of the same quality as the same product made elsewhere. Membership of the CAC is open to all member nations and associate members of the FAO and/or WHO. The CAC currently has 188 Member Countries and one Member Organisation (the European Union). In recent years there has been a significant increase in the membership. Developing countries now constitute a significant proportion of total membership. However, many countries are still faced with resource constraints to effective participation in CAC activities. FAO and WHO technical assistance programmes support the efforts of developing countries to strengthen their national food safety systems to protect local consumers and to take advantage of international food trade opportunities. In addition, the FAO/WHO Codex Trust Fund supports the participation of countries in Codex technical committee meetings, and countries have been funded to attend sessions of the CAC.

CAC meetings are held yearly and alternately at the FAO headquarters in Rome and the WHO headquarters in Geneva. At these meetings draft and final standards, guidelines, and codes of practice are adopted. Each member of the Commission has one vote. Decisions of the Commission are taken by a majority of votes cast. Representation is on a country basis. National delegations are led by senior officials appointed by their governments. Delegations may include representatives of industry, consumers' organisations, and academic institutions. Countries not members of the Commission sometimes attend in an observer capacity. A number of international governmental organisations and international NGOs also attend in an observer capacity. These organisations may put forward their points of view at every stage except in the final decision, which is taken by member governments. The Commission and member governments have established country Codex Contact Points and many member countries have National Codex Committees to coordinate activities nationally.

The main standard setting work of the CAC is carried out in more than 20 Codex Committees and Task Forces. These include committees dealing with "vertical" and "horizontal" standards; task forces dedicated to a particular task of limited duration; and regional coordinating committees. This work is also carried out in combination with, and the support of the work of a number of joint FAO/WHO expert scientific groups:

- the Joint FAO/WHO Expert Committee on Food Additives (JECFA) was established in 1956, whose remit now covers the evaluation of contaminants, naturally occurring toxicants and residues of veterinary drugs in food;
- the Joint FAO/WHO Meeting on Pesticide Residues (JMPR) has met regularly since 1963 and was set up to provide independent scientific advice to the FAO and WHO with recommendations from panels of independent experts on the use of pesticides in agriculture and safe levels of residues in foods;
- The Joint FAO/WHO Meeting on Microbiological Risk Assessment (JEMRA) began in 2000. The aim of JEMRA is to optimise the use of microbiological risk assessment as the scientific basis for risk management decisions that address microbiological hazards in foods.

At first, the CAC concentrated on commodity standards called "vertical standards," standards that apply to specific categories of foods such as cereals; fats and oils; fish and fish products; fresh fruits and vegetables; processed and quick-frozen fruits and vegetables; fruit juices; meat and meat products; milk and milk products; sugars, cocoa products, and chocolate. However, by the 1980s it was generally agreed that the diversification of food products was accelerating so rapidly that the setting of these types of specific standards was in fact hindering trade. Thus, a move toward "horizontal" standards began. "Horizontal standards" are general standards and principles that have application across a wide range of foods, for example, rules relating to food additives and contaminants; food labelling; food hygiene, methods of analysis and sampling; pesticide residues, residues of veterinary drugs in foods; food import and export inspection and certification systems; nutrition and foods for special dietary uses, etc. These standards are then published in one of the Codex's 13 volumes. Codex standards pass through various stages of ratification by members – the eight-step process – the final one being that of acceptance. When members accept a Codex standard they are committed to allowing products conforming to that standard on to their market.

Codex Alimentarius and WTO Dispute Settlement Process

In order to protect their citizens, national governments of importing countries introduce laws and regulations to ensure that food imported from other countries is safe and does not jeopardise the health of consumers or pose a threat to health and safety of their indigenous animal and plant populations. However, in terms of international trade, these measures can also be used as disguised barriers to trade that discriminate against imported products in favour of domestic ones. Codex standards have therefore become critical as they are used as guidelines for the resolution of disputes under the enhanced WTO dispute settlement procedure. Annex 2 of the WTO covers all disputes arising from the GATT and WTO agreements. A dispute is triggered when a WTO member complains that another member has failed to live up to the obligations of the GATT or WTO agreements, i.e., a benefit guaranteed under one or other of these agreements has been "nullified or impaired" by another member(s). The dispute settlement procedure encourages the governments involved to discuss their problems and settle the dispute by themselves. The first stage is therefore consultations between the governments concerned. If the governments cannot resolve their dispute they can ask the WTO director-general to mediate or try to help. If consultations fail, the complaining country can ask for a panel to be appointed. If the panel decides that the disputed trade measure does break a WTO agreement or an obligation, it recommends that the measure be made to conform with WTO rules. The panel may suggest how this could be done. Either side can appeal a panel's ruling. Appeals are limited to points of law and legal interpretation — they cannot re-examine existing evidence or examine new issues. The appeal can uphold, modify, or reverse the panel's legal findings and conclusions. If a member does not comply with WTO recommendations on bringing its practice in line with WTO rules, then trade compensation or sanctions, for example in the form of duty increases or suspension of WTO obligations, may follow.

Europe

Having considered the global agencies and institutions that impact on food and nutrition regulation, the EU will be considered as an example of evolution towards a modern system of food and nutrition regulation.

The EU is currently an association of 28 Member States that have agreed to integrate and coordinate much of their economic policy and some other policy areas. The original European Economic Community (EEC) was formed following the signing of the Treaty of Rome in 1957 and consisted of six Member States, increasing over time to 9, 12, 15, 25, 27 and then 28 Member States in 2013 following the accession of Croatia. At first, Member States concentrated on the free movement of foodstuffs through the common market.

Three institutions, the European Commission, the Council of the European Union, and the European Parliament take decisions in the legislative field. The prompt for political action in any given policy area can come from particular Member States, the Council of Ministers, the European Parliament, lobbying by trade associations, research on risks and hazards, and/or technical developments, etc.

During the first 40 years of what came to become the EU, European food regulation developed in an uncoordinated fashion. This resulted in a fragmented framework of rules and regulations with different national policies relating to food overlapping across a variety of related but separate policy areas such as trade and agriculture to which food production, trade and consumption was linked.

In 1974, a Scientific Committee for Food (SCF) was established by the European Commission "to advise the Commission on any problem relating to the protection of the health and safety of persons arising or likely to arise from the consumption of food, in particular on nutritional, hygienic and toxicological issues." However, various scientific committees established by the European Commission (including the SCF) were continually criticised on a number of grounds by the European Parliament and by industry and consumer NGOs. Following the bovine spongiform encephalopathy (BSE) crisis in the UK, there was a further decrease in confidence in these scientific committees and, with the new powers in public health granted by the Maastricht Treaty, the European Parliament forced the Commission to totally revise their structure. A major reorganisation of the Commission's services ensued.

The responsibility for monitoring the implementation of food safety legislation and for providing scientific advice, hitherto jointly shared by the Commissioners for Agriculture and Industry, was transferred to the Commissioner for Consumer Affairs. The rationale at the time was that it was necessary to separate monitoring, compliance with and enforcement of the law, from the law-making function itself. This latter function remained for a time with the Agriculture and Industry Commissioners, however the legislation function on food safety was later transferred to the Health and Consumer Protection Commissioner (presently Directorate General SANTE Health and Food Safety). The Commission also announced that the way in which scientific advice on food safety was provided at European level would be re-organised and strengthened. A Scientific Steering Committee to oversee the work of the eight regrouped scientific committees was created. In 1997, The Green Paper on the General Principles of Food Law was published in order to launch a debate on the future development of EU food law. Its aim was to provide the Commission with a solid background for a major programme of new or amending legislation that it would later propose in the 2000 White Paper on Food Safety.

In January 2002, Regulation (EC) No. 178/2002, otherwise known as the General Food Law, was adopted. The Regulation set out the general principles of EU food law and established a European Food Safety Authority. It also strengthened the Rapid Alert System for Food and Feed (RASFF) created in 1979 for the notification of direct or indirect risks to human health deriving from feed or food, and set down clear procedures for the handling by the Commission and the Member States of food safety emergencies and crises.

This Regulation, for the first time, set out the following main principles of EU food law, which were intended to cover all food and feed at all stages of production, processing, and distribution:

- A requirement that food law must be based on a system of **risk analysis** founded on risk assessment, risk management, and risk communication;
- A requirement that **the precautionary principle** will be applied in the case of a potential risk to human health where there is scientific uncertainty as to what measures to take;
- A requirement that public authorities at all levels will apply the principle of **transparency** in consulting with and informing the public on actual or potential risks and the actions that are taken or proposed to deal with them.

The Regulation also provided for a system to ensure **"farm to fork" traceability** of all food and feed at all stages of the food and feed chain.

European Food Safety Authority

The primary responsibility of the European Food Safety Authority (EFSA) is to provide independent scientific advice on all matters with a direct or indirect impact on food safety. The Authority has been given a wide brief, so that it can cover all stages of food production and supply, from primary production to the safety of animal feed, right through to the supply of food to consumers. It gathers information from all parts of the globe, keeping an eye on new developments in science. Although the Authority's main "customer" is the Commission, it is open to respond to scientific questions from the European Parliament and the Member States and it can also initiate risk assessments on its own behalf. The Authority carries out assessments of risks to the food chain and indeed can carry out scientific assessment on any matter that may have a direct or indirect effect on the safety of the food supply, including matters relating to animal health, animal welfare, and plant health. The Authority also gives scientific advice on non-food and feed, genetically modified organisms (GMOs), and on nutrition in relation to Community legislation.

Nutrition and Public Health in the EU

It is up to national governments to develop and implement their own healthcare policy and ensure that healthcare is provided to citizens. The EU's role is to complement those national policies by helping Member State governments achieve shared objectives, generating economies of scale by pooling resources helping to tackle shared challenges such as pandemics and the prevention and treatment of chronic diseases.

Provisions of the EU Treaties on health policy have consistently envisaged that measures designed to promote health be complementary to national policies, the most recent manifestation of this being found in Article 168 of the Treaty on the functioning of the European Union (TFEU).

Under Article 4 TFEU, the EU shares competence with Member States in several areas. Shared competence means that both the EU and its member states may adopt legally binding rules and regulations in the area concerned. However, the member states can do so only where the EU has not exercised its competence or has explicitly ceased to do so. Most importantly in terms of taking action to minimise the health effects of poor diet, legislative action addressing this issue would likely be deemed to be contrary to Article 34 TFEU and EU Treaty rules on the free movement of food – any measures adopted would be deemed to be equivalent to a quantitative restriction on trade, with little chance of justification under Article 36 TFEU. Therefore, while EU policy documents support policy decision making at Member State level, EU law prevents national policy from becoming national law where this would inhibit, directly or indirectly, actually or potentially, interstate trade.

EU consumer policy guarantees a high level of consumer safety with respect to food, the EU also shares competence with member States in common safety concerns in public health matters which are limited to aspects defined in TFEU. Under Article 6 of TEFU the EU has competence to support, coordinate, or supplement actions of the member states in the protection and improvement in human health. In these areas the EU may not adopt legally binding acts that require the member states to harmonise their laws and regulations. EU health policy, implemented though the Health Strategy, focuses on: prevention – especially by promoting healthier lifestyles; equal chances of good health and quality healthcare for all; tackling serious health threats involving more than one EU country; keeping people healthy into old age; supporting dynamic health systems; and new technologies. The EU gives EU countries tools to help them cooperate and identify best practice, e.g., health promotion activities, tackling risk factors, disease management and health systems. By funding health projects through the EU health programme, the EU backs preventive action against diseases, e.g., through responsible food labelling – so consumers know what they are eating. The EU also funds measures to promote healthy diet and exercise – encouraging governments, NGOs and industry to work together, making it easier for consumers to change their lifestyles. The European Centre for Disease Prevention and Control in Stockholm assesses emerging threats, so the EU can respond rapidly. It pools knowledge on current and emerging threats and works with national counterparts to develop disease monitoring across Europe.

In 2000, the European Commission adopted a Communication on the Health Strategy of the European Community. This described how the Commission was working to achieve a coherent and effective approach to health issues across all the different policy areas and emphasised that health services must meet the population's needs and concerns, in a context characterised by the challenge of aging and the growth of new medical techniques, as well as the more international dimension of health care (contagious diseases, environmental health, increased mobility of persons, services and goods). A new Health Strategy for the EU 2008–2013 was adopted in 2007.

In 2005, the Commission also launched a new forum, called "Diet, Physical Activity and Health – a European Platform for Action." The platform brought together all relevant players active at European level that were willing to enter into binding and verifiable commitments that could help to halt and reverse current obesity trends. This included retailers, food processors, the catering industry, the advertising business, consumer and health NGOs, the medical professions, and the EU presidency. In 2005, the Commission also published a Green Paper called "Promoting healthy diets and physical activity: a European dimension for the prevention of overweight, obesity and chronic diseases." This was followed in May 2007 by the Commission's White Paper outlining strategies/initiatives in the area of diet, physical activity, and health aimed at promoting good health and quality of life and reducing risks of disease.

The White Paper identified four ways in which obesity could be addressed at EU level:

- Actions should aim to address the root causes of health-related risks, extending to those associated with both poor diet and limited physical activity;
- Actions identified in the White Paper should apply horizontally across government policy

areas and at different levels of government, using a range of instruments such as legislation, networking, and public-private initiatives;
- Action would be required on the part of the private actors, the food industry, civil society, and local actors such as schools and community organisations.
- Close monitoring of the impact of measures adopted would be required to ascertain the actual effect of those measures on diet and physical activity levels.

The White Paper also identified three ways in which existing EU laws could be used to help tackle nutrition related illness and disease:

- Development of nutrition labelling requirements so as to allow consumers to make better decisions about what they eat. The EU Regulation on the Provision of Food Information to Consumers (FIC) made provision for this.
- Exerting proper controls over the use of nutrition and health claims, which became the subject of specific EU regulation in 2006.
- Tailored regulation regarding the advertisement and marketing of food, especially to children, would also be required.

More recently, through its research programme, Horizon 2020, the EU will spend almost €7.5 billion on research to improve European healthcare between 2014 and 2020.The EU works closely with strategic partners, such as the World Health Organization, to improve healthcare worldwide through research, development aid, greater access to medicines, and so on.

UK and Public Health Bodies

Several government departments in the UK play a role in devising, implementing, and enforcing food law and policy. Foremost amongst these is the Department for the Environment, Food and Rural Affairs (DEFRA). Other state agencies, such as the Food Standards Authority (FSA), also play an important role in protecting the public from risks to their health that can arise through the consumption of unsafe food. The FSA also plays an increasing role in the development of national policy.

Food law enforcement activity occurs primarily at local level through the operations of various designated competent authorities. It is the individual units and officers making up these competent authorities that interface directly with food business operators, ensuring compliance with regulatory requirements and taking appropriate action where necessary. Determining which food authority has specific responsibility for the enforcement and oversight of any particular aspect of English food law depends on which legislative act applies in the circumstances. In general, however, the designated food authority is often the local borough, district or county council.

The use of agencies such as the FSA, the Health Protection Agency, the Environmental Agency, and the Intellectual Property Office to oversee the implementation of food law, as opposed to government departments, have also become much more common since the BSE crisis of the 1990s.

DEFRA

Of all UK government departments, DEFRA holds most of the responsibility for the oversight of law and policy on food and related environmental and rural issues. Although DEFRA only has direct responsibility for policy areas such as farming, fishing, animal health and welfare, and environmental protection in England, it also works with the devolved administrations in other parts of the UK. DEFRA has its headquarters in London, but also has offices throughout England. It is also supported and assisted in its work by a plethora other agencies and public bodies such as the Animal Health and Veterinary Laboratories Agency, the Food and Environment Research Agency, the Agriculture and Horticulture Development Board, and the Sea Fishery Industry Authority, to name a few.

It should be noted that other government departments such as the Department of Health and the Department of Energy and Climate Change also have a significant, but perhaps less obvious role in the formulation and application of food policy and law.

The Food Standards Agency (FSA)

The FSA, for example, is responsible for overseeing a wide range of food safety related matters across the UK, the idea being that of an independent body which can direct industry, advise consumers, and connect the producing, scientific, and regulating sectors more effectively.

Although it lacks the power to formulate policy, the FSA does have a significant degree of influence arising from its dealings with both government and the public. In terms of enforcement of food standards, the FSA has the power to order food authorities to take action to ensure compliance with food standards, including the duty to appoint a public analyst. It is also tasked with monitoring the performance of the various local authorities that enforce food law "on the ground". This function includes setting standards in relation to enforcement.

While the FSA has the flexibility to operate independently, it remains a state agency, and the government retains a significant degree of control through its establishing legislation, the Food Standards Act, 1999. For example, the Secretary of State reserves the power issue enforcement functions set out in other pieces of legislation, such as the Food Safety Act, 1990.

The FSA also coordinates closely with food safety agencies in other parts of the UK such as Food Standards Scotland and the Food Standards Agency Northern Ireland.

The Health Protection Agency

The Health Protection Agency has a range of functions directly related to the prevention of ill-health arising out of the production and consumption of food, such as setting of guidelines for certain types of food sampling and testing. It also implements a national programme of studies on foods in association with Local Government Regulation, which elaborate on issues identified by environmental health officers and HPA public health microbiologists as a source of risk from a food safety perspective. This agency also provides support to a number of national (Department of Health) scientific advisory committees, a number of which are contributed to jointly by the FSA.

The Association for Nutrition

The Association for Nutrition (AfN) regulates nutrition in the UK through its governance of the UK Voluntary Register of Nutritionists (UKVRN). The UKVRN distinguishes nutritionists who "meet rigorously applied training, competence and professional practice criteria" and includes nutrition practitioners working a wide range of professions and industries. There are two types of Registrants; Registered Associate Nutritionists (ANutr), usually graduate from a BSc (Hons) or MSc in nutrition science; and Registered Nutritionist (RNutr), qualified professionals with demonstrable experience of evidence-based practice. In addition, the AfN accredit undergraduate and postgraduate degree programmes in the UK and Ireland (and internationally where the criteria are met) and endorse evidence-based training courses.

Public Health England

Public Health England (PHE) is an agency of the Department of Health and Social Care. PHE is responsible for promoting better public health by promoting healthier lifestyles, advising government, the NHS and the public.

16.8 Looking to the future

The food we eat is an area of everyday life that is very heavily regulated from the food safety point of view, including chemical and microbial hazards, but increasingly from the nutritional point of view. The bedrock of sensible nutrition regulation planning is the availability of good data and the intelligent use of that data to both inform and challenge policymakers. At the same time, globalisation of the food supply has been accompanied by evolving governance issues that have produced a regulatory environment at the national and global level led by large national, and international agencies that must regulate effectively by facilitating trade while also preserving the confidence of consumers in the food supply chain.

Although new technologies, lengthening supply chains, growing populations, climate change, and international development are all issues that modern food regulatory frameworks must contend with, the UK's decision to leave the European Union in June 2016 is perhaps the most important recent development that will have possibly significant, but as yet unknown consequences in terms of food regulation and public health and nutrition in the UK and the EU. Pursuant to Article 50 of the Lisbon Treaty /

Treaty on European Union ("TEU"), "*Any member state may decide to withdraw from the union in accordance with its own constitutional requirements*.". On 29 March 2017, the United Kingdom notified the European Council of its intention to do so. On 29 April 2017, the European Council – made up of the heads of state or government of the EU countries – adopted guidelines, which defined the framework for the negotiations and set out the EU's overall positions. At the time of writing, a deal on withdrawal and the legal grounds for a future relationship with the EU are being negotiated. The nature of this future relationship remains uncertain at the time of writing. However, regulatory divergence and the possibility of a shift from EU-based food regulatory norms and practices remains possible. This will have an impact on the formulation, implementation, and enforcement of public health and nutrition policies into the future.

Acknowledgement

This chapter has been revised and updated by Aideen McKevitt, James Gallagher, and Cassandra Ellis, based on the original chapter by Michael Gibney and Aideen McKevitt.

References

Advertising Standards Agency (2017) https://www.asa.org.uk/advice-online/food-hfss-overview.html (Accessed August 2018).

Backholer, K., Blake, M., and Vandevijvere, S. (2017). Sugar-sweetened beverage taxation: An update on the year that was 2017. *Public Health Nutrition* **20**(18), 3219–3224.

Breda, J.J., Whiting, S.H., Encarnação, R. *et al.* (2014). Energy Drink Consumption in Europe: A Review of the Risks, Adverse Health Effects, and Policy Options to Respond. *Frontiers in Public Health.* **2**, 134, 1–5.

Colchero, M.A., Guerrero-López, C.M., Molina, M. *et al.* (2016). Beverages Sales in Mexico before and after Implementation of a Sugar Sweetened Beverage Tax. *PLoS ONE.* **11**(9): e0163463).

Crockett, R.A., King, S.E., Marteau, T.M. *et al.* (2018). Nutritional labelling for healthier food or non-alcoholic drink purchasing and consumption. *Cochrane Database of Systematic Reviews.* Issue 2.

Draper, A., Adamson, A.J., Clegg, S. *et al.* (2013). Front-of-pack nutrition labelling: are multiple formats a problem for consumers? *European Journal of Public Health.* **23**, 3, 517–521.

Food information to consumers. (2016). Legislation December 2016. https://ec.europa.eu/food/safety/labelling_nutrition/labelling_legislation_en (Accessed August 2018).

Food Safety Authority Ireland. (2016). Information on Nutrition and Health Claims. https://www.fsai.ie/science_and_health/nutrition_and_health_claims.html (Accessed August 2018)

Garde, A. and Xuereb, G. (2017). WHO Recommendations on the Marketing of Food and Non-Alcoholic Beverages to Children. *European Journal of Risk Regulation.* **8**(2), 211–223.

Guide to creating a front of pack (FoP) nutrition label for pre-packed products sold through retail outlets https://assets.publishing.service.gov.uk/government/uploads/system/uploads/attachment_data/file/566251/FoP_Nutrition_labelling_UK_guidance.pdf (Accessed August 2018).

Hieke, S., Kuljanic, N., Fernandez, L. *et al.* (2016). Country Differences in the History of Use of Health Claims and Symbols. *European Journal of Nutrition & Food Safety.* **6**(3): 148–168.

Janssen, H., Davies, I., Richardson, L. *et al.* (2018). Determinants of takeaway and fast food consumption: A narrative review. *Nutrition Research Reviews.* **31**(1), 16–34.

Kanter, R., Vanderlee, L., and Vandevijvere, S. (2018). Front-of-package nutrition labelling policy: global progress and future directions; *Public Health Nutrition.* **21**(8), 1399–1408.

Obesity Australia: understanding and action. (2013). Action Agenda. https://static1.squarespace.com/static/57e9ebb16a4963ef7adfafdb/t/580ec0ba9de4bb7cf16fff29/1477361853047/Obesity%2BAustralia%2BAction%2BAgenda%2BApril%2B2013.pdf (Accessed August 2018).

Pieroni, L. and Salmasi, L. (2014). Fast-food consumption and body weight. Evidence from the UK. *Food Policy.* **46**, 94–105.

Regulation (ec) no 1924/2006 of the European Parliament and of the Council 2006R1924 — EN — 13.12.2014 — 00 4.001 — 1 of 20 December 2006 on nutrition and health claims made on foods (OJ L 404, 30.12.2006, p. 9) https://eur-lex.europa.eu/legal-content/EN/TXT/PDF/?uri=CELEX:02006R1924-20141213 (accessed August 2018).

Scottish Government. (2014). Beyond the School Gate - Improving Food Choices in the School Community. https://www.gov.scot/Publications/2014/05/4143/4 (accessed August 2014).

WHO Marketing of foods and non-alcoholic beverages to children: recommendations and framework http://www.who.int/dietphysicalactivity/marketing-food-to-children/en/ (accessed August 2018b).

World Health Organization. (2010). Nutrient profiling: report of a technical meeting. http://www.who.int/nutrition/publications/profiling/WHO_IASO_report2010/en/ (accessed August 2018).

Further reading

Websites

BEUC European Consumers Organisation: http://www.beuc.org/Content

CIAA: http://www.ciaa.be/asp/index.asp/

DG-SANCO: www.europa.eu.int/comm/dg24

EUROPA: http://europa.eu

European Commission: http://ec.europa.eu/index_en.htm

European Court of Justice: http://curia.europa.eu/en/index.htm

European Food Safety Authority: http://www.efsa.europa.eu

EUROPA Food and Feed Safety: http://ec.europa.eu/food/index_en.htm
European Food Information Council: http://www.eufic.org
Eur-Lex The portal to European Union Law: http://eur-lex.europa. eu/en/index.htm
European Parliament: http://www.europarl.europa.eu
International Life Sciences Institute: http://www.ilsi.org
Institute of Food Science and Technology (IFST): http://www.ifst. org
Food Standards Agency (FSA): http://www.foodstandards.gov.uk
European Food Information Council: http://www.eufic.org
European Union: http://.europa.eu

UK

Association for Nutrition http://www.associationfornutrition.org
Food Standards Agency: http://www.foodstandards.gov.uk
NHS Health Scotland http://www.healthscotland.scot
Public Health England https://www.food.gov.uk
Scientific Advisory Committee on Nutrition https://www.gov.uk/government/groups/scientific-advisory-committee-on-nutrition
HM Government (2016) Childhood Obesity: A Plan for Action. https://assets.publishing.service.gov.uk/government/uploads/system/uploads/attachment_data/file/546588/Childhood_obesity_2016__2__acc.pdf (accessed August 2018)
HM Government (2018) Childhood Obesity: A Plan for Action: Chapter 2. https://assets.publishing.service.gov.uk/government/uploads/system/uploads/attachment_data/file/718903/childhood-obesity-a-plan-for-action-chapter-2.pdf (accessed August 2018)
PHE (2015) Sugar Reduction: The evidence for action, Public Health England, London, https://assets.publishing.service.gov.uk/government/uploads/system/uploads/attachment_data/file/470179/Sugar_reduction_The_evidence_for_action.pdf (accessed August 2018).
The Food Foundation (2017) UK's restrictions on junk food advertising to children, international learning series / 3 https://foodfoundation.org.uk/wp-content/uploads/2017/07/3-Briefing-UK-Junk-Food_vF.pdf (accessed August 2018)

European food agencies

France – L'Agence Française de Sécurité Sanitaire des Aliments: http://www.afssa.fr
Ireland – Food Safety Authority of Ireland: http://www.fsai.ie
Sweden – National Food Administration: http://www.slv.se

US sites

Arbor Nutrition Guide: http://www.arborcom.com/
Centre for Disease Control and Prevention, Atlanta (CDC): http://www.cdc.gov
Centre for Food Safety and Applied Nutrition: http://www.cfsan. fda.gov/list.html
Centre for Nutrition Policy and Promotion: http://www.usda.gov/cnpp
Environmental Protection Agency (EPA): http://www.epa.gov
Food and Drug Administration (FDA): http://www.fda.gov/default.htm
Food and Nutrition Information Center, USDA: http://www.nal.usda.gov/fnic
Food and Safety Inspection Service (FSIS): http://www.fsis.usda.gov
Iowa State University Extension, including a Food Safety Project: http://www.extension.iastate.edu/foodsafety
Institute of Food Technologists – a non-profit scientific society: http://www.ift.org
United States Department of Health and Human Services: http://www.os.dhhs.gov
United States Department of Agriculture (USDA): http://www.usda.gov

Worldwide

Codex Alimentarius: http://www.codexalimentarius.net
Consumers International: http://www.consumersinternational.org
Dept. of Plant Agriculture, University of Guelph, Ontario, Canada: http://www.plant.uoguelph.ca/safefood
Food and Agriculture Organization of the United Nations (FAO): http://www.fao.org
Food Standards Australia New Zealand: http://www.foodstandards.gov.au
International Food Information Council (IFIC): http://www.ific.org
International Standards Organization (ISO): http://www.iso.ch
World Health Organization (WHO): http://www.who.int
World Trade Organization: http://www.wto.org

Papers

Advertising Standards Authority. Food: Nutrition Claims https://www.asa.org.uk/advice-online/food-nutrition-claims.html
Brent Bernell, The History and Impact of the New York City Menu Labelling Law, 65 Food & Drug L.J. 839 (2010)
EU Nutrition and Health Claims https://ec.europa.eu/food/safety/labelling_nutrition/claims_en (Accessed August 2018)
Food Standards Agency. (2017). Guidance on voluntary energy (kj/kcal) labelling for out of home businesses. https://www.food.gov.uk/sites/default/files/media/document/caloriewisetechnicalguidance_1.pdf (accessed August 2018)
Keyhole – Sweden https://www.livsmedelsverket.se/en/food-and-content/labelling/nyckelhalet
Obesogenic Neighbourhood Food Environments, p 327-338. In: (Ed. J.L. Buttriss, A.A. Welch, J. M. Kearney, Dr. S.A. Lanham-New) *Public Health Nutrition* 2e. ISBN: 978-1-118-66097-3; Jun 2017, Wiley Blackwell.
Swan G, Powell N, Knowles B, *et al.* (2018). A definition of free sugars for the UK. *Public Health Nutrition.* **21**(9), 1636–1638.
The Health Star Rating – Australia http://www.healthstarrating.gov.au/internet/healthstarrating/publishing.nsf/Content/home

17
Food and Nutrition-Related Diseases: The Global Challenge

Thomas R. Hill and Georg Lietz

Key messages

- This chapter provides an update on trends and types of nutrition-related diseases in developed and developing countries.
- In developed countries excessive intakes of macronutrients (overnutrition) and suboptimal intakes of micronutrients (hidden hunger), mainly because of low fruit and vegetable consumption, lead to obesity and related non-communicable diseases (NCDs).
- Developing countries are suffering from a double burden of malnutrition due to the persistence of undernutrition, related deficiency and infectious diseases, and the emergence of NCDs as a result of the nutrition transition. The chapter explains the vicious cycle of poverty and undernutrition and how this is related to underdevelopment and increased risk of NCDs in the developing world.
- Current global challenges for food and nutrition interventions on different levels are highlighted.

17.1 Introduction

Nutrition has profound effects on health throughout the human life course and is inextricably linked with cognitive and social development, especially in early childhood. The relationship between nutrition and health was summarised in Figure 1.2, illustrating that the nutritional quality and quantity of foods eaten, and therefore nutritional status, are major modifiable factors in promoting health and well-being, in preventing disease, and in treating some diseases. It is now accepted that our nutritional status influences our health and risk of both infectious and non-communicable diseases.

Indeed, billions of people in both developed and developing countries suffer from one or more forms of malnutrition, contributing to the global burden of disease. Malnutrition remains an immense and universal problem, with at least one in three people globally experiencing malnutrition in some form, with almost every country in the world facing a serious nutrition-related challenge (Global Nutrition Report 2017). The Global Burden of Disease study in 1990 provided for the first time a comparative assessment of mortality at a global level and identified that maternal and child undernutrition contributed to 11% of the global burden of disease (Murray and Lopez, 1996). The findings of this report created the most successful anti-poverty movement in history, the establishment of the Millenium Goals by the United Nations General Assembly in 2000, which resulted in a reduction of mortality rates from nutritional deficiencies by 33·6% (Global Burden of Disease 2017 cause of death; for more detail see chapter 25 in Public Health Nutrition). However, at the same time,

Introduction to Human Nutrition, Third Edition. Edited on behalf of The Nutrition Society by Susan A. Lanham-New, Thomas R. Hill, Alison M. Gallagher and Hester H. Vorster.

Companion website: www.wiley.com/go/lanham-new/humannutrition

non-communicable diseases (NCDs) comprise the greatest fraction of deaths world-wide, contributing to 73.4% in 2017, with the total numbers of deaths from NCDs increasing from 33.5 million in 2007 to 41.1 million in 2017 (Global Burden of Disease, 2017).

Obesity, one of the main risk factors of NCDs, is increasing in almost every country in the world, due to complex changes in food systems, food quality, nutrition, technology, and levels of physical activity. Indeed, consumption of high energy-dense foods at increasingly affordable prices has led to changes in food consumption patterns, which unfortunately coincided with more sedentary, less active lifestyles. The resultant over-nutrition of especially macronutrients has resulted in a nutrition transition in the developed world, leading to an accelerated emergence of NCDs. However, globalisation characterised by urbanisation, acculturation, global trade, and information exchange has led to a very rapid nutrition transition in developing countries, with the consequence that obesity and NCDs emerged before the problems of undernutrition and specific nutritional deficiencies have been solved. Thus, developing countries now suffer from a double burden of nutrition-related diseases because of the coexistence of under- and over-nutrition.

In high-income countries, the incidence of diet-related NCD risk factors such as obesity is highest among poorer, less-educated groups. More complex inequality patterns for obesity and associated health conditions are seen in low and middle-income countries, since groups of lower socioeconomic status eat less fruit, vegetables, fish and fibre than those of higher socioeconomic status (Global Nutrition Report, 2017). Importantly, unlike undernutrition, economic growth is positively associated with an increase of obesity, since a 10% rise in income per capita translates into a 4.4% increase in obesity. Thus, developing countries need to employ public health measures to counteract this risk as their economies develop.

The purpose of this chapter is to describe the major nutrition-related diseases in the developed and developing world, highlighting obesity and type 2 diabetes, to show the interrelationships between the causes and consequences of under- and over-nutrition, and to identify the global challenges in addressing the heavy burden of malnutrition that contribute to underdevelopment, disability, and premature death.

17.2 Nutrition-related diseases in developed countries

The current situation

Economic development, education, food security, and access to health care and immunisation programs in developed countries have resulted in dramatic decreases in undernutrition-related diseases. Unfortunately, many of these factors have also led to unhealthy behaviours, inappropriate diets, and lack of physical activity, which has exacerbated the development of chronic diseases, also known as noncommunicable diseases (NCDs). In 2017, NCDs accounted for 73% of all global deaths, with over half of all deaths (28.8 million) attributable to just four risk factors: high blood pressure, smoking, high blood glucose, and high body-mass index. Obesity prevalence has risen in almost every country in the world-leading to more than a million deaths from type 2 diabetes, half a million deaths from diabetes-related chronic kidney disease, and 180 000 deaths related to non-alcoholic steatohepatitis. Thus, the increasing prevalence of obesity might explain why death rates for cardiovascular disease are no longer declining in Australia, Austria, Brazil, Germany, Netherlands, the UK, and the USA. Indeed, at a global level, total deaths from cardiovascular diseases increased by 21·1% between 2007 and 2017, with ischaemic heart disease and stroke accounting for 84.9% of cardiovascular disease deaths in 2017 (Global Burden of Disease, 2017).

Definition, terminology and characteristics

The NCDs that are related to diet and nutrient intakes are obesity, hypertension, atherosclerosis, ischemic heart disease, myocardial infarction, cerebrovascular disease, stroke, diabetes mellitus (type 2), osteoporosis, liver cirrhosis, dental caries, and nutrition-induced cancers of the breast, colon, and stomach. They develop over time because of exposure to interrelated societal, behavioural, and biological risk factors. Together with tobacco use, alcohol abuse, and physical inactivity, an unhealthy or inappropriate diet is an important modifiable risk factor for NCDs. Diet, therefore, plays a major role in prevention and treatment of NCDs. NCDs are sometimes called "chronic diseases," but some infectious diseases such as HIV/AIDS and tuberculosis are also chronic. The risk factors for NCDs accumulate throughout the life course – from infancy to adulthood, and manifest after decades of exposure. The increase in childhood obesity is especially of concern because it has long-term implications for NCDs. NCDs account for 18 of the leading 20 causes of age-standardised years lived with disability (YLD) on a global scale (Global Burden of Disease, 2015). Iron deficiency anaemia decreased from being the second leading cause of YLD in 1990 to the fourth leading cause of YLD in 2015, whereas diabetes increased from the ninth to the sixth leading cause of YLD from 1990 to 2015 (Global Burden of Disease, 2015).

Risk factors for NCDs

Table 17.1 lists the risk factors for NCDs. The factors are interrelated and form a chain of events starting with societal factors such as socioeconomic status and environments that influence behavior, leading to the development of biological risk factors that cause the NCDs. The biological risk factors often cluster together. For example, obesity (abnormal body composition) is associated with insulin resistance, hyperlipidaemia, and hypertension, which all contribute to the development of both cardiovascular disease and diabetes. Cardiovascular disease is furthermore one of the complications of untreated diabetes. The mechanisms through which these risk factors contribute to the development of NCDs are discussed in detail in appropriate chapters and sections of this series of textbooks.

Case study: The rise of type 2 diabetes (WHO, 2016)

The aetiology and treatment of diabetes will be discussed in Chapter 13 of the Clinical Nutrition textbook. The aim of this section is to highlight the growing burden of diabetes worldwide and outline some of the iniatives which could reduce this global burden. The WHO estimated in 2014, that 8.5% of adults had diabetes. In 2016, 1.6 million deaths globally were directly attributed to diabetes while high blood glucose alone was the cause of another 2.2 million deaths (WHO, 2016). One in 3 adults aged over 18 years are overweight and 1 in 8 are obese. The number of people with diabetes has risen from 108 million in 1980 to 422 million in 2014. The global prevalence of diabetes among adults over 18 years of age has risen from 4.7% in 1980 to 8.5% in 2014. Diabetes of all types can lead to various complications and can increase the overall risk of dying prematurely. Possible complications include heart attack, stroke, kidney failure, leg amputation, vision loss, and nerve damage. In pregnancy, poorly controlled diabetes increases the risk of fetal death and other complications.

Prevention

Based on current knowledge, Type 1 diabetes cannot be prevented. Effective approaches to prevent

Table 17.1 Risk factors for nutition-related noncommunicable diseases (NCDS)

Societal	Behavioral	Biological	NCDs
Socioeconomic status	Smoking	Tobacco addiction	Lung disease
Cultural habits	Alcohol abuse	Alcohol addiction	Cardiovascular disease
Environmental factors	Lack of physical activity	Dyslipidemia	Atherosclerosis
	Inappropriate diets:	Hyperlipidemia	Cerebrovascular disease
	inadequate	Insulin resistance	Stroke
	fiber	Hypertension	Ischemic heart disease
	micronutrients	Obesity (body composition)	Myocardial infarction
	excess		Diabetes
	total fat		Osteoporosis
	saturated fat		Dental caries
	trans fat		Cirrhosis
	cholesterol		Diet-induced cancers
	salt (NaCl)		
	energy		

type 2 diabetes and it's associated complications include policies and practices across whole populations and within specific settings (such as in schools, the home, and in the workplace) that contribute to good health for everyone, regardless of whether they have diabetes, such as taking regular exercise, eating a balanced diet, avoiding smoking, and controlling blood pressure and blood lipids. Adopting a life-course approach is essential for preventing type 2 diabetes should be a stong feature of preventive strategies. Early in life, when eating and physical activity habits are formed, and when the long-term regulation of energy balance may be programmed, there is a critical window for intervention to mitigate the risk of obesity and type 2 diabetes later in life. A successful strategy requires a multifaceted approach including a whole-of-government and whole-of-society approach, in which all sectors systematically consider the health impact of policies in trade, agriculture, finance, transport, education and urban planning – recognising that health is enhanced or obstructed as a result of policies in these and other areas.

Management

The starting point for living well with diabetes is an early diagnosis – the longer a person lives with undiagnosed and untreated diabetes, the worse their health outcomes are likely to be. Easy access to basic diagnostics, such as blood glucose testing, should therefore be available in primary health-care settings. Established systems for referral and back-referral are needed, as patients will need periodic specialist assessment or treatment for complications. For those who are diagnosed with diabetes, a series of cost-effective interventions can improve their outcomes, regardless of what type of diabetes they may have. These interventions include regular monitoring and control of blood glucose, through a combination of diet, physical activity and, if necessary, medication; control of blood pressure and blood lipids to reduce cardiovascular risk and other complications; and regular screening for damage to the eyes, kidneys and feet, to facilitate early treatment. Diabetes management can be strengthened through the use of standards and protocols. Efforts to improve capacity for diagnosis and treatment of diabetes should occur in the context of integrated noncommunicable disease (NCD) management to yield better outcomes. At a minimum, diabetes and cardiovascular disease management can be combined. Integrated management of diabetes and tuberculosis and/or HIV/AIDS [discussed later in this chapter] can be considered where there is high prevalence of these diseases. Although dietary factors are of paramount importance in the management and prevention of type 2 diabetes, nutrition is also one of the most controversial and difficult aspects of the management of this disease. For example, there is wide variation in the use of dietary modification alone to manage type 2 diabetes as fewer than 5–10% of patients with type 2 diabetes in India and 31% in the UK are reported. Furthermore, these patients are often less closely managed than patients on medication, and dietary information is often neglected, even though attention to diet is needed to achieve adequate glycaemic control (Forouhi *et al.*, 2018). However, deterioration of type 2 diabetes is not inevitable as fasting plasma glucose can be normalised following a low calorie diet, despite simultaneous withdrawal of metformin therapy (Forouhi *et al.*, 2018). Importantly, 46% of a UK primary care cohort remained free of diabetes at one year during a structured low calorie weight loss programme (the DiRECT trial), and a return to the non-diabetic state brings an improvement in cardiovascular risk, resolution of painful neuropathy and a halt in progression of retinal complications (Forouhi *et al.*, 2018).

National capacity for prevention and control of diabetes

National capacity to prevent and control diabetes as assessed in the 2015 NCD Country Capacity Survey varies widely by region and country-income level. Most countries report having national diabetes policies, as well as national policies to reduce key risk factors and national guidelines or protocols to improve management of diabetes. In some regions and among lower-income countries, however, these policies and guidelines lack funding and implementation. In general, primary health-care practitioners in low-income countries do not have access to the basic technologies needed to help people with diabetes properly manage their disease. Only one in three low- and middle-income countries report that the most basic technologies for diabetes diagnosis and management are generally available in primary health-care facilities. Many countries have conducted national population-based surveys of the prevalence of physical inactivity and overweight and obesity in the past five years, but less than half have included blood glucose measurement in these surveys. The lack of access to affordable insulin remains a key impediment to successful treatment and results in needless complications and premature deaths. Insulin and oral hypoglycaemic agents are reported as generally available in only a minority of low-income countries. Moreover, essential medicines critical to gaining control of diabetes, such as agents to lower blood pressure and lipid levels, are frequently unavailable in low- and middle-income countries. Policy and programme interventions are needed to improve equitable access.

Important key points are:

- Diabetes prevalence has been rising more rapidly in middle- and low-income countries.
- Diabetes is a major cause of blindness, kidney failure, heart attacks, stroke and lower limb amputation.
- In 2016, an estimated 1.6 million deaths globally were directly caused by diabetes. Another 2.2 million deaths globally were attributable to high blood glucose in 2012.
- Nearly half of all deaths attributable to high blood glucose occur before the age of 70 years. WHO estimates that diabetes was the seventh leading cause of death in 2016.
- Regular physical activity, adopting a healthy diet, maintaining a normal body weight and avoiding smoking are ways to prevent or delay the onset of type 2 diabetes.
- Diabetes can be treated and its consequences avoided or delayed with diet, physical activity, medication and regular screening and treatment for complications.

The role of nutrition in reducing the burden of NCD's

The evidence that diets, specific nutrient deficiencies and excesses influence the development of NCDs is solid. It comes from extensive research, which collectively gave convincing evidence of the relationships between nutrition and NCDs: first, from ecological studies that compared different populations, the effects of migration of populations, food availability during economic development, and differences in dietary and nutrient intakes. Second, numerous epidemiological studies have established the associations between diet and biological risk factors of NCDs. Third, interventions with specific nutrients and foods in placebo-controlled trials using both healthy and diseased subjects confirmed the relationships seen in epidemiological studies. And last, molecular and genetic research has elucidated many mechanisms through which diet and nutrients affect genetic mutation and expression, adding to our knowledge of how nutrition influences NCD development. This body of knowledge has led to several sets of international dietary recommendations and guidelines to reduce the burden of nutrition-related NCDs. An example of one such set of guidelines from the World Health Organization (WHO) is shown in Box 17.1. These generic recommendations could be used as the basis for the development of country-specific strategies and food-based guidelines for dietary prevention of NCDs. However, according to the Institute for Health Metrics and Evaluation's 2016 Financing Global Health report, only 1.7% of the total US $37.6 billion in Development Assistance for Health went to NCDs and mental health, compared with almost 30% to maternal and child health and 25% to HIV and AIDS. Furthermore, whilst funding for NCDs increased annually by 5.2% from 2010 to 2016, it remained the health area with the least funding (Global Nutrition Report, 2017).

Prevention of NCDs in developed countries

The complex chain of events where behavioural and lifestyle factors influence the development of the biological risk factors for NCDs, emphasises the need for a multisectorial approach in which all factors in the chain are targeted throughout the life course. In addition to the medical treatment of some biological risk factors (such as pharmacological treatment of hypercholesterolaemia) and of the NCD itself (such as blood glucose control in diabetes) there is

Box 17.1 The WHO population nutrient intake goals for prevention of death and disability from NCDs[a]

Dietary factor (food or nutrient)	Recommended goal (range)
Total fat	15–30% of total energy
Saturated fatty acids	<10% of total energy
Polyunsaturated fatty acids (PUFAs)	6–10% of total energy
n-6 PUFAs	5–8% of total energy
n-3 PUFAs	1–2% of total energy
Trans fatty acids	<1% of total energy
Monounsaturated fatty acids (MUFAs)	By difference[b]
Total carbohydrate	55–75% of total energy[c]
Free sugars[d]	<10% of total energy
Protein	10–15% of total energy
Cholesterol	<300 mg per day
Sodium chloride (sodium)	<5 g per day (<2 g per day)
Fruits and vegetables	≥400 g per day
Total dietary fiber	>25 g per day
Non-starch polysaccharides	>20 g per day

[a] WHO Technical Support Series No. 916.

[b] MUFAs are calculated as total fat minus saturated plus polyunsaturated plus trans fatty acids).

[c] Energy from carbohydrate is the percentage energy available after taking into account that consumed as fat and protein.

[d] Free sugars refers to all monosaccharides and disaccharides added to foods by the manufacturer, cook, or consumer, plus sugars naturally present in honey, syrups, and fruit juices. It does not include sugars present in milk, fruit and vegetables.

convincing evidence that primary prevention is possible, cost-effective, affordable, and sustainable. In the developed world, early screening and diagnosis, and access to health care make primary prevention more feasible than in many developing countries. However, overcoming the barriers to increase physical activity and changing dietary behavior towards more prudent, low-fat, high-fiber diets may be more difficult. The strategies and programs to prevent NCDs would be similar in developed and developing countries, although the context and specific focus of different interventions may vary. Because the future burden of NCDs will be determined by the accumulation of risks over a lifetime, the life course approach is recommended. This will include optimising the nutritional status of pregnant women (see Box 17.3), breastfeeding of infants, ensuring optimal nutrition status and growth of children, preventing childhood obesity and promoting "prudent" diets for adolescents, adults, and older people. Addressing childhood obesity in developed countries is one of the biggest nutritional challenges these countries are facing today. Increases in the prevalence of childhood obesity have been documented for most developed countries. For example, in the USA, the National Health and Nutrition Examination Surveys (NHANES) showed that between 2007–2008 and 2015–2016, increases in obesity and severe obesity prevalence persisted among adults, whereas there were no overall significant trends among youth. For example, age-standardised prevalence of obesity among adults increased from 33.7% in 2007–2008 to 39.6% in 2015–2016. Among 7–17 year-olds, obesity prevalence was 16.8% and 18.5% in 2015–2016, whereas in children aged 2 to 5 years prevalence increased from 10.1% in 2007–2008 to 13.9% in 2015–2016. The World Health Organization estimated in 2016 that at least 41 million of the world's children under 5 years of age are overweight or obese.

Overweight and obesity have dire consequences in children, particular if other biological risk factors of NCDs occur alongside obesity. There are also immediate health consequences such as risks to develop gallstones, hepatitis, sleep apnoea, and others. Moreover, obese children have a lack of self-esteem, are often stigmatised and have difficulties with body image and mobility. Overweight and obese children often become overweight or obese adults and carry the long-term risk of premature morbidity and mortality from NCDs. Children in the developed world are exposed to a food environment in which high energy-dense and micronutrient-poor foods, beverages, and snacks are available, affordable, and aggressively marketed. This illustrates that to address the problem of childhood obesity, active and responsible partnerships and common agendas should be formed between all stakeholders (for example between governments, NGOs and the food industry). There are indications that dialogue with the food industry is not sufficient, and that many countries are now considering or already implementing legislation to create a more healthy food environment for children. The problems of childhood overweight and obesity and consequent increases in NCDs are not only seen in developed countries. They are emerging in developing countries and in some the total number of children affected exceeds those in developed countries. Timely interventions are needed to prevent the escalation experienced in developed countries.

17.3 Nutrition-related diseases in developing countries

The poverty–malnutrition cycle

Malnutrition in developing countries affects individuals throughout the life course: from birth to infancy and childhood, through adolescence into adulthood, and into old age. Malnutrition affects, therefore, critical periods of growth and mental development, maturation, active reproductive as well as economical productive phases. To capture the impact of this life-long exposure to malnutrition, the Global Burden of Disease (GBD) Study uses the disability adjusted life-year (DALY), which combines years of life lost (YLLs) due to mortality and years lived with disability (YLDs) into a single metric. One DALY can be thought of as one lost year of healthy life. In a population, the sums of DALYs represent the gap between the population's present health status and an ideal situation where the entire population lives to an advanced age, free of disease. Worldwide, DALYs decreased for communicable, maternal, neonatal, and nutritional disorders between 1990 and 2013, whereas for non-communicable diseases, global DALYs have been increasing (Murray *et al.*, 2015). The leading causes of DALYs vary substantially across regions, with chronic obstructive pulmonary disease being the leading cause in east Asia, malaria in west Africa, and HIV/AIDS in eastern and southern sub-Saharan Africa.

The health of populations in developing countries is largely determined by their environment. "Environmental" factors include social and economic conditions depending on and influencing availability and distribution of resources, agricultural and food systems, availability and access to nutritious food and safe drinking water, implementation of immunisation programs, exposure to unhygienic surroundings and toxins, women's status and education, as well as the "political" milieu including dictatorships, conflict and war, which often determine the availability of health services. There is a close, interrelated association between undernutrition and poverty in developing countries. A fifth of the global population (767 million people in 2017) live in extreme poverty. Importantly, poor nutrition elevates risk of poverty. Indeed, 43% of children under the age of 5 years in low and middle-income countries are at elevated risk of poverty because of stunting. Well-nourished children are 33% more likely to escape poverty as adults, whereas stunted children earn 20% less as adults than non-stunted children. Both stunting and wasting are associated with GDP growth: the prevalence of stunting and wasting declines by an estimated 3.2% and 7.4% for every 10% increase in income per capita, respectively (Global Nutrition Report 2017). Although the number of stunted and wasted children have fallen in many countries, the global progress to reduce these forms of malnutrition is not rapid enough to meet internationally agreed nutrition targets, including Sustainable Development Goal (SDG) target 2.2 to end all forms of malnutrition by 2030 Global Nutrition Report 2017).

Figure 17.1 illustrates this relationship, also showing some of the mechanisms responsible for perpetuating the relationship over generations.

Figure 17.1 also shows that these physically and mentally underdeveloped children eventually develop into adults with "decreased human capital" and decreased competence. These adults are often not able to create enabling environments for themselves or their children to escape poverty and undernutrition in the next generation. But moreover, these "underdeveloped" adults are at increased risk of obesity and other NCDs because of early programming (possibly through epigenetic or DNA methylation changes) in the undernourished fetus. It is especially when these adults are exposed to low micronutrient quality and high energy-dense diets that they rapidly become overweight and obese. This phenomenon explains to a certain extent the coexistence of under- and overnutrition in the same household with undernourished, wasted, and stunted children being cared for by an overweight or obese mother or care-giver.

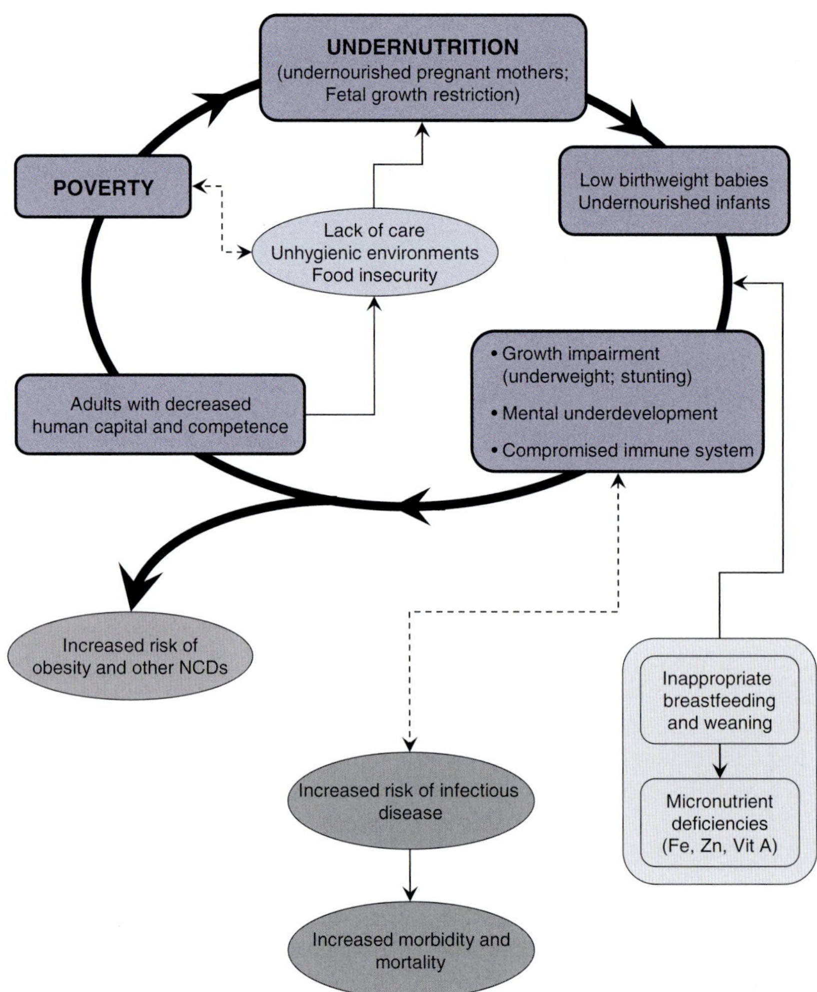

Figure 17.1 The intergenerational vicious cycle between undernutrition and poverty.

Obesity and noncommunicable diseases in developing countries

Obesity and other NCDs are increasingly becoming major public health problems in the developing world. In 2014, approximately 1.9 billion adults worldwide were overweight or obese, whereas an estimated 41 million children under the age of 5 years were overweight or obese in 2016 (WHO 2017). Maternal overweight and obesity at the time of pregnancy increases the risk for childhood obesity that continues into adolescence and early adulthood, thus increasing the risk of generational transmission of obesity (Black *et al.*, 2013). Although Oceania, Europe, and the Americas had the highest proportion of overweight and obese women, high prevalences are also seen in northern and southern Africa, and central and west Asia. Maternal obesity leads to several adverse maternal and fetal complications during pregnancy, delivery, and post-partum. Obese pregnant women are four times more likely to develop gestational diabetes mellitus and two times more likely to develop pre-eclampsia compared with women with a BMI 18–24.9 kg/m^2 (Black *et al.*, 2013). Furthermore, underdevelopment and a lack of resources in developing countries limit the availability of diagnostic and therapeutic care of people suffering from NCDs, leading to increased morbidity and mortality.

Major nutrient deficiency diseases in developing countries

Globally, 165 million children were stunted in 2013. Undernutrition leading to fetal growth restriction, stunting, wasting, deficiencies of vitamin A and zinc along with suboptimum breastfeeding caused 3·1 million child deaths (45% of all child deaths) in 2011 (Black *et al.*, 2013). Maternal undernutrition contributed to 800 000 neonatal deaths through small for gestational age births (Bhutta *et al.*, 2013). Although childhood stunting is still very high, the global prevalence of childhood stunting declined from 32.7% to 22.9% between 2000 and 2016, and the total number of stunted children less than 5 years of age declined from 198.4 million to 154.8 million (WHO, 2017). However, prevalence of stunting is higher in south Asia and sub-Saharan Africa than elsewhere. The amount of people going hungry has increased since 2015, and an estimated 38 million people are facing severe food insecurity in Nigeria, Somalia, South Sudan, and Yemen while Ethiopia and Kenya are experiencing significant droughts (Global Nutrition Report, 2017). In addition to the undernutrition related to poverty, hunger, and food insecurity, leading to stunted physical and mental development, specific nutrient deficiencies are causes of specific diseases (as discussed in Chapters 7, 8 10, and 11 of this textbook).

The major nutrient deficiency diseases prevalent in developing countries are briefly summarised in Box 17.2, to illustrate the scope of the problem and to identify the nutrition challenges in the developing world for the twenty-first century.

Nutrition-related infectious disease in developing countries

Nutrition is a major determinant of the human body's defense against infectious diseases. Optimal nutrition is necessary for the integrity of the physical barriers (skin, epithelium) against pathogens. Specific nutrients furthermore play important roles in defining acquired immune function (both humoral and cell-mediated responses) and to influence, modulate, or mediate inflammatory processes, the virulence of the infectious agent, and the response of cells and tissues to hypoxic and toxic damage.

The immune system and the influence of malnutrition on its functions are discussed in detail in the clinical nutrition textbook of the series. Given the high prevalence of malnutrition (undernutrition) in developing countries, it is not surprising that infectious diseases are still dominating mortality statistics in these countries. In children under 5 years of age these are diarrhoea and common childhood illnesses in which malnutrition could lead to premature childhood deaths. Of all infectious and parasitic child deaths, 34% can be attributed to underweight; 26% to unsafe water, hygiene and sanitation; and 15% to smoke from indoor use of solid fuels (WHO, 2009).

17.4 HIV/AIDS

Introduction

Infection with HIV and the consequent development of AIDS is a global pandemic already responsible for a large proportion of total deaths in some developing countries. Despite the expanded access to antiretroviral therapy (ART)

Box 17.2 Nutrient deficiency diseases in developing countries: prevalence (Black *et al.*, 2013)

Nutrient	Consequence: disease	Estimated: 1995–2013
Iron	Anemia; poor brain development in infancy	19.2% of pregnant women, 18.1% of children under 5 years of age
Vitamin A	Blindness; increased mortality from infectious diseases (children under 5 years especially vulnerable)	15.3% of pregnant women, 33.3% of children under 5 years of age
Iodine	Goiter, cretinism (infants) with severe brain damage and mental retardation	28.5% Globally, 40.0% in Africa, 44.2% in Europe
Zinc	Its role in stunting and life-threatening childhood illnesses is only now becoming clear	17.3% Globally, 23.9% in Africa, 7.6% in Europe

and a declining incidence of HIV infection approximately 940 000 people died from HIV globally in 2017 [52% fewer than in 2004 (the peak) and 34% fewer than in 2010 in spite of a period of substantial population growth in many high burden countries]. The pandemic has a devastating and tragic social, economic and demographic impact on previous development and health gains in developing countries. It affects mostly young, sexually active adults in their reproductive years as well as babies born from infected mothers. To understand the nutritional challenges of HIV/AIDS it is necessary to understand how the virus is transmitted and to follow the clinical course of the infection. The virus characteristics, its binding to cell surface receptors, its entry into cells of the immune system, its replication and transcription, as well as its genetic variability, and different classes of the virus have been intensively researched and described, forming the basis for the development of antiretroviral drugs to treat HIV/AIDS. More about this can be found in the clinical nutrition textbook of this series or at http://en.wikipedia.org/wiki/HIV.

Transmission of HIV

Because there is still no vaccine against HIV and no cure available, the emphasis is on prevention of transmission of the virus. It is transmitted from person to person via certain body fluids: blood (and blood products), semen, pre-seminal fluid, vaginal secretions, and breast milk.

The majority of HIV infections are acquired through unprotected sexual contact when sexual secretions of one partner come into contact with genital, oral, or rectal mucous membranes of another. The estimated infection risk per 10 000 exposures (without a condom) to an infected source varies from 0.5 to 50, depending on the type of exposure.

The blood transmission route is responsible for infections in intravenous drug users when they share needles with contaminated persons. Although blood and blood products are these days mostly checked for HIV, unhygienic practices in some developing countries, needle prick injuries of nurses and doctors, as well as procedures such as tattoos, piercings, and scarification rituals pose some risk for infection.

Transmission of the virus from an infected mother to her child can occur *in utero* during pregnancy, during childbirth (intrapartum), or during breastfeeding. The transmission rate between untreated infected mothers and children is approximately 25%. This risk can be reduced to 1% with combination antiretroviral treatment of the mother and cesarean section. The overall risk of a breastfeeding mother to child is between 20% and 45%. Recent studies have shown that this risk can be reduced three- to fourfold by exclusive breastfeeding for up to 6 months. Exclusive breastfeeding for 6 months is therefore the present recommendation from the WHO for infected mothers in developing countries "unless replacement feeding is acceptable, feasible, affordable, sustainable and safe for them and their infants before that time."

The clinical course of HIV infection: progression to AIDS

The different stages of HIV infection dictate different types of nutritional intervention. Even before infection, the vicious cycle of undernutrition and poverty in developing countries may increase vulnerability to infection: the hopelessness and despair of poverty could lead to alcohol abuse, violence, rape, and irresponsible sexual behaviours, increasing exposure to the virus. In addition, malnutrition could compromise the integrity of the immune system, increasing vulnerability to infection. Breaking this cycle by appropriate public health nutrition interventions in poverty alleviation programs may indirectly also impact on HIV transmission.

- Stage 1: Incubation period
- There are no symptoms during this stage and its duration is usually 2–4 weeks.
- Stage 2: Acute infection (seroconversion)
- There is rapid viral replication during this stage. It may last from a week to several months with a mean duration of 28 days. The symptoms in this stage include fever, lymphadenopathy, pharyngitis, rash, myalgia, malaise, headache, and mouth and esophageal sores.
- Stage 3: Asymptomatic or latency stage
- This stage may last from a few weeks up to 10 or 20 years, depending on the nutritional

status and drug treatment of the individual. It is characterised by none or only a few symptoms, which may include subclinical weight loss, vitamin B_{12} deficiency, changes in blood lipids and liver enzymes, and an increased susceptibility to pathogens in food and water.

- Stage 4: Symptomatic HIV infection
- CD4+ cell counts (the immune cells containing the CD4 receptor, which binds the virus and which is destroyed during viral replication) have decreased from normal values of 1200, to between 200 and 500 cells/μl. Wasting is a characteristic symptom and is defined as an involuntary loss of more than 10% of baseline body weight. Other symptoms include loss of appetite, white plaques in the mouth, skin lesions, fever, night sweats, TB, shingles, and other infections. Nutrition interventions may help to preserve lean body mass, "strengthen" the immune system and slow progression to stage 5.
- Stage 5: AIDS
- The CD4+ counts are now below 200 cells/μL. The immunosuppression is severe and leads to many possible opportunistic or secondary infections with fungi, protozoa, bacteria and/or other viruses.

Malignant diseases and dementia may develop. This is the final stage, and if not treated by antiretroviral drugs and specific drugs for the secondary infections it invariably leads to death.

Nutrition and HIV/AIDS

The role of nutrition in HIV/AIDS is complex. As mentioned above, malnutrition could contribute to increased vulnerability to infection in developing countries. The virus probably increases nutritional needs, while its effects on the nervous and digestive system lead to decreased appetite and intakes, impaired digestion, and malabsorption. The consequent loss of lean body mass gave the infection its original African name of "thin disease". There are indications that improved nutrition may slow the progression of HIV infection to AIDS. There is evidence that nutritional support can help in the tolerance of antiretroviral drugs and their side-effects and assist in the management of some of the secondary infections of AIDS.

The optimal diet for people living with HIV/AIDS is not known. At least one study (the THUSA study in South Africa) indicated that asymptomatic infected subjects who regularly included animal-derived foods in their diets had better health outcomes than those on plant-based diets and with high omega-6 polyunsaturated fat intakes. The nutritional recommendations for people living with HIV/AIDS are therefore evidence informed and not totally evidence based at this stage. Global recommendations have recently been evaluated by the Academy of Science of South Africa, and some of their conclusions are summarised in Box 17.3.

The transmission of the virus and the different stages in the progression of infection to AIDS indicate that different levels of nutrition intervention and support are needed, as illustrated in Box 17.3. Specific nutrient requirements during HIV infection are discussed in the clinical nutrition textbook of this series.

Box 17.3 Nutritional recommendations for HIV/AIDS

1 Nutrition recommendations should do no harm
2 Optimum nutrition at population level is necessary as part of a set of general measures to reduce the spread of HIV and TB
3 The focus should be on diversified diets including available, affordable and traditional foods. However, fortified foods as well as macro- and micronutrient supplements at safe levels (not more than twice daily recommended level) may be helpful
4 Ready-to-use therapeutic food supplements are effective in reversing poor nutritional status found in severely affected individuals
5 Because micronutrient deficiencies may hasten disease progression and facilitate mother-to-child transmission of HIV, multivitamin, zinc and selenium supplementations are indicated, but vitamin A supplementation may increase mother-to-child transmission and zinc supplementation may be harmful in pregnant women
6 HIV-infected pregnant women, lactating mothers and their babies need special advice and care to ensure best possible outcomes
7 Established, well-described steps and protocols should be followed in public health nutrition interventions and in the therapeutical (medical) nutritional support of patients

General Principles from ASSAf (2007).

17.5 The global challenge to address malnutrition

Background

The nutritional problems and diseases facing mankind at the beginning of the twenty-first century have been identified and briefly discussed in this chapter. In developed countries these are mainly childhood and adult obesity and the NCDs related to a combination of overnutrition, lack of activity, smoking, alcohol abuse, and stressful lifestyles. In developing countries the magnitude of undernutrition is staggering. Moreover, obesity and NCDs have emerged in these countries and are increasingly becoming major causes of mortality. This double burden is further exacerbated by the HIV/AIDS pandemic.

Currently, progress on global nutrition targets is not on track: For stunting, the current rate of reduction is not rapid enough to attain 100 million by 2025; for wasting, the current rate of reduction is not rapid enough to reach below 5% by 2025; for overweight, the current rate indicates rise in overweight in Africa and Asia; for anaemia, the global average of the prevalence in women of reproductive age increased from 30.3% (2012 baseline) to 32.8% in 2016 (see also Box 17.4 for more detail). Thus, it is becoming clear that actions delivered through the "nutrition sector" alone cannot achieve the global nutrition targets, but that action throughout the Sustainable Development Goals (SDGs) is needed to address the causes of malnutrition. Deep, embedded political commitment to nutrition will be key to progress. If more than one form of malnutrition is tackled, this will increase the effectiveness and efficiency of investment of time, energy and resources to improve nutrition.

Box 17.4 The Global Nutrition situation

12 billion people lack key micronutrients like iron and vitamin A
155 million children are stunted
52 million children are wasted
2 billion adults are overweight or obese
41 million children are overweight
88% of countries face a serious burden of either two or three forms of malnutrition
The world is off track to meet all global nutrition targets for improving nutrition

Suggestions to meet the challenge

Clearly, the time for individual, separate programs to address undernutrition in one way and overnutrition and NCDs in another is past. What is needed is a holistic, integrated approach that will promote and make optimum nutrition possible. Several UN agencies, separately or in combination have developed "strategic directions" and described policy principles, strategies to introduce this on different levels in different settings, as well as actions to promote healthy diets. The challenge is huge, for there are many barriers to overcome: from war, to uncommitted political agendas, to the "unhealthy" food preferences of individuals. The lessons learned from the failure of many developing countries to be on-track in reaching the Millennium Development Goals by 2015 plead for a new approach and global leadership. This could be possible in partnerships in which there is recognition and respect for different agendas, but where partners are willing to develop a common nutrition agenda and agree on steps to reach common goals.

The Global Nutrition Report (2017) has indicated that the causes of malnutrition can only be addressed through tackling problems in relation to a) sustainable food production, b) safe water, c) reducing food waste, d) a strong and robust health system, e) equity in the distribution of wealth and education, f) peace and stability and g) rigorous data collection.

a Sustainable food production is key to nutrition outcomes. Agricultural yields are predicted to decrease as temperatures increase resulting in decreased protein, iron, zinc and other micronutrients in major crops. Furthermore, unsustainable fishing threatens 17% of the world's protein and a source of essential micronutrients. Policies and investments to maintain and increase the diversity of agricultural landscapes are needed to ensure small and medium-sized farms can continue to produce the key micronutrients they do now.
b Strong systems of infrastructure play key roles in providing safe, nutritious and healthy diets

and clean water and sanitation. It will be essential to reduce food waste (currently at 30% of production) and the contamination of food which leads to diarrhoea and underweight and death among young children. Current infrastructure has made it easier to deliver foods that increase the risk of obesity and diet-related non-communicable diseases (NCDs).

c Health systems have an important role in promoting infant and young child feeding, supplementation, therapeutic feeding, nutrition counselling to manage overweight and underweight, and screening for diet-related NCD in patients. Essential nutrition actions with substantive evidence need to ensure they are reaching those who need it most.

d Equity and inclusion matter for nutrition outcomes: ignoring equity in the distribution of wealth and education will make it impossible to end malnutrition in all its forms. A fifth of the global population live in extreme poverty and 46% of all stunting falls in this group. At the same time, measures must be put into place to counteract the risk of growing obesity as economies develop, particularly since the burden of obesity is rising at lower levels of economic development. Severe food insecurity remains a problem across the world – from 30% in Africa to 7% in Europe. Actions to ensure women are included and treated equitably are needed to ensure they can breastfeed and look after their own nutrition.

e Peace and stability are vital to ending malnutrition. Long-term instability can exacerbate food insecurity and can lead to famines. When conflict or emergencies occur, nutrition must be included in disaster risk reduction and post-conflict rebuilding.

f To improve nutrition more regular, detailed and disaggregated data is needed. Currently, there is a particular lack of data that is disaggregated by wealth, gender, geography, age and disability. National averages are not enough as nutritional levels can vary even within households. Two notable data gaps are around adolescents and dietary intake.

Although addressing malnutrition has a high economic and health cost return ($16 gained for every $1 invested), the global spending by donors on undernutrition or NCDs and obesity is 0.5% or 0.01% of global ODA, respectively. Therefore, commitment and data gaps are hindering accountability and progress. To improve nutrition universally we need better, more regular, disaggregated data and clear commitment from all international agencies. There is total agreement in the body of literature on the nutrition challenges of the twenty-first century that the focus should be on prevention of nutrition-related diseases to minimise their serious economic and social consequences.

Further reading

ASSAf. (2007). *HIV/AIDS, TB and Nutrition*. Scientific enquiry into nutritional influences on human immunity with special refeference to HIV infection and active TB IN South Africa. Pretoria, Academy of Science of South Africa. 1–282 (www.assaf.org.za).

Bhutta, Z.A., Das, J.K., Rizvi, A. *et al.* (2013). Lancet Nutrition Interventions Review Group, the Maternal and Child Nutrition Study Group. Evidence-based interventions for improvement of maternal and child nutrition: what can be done and at what cost? *Lancet*. Aug 3;**382**(9890):452–477.

Black, R.E., Victora, C.G., Walker, S.P. *et al.* (2013). Maternal and Child Nutrition Study Group. Maternal and child undernutrition and overweight in low-income and middle-income countries. *Lancet*. Aug 3;**382**(9890):427–451.

Development Initiatives. (2017). *Global Nutrition Report 2017: Nourishing the SDGs*. Bristol, UK: Development Initiatives.

Forouhi, N.G., Misra, A., Mohan, V. *et al.* (2018). Dietary and nutritional approaches for prevention and management of type 2 diabetes. *BMJ*. Jun 13;**361**:k2234. doi: 10.1136/bmj.k2234.

Global Burden of Disease (GBD) 2015. (2016). Disease and Injury Incidence and Prevalence Collaborators, Global, regional, and national incidence, prevalence, and years lived with disability for 310 diseases and injuries, 1990-2015: a systematic analysis for the Global Burden of Disease Study, national incidence, prevalence, and years lived with disability for 310 diseases and injuries, 1990–2015: a systematic analysis for the Global Burden of Disease Study 2015, *Lancet* **388**: 1545–1602

Global Burden of Disease (GBD) 2017. (2018). Causes of Death Collaborators, Global, regional, and national age-sex-specific mortality for 282 causes of death in 195 countries and territories, 1980–2017: a systematic analysis for the Global Burden of Disease Study 2017; *Lancet* **392**: 1736–1788.

Murray, C.J.L. and Lopez, A.D. (2017). Global Burden of Disease: A comprehensive Assessment of Mortality and Disability from Diseases, Injuries and Risk Factors in 1990 and projected to 2020. The Global Burden of Disease and Injury 1. 1996. Harvard School of Public Health, Boston, MA. The double burden of malnutrition. Policy brief. Geneva: World Health Organization.

Murray, C.J.L., Barber, R.M., Foreman, K.J. *et al.* (2015). Global, regional, and national disability-adjusted life years (DALYs) for 306 diseases and injuries and healthy life expectancy (HALE) for 188 countries, 1990–2013: quantifying the epidemiological transition. *Lancet.* **386**: 2145–2191.

World Health Organization. (2017). *Global Nutrition Monitoring Framework: operational guidance for tracking progress in meeting targets for 2025*. Geneva: World Health Organization.

World Health Organization. (2016). *Global Burden of Diabetes Report*. Geneva: World Health Organization. ISBN 978 92 4 156525 7 (NLM classification: WK 810). (https://www.who.int/diabetes/global-report/en/)

World Health Organization. (2009). *Global health risks: mortality and burden of disease attributable to selected major risks*. Geneva: World Health Organization. ISBN 978 92 4 156387 1 (NLM classification: WA 105) (https://www.who.int/healthinfo/global_burden_disease/GlobalHealthRisks_report_full.pdf)

Introduction to Human Nutrition, Editor Biographies

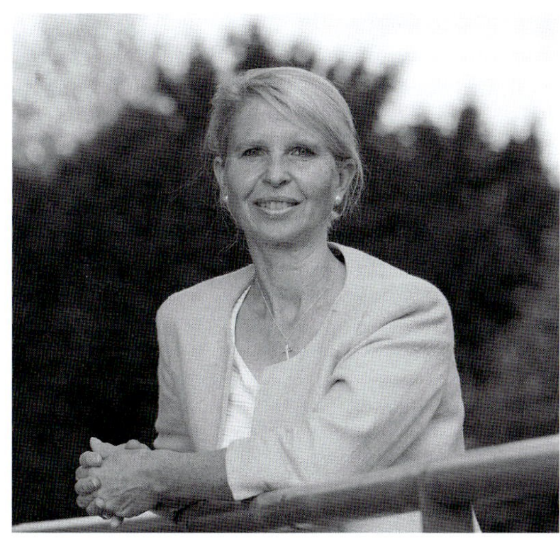

Professor Susan A. Lanham-New RNutr, FAfN, FSB
Professor of Human Nutrition & Department Head, University of Surrey

Professor Susan Lanham-New is Professor of Human Nutrition and has been Head of the Nutritional Sciences Department at the University of Surrey since 2010. She led a successful *Nutritional Sciences at Surrey* application for the 2017/2018 Queen's Anniversary Prize (QAP) for Further & Higher Education. She is a Member of the Scientific Advisory Committee on Nutrition (SACN) and is Editor in Chief of the Nutrition Society Textbook Series since 2009. She is also co-Editor of the first academic textbook on Nutritional Aspects of Bone Health. Her research focuses on the area of nutrition and bone health, for which she has won a number of awards including the 2001 Nutrition Society Medal for her work on the role of the skeleton in acid-base homeostasis as well as Young Investigator Awards at the World Congress of Osteoporosis (Amsterdam, 1996); the joint IBMS/ECTS Osteoporosis Conference (Madrid, 2001) and the National Osteoporosis Society (Bath, 2000). She has just been announced as winner of the prestigious 2018/2019 British Nutrition Foundation Prize for her work on nutrition and bone health and in particular vitamin D. She has published more than 150 peer-reviewed original papers, book chapters and reviews and raised more than £6.5M in research grants and has supervised 23 PhD students. She is a member of the Nutrition Forum for the Royal Osteoporosis Society and the Scientific Advisory Group and Governor of the British Nutrition Foundation. She has recently been given Fellowship status of the Royal Society of Biology and the Association for Nutrition and is the new Honorary Secretary of the Nutrition Society, having served as Honorary Communications Officer from 2000–2006.

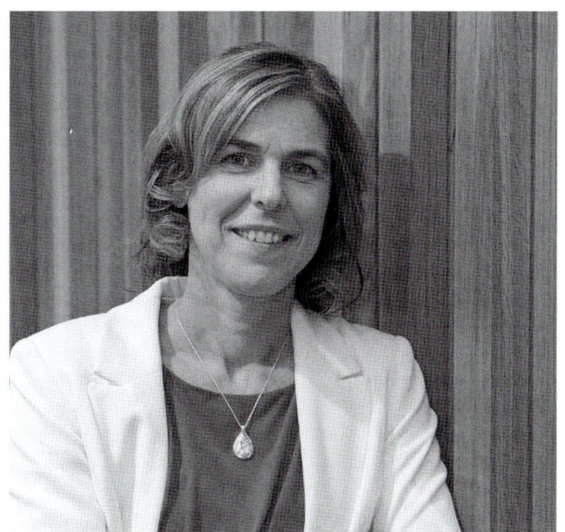

Professor Alison M. Gallagher RNutr FAfN
Professor of Public Health Nutrition, Ulster University

Introduction to Human Nutrition, Third Edition. Edited on behalf of The Nutrition Society by Susan A. Lanham-New, Thomas R. Hill, Alison M. Gallagher and Hester H. Vorster.

Companion website: www.wiley.com/go/lanham-new/humannutrition

Professor Alison Gallagher is Professor of Public Health and has been Head of Doctoral College since 2017. She contributes to the research conducted within the Nutrition Innovation Centre for Food and Health (NICHE) at Ulster University. She has published over 100 peer-reviewed original papers, book chapters and reviews and raised more than £2M in research grants and has supervised 14 PhD researchers. Her research is focused on obesity, particularly risk factor development, low-energy/non-nutritive sweeteners and their potential health impacts, physical activity and the implementation of lifestyle interventions at key stages across the lifecycle. A Registered Nutritionist (Public Health) and Fellow of the Association of Nutrition, she remains an active member of the Nutrition Society, being Treasurer of the Nutrition Society (Irish Section) 2007–2015, Honorary Programmes Secretary of the Nutrition Society 2010–2017 and co-Chair of the Scientific Committee for the Federation of Nutritional Sciences 13th European Nutrition Conference held in Dublin, October 2019. She is a member of NICHS Scientific Research Committee and the ISA Scientific Advisory Panel. She is a passionate advocate for the European Nutrition Leadership Platform (ENLP), having participated in the ENLP seminar in 1997 and being involved since with this international leadership programme, currently as Chair/President of the ENLP Board (www.enlp.eu.com).

Professor Thomas Hill is Professor of Nutrition at the Human Nutrition Research Centre in the Faculty of Medical Sciences, Newcastle University. In 2004, he completed his PhD at University College, Cork where he studied the seasonal effect of vitamin D status on bone metabolism in older women. Professor Hill's research focuses on the role of dietary factors in musculoskeletal ageing and his widely cited vitamin D research has informed global vitamin D recommendations in North America, Europe and the UK. He has published widely in nutrition and medical science journals and has co-authored a number book chapters on vitamins in prestigious textbooks including the Oxford Textbook of Medicine 6th Edition and the Encyclopedia of Dairy Sciences. Professor Hill served on the editorial board of the British Journal of Nutrition and Nutrition Research Reviews from 2012–2018 and was membership secretary of the Nutrition Society, Irish section from 2006–2011. He served on the Public Health Nutrition sub-committee of the Food Safety Authority of Ireland from 2012–2016 and is a current member of the Royal Osteoporosis Society Nutrition and Lifestyle forum. His teaching roles include head of undergraduate Nutrition programmes at Newcastle University and he has external examiner appointments for a number of undergraduate and postgraduate Nutrition programmes in the UK, Ireland and Australia.

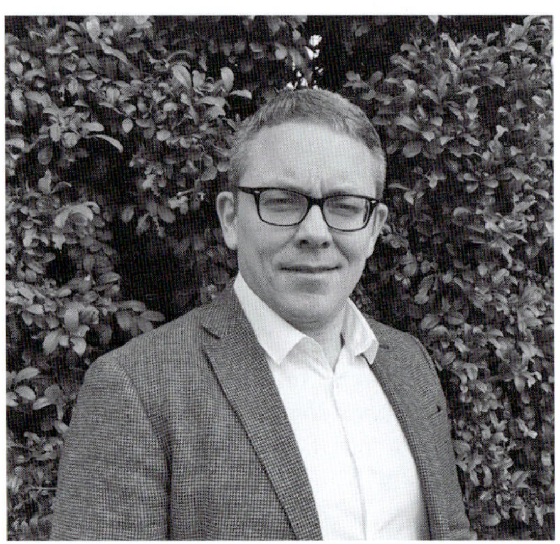

Professor Thomas R. Hill RNutr
Professor of Nutrition, Newcastle University

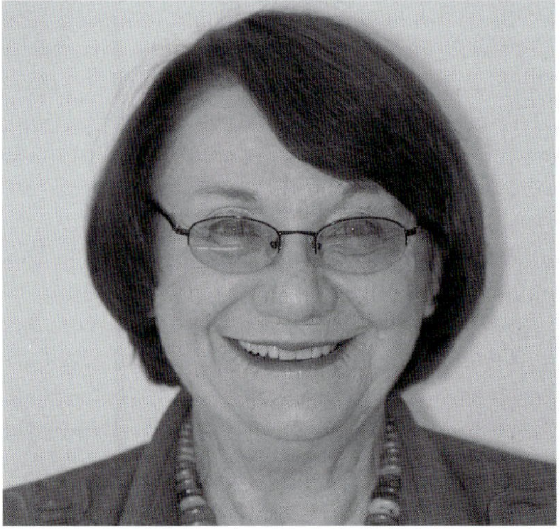

Hester H. Vorster
Emeritus Research Professor, North-West University

HH (Esté) Vorster is an Emeritus Research Professor in the Faculty of Health Sciences of the North-West University (NWU), Potchefstroom, South Africa, appointed after her retirement as director of the Centre of Excellence for Nutrition at the same University. She obtained a D.Sc. in 1989 in Physiology from the NWU with a thesis on the effects of dietary fibre on lipid and haemostatic risk factors of non-communicable diseases.

Vorster started Nutrition Research at Potchefstroom in the 1980's. She conceptualized Nutrition as a multidisciplinary domain, from molecules to society, and structured research and infrastructure to address **malnutrition problems in Africa on basic (molecular and genetic), clinical and epidemiological levels**. Vorster has supervised 33 Ph.D. and numerous M.Sc. students, and has published more than 300 research outputs as papers in scientific journals, books, chapters in books, editorials and research reports.

Vorster has served as Chair and President of the Nutrition Society of South Africa (NSSA) and received the NSSA award for "Outstanding Contributions to Nutrition Research" in 1996. She is a member of "Die Suid-Afrikaanse Akademie vir Wetenskap en Kuns", and received their prestigious "Havenga Medalje vir Geneeskunde" in 2007 for scientific outputs in Medical Sciences, and their prize for the best paper in Natural Science in 2014. She received the Nevin Scrimshaw award for "vision and leadership in nutrition training and service to international nutrition" in 2012 from the African Nutrition Society. She received Fellowship from the International Union of Nutritional Sciences (IUNS) in 2013, and is the recipient of numerous research awards from her University.

She served on the Council of the Academy of Science of South Africa as Secretary General, was on the board of the South Africa-Netherlands Programme for Alternatives in Development, a director of the Women's Outreach Foundation, and trustee and scientific advisor of the "5-a-day for Better Health Trust". She often serves as consultant and scientific advisor for the National Department of Health, as well as for international agencies such as the WHO, FAO, and UNICEF.

Vorster organised and chaired the IUNS in Durban in 2005. She is regularly invited as plenary, keynote or guest speaker at international, regional and national Nutrition congresses, symposia and workshops to talk on her experiences researching the "***Nutrition transition and its determinants and consequences in Africa***". She is on the editorial board of a number of International Journals of Nutrition and Health.

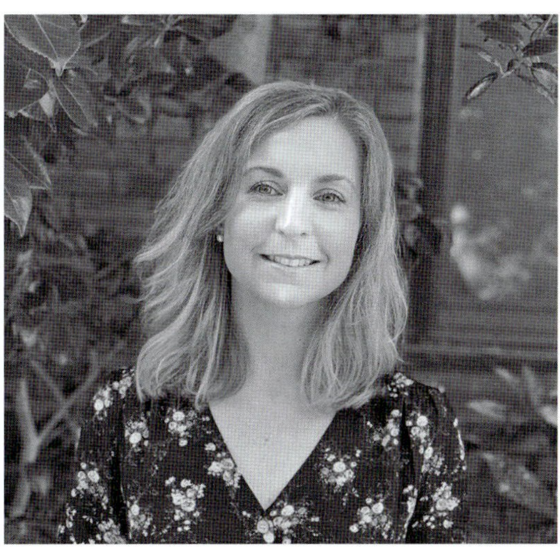

Cassandra H. Ellis MSc RNutr (Public Health)
Deputy Editor, The Nutrition Society

Cassandra is the Nutrition Society's Science Communications Manager and acts as a Deputy Editor on the Textbook Series.

In her role as Deputy Editor, Cassandra works closely with the Editor in Chief and the publisher, Wiley Blackwell, to protect and enhance the reputation of the textbooks for excellence, high standards, relevance and applicability to nutritional science. Cassandra has internal responsibility for the successful planning and execution of the Textbook Series, ensuring they are brought to publication on time and on budget. She supports the Editors in the successful delivery of revisions and new titles within the Series leading on the scoping, planning and collaborating with external partners.

Index

Page numbers in *italics* indicate figures; page numbers in **bold** indicate tables.

Introduction to Human Nutrition, Third Edition. Edited on behalf of The Nutrition Society by Susan A. Lanham-New, Thomas R. Hill, Alison M. Gallagher and Hester H. Vorster.

Companion website: www.wiley.com/go/lanham-new/humannutrition